Dermatoanthropology of Et

Neelam A. Vashi · Howard I. Maibach
Editors

Dermatoanthropology of Ethnic Skin and Hair

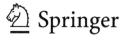 Springer

Editors
Neelam A. Vashi, MD
Department of Dermatology,
  Center for Ethnic Skin
Boston University
Boston, MA
USA

Howard I. Maibach, MD
University of California, San Francisco
San Francisco, CA
USA

and

Boston University School of Medicine
Boston Medical Center
Boston, MA
USA

ISBN 978-3-319-53960-7   ISBN 978-3-319-53961-4   (eBook)
DOI 10.1007/978-3-319-53961-4

Library of Congress Control Number: 2017934311

Printed on acid-free paper

This Springer imprint is published by Springer Nature
The registered company is Springer International Publishing AG
The registered company address is: Gewerbestrasse 11, 6330 Cham, Switzerland

This book is dedicated to Ava, my precious little baby, whose smiles and giggles forever fill my heart with joy. And to my husband, Eric, whose endless love and unwavering support have made my life's endeavors possible.

Neelam A. Vashi

Preface

Vashi and Maibach's *Dermatoanthropology of Ethnic Skin and Hair* is a comprehensive text that extensively examines cutaneous disease in persons with skin of color. The breadth of knowledge in this book encompasses the wide scope of dermatologic disease with 26 distinct and unique chapters. It serves as a guide to the diagnosis and treatment of skin disorders for those populations with darker skin types.

This book provides an overview of medical, surgical, and cosmetic dermatology in addition to providing an extensive anthropological and basic science background to fully understand skin disorders in persons of color. Topics of discussion include anthropology of skin and hair, biophysical properties of ethnic skin, structure and function of the skin, physiologic pigmentation, mucosal lesions, acne, rosacea, inflammatory disorders, infections, autoimmune disorders, connective tissue disease, hyperpigmentation, hypopigmentation and depigmentation, keloids, scarring, pediatric disease, alopecias, adnexal disorders, common cosmetic concerns and treatments, and cultural considerations.

As the domestic and worldwide populations evolve, dermatologists will increasingly have to recognize nuances in skin disorders that occur in darker skin. We hope that this book helps dermatologists with the challenges involved in treating those with darker skin tones in culturally appropriate ways. It has been a great honor to have leaders in the field of dermatology and ethnic skin contribute to this book. We are forever grateful for the hard work and insights that were shared for this important contribution to dermatologic literature.

Boston, USA   Neelam A. Vashi, MD
San Francisco, USA   Howard I. Maibach, MD

Contents

Contributors

Lisa Akintilo, BA Department of Dermatology, Northwestern University Feinberg School of Medicine, Chicago, IL, USA

Ali Al-Haseni, MD Department of Dermatology, Boston University Medical Center, Boston, MA, USA

Andrew F. Alexis, MD, MPH Department of Dermatology, Mount Sinai St. Luke's and Mount Sinai West, New York, NY, USA

Umer A. Ansari, BS Eastern Virginia Medical School, Norfolk, VA, USA

E. Berardesca, MD Department of Dermatology, San Gallicano Dermatological Institute, IRCCS, Rome, Italy

Daniel J. Callaghan III., MD Department of Dermatology, Boston University Medical Center, Boston, MA, USA

Valerie D. Callender, MD, FAAD Callender Dermatology and Cosmetic Center, Glenn Dale, MD, USA

N. Cameli, MD San Gallicano Dermatological Institute, IRCCS, Rome, Italy

Yunyoung C. Chang, MD Department of Dermatology, Boston University School of Medicine, Boston, MA, USA

Judy Cheng, MD, MPH Department of Dermatology, Boston University Medical Center, Boston, MA, USA

Ophelia E. Dadzie, BSc (Hons), MBBS, FRCP, DipRCPath (Dermpath) Departments of Dermatology and Histopathology, The Hillingdon Hospitals NHS Foundation Trust, Uxbridge, UK; Imperial College London, University of London, London, UK

Yasin A. Damji, BA Boston University School of Medicine, Boston, MA, USA

Nada Elbuluk, MD, MSc The Ronald O. Perelman Department of Dermatology, NYU School of Medicine, New York, NY, USA

Steven R. Feldman, MD, PhD Department of Dermatology, Pathology and Public Health Sciences, Wake Forest University School of Medicine, Winston-Salem, NC, USA

Lynne J. Goldberg, MD Department of Dermatology, Boston University School of Medicine, Boston, MA, USA

Rebat M. Halder, MD Department of Dermatology, Howard College of Medicine, Washington, DC, USA

Valerie M. Harvey, MD, MPH Department of Dermatology, Eastern Virginia Medical School, Norfolk, VA, USA; Hampton University Skin of Color Research Institute, Hampton, VA, USA

Catherine M. Higham, MD Boston University Medical Center, Boston, MA, USA

Nina G. Jablonski, AB, PhD Evan Pugh University Professor of Anthropology, Department of Anthropology, Center for Human Evolution and Diversity, The Huck Institutes of the Life Sciences, The Pennsylvania State University, University Park, PA, USA

Bridget P. Kaufman, MD Department of Dermatology, Mount Sinai St. Luke's and Mount Sinai West, New York, NY, USA

Roopal V. Kundu, MD Department of Dermatology, Northwestern University Feinberg School of Medicine, Chicago, IL, USA

Christina Lam, MD Department of Dermatology, Boston University Medical Center, Boston, MA, USA

Allison R. Larson, MD Department of Dermatology, Boston Medical Center, Boston, MA, USA

Tina Lasisi, BA, PhD Cand. Department of Anthropology, The Pennsylvania State University, State College, PA, USA

Christina N. Lawson, MD, FAAD Dermatology Associates of Lancaster, Lancaster, PA, USA

Stephanie T. Le, MS Eastern Virginia Medical School, Norfolk, VA, USA

Margaret S. Lee, MD, PhD Department of Dermatology, Boston University School of Medicine, Boston, MA, USA

Porcia Bradford Love, MD River region Dermatology and Laser, University of Alabama School of Medicine, Montgomery, AL, USA

Neeta Malviya, BS Department of Dermatology, University of Texas Southwestern Medical Center, Dallas, TX, USA

M. Mariano, MD San Gallicano Dermatological Institute, IRCCS, Rome, Italy

Mayra B.C. Maymone, PhD Cand. Department of Dermatology, Boston Medical Center, Boston, MA, USA

Temitayo Ogunleye, MD Philadelphia, PA, USA

Jennifer Paek, BS Boston University School of Medicine, Boston, MA, USA

Amit Pandya, MD Department of Dermatology, UT Southwestern Medical Center, Dallas, TX, USA

Trisha J. Patel, MD Department of Dermatology, Howard College of Medicine, Washington, DC, USA

Stavonnie Patterson, MD Department of Dermatology, Northwestern University Feinberg School of Medicine, Chicago, IL, USA

Kavitha K. Reddy, MD Department of Dermatology, Boston University Medical Center, Boston, MA, USA

Shalini B. Reddy, MD Department of Dermatology, Boston University Medical Center, Boston, MA, USA

Dimitrios Rigopoulos, MD 2nd Department of Dermatology and Venereology, Medical School, 'Attikon' General University Hospital, National and Kapodistrian University of Athens, Haidari, Greece

Ife J. Rodney, MD Department of Dermatology, Howard College of Medicine, Washington, DC, USA

Debjani Sahni, MD Department of Dermatology, Boston University Medical Center, Boston, MA, USA

Babu Singh, MD Department of Dermatology, Boston University Medical Center, Boston, MA, USA

Lubna H. Suaiti, MCChB, MS Department of Dermatology, Boston University Medical Center, Boston, MA, USA

Susan C. Taylor, MD Department of Dermatology, Hospital of the University of Pennsylvania, Penn Medicine, Philadelphia, PA, USA

Shalini Thareja, BA Emory School of Medicine, Atlanta, GA, USA

Ekaterini Tiligada, PhD Department of Pharmacology, Medical School, National and Kapodistrian University of Athens, Athens, Greece

Rechelle Z. Tull, BA, BS Department of Dermatology, Wake Forest University School of Medicine, Winston-Salem, NC, USA

Neelam A. Vashi, MD Department of Dermatology, Center for Ethnic Skin, Boston University, Boston, MA, USA; Boston University School of Medicine, Boston Medical Center, Boston, MA, USA

Scott Walter, MD Department of Dermatology, Boston University Medical Center, Boston, MA, USA

Lauren E. Wiznia, MD The Ronald O. Perelman Department of Dermatology, NYU School of Medicine, New York, NY, USA

Pedro Zancanaro, MD Department of Dermatology, Boston University Medical Center, Boston, MA, USA

Chapter 1
The Anthropology of Skin Colors: An Examination of the Evolution of Skin Pigmentation and the Concepts of Race and Skin of Color

Nina G. Jablonski

Skin color is a conspicuous trait of biological and social importance. The associations of skin color with concepts of human races and social privilege in recent human history have added to the significance, as well as to the misunderstanding of the trait, in general society and in medicine. In this chapter, I present a short review of what we know about human skin color in its evolutionary and social contexts. Examination of the evolution of the diversity of skin color is an essential foundation because it informs our understanding of biological and social concepts of race, and of the validity of the concept of skin of color.

The Evolution of "Naked" Skin and Skin Pigmentation in the Human Lineage

Most of the surface area of the human body except for the scalp, axillae, and groin is covered with functionally naked skin. The vellus hairs that emerge from hair follicles are placeholders in maintaining the integrity of the follicle, but do not serve the purposes of the terminal hairs that covered our distant hominin (Hominin refers to the group consisting of modern humans, extinct human species, and all immediate ancestors belonging to the genera *Homo*, *Australopithecus*, *Paranthropus*, and *Ardipithecus*.) and primate ancestors. The evolution of hair loss in the human

N.G. Jablonski (✉)
Evan Pugh University Professor of Anthropology, Center for Human
Evolution and Diversity, The Huck Institutes of the Life Sciences,
The Pennsylvania State University, 409 Carpenter Building,
University Park, PA 16802, USA
e-mail: ngj2@psu.edu

© Springer International Publishing AG 2017
N.A. Vashi and H.I. Maibach (eds.), *Dermatoanthropology of Ethnic Skin and Hair*, DOI 10.1007/978-3-319-53961-4_1

lineage has been discussed extensively in the literature and is reviewed elsewhere [1]. Direct evidence for the evolution of functionally significant novelties of the soft tissues, including skin, is rare because of the nature of the fossil record. Thus, most arguments about evolutionary causation rely on critical examination of pertinent comparative anatomical, physiological, paleoecological, and climatological evidence and the advancing of "most likely" scenarios, which are consistent with available evidence. Using these criteria, the most likely reason for the evolution of the loss of body hair in the human lineage was because of the increased importance of eccrine sweating in thermoregulation under conditions of high environmental heat and high activity levels [2–5]. The considerable advantages of the loss of body hair were accompanied by notable disadvantages, namely, the loss of some protection against abrasion, ultraviolet radiation (UVR), chemicals, pathogens, and parasites. Compensatory changes evolved quickly in hominin skin, as evidenced by genomic comparisons between humans and our closest relative, the chimpanzee. These comparisons have revealed that the human lineage is characterized by accelerated evolution of keratinization and epidermal differentiation genes that contribute to enhanced barrier functions of the epidermis [6–8]. Accompanying changes in constitutive pigmentation were inferred to have occurred before genomic evidence was available [2, 3], and these were substantiated quickly when it was. Comparative study of the human melanocortin 1 receptor (*MC1R*) locus demonstrated that the timing of evolution of permanent, dark, eumelanin-rich, skin pigmentation coincided with the evolution of functional hairlessness and increased density of eccrine sweat glands early in the history of the genus *Homo*, approximately 1.2 million years ago or earlier [9]. Adaptive evolution for sun-resistant alleles of the *MC1R* locus appears to have occurred, therefore, when early members of the genus *Homo* became mostly hairless and highly physically active inhabitants of open savannah environments in Africa. For members of the *Homo* lineage evolving since then in sub-Saharan Africa—including the earliest modern people, *Homo sapiens*—the absence of polymorphism in the *MC1R* gene has been maintained by purifying selection [10, 11]. This denotes that protective eumelanin-rich constitutive pigmentation has persisted because of its contribution toward the survival and successful reproduction of populations living under high UVR at low latitudes.

Extremely high correlations exist between skin pigmentation (as measured by skin reflectance) and levels of minimal erythema dose UVR (UVMED), with skin color being almost fully modeled as an effect of autumn UVMED alone ($r = 0.927$; $P < 0.0001$) [3, 12]. The strength of these correlations invites causal explanations that demonstrate real or probable enhanced reproductive success as a result of the possession of specific skin pigmentation phenotypes under specific conditions of environmental UVR. Many adaptive explanations for the evolution of variation in human skin color have been put forward in the past century, as reviewed elsewhere [1], and most have suffered from the fact that they cannot demonstrate likely differences in survivorship and reproduction of different skin color phenotypes under the same environmental conditions. The "skin cancer hypothesis" has been the most popular of these, invoking dark pigmentation as protection against sunburn, DNA damage, and skin cancer. Blum pointed out decades ago that dark skin pigmentation could not have evolved primarily as protection against skin cancers because such cancers rarely cause death or affect reproductive success during the peak reproductive years [13]. This has not prevented the skin cancer hypothesis from being revived, based on the argument that ancestral hominins had pale or lightly pigmented skin and that modern Africans with *OCA2* albinism are a suitable model for the ancestral state [14]. There is no evidence from comparative anatomy or genetics to indicate that this was the case, and that skin cancer was a potent selective force for the evolution of dark pigmentation in early hominins [15]. Many other explanations have been similarly weak or insufficiently explanatory, including ideas that the eumelanin was most important in affording protection against tropical parasites and tropical skin diseases because of its potent antimicrobial properties [16–18], or that the primary function of eumelanin was augmentation of epidermal barrier function by increasing the skin's resistance to desiccation under arid conditions [19–21].

The most strongly and consistent supported hypothesis is that dark pigmentation evolved in the functionally naked skin of early *Homo* to help protect against photodegradation of cutaneous and systemic folate under high UVR conditions. The physiological effects of photodegradation of folate were explored long before the full extent of folate's roles in DNA biosynthesis, repair, DNA methylation, amino acid metabolism, and melanin production were appreciated [22]. The original enunciation of the nutrient photolysis theory for the evolution of dark pigmentation set forth the hypothesis that protective eumelanin-rich pigmentation evolved in early *Homo* primarily to prevent reduction of fertility due to photodegradation of folate in cutaneous blood vessels and the systemic circulation [3]. Folate depletion by UVR would precipitate folate deficiencies which would, in turn, lead to potentially fatal birth defects such as neural tube defects (NTDs). Investigations of the photosensitivity of folate under different conditions in vitro and in vivo have demonstrated that the relationship between skin pigmentation and folate metabolism is complicated, and it involves direct photodegradation of folate (in its main form of 5-methyltetrahydrofolate or 5-MTHF) as well as its photodegradation in the presence of flavins and porphyrins by reactive oxygen species (ROS) [23–26]. Folate metabolism is also regulated by genes and epigenomic factors, which favors conservation of folate under conditions of longer day length and greater potential UVR-related folate loss [27, 28]. Recent physiological evidence also indicates the importance of folate (in the form of 5-MTHF) in thermoregulation, via its effect on controlling nitric oxide-mediated cutaneous vasodilation [29–32]. Maintaining the integrity of folate metabolism is important with respect to evolution because it directly affects reproductive success and survival early in life. Natural selection has, thus, affected varied genetic and physiological mechanisms in order to protect folate and 5-MTHF in the face of high UVR. The primary role of dark constitutive skin pigmentation in hominin and modern human evolution is that of a natural sunscreen to conserve folate.

The Evolution and Dispersal of *Homo sapiens* and Its Consequences for Skin Pigmentation

The key events in the human lineage occurred in equatorial Africa under conditions of intense and relatively invariant sunlight and UVR. Dispersal of hominins into non-equatorial Africa and Eurasia involved movements out of UVR-saturated environments into habitats that were more mixed with respect to the seasonal pattern, intensity, and wavelength mixture of UVR [33]. Two distinct species of hominin engaged in widespread dispersals throughout the Old World: early *Homo erectus* beginning around 1.8 million years ago [34] and *Homo sapiens*, beginning around 55,000 years [35]. The details of the first radiation are fascinating, but beyond the scope of this chapter. Suffice it to say that most of the non-African descendants of the first dispersal event went extinct without a trace; a limited amount of genetic admixture between Neanderthals and modern humans occurred, and the functional significance of this is a matter of continuing research [36, 37]. There is no evidence to suggest that *Homo erectus* or early *Homo sapiens* used sewn clothing or other methods of full-coverage protection against the sun and elements. Thus, apart from the time they spent in the shade or in natural shelters, their bodies were subjected to the full force of UVR wherever they went. Skin was the primary interface with the environment for most of human evolution.

In order to understand the nature of the selective pressures facing hominins as they dispersed out of the tropics, some more information on UVR is needed. The biological activity of UVR varies according to wavelength [38, 39]. Only some wavelengths of UVB catalyze production of vitamin D in the skin. The process can occur with exposure to wavelengths between 270 and 300 nm, but peak synthesis occurs between 295 and 297 nm only. Much less UVB than UVA reach the earth's surface because of scattering and absorption by oxygen, ozone, and water molecules in the atmosphere. Because of this and the geometry of sunlight reaching different places in different seasons, UVB is more variable in its intensity and distribution than UVA [33]. At the equator and within the tropics, average UVB is high, with two seasonal peaks at the equinoxes [33]. Outside of the tropics, average UVB levels are much lower and exhibit a single peak at the Summer Solstice [33]. Average UVB in northern Eurasia and North America is extremely low and highly variable. The Southern Hemisphere lacks a comparable, habitable, low-UVB land mass except for the southern tip of South America [40].

The eumelanin in skin is a highly effective sunscreen, and the potential for cutaneous vitamin D_3 production is reduced by dark skin. Other things being equal, the higher the eumelanin content, the lower the rate of pre-vitamin D_3 production in the skin [3, 41–44]. Darkly pigmented hominins dispersing out of equatorial Africa thus faced conditions that significantly affected their physiology. Penetration of UVR into the skin is related to the amount and the distribution of melanin; large, more superficial, melanin-filled melanosomes and "melanin dust" present in the stratum corneum are highly effective at reducing transmission [45]. The penetration of UVB into the skin is minimal compared to UVA because UVB typically travels only a few microns. Eumelanin in the skin competes with pre-vitamin D_3 precursor (7-dehydrocholesterol) UVB photons and prevents its penetration into the basal and spinosal layers deep in the epidermis, where pre-vitamin D_3 production takes place [43, 44]. Pre-vitamin D_3 production occurs in skins of all colors, but in eumelanin-rich skin low doses of UVB do not raise 25(OH)D levels to physiologically adequate levels at which storage can take place; higher doses over longer periods of time are required for this, and these conditions are not met outside of the equatorial latitudes. The nonlinearity of pre-vitamin D_3 production results in lighter skinned individuals achieving greater effect from higher doses of UVB than darker skinned individuals [46, 47]. For people with darkly pigmented skin, these "vitamin-D-safe zones" are smaller and shifted toward the equator because of the efficacious sunscreening action of eumelanin [3]. For people with dark skin living outside of the tropics, there is insufficient UVB available in the sunlight outside of the time immediately around the summer solstice to satisfy the body's vitamin D requirements under conditions of casual sun exposure. This is especially true in latitudes north and south of 45° where the availability of UVB in sunlight is greatly foreshortened [3, 33, 48–50]. Thus, when we consider the evolution of skin pigmentation, it is clear that long-term occupation of non-tropical latitudes would not have been possible without loss of some constitutive eumelanin pigmentation in order to prevent the serious sequelae of hypovitaminosis D [3].

The importance of the evolution of depigmentation for hominins living under non-tropical regimes was inferred before genomic evidence was available [3] and has been reinforced many times since, as summarized elsewhere [51–53]. As discussed above, the near absence of variation in *MC1R* was established in the early history of the *Homo* lineage and has been maintained in ancestral and modern *Homo sapiens* in Africa because of the importance of dark pigmentation to survival and reproductive success. In contrast, the *MC1R* gene is highly variable outside of Africa, especially in northern Europe, where it is associated with red or blonde hair and lightly pigmented skin. Depigmented skin did not evolve solely because of changes in the *MC1R* locus, however. Rather, a variant form the *SLC24A5* gene homologous to that which produces the golden variant in zebrafish appears to have been more functionally significant in the evolution of depigmentation in the ancestors of modern Europeans because of its effect on melanosome size [54]. Depigmentation in the ancestors of eastern Asians was not achieved through mutations at the SLC24A5 locus, however [54], indicating that the skin of East Asians underwent loss of pigmentation via a different set of genetic mechanisms. These are not yet well characterized [55, 56]. The finding that depigmented skin evolved independently in the ancestors of modern Europeans and East Asians suggests that at least two (and probably more) distinct genetic mutations occurred and underwent positive selection in two regions of the world that receive relatively low levels of UVB [53, 57, 58]. The most likely reason for this was that it was associated with a loss of skin pigment that favored vitamin D production under conditions of low UVB [49, 51, 53].

There has been a cause and effect relationship between UVR and skin pigmentation in human evolution. Skin pigmentation phenotypes have been modified under the action of natural selection to maintain an optimum balance between photoprotection and photosynthesis over spatially varying conditions of UVR. Skin color thus evolved as the product of two opposing clines, one emphasizing dark pigmentation and photoprotection against high loads of UVA and UVB near the equator, the other favoring depigmented skin to promote seasonal, UVB-induced photosynthesis of vitamin D_3 nearer the poles [33]. Intermediate latitudes with seasonally high loads of UVB favored the evolution of people with intermediate pigmentation, who are capable of tanning. The genetic basis for "tannability" is tremendously varied and is the subject of considerable research [59, 60]. The most important points to reinforce here are that the geographical gradient of human skin color evolved under the influence of natural selection, and that the very similar skin color phenotypes (dark, light, and intermediate) have evolved independently numerous times under similar UVR conditions. The extensive "palette" of skin color genes has made possible the evolution of remarkably similar skin color from different combinations of genes and genetic polymorphisms. Diverse combinations of skin color genes occurred during the course of prehistory as the combined result of natural selection, gene flow due to migration, and founder effect or genetic drift due to population bottlenecks occurring in the course of dispersal events [61]. New combinations of pigmentation genes are being made every day as modern people move around the world over long distances and mate with one another. Many of the resulting skin color phenotypes are visually indistinguishable from one another. This does not mean that there may not be minor differences discernible by reflectometry or in physiological response to UVR challenge. But the palette of skin color genes in humans is highly redundant, and there are many genetic ways to produce virtually identical phenotypes. This fact has profound implications for our understanding of the concepts of race and skin of color.

Skin Pigmentation Evolution Invalidates the Concept of Color-Based Race and Suggests That "Skin of Color" Is an Outdated and Inaccurate Concept

The question is often asked, "how does an understanding of the biology and the evolutionary basis of skin color diversity contribute to our understanding of the concepts of race and skin of color?" The answer is simple, but it is sometimes not what questioners expect or want to hear.

For as long as the concept of race has existed, it has been messy and ill defined. From its beginnings in the sixteenth century, race was a concept that was associated with some characteristics of physical difference, primarily those of skin color, along with characteristics of temperament and capacity for culture and moral judgement [62]. Early proponents of strict racial categories such as the eighteenth century philosophers Immanuel Kant and David Hume held tremendous sway over public opinion in Europe and the Americas, even though their writings on human diversity were based on no methodical personal observations and despite the fact that some of their contemporaries openly and vigorously disputed their conclusions with empirical data [62]. Beliefs in the scientific validity of race, and of a naturally defined racial hierarchy, grew in the nineteenth and early twentieth centuries. The reasons for this have been well reviewed elsewhere [62–64] and what is clear is that so-called scientific theories of race were anything but. They were pseudoscientific justifications for racism and rationalizations for the maintenance of the lucrative transatlantic slave trade.

Biologists and anthropologists long recognized the inutility and invalidity of the biological race concept [62, 65], and new genetic and genomic evidence continues to support this conclusion [66, 67]. The evidence presented in this review indicates that color-based concepts of race are entirely obsolete because people with identical skin color phenotypes can be genetically entirely different. Despite these facts, clinicians and forensic scientists generally have retained racial categories—along with a belief in the validity of races—because race labels have been a part of medical and legal practice in the U.S. and many other countries for more than a century. Many health-related granting organizations require that human subjects be identified by race or ethnicity in order to be entered into clinical studies or trials, and also stipulate that investigators report results accordingly. Race and ethnicity lack inherent biological meaning because they are nonexclusive and are defined by cultural and linguistic characteristics, but they continue to be recycled and revalidated in the medical, forensic, and pharmacological literature, out of habit and usually without question or justification.

The absence of scientific justification for races as "biological real" does not mean that they are not socially real. Race is a lived reality for many people in the world because opportunities in education, housing, and employment have been defined by race in the past, and because the legacies of these inequalities continue. If there is a biological reality to race it is in the socioeconomic determinants of health outcomes that people using the same racial labels share. Race thus becomes synonymous with class, and a determinant of educational opportunities and earning potential, a predictor of the availability of healthy foods and lifestyles, and an indicator of the likelihood of the presence or absence of chronic social stress. Races have a social reality, and that social reality often has health consequences.

The concepts of "ethnic skin" or "skin of color" are similarly misleading. They exist only because descriptions of human skin by anatomists, histologists, and early dermatologists were based on the skin of lightly pigmented European people, with other skin types described later as deviations from a European norm [68]. This is ironic especially because when the skin of most Europeans—and especially that of northern Europeans—is compared to a global array of human skin, it is numerically uncommon and physiologically unusual [68]. There is no biological or evolutionary unity or identity to "ethnic skin" or "skin of color." The only important shared functional characteristic of skin of color is that the presence of more eumelanin renders it less susceptible to photoaging and skin cancer than lightly pigmented or depigmented European skin. As this review (and many of its supporting references) makes clear, the presence of more eumelanin in the skin does not imply shared ancestry or genetics, and can even be potentially misleading if it is assumed that darker-than-European skin denotes particular disease susceptibilities or physiological responses with respect to the skin or the whole body. The labels, "ethnic skin" and "skin of color" have limited usefulness other than to designate skin that has been mostly ignored in the history of medicine and science. The study of cutaneous diversity is extremely important, especially as increasing amounts of genetic admixture between once widely separated human groups are creating new skin colors, new pigment gene combinations, and new potentials for genetic interactions of unknown functional significance.

References

1. Jablonski NG. The evolution of human skin and skin color. Annu Rev Anthropol. 2004;33:585–623.
2. Zihlman AL, Cohn BA. The adaptive response of human skin to the savanna. Hum Evol. 1988;3(5):397–409.
3. Jablonski NG, Chaplin G. The evolution of human skin coloration. J Hum Evol. 2000;39 (1):57–106.
4. Wheeler PE. The evolution of bipedality and loss of functional body hair in hominids. J Hum Evol. 1984;13(1):91–8.
5. Bramble DM, Lieberman DE. Endurance running and the evolution of *Homo*. Nature. 2004;432(7015):345–52.
6. The Chimpanzee Sequencing and Analysis Consortium. Initial sequence of the chimpanzee genome and comparison with the human genome. Nature. 2005;437(7055):69–87.
7. Toulza E, Mattiuzzo N, Galliano M-F, Jonca N, Dossat C, Jacob D, et al. Large-scale identification of human genes implicated in epidermal barrier function. Genome Biol. 2007;8 (6):R107.
8. Gautam P, Chaurasia A, Bhattacharya A, Grover R, Consortium IGV, Mukerji M, et al. Population diversity and adaptive evolution in keratinization genes: impact of environment in shaping skin phenotypes. Mol Biol Evol. 2014;32(3):555–73.
9. Rogers AR, Iltis D, Wooding S. Genetic variation at the MC1R locus and the time since loss of human body hair. Curr Anthropol. 2004;45(1):105–24.
10. Hudjashov G, Villems R, Kivisild T. Global patterns of diversity and selection in human tyrosinase gene. PLoS ONE. 2013;8(9):e74307.
11. Harding RM, Healy E, Ray AJ, Ellis NS, Flanagan N, Todd C, et al. Evidence for variable selective pressures at MC1R. Am J Hum Genet. 2000;66:1351–61.
12. Chaplin G, Jablonski NG. Environmental correlates of human skin color, revisited. Am J Phys Anthropol. 2002;117(S34):53.
13. Blum HF. Does the melanin pigment of human skin have adaptive value? Quart Rev Biol. 1961;36(1):50–63.
14. Greaves M. Was skin cancer a selective force for black pigmentation in early hominin evolution? Proc R Soc B: Biol Sci. 2014;281(1781):1–10.
15. Jablonski NG, Chaplin G. Skin cancer was not a potent selective force in the evolution of protective pigmentation in early hominins. Proc R Soc B: Biol Sci. 2014;281(1789).
16. Mackintosh JA. The antimicrobial properties of melanocytes, melanosomes and melanin and the evolution of black skin. J Theor Biol. 2001;211(2):101–13.

17. Wassermann HP. Human pigmentation and environmental adaptation. Arch Environ Health. 1965;11(5):691–4.
18. Wassermann HP. Ethnic pigmentation: historical, physiological, and clinical aspects. Amsterdam: Excerpta Medica; 1974. 284 p.
19. Elias PM, Menon G, Wetzel BK, Williams JW. Evidence that stress to the epidermal barrier influenced the development of pigmentation in humans. Pigm Cell Melanoma Res. 2009;22 (4):420–34.
20. Elias PM, Menon G, Wetzel BK, Williams JW. Barrier requirements as the evolutionary "driver" of epidermal pigmentation in humans. Am J Hum Biol. 2010;22(4):526–37.
21. Elias PM, Williams ML. Basis for the gain and subsequent dilution of epidermal pigmentation during human evolution: the barrier and metabolic conservation hypotheses revisited. Am J Phys Anthropol. 2016;Early View:1–19.
22. Branda RF, Eaton JW. Skin color and nutrient photolysis: an evolutionary hypothesis. Science. 1978;201(4356):625–6.
23. Off MK, Steindal AE, Porojnicu AC, Juzeniene A, Vorobey A, Johnsson A, et al. Ultraviolet photodegradation of folic acid. J Photochem Photobiol, B. 2005;80(1):47–55.
24. Steindal AH, Juzeniene A, Johnsson A, Moan J. Photodegradation of 5-methyltetrahydrofolate: biophysical aspects. Photochem Photobiol. 2006;82(6):1651–5.
25. Steindal AH, Tam TTT, Lu XY, Juzeniene A, Moan J. 5-Methyltetrahydrofolate is photosensitive in the presence of riboflavin. Photochem Photobiol Sci. 2008;7(7):814–8.
26. Tam TTT, Juzeniene A, Steindal AH, Iani V, Moan J. Photodegradation of 5-methyltetrahydrofolate in the presence of uroporphyrin. J Photochem Photobiol, B. 2009;94(3):201–4.
27. Lucock MD, Glanville T, Ovadia L, Yates Z, Walker J, Simpson N. Photoperiod at conception predicts C677T-MTHFR genotype: a novel gene-environment interaction. Am J Hum Biol. 2010;22(4):484–9.
28. Lucock MD, Yates Z, Martin C, Choi J-H, Boyd L, Tang S, et al. Vitamin D, folate, and potential early lifecycle environmental origin of significant adult phenotypes. Evol Med Public Health. 2014;2014(1):69–91.
29. Stanhewicz AE, Bruning RS, Smith CJ, Kenney WL, Holowatz LA. Local tetrahydro-biopterin administration augments reflex cutaneous vasodilation through nitric oxide-dependent mechanisms in aged human skin. J Appl Physiol. 2012;112(5):791–7.
30. Alexander LM, Kutz JL, Kenney WL. Tetrahydrobiopterin increases NO-dependent vasodilation in hypercholesterolemic human skin through eNOS-coupling mechanisms. Am J Physiol Regul Integr Comp Physiol. 2013;304(2):R164–9.
31. Smith CJ, Kenney WL, Alexander LM. Regional relation between skin blood flow and sweating to passive heating and local administration of acetylcholine in young, healthy humans. Am J Physiol Regul Integr Comp Physiol. 2013;304(7):R566–73.
32. Stanhewicz Anna E, Alexander Lacy M, Kenney WL. Folic acid supplementation improves microvascular function in older adults through nitric oxide-dependent mechanisms. Clin Sci. 2015;129(2):159–67.
33. Jablonski NG, Chaplin G. Human skin pigmentation as an adaptation to UV radiation. Proc Natl Acad Sci. 2010;107(Supplement 2):8962–8.
34. Antón SC, Potts R, Aiello LC. Evolution of early *Homo*: an integrated biological perspective. Science. 2014;345(6192).
35. Hershkovitz I, Marder O, Ayalon A, Bar-Matthews M, Yasur G, Boaretto E, et al. Levantine cranium from Manot Cave (Israel) foreshadows the first European modern humans. Nature. 2015;520:216–9.
36. Wang S, Lachance J, Tishkoff SA, Hey J, Xing J. Apparent variation in Neanderthal admixture among African populations is consistent with gene flow from non-African populations. Genome Biol Evol. 2013;5(11):2075–81.
37. Sankararaman S, Mallick S, Dannemann M, Prufer K, Kelso J, Paabo S, et al. The genomic landscape of Neanderthal ancestry in present-day humans. Nature. 2014;507:354–7.

38. Madronich S, McKenzie RL, Bjorn LO, Caldwell MM. Changes in biologically active ultraviolet radiation reaching the Earth's surface. J Photochem Photobiol, B. 1998;46(1–3): 5–19.

39. Grifoni D, Zipoli G, Sabatini F, Messeri G, Bacci L. Action spectra affect variability of the climatology of biologically effective ultraviolet radiation on cloud-free days. Radiat Prot Dosimetry. 2013;157(4):491–8.

40. Chaplin G, Jablonski NG. Hemispheric difference in human skin color. Am J Phys Anthropol. 1998;107(2):221–4.

41. Webb AR, Kline L, Holick MF. Influence of season and latitude on the cutaneous synthesis of vitamin D_3: exposure to winter sunlight in Boston and Edmonton will not promote vitamin D_3 synthesis in human skin. J Clin Endocrinol Metab. 1988;67(2):373–8.

42. Webb AR. Who, what, where and when—influences on cutaneous vitamin D synthesis. Prog Biophys Mol Biol. 2006;92(1):17–25.

43. Clemens TL, Henderson SL, Adams JS, Holick MF. Increased skin pigment reduces the capacity of skin to synthesise vitamin D_3. Lancet. 1982;319(8263):74–6.

44. Chen TC, Chimeh F, Lu Z, Mathieu J, Person KS, Zhang A, et al. Factors that influence the cutaneous synthesis and dietary sources of vitamin D. Arch Biochem Biophys. 2007;460 (2):213–7.

45. Nielsen KP, Zhao L, Stamnes JJ, Stamnes K, Moan J. The importance of the depth distribution of melanin in skin for DNA protection and other photobiological processes. J Photochem Photobiol, B. 2006;82(3):194–8.

46. Armas LAG, Dowell S, Akhter M, Duthuluru S, Huerter C, Hollis BW, et al. Ultraviolet-B radiation increases serum 25-hydroxyvitamin D levels: the effect of UVB dose and skin color. Am Acad Dermatol. 2007;57(4):588–93.

47. Harris SS, Dawson-Hughes B. Seasonal changes in plasma 25-hydroxyvitamin D concentrations of young American black and white women. Am J Clin Nutr. 1998;67(6):1232–6.

48. Chaplin G, Jablonski NG. Vitamin D and the evolution of human depigmentation. Am J Phys Anthropol. 2009;139(4):451–61.

49. Jablonski NG, Chaplin G. Human skin pigmentation, migration and disease susceptibility. Philos Trans R Soc B Biol Sci. 2012;367(1590):785–92.

50. Jablonski NG, Chaplin G. Epidermal pigmentation in the human lineage is an adaptation to ultraviolet radiation. J Hum Evol. 2013;65(5):671–5.

51. Saternus R, Pilz S, Graber S, Kleber M, Marz W, Vogt T, et al. A closer look at evolution: variants (SNPs) of genes involved in skin pigmentation, including EXOC2, TYR, TYRP1, and DCT, are associated with 25(OH)D serum concentration. Endocrinology. 2015;156 (1):39–47.

52. Rossberg W, Saternus R, Wagenpfeil S, Kleber M, Marz W, Reichrath S, et al. Human pigmentation, cutaneous vitamin D synthesis and evolution: variants of genes (SNPs) involved in skin pigmentation are associated with 25(OH)D serum concentration. Anticancer Res. 2016;36(3):1429–37.

53. Norton HL, Kittles RA, Parra E, McKeigue P, Mao X, Cheng K, et al. Genetic evidence for the convergent evolution of light skin in Europeans and East Asians. Mol Biol Evol. 2007;24 (3):710–22.

54. Lamason RL, Mohideen M-APK, Mest JR, Wong AC, Norton HL, Aros MC, et al. SLC24A5, a putative cation exchanger, affects pigmentation in zebrafish and humans. Science. 2005;310(5755):1782–6.

55. Maria de Gruijter J, Lao O, Vermeulen M, Xue Y, Woodwark C, Gillson CJ, et al. Contrasting signals of positive selection in genes involved in human skin-color variation from tests based on SNP scans and resequencing. Invest Genet. 2011;2(1):1–12.

56. Yin L, Coelho SG, Ebsen D, Smuda C, Mahns A, Miller SA, et al. Epidermal gene expression and ethnic pigmentation variations among individuals of Asian, European and African ancestry. Exp Dermatol. 2014;23(10):731–5.

57. Wilde S, Timpson A, Kirsanow K, Kaiser E, Kayser M, Unterlander M, et al. Direct evidence for positive selection of skin, hair, and eye pigmentation in Europeans during the last 5000 y. Proc Natl Acad Sci. 2014;Early Edition:1–6.
58. Allentoft ME, Sikora M, Sjogren K-G, Rasmussen S, Rasmussen M, Stenderup J, et al. Population genomics of Bronze Age Eurasia. Nature. 2015;522(7555):167–72.
59. Quillen EE. The evolution of tanning needs its day in the sun. Hum Biol. 2015;87(4):352–60.
60. Nan H, Kraft P, Qureshi AA, Guo Q, Chen C, Hankinson SE, et al. Genome-wide association study of tanning phenotype in a population of European ancestry. J Invest Dermatol. 2009;129(9):2250–7.
61. Henn BM, Cavalli-Sforza LL, Feldman MW. The great human expansion. Proc Natl Acad Sci. 2012;109(44):17758–64.
62. Jablonski NG. Living color: the biological and social meaning of skin color. Berkeley, CA: University of California Press; 2012: 260 p.
63. Samson J. Race and empire. In: Emsley C, Martel G, editors. Harlow, UK: Pearson Education Limited; 2005. 165 p.
64. Sanjek R. The enduring inequalities of race. In: Gregory S, Sanjek R, editors. race. New Brunswick, NJ: Rutgers University Press; 1994. p. 1–17.
65. Lewontin RC. Human diversity. W.H. Freeman & Company; 1995.
66. Long JC, Kittles RA. Human genetic diversity and the nonexistence of biological races. Hum Biol. 2009;81(5–6):777–98.
67. Barbujani G, Ghirotto S, Tassi F. Nine things to remember about human genome diversity. Tissue Antigens. 2013;82(3):155–64.
68. Jablonski NG. 'Ethnic skin' and why the study of human cutaneous diversity is important. Br J Dermatol. 2013;169 Suppl 3.

Chapter 2
The Impact of Skin and Hair Disease in Ethnic Skin

Temitayo Ogunleye and Susan C. Taylor

The ethnic/racial demographic of the United States is in the midst of significant change and physicians must be adept at recognizing and effectively treating dermatologic disease states in patients with skin of color. Inherent in effectively treating these cutaneous diseases is sufficiently understanding the patient's viewpoint about his/her disease, as well as hindrances to treatment, compliance, patient satisfaction, and access to leading treatment modalities. Information about the physical and psychosocial impact of a disease can be used to guide treatment practices and appropriately address patient expectations. Additionally, the recognition of psychosocial and physical burdens associated with cutaneous diseases (i.e., health-related quality of life) will become paramount to support treatment appeals as reimbursement for treatment of various conditions is becoming more limited, while some diseases are deemed purely cosmetic and coverage for treatment is denied.

Health-Related Quality of Life

Health-related quality of life (HRQL, HRQoL) instruments assess disease burden using physical, social, and psychological measures [1, 2]. These broadly encompassing measures are important in dermatologic diseases in particular, as health status or physical impairment may not fully correlate with the impact of the disease on the patient's life, nor correlate with severity of disease [3, 4]. Several

S.C. Taylor (✉)
Department of Dermatology, Hospital of the University of Pennsylvania, Penn Medicine, Washington Square, 16th Floor, 800 Walnut Street, Philadelphia, PA 19107, USA
e-mail: drstaylor1@aol.com

T. Ogunleye
3737 Market St. 11th Floor, Philadelphia, PA 19104, USA

© Springer International Publishing AG 2017
N.A. Vashi and H.I. Maibach (eds.), *Dermatoanthropology of Ethnic Skin and Hair*, DOI 10.1007/978-3-319-53961-4_2

13

dermatology-specific quality of life (QOL) questionnaires have been developed, including the Short Health Form 36 (SF-36) [5], the Skindex-29 [6] and the Dermatology Life Quality Index (DLQI) [7] that assess disease burden in general dermatologic disease (Table 2.1). Recently, disease-specific QOL questionnaires have been developed such as the Cardiff Acne Disability Index [8], Psoriasis Disability Index [1], Quality of Life Index for Atopic Dermatitis [9], Chronic Urticaria Quality of Life Questionnaire [10], and Melasma Quality of Life scale (MELASQOL) [3].

The DLQI, developed in 1994, was the first dermatology-specific QOL instrument [7] (Table 2.1). It is a widely used 10-question validated questionnaire that has been used in over 40 different skin conditions in over 80 countries. The SF-36 questionnaire consists of 36 items forming 8 domains (Table 2.1) [11]. Several versions of this questionnaire with fewer questions also exist. The Skindex-29 consists of 29 items forming 3 scales: symptoms, emotions, and functioning [6, 12] (Table 2.1). Higher scores in the DLQI and Skindex 29 correlate with decreased quality of life, while higher scores in the Skindex-29 instrument correlate with increased quality of life. Clinical meaning of scores is usually determined via a statistically significant difference of scoring after some intervention or comparison of mean scores to other diseases or the general population, although some have created banding of scores to assign clinical meaning to absolute scores [13] (Table 2.2). Issues with the banding scoring method include wide variability of bands created in various studies, and possible lack of generalizability based on population or disease states studied [13].

Table 2.1 Dermatology specific quality of life questionnaires

Name of survey instrument	DLQI	SF-36	Skindex 29
Areas examined	Symptoms Feelings Daily activities Leisure Work/school Personal relationships Treatment	Physical functioning Social functioning Role physical (limitations in usual activities because of physical problems) Role emotional (limitations in usual activities because of emotional problems) Bodily pain Mental health Vitality General health perception	Symptoms (e.g., itch, pain, and irritation) Emotions (e.g., worry, shame, embarrassment, frustration, and depression) Functioning (e.g., sleep, social life, social isolation, sexuality, work, and hobbies
Number of questions	10	36	29
Scoring	0–30	0–100	0–100

Table 2.2 Sample of proposed scoring interpretation

DLQI (Hongbo) [13, 65]	Skindex 29 (Chen) [13]	QoL effect
0–1	0–10	None/very little
2–5	11–25	Mild
6–10	26–50	Moderate
11–20	51–70	Severe
21–30	71–100	Very severe

In this chapter, we examine QOL studies that target conditions specific to or more common in skin of color patients and in particular those improperly deemed as aesthetic in nature. Providing a better understanding of the extent of disease burden will result in improved care of these patients.

Disorders of Pigmentation

Disorders of pigmentation occur commonly in individuals with skin of color and practice surveys reveal that they are the third most common presenting complaint in darker skinned individuals [14]. Although some physicians and insurance companies may consider these issues cosmetic, pigmentary disorders can be very distressing to the affected individual and can have long-lasting psychosocial implications. Disorders of hypopigmentation, specifically vitiligo, and of hyperpigmentation, including melasma and postinflammatory hyperpigmentation, have been examined to understand the associated psychosocial and physical burdens on patients.

Vitiligo

Vitiligo is an autoimmune disorder involving melanocytes, leading to loss of pigmentation in areas of skin and mucous membranes (Fig. 2.1). Depigmented or hypopigmented well-demarcated patches are seen most frequently on the hands, forearms, feet and face, but may be found anywhere. Involvement varies and may be localized, generalized or universal. In individuals with skin of color, the contrast between the normal darkly pigmented skin and the depigmented or white vitiliginous skin makes it a highly visible disorder.

The lesions of vitiligo are asymptomatic, contributing to the labeling of the disease as a cosmetic concern in some Western countries, which subsequently has led to undertreatment and decreased insurance coverage for treatments [15–17]. However, altered skin color as well skin color that is not uniform can negatively affect the perception of general health, wealth, worth, and desirability of an

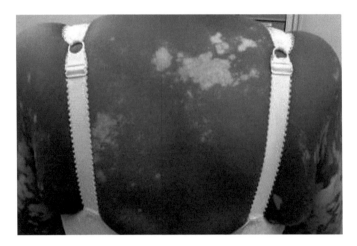

Fig. 2.1 Vitiligo on the back of an affected individual. Note the large patches of depigmentation, with scattered small confetti macules

individual [18]. Vitiligo can lead to social exclusion and is a major medical problem in India [19, 20]. In that society, vitiligo has been mistaken for infectious diseases such as leprosy, leading to shunning [19]. Additionally, it can affect marriageability and render a young woman unable to get married [21, 22]. Hence, the burden of illness for vitiligo can have far-reaching implications beyond the cosmetic appearance.

Gender differences in quality of life have been demonstrated in women with vitiligo where there is evidence of increased depression, anxiety, and community isolation [23]. In a 2016 review of 21 studies assessing the DLQI score of 4721 patients with vitiligo, ten of these studies revealed impaired quality of life for both genders, but female patients had more QoL impairment (total mean 8.03) than males (5.99) [23].

A Netherlands study of 245 patients using the Skindex 29 and SF-36 found that adult patients with generalized vitiligo had a low mental HRQL [11], comparable with that of patients with symptomatic skin diseases such as eczema [24, 25], psoriasis [24, 26, 27], and hand eczema [28]. Patients with dark skin (skin type IV–VI) and those who had treatment in the past had significantly more impairment in psychosocial functioning ($P < 0.01$) [11]. This difference may be attributable to the ease of visibility of vitiligo in darker skinned patients. Authors also propose that patients who have been treated in the past may have less hope regarding future treatment of their disorder, and have overall less acceptance of their disease [11]. A 2015 cross-sectional study of 300 patients also found that darker skinned patients felt '(their) vitiligo ha(d) repercussions on (their) physical appearance' ($P = 0.042$) and 'managing (their) vitiligo on a daily basis (wa)s a burden' ($P = 0.037$) [29]. Fair skinned individuals were more concerned about skin cancer risks from vitiligo ($P = 0.039$) [29].

Overall, these studies suggest that regardless of skin type, patients with vitiligo experience significant disease-related burden and self-perceived stress [11, 29]. However, patients with darker skin may have increased emotional burden in comparison with their lighter skinned counterparts [29]. In addition, treatment of vitiligo was also found to be an independent stressor that interfered negatively with quality of life [11]. Lastly, fair-skinned vitiligo patients had increased concern about skin cancer development, highlighting an opportunity for education as recent research indicates that patients with vitiligo have a decreased risk of melanoma and nonmelanoma skin cancer [29–31].

Melasma

Melasma is a relatively common disorder of acquired hyperpigmentation characterized by symmetric, poorly demarcated brown macules and patches that occur primarily on sun-exposed areas on the face and neck (Fig. 2.2). The three clinical patterns of melasma are centrofacial (most common), malar, and mandibular. Risk factors include exposure to ultraviolet radiation, genetics, hormonal therapy and pregnancy, phototoxic drugs, and anticonvulsant medications [32].

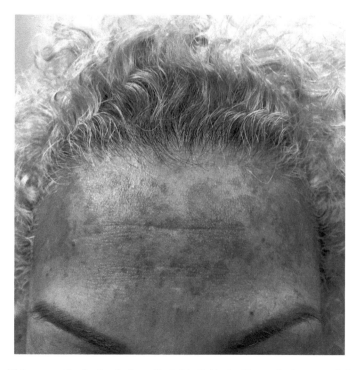

Fig. 2.2 Melasma on the forehead of an affected individual with poorly demarcated *dark brown macules* coalescing into patches

Melasma affects all races but is especially prevalent in those with darker skin types (Fitzpatrick skin types III–VI) and has been frequently reported in patients of Hispanic, African American, Arab, South Asian, Southeast Asian, and East Asian descent [32]. Additionally, melasma is more prevalent in women, with men comprising only 10% of all cases [33].

In 2003, Balkrishnan et al. developed a new health-related quality of life (HRQL) instrument for women with melasma by merging Skindex-16 and other skin pigmentation questionnaires [3]. This questionnaire differed from previous dermatological HRQL instruments such as the DLQI and Skindex-16, which placed equal weight on physical and psychological effects of skin disease [6, 7]. However, since the physical discomfort from melasma is negligible, but psychosocial effects may be severe, a more targeted questionnaire was necessary to adequately measure the burden of this disease. MELASQoL was developed from questions more relevant to melasma-specific QoL issues and with greater emphasis on the emotional and psychosocial aspects [3].

The MELASQoL by Balkrishnan et al. [3] identified social life, leisure and recreation, and emotional well-being as being most affected by melasma, whereas, a 2006 validation study of the MELASQoL in Latino patients, reported the QOL domains most affected by melasma were emotional well-being, social life, physical health, and finances [4]. In Asian patients in a 2016 Singapore study of 49 women, the strongest predictors of decreased HRQoL in women with melasma were increased disease severity ($P < 0.05$), increased fear of negative evaluation ($P < 0.01$), and the belief that their HRQoL would be better if they did not have melasma ($P < 0.01$) [34].

In summary, the MELASQoL questionnaire has been helpful in more accurately elucidating the psychosocial burden of melasma. Patients report difficulties in interpersonal relationships, ability to enjoy leisure and recreational activities, and a financial burden, likely from failed attempts from treatment [3, 35, 36]. These studies reinforce the need for more successful treatments of this condition that can have impact that reaches beyond cosmetic disfigurement. This tool has been successfully adapted and validated in multiple languages including Spanish, Brazilian Portuguese, Hindi and French. Since melasma is common worldwide, particularly in individuals with skin of color, translation to other languages will be helpful in understanding the impact of melasma in difference countries and to increase the body of HrQoL data for this condition.

Acne and Postinflammatory Hyperpigmentation

Acne is one of the most frequently encountered diseases in dermatology for individuals 15–40 years of age in the United States [37] Acne is also the most common dermatological diagnosis in non-Caucasian patients [38–41]. In a community-based photographic study, clinical acne was found to occur most commonly in Black/African American (37%), Hispanic/Latina (32%), and Asian (30%) women, more so than in Continental Indian (23%) and White/Caucasian (24%) women [42].

Clinically, acne may present with open and closed comedones and/or a mixture of inflammatory papules, pustules, and nodules most commonly on the face, chest, and back of varying severity. In particular, postinflammatory hyperpigmentation (PIH) is a prominent sequelae of acne in darker skin tone, and can be a source of increased quality of life burden in skin of color patients. Acne is likely the most common cause of PIH in patients with skin of color, especially in Black patients where up to two-thirds of patients may experience PIH [42, 43]. If the inciting inflammatory condition improves or resolves but postinflammatory hyperpigmentation remains unaddressed, the patient will often consider the treatment to be a failure [44].

Callender et al. surveyed a diverse sampling of 208 women and found that 70% non-White/Caucasian women surveyed felt that their skin type required targeted attention and two-thirds (66.3%) desired an acne treatment that was designed to meet the needs of their skin [43]. More than 75% preferred to visit a healthcare professional who had experience treating acne in non-White/Caucasian women [43]. In addition, the majority of the women surveyed (85.1%) would be interested in an acne treatment that had been proven effective in treating acne for their race, ethnicity, or skin type [43]. The types of information considered most convincing in proving the efficacy of an acne treatment were scientific data or statistics (33.7%), recommendation by a dermatologist (17.8%) or friend/family member (15.8%), photographs (13.9%), primary care physician recommendation (10.9%), and other types of information (8.0%) [43].

Acne was shown to be burdensome and associated with low QoL, negative self-perceptions and symptoms of depression/anxiety in the Callender study [43]. Levels of social and emotional problems in acne patients were similar to that of psoriasis patients [45], and even those with severe chronic disabling diseases, such as arthritis and diabetes [46].

Acne in skin of color patients has the potential sequelae of postinflammatory hyperpigmentation that can add to the burden of disease. Clearing PIH was most important for many of the non-White/Caucasian women studied by Callender (41.6%; $p < 0.0001$) but was a lesser concern for White/Caucasian women (8.4%) [43]. Surveys also suggest that this patient population views a dearth of appropriate treatments and understanding of acne in their skin type, indicating a potential need for better products made for darker skin types [43]. Improved education of dermatologists regarding their approach in darker skin types including aggressive treatment of inflammatory lesions to decrease PIH and concomitant treatment of PIH may improve both clinical and QoL outcomes.

Keloids

Keloids represent an exaggerated healing response to trauma, resulting in irregular deposition of collagen beyond the boundaries of the original injury. Erythematous to hyperpigmented firm or rubbery nodules/plaques are seen, extending beyond the original trauma, and sometimes with no known antecedent trauma. Although sometimes considered a cosmetic issue, keloids are often painful, itchy, and cause a burning sensation. Keloid scarring is more prevalent in those of African, Asian, and Hispanic descent [47]. Most studies regarding keloids focus on the efficacy of available treatment options, but keloids have a significant effect on the quality of life.

A 2015 study of 108 keloid patients revealed that keloid disease had a large impact on the emotional well-being of patients [48]. Nearly half of the patients (48%) had severe emotional symptoms and about a quarter reported severe problems on the symptomatic and functional scale of the Skindex-29 questionnaire, such as itching and pain [48]. HRQL reduction was similar to the burden of diseases such as psoriasis, dermatitis, arthritis, and cancer [49]. Importantly, itching and pain were associated with the largest HRQL impairment, while cosmetic factors such as color, thickness, pliability, and irregularity of the scar were less related [48].

Another study of 130 patients with scars stratified based on type found that physiological and hypertrophic scars had little impact on the quality of life, while keloidal scars and atrophic scars more strongly decreased quality of life not only related to symptoms but also due to influences on daily activities, leisure and personal relationships [50].

Keloid scars can be disfiguring, but are a significant source of physical and psychosocial impairment. Importantly, QoL studies suggest that physical impairment is more burdensome than cosmetic appearance, highlighting the non-cosmetic and necessary nature of treatment [49, 50].

Alopecia

Hair loss is a common complaint in skin of color patients and several studies have shown that patients with alopecia have psychological sequelae [51–53]. Since alopecia is largely considered to be an aesthetic condition, ill feelings can be exacerbated by health care providers who may underestimate the impact of hair loss on such patients.

Alopecia can be categorized into scarring or non-scarring subtypes based on the clinical finding of loss of follicular ostia in areas of involvement, and the pathologic presence of decreased number of viable follicles and follicular scarring. Alopecia areata, androgenetic alopecia, telogen effluvium and early traction alopecia are the main types of non-scarring alopecia, while lichen planopilaris, central centrifugal cicatricial alopecia, dissecting cellulitis, acne keloidalis nuchae and late stage traction alopecia are the main types of scarring alopecia. Certain types of scarring hair loss such as traction alopecia or central centrifugal scarring alopecia occur with increased frequency in darker skinned populations, particularly women. However, quality of life studies specific to these conditions are few.

A study of 50 South African women with alopecia found on a scale ranging from 0 (high QoL) to 100 (severely decreased QoL) a mean QLI of 67, indicating notable disease burden [54]. The factors with the highest impact were those relating to self-image (56.3%) and relationships and interaction with other people (34.8%) [54]. Specifically, subjects expressed concern that their children may develop alopecia or that their own condition would worsen, not being able to forget about the presence their alopecia, and worries about cost. The presence of symptoms such as itching were of less importance (8.9%) [54].

Another study examining 105 British men and women with primary cicatricial alopecia found that 19% of patients demonstrated a severe impact (DLQI score ≥ 11) on their QoL [55]. Interestingly, increasing age, being female and having <25% of hair loss were associated with better illness perceptions, less psychological distress, and higher QoL [55]. Based on these results, practitioners may consider more thorough evaluation for psychosocial issues in male patients with primary cicatricial alopecia who may have higher disease burden than some practitioners would anticipate.

Similar impact on quality of life was seen in patients with non-scarring hair loss including alopecia areata, androgenic alopecia, and telogen effluvium [56]. A 2012 study of 104 subjects with these conditions using the Skindex-16 instrument found a mean score of 57.3 (SD $\pm$ 16.2), indicative of moderately decreased quality of life [56]. The emotions domain reflected the lowest QoL (mean = 83.8 $\pm$ 15.2), followed by function domain (mean = 50.2 $\pm$ 30.0) and symptoms domain (mean = 19.9 $\pm$ 19.9), again suggesting that the emotional burden can be more influential to the well-being of the patient than the physical burden of these conditions [56].

In general, these studies confirm the emotional impact of hair loss in patients in a quantitative fashion. As the primary caretakers of these conditions in medicine, dermatologists should continue to treat both the hair disease process, as well as the psychosocial distress of the patients. By addressing both, we may be able to alleviate unnecessary fears of patients, increase patient satisfaction, and improve patients' overall quality of life.

Sarcoidosis

Sarcoidosis is a granulomatous disease that may involve any organ. The disease course is highly variable, ranging from an asymptomatic state to a progressive condition that may, occasionally, be life-threatening. The pathologic hallmark of sarcoidosis is the granuloma that may resolve spontaneously or with anti-sarcoidosis therapy. The typical cutaneous findings are reddish brown papules and plaques found anywhere on the body, including the face, but are highly variable and include subcutaneous, ulcerative, lichenoid, psoriasiform, verrucous, and hypopigmented forms.

Sarcoidosis affects all races, but African-American women have the highest rates of sarcoidosis in the United States, including the highest rates of chronic cutaneous sarcoidosis [57]. Particularly in cutaneous cases with quiescent lung disease, sarcoidosis may be treated less aggressively secondary to the nonlife-threatening nature of cutaneous disease [58]. However, an important alternative indication for treatment includes decreased quality of life.

Previous studies have shown that sarcoidosis experts are relatively poor judges of the impact of the disease on the patient's quality of life [59], and initiate treatment based on increases in serum angiotensin-converting enzyme levels or nodularity on chest imaging, which may not translate into appreciable impact on patient quality of life [58]. However, studies examining HRQL as a primary outcome in sarcoidosis studies are scarce. The Sarcoidosis Health Questionnaire (SHQ) is a 29-item validated sarcoidosis-specific survey assessing the impact of sarcoidosis involvement of multiple organ systems, but only has one question relating to the skin, and therefore may not adequately capture cutaneous burden on quality of life [60]. The Sarcoidosis Assessment Tool (SAT) is a new quality of life instrument developed specifically for sarcoidosis that includes cutaneous disease in addition to pulmonary and ophthalmic involvement [61–63]. Skin Concerns and Skin Stigma scores of the SAT range from 0 to 40 and 0 to 20, respectively, with higher scores correlating with greater burden [63].

In a small cross-sectional study of 13 patients designed to examine the validity and reliability of other cutaneous sarcoidosis outcome instruments, the Skindex-29, DLQI, and the SAT were given [64]. The mean Skindex-29 Emotions, Symptoms, and Functioning domain scores were 65.8, 44.6, and 42.9, respectively, indicating that patients were severely impacted emotionally by their disease, and their symptoms of itch/pain at least moderately affected their lives. The mean SAT Skin Concerns and Skin Stigma raw sum scores were 13.3 and 11.1, respectively, again confirming negatively impacted quality of life. These questionnaires all suggest some level of burden on skin-specific disease, but larger scale studies with quality of life as the primary outcome are needed.

Conclusion

Inflammatory, granulomatous, scarring, and pigmentary skin and hair diseases that are specific to or more common in skin of color patients have been shown to significantly and negatively impact the quality of life of these patients. Thus, examining the burden of disease on quality of life in the skin of color patients is important, especially when many conditions may be improperly labeled as purely aesthetic. Health-related quality of life studies play a pivotal role in highlighting the psychosocial effects of disease that at times may even be greater than the physical impact of the disorder. As healthcare providers, we can utilize quality of life research to assure that we are not underestimating disease burden and treating single facets of multifaceted disease in order to provide complete care. In addition, we may be able to use these instruments to provide data for improved advocacy for the health coverage of some of these disorders.

References

1. Finlay AY, Kelly SE. Psoriasis—an index of disability. Clin Exp Dermatol. 1987;12(1):8–11.
2. Finlay AY. Quality of life assessments in dermatology. Sem Cutaneous Med Surg. 1998;17(4): 291–6.
3. Balkrishnan R, McMichael AJ, Camacho FT, Saltzberg F, Housman TS, Grummer S, et al. Development and validation of a health-related quality of life instrument for women with melasma. Br J Dermatol. 2003;149(3):572–7.
4. Dominguez AR, Balkrishnan R, Ellzey AR, Pandya AG. Melasma in Latina patients: cross-cultural adaptation and validation of a quality-of-life questionnaire in Spanish language. J Am Acad Dermatol. 2006;55(1):59–66.
5. McHorney CA, Ware JE Jr, Raczek AE. The MOS 36-Item Short-Form Health Survey (SF-36): II. Psychometric and clinical tests of validity in measuring physical and mental health constructs. Med Care. 1993;31(3):247–63.
6. Chren MM, Lasek RJ, Quinn LM, Mostow EN, Zyzanski SJ. Skindex, a quality-of-life measure for patients with skin disease: reliability, validity, and responsiveness. J Invest Dermatol 1996;107(5):707–13.
7. Finlay AY, Khan GK. Dermatology Life Quality Index (DLQI)—a simple practical measure for routine clinical use. Clin Exp Dermatol. 1994;19(3):210–6.
8. Motley RJ, Finlay AY. Practical use of a disability index in the routine management of acne. Clin Exp Dermatol. 1992;17(1):1–3.
9. Whalley D, Mckenna SP, Dewar AL, Erdman RA, Kohlmann T, Niero M, et al. A new instrument for assessing quality of life in atopic dermatitis: international development of the Quality of Life Index for Atopic Dermatitis (QoLIAD). Br J Dermatol. 2004;150(2):274–83.
10. Baiardini I, Pasquali M, Braido F, Fumagalli F, Guerra L, Compalati E, et al. A new tool to evaluate the impact of chronic urticaria on quality of life: chronic urticaria quality of life questionnaire (CU-Q2oL). Allergy Eur J Allergy Clin Immunol. 2005;60(8):1073–8.
11. Linthorst Homan MW, Spuls PI, de Korte J, Bos JD, Sprangers MA, van der Veen JPW. The burden of vitiligo: patient characteristics associated with quality of life. J Am Acad Dermatol. 2009 9;61(3):411–20.
12. Chren MM, Lasek RJ, Flocke SA, Zyzanski SJ. Improved discriminative and evaluative capability of a refined version of Skindex, a quality-of-life instrument for patients with skin diseases. Arch Dermatol 1997;133(11):1433–40.
13. Rogers A, DeLong LK, Chen SC. Clinical meaning in skin-specific quality of life instruments: a comparison of the dermatology life quality index and skindex banding systems. Dermatol Clin. 2012 4;30(2):333–42.
14. Halder RM, Grimes PE, McLaurin CI, Kress MA, Kenney JA Jr. Incidence of common dermatoses in a predominantly black dermatologic practice. Cutis. 1983;32(4):388–90.
15. Ongenae K, Van Geel N, De Schepper S, Haeghen YV, Naeyaert J-M. Management of vitiligo patients and attitude of dermatologists towards vitiligo. Eur J Dermatol. 2004;14(3): 177–81.
16. Njoo MD, Bossuyt PMM, Westerhof W. Management of vitiligo. Results of a questionnaire among dermatologists in the Netherlands. Int J Dermatol. 1999;38(11):866–72.
17. Ongenae K, Beelaert L, van Geel N, Naeyaert J-M. Psychosocial effects of vitiligo. J Eur Acad Dermatol Venereol. 2006;20(1):1–8.

18. Grimes PE. White patches and bruised souls: advances in the pathogenesis and treatment of vitiligo. J Am Acad Dermatol. 2004 7;51(1, Supplement):5–7.
19. Chaturvedi SK, Singh G, Gupta N. Stigma experience in skin disorders: an Indian perspective. Dermatol Clin. 2005;23(4 SPEC. ISS.):635–42.
20. Parsad D, Dogra SF, Kanwar AJ. Quality of life in patients with vitiligo. Health and quality of life outcomes JID - 101153626 0630.
21. Kaur H, Ramesh V. Social problems of women leprosy patients—a study conducted at 2 urban leprosy centres in Delhi. Lepr Rev. 1994;65(4):361–75.
22. Rao S, Garole V, Walawalkar S, Khot S, Karandikar N. Gender differentials in the social impact of leprosy. Lepr Rev. 1996;67(3):190–9.
23. Amer AAA, Gao X. Quality of life in patients with vitiligo: an analysis of the dermatology life quality index outcome over the past two decades. Int J Dermatol. 2016:n/a-n/a.
24. Lundberg L, Johannesson M, Silverdahl M, Hermansson C, Lindberg M. Health-related quality of life in patients with psoriasis and atopic dermatitis measured with SF-36, DLQI and a subjective measure of disease activity. Acta Derm-Venereol. 2000;80(6):430–4.
25. Holm EA, Wulf HC, Stegmann H, Jemec GBE. Life quality assessment among patients with atopic eczema. Br J Dermatol. 2006;154(4):719–25.
26. Wahl A, Hanestad BR, Wiklund I, Moum T. Coping and quality of life in patients with psoriasis. Qual Life Res. 1999;8(5):427–33.
27. Wahl A, Moum T, Hanestad BR, Wiklund I. The relationship between demographic and clinical variables, and quality of life aspects in patients with psoriasis. Qual Life Res. 1999;8(4):319–26.
28. Wallenhammar L-M, Nyfjäll M, Lindberg M, Meding B. Health-related quality of life and hand eczema—a comparison of two instruments, including factor analysis. J Invest Dermatol. 2004;122(6):1381–9.
29. Ezzedine K, Grimes PE, Meurant J-, Seneschal J, Léauté-Labrèze C, Ballanger F, et al. Living with vitiligo: results from a national survey indicate differences between skin phototypes. Br J Dermatol. 2015;173(2):607–9.
30. Teulings HE, Overkamp M, Ceylan E, Nieuweboer-Krobotova L, Bos JD, Nijsten T, et al. Decreased risk of melanoma and nonmelanoma skin cancer in patients with vitiligo: a survey among 1307 patients and their partners. Br J Dermatol. 2013;168(1):162–71.
31. Paradisi A, Tabolli S, Didona B, Sobrino L, Russo N, Abeni D. Markedly reduced incidence of melanoma and nonmelanoma skin cancer in a nonconcurrent cohort of 10,040 patients with vitiligo. J Am Acad Dermatol. 2014 12;71(6):1110–6.
32. Sheth VM, Pandya AG. Melasma: a comprehensive update: Part i. J Am Acad Dermatol. 2011;65(4):689–97.
33. Sarkar R, Puri P, Jain Jr RK, Singh AF, Desai A. Melasma in men: a clinical, aetiological and histological study. J Eur Acad Dermatol Venereol: JEADV JID - 9216037 1108.
34. Harumi O, Goh CL. The effect of melasma on the quality of life in a sample of women living in Singapore. J Clin Aesthetic Dermatol. 2016;9(1):21–4.
35. Freitag FM, Cestari TF, Leopoldo LR, Paludo P, Boza JC. Effect of melasma on quality of life in a sample of women living in southern Brazil. J Eur Acad Dermatol Venereol: JEADV JID - 9216037 0811.
36. Ikino JK, Nunes DH, Silva VP, Frode TS, Sens MM. Melasma and assessment of the quality of life in Brazilian women. An Bras Dermatol. 2015;90(2):196–200.
37. Stern RS. Medication and medical service utilization for acne 1995–1998. J Am Acad Dermatol. JID - 7907132 0125.
38. Shah SK, Bhanusali DG, Sachdev A, Geria AN, Alexis AF. A survey of skin conditions and concerns in South Asian Americans: a community-based study. J Drugs Dermatol. 2011;10(5):524–8.
39. Alexis AF, Sergay AB, Taylor SC. Common dermatologic disorders in skin of color: a comparative practice survey. Cutis. 2007;80(5):387–94.
40. Poli F. Acne on pigmented skin. Int J Dermatol. 2007;46(Suppl 1):39–41.

41. Child FJ, Fuller LC, Higgins EM, Du Vivier AW. A study of the spectrum of skin disease occurring in a black population in south-east London. Br J Dermatol. 1999;141(3):512–7.
42. Perkins AC, Cheng CE, Hillebrand GG, Miyamoto K, Kimball AB. Comparison of the epidemiology of acne vulgaris among Caucasian, Asian, Continental Indian and African American women. J Eur Acad Dermatol Venereol. 2011;25(9):1054–60.
43. Callender VD, Alexis AF, Daniels SR, Kawata AK, Burk CT, Wilcox TK, et al. Racial differences in clinical characteristics, perceptions and behaviors, and psychosocial impact of adult female acne. J Clin Aesthet Dermatol. 2014;7(7):19–31.
44. Alexis AF. Acne in patients with skin of color. J Drugs Dermatol. 2011;10(6):s13–6.
45. Lasek RJ, Chren MM. Acne vulgaris and the quality of life of adult dermatology patients. Arch Dermatol. 1998;134(4):454–8.
46. Mallon E, Newton JN, Klassen A, Stewart-Brown SL, Ryan TJ, Finlay AY. The quality of life in acne: a comparison with general medical conditions using generic questionnaires. Br J Dermatol. 1999;140(4):672–6.
47. Chike-Obi CJ, Cole PD, Brissett AE. Keloids: pathogenesis, clinical features, and management. Semin Plast Surg. 2009;23(3):178–84.
48. Kouwenberg CA, Bijlard E, Timman R, Hovius SE, Busschbach JJ, Mureau MA. Emotional quality of life is severely affected by keloid disease: pain and itch are the main determinants of burden. Plast Reconstr Surg. 2015;136(4 Suppl):150–1.
49. Aaronson NK, Muller M, Cohen PD, Essink-Bot ML, Fekkes M, Sanderman R, et al. Translation, validation, and norming of the Dutch language version of the SF-36 Health Survey in community and chronic disease populations. J Clin Epidemiol. 1998;51(11): 1055–68.
50. Reinholz M, Poetschke J, Schwaiger H, Epple A, Ruzicka T, Gauglitz GG. The dermatology life quality index as a means to assess life quality in patients with different scar types. J Eur Acad Dermatol Venereol. 2015;29(11):2112–9.
51. van der Donk J, Passchier J, Knegt-Junk C, Van der Wegen-Keijser MH, Nieboer C, Stolz E, et al. Psychological characteristics of women with androgenetic alopecia: a controlled study. Br J Dermatol. 1991;125(3):248–52.
52. Van Der Donk J, Hunfeld JA, Passchier J, Knegt-Junk KJ, Nieboer C. Quality of life and maladjustment associated with hair loss in women with alopecia androgenetica. Soc Sci Med. 1994;38(1):159–63.
53. Camacho F, García-Hernández M. Psychological features of androgenetic alopecia1. J Eur Acad Dermatol Venereol. 2002;16(5):476–80.
54. Dlova NC, Fabbrocini G, Lauro C, Spano M, Tosti A, Hift RH. Quality of life in South African Black women with alopecia: a pilot study. Int J Dermatol. 2015.
55. Chiang YZ, Bundy C, Griffiths CEM, Paus R, Harries MJ. The role of beliefs: lessons from a pilot study on illness perception, psychological distress and quality of life in patients with primary cicatricial alopecia. Br J Dermatol. 2015;172(1):130–7.
56. Reid EE, Haley AC, Borovicka JH, Rademaker A, West DP, Colavincenzo M, et al. Clinical severity does not reliably predict quality of life in women with alopecia areata, telogen effluvium, or androgenic alopecia. J Am Acad Dermatol. 2012 3;66(3):e97–102.
57. Wanat KA, Rosenbach M. Cutaneous sarcoidosis. Clin Chest Med. 2015 12;36(4):685–702.
58. Judson MA. Quality of life assessment in sarcoidosis. Clin Chest Med. 2015 12;36(4):739–50.
59. Cox CE, Donohue JF, Brown CD, Kataria YP, Judson MA. Health-related quality of life of persons with sarcoidosis. Chest. 2004;125(3):997–1004.
60. Cox CE, Donohue JF, Brown CD, Kataria YP, Judson MA. The Sarcoidosis Health Questionnaire: a new measure of health-related quality of life. Am J Respir Crit Care Med. 2003;168(3):323–9.
61. Victorson DE, Cella D, Grund H, Judson MA. A conceptual model of health-related quality of life in sarcoidosis. Qual Life Res. 2013;23(1):89–101.
62. Victorson DE, Choi S, Judson MA, Cella D. Development and testing of item response theory-based item banks and short forms for eye, skin and lung problems in sarcoidosis. Qual Life Res. 2013;23(4):1301–13.

63. Judson MA, Mack M, Beaumont JL, Watt R, Barnathan ES, Victorson DE. Validation and important differences for the Sarcoidosis Assessment Tool. A new patient-reported outcome measure. Am J Respir Crit Care Med. 2015 04/01; 2016/04;191(7):786–795.
64. Yeung H, Farber S, Birnbaum BK, et al. REliability and validity of cutaneous sarcoidosis outcome instruments among dermatologists, pulmonologists, and rheumatologists. JAMA Dermatol. 2015;151(12):1317–22.
65. Hongbo Y, Thomas CL, Harrison MA, Salek MS, Finlay AY. Translating the science of quality of life into practice: What do dermatology life quality index scores mean? J Invest Dermatol. 2005;125(4):659–64.

Chapter 3
Biophysical Properties of Ethnic Skin

E. Berardesca, M. Mariano and N. Cameli

Even though it is well established that all humans belong to the same species, many physical differences exist among human populations. The use of bioengineering techniques is useful to investigate these differences that could be due both to genetic, socioeconomic, and environmental factors [1].

Barrier Function

Stratum corneum is equally thick in different races [2–5]. However, Weigand et al. demonstrated that the stratum corneum in Blacks contains more cell layers and requires more cellophane tape strips to be removed than the stratum corneum of Caucasians [6], while Kampaore and Tsuruta showed that Asian skin was significantly more sensitive to stripping than Black skin [7]. Weigand also found great variance in values obtained from Black subjects, whereas data from White subjects were more homogeneous. No correlation was found between the degree of pigmentation and the number of cell layers. These data could be explained due to the greater intercellular cohesion in Blacks, resulting in an increased number of cell layers and an increased resistance to stripping. This mechanism may involve lipids [8], because the lipid content of the stratum corneum, ranges from 8.5 to 14%, with higher values in Blacks [5, 9]. This result was confirmed by Weigand et al. who showed that delipidized specimens of stratum corneum were equal in weight in the

E. Berardesca (✉)
Department of Dermatology, San Gallicano Dermatological Institute,
IRCCS, via Chianesi 53, 00144 Rome, Italy
e-mail: berardesca@berardesca.it

M. Mariano · N. Cameli
San Gallicano Dermatological Institute, IRCCS, via Chianesi 53,
00144 Rome, Italy

© Springer International Publishing AG 2017
N.A. Vashi and H.I. Maibach (eds.), *Dermatoanthropology of Ethnic Skin and Hair*, DOI 10.1007/978-3-319-53961-4_3

two races [6]. Johnson and Corah found that the mean electrical resistance of an adult Black skin is doubled when compared to adult White skin, suggesting an increased cohesion of the stratum corneum [10]. In fact, La Ruche and Cesarini found that, in comparison with White skin, the Black skin stratum corneum is equal in thickness but more compact: about twenty cell layers are observed in Blacks versus sixteen layers in Whites [5].

Corcuff et al. [11] investigated the corneocyte surface area and the spontaneous desquamation and found no differences between Black, White, and oriental skin. However, an increased desquamation (up to 2.5 times) was found in Blacks. Overall, the data is still controversial. They concluded that the differences may be related to a different composition of the intercellular lipids of the stratum corneum. Sugino et al. [12] found significant differences in the amount of ceramides in the stratum corneum, with the lowest levels in Blacks followed by Caucasian, Hispanics, and Asians. In this experiment, ceramide levels were inversely correlated with transepidermal water loss (TEWL) and directly correlated with water content. Meguro et al. [13] confirmed these correlations. These data may partially explain the controversial findings in the literature on the mechanisms of skin sensitivity.

Changes in skin permeability and barrier function have been reported: Kompaore et al. [7, 14] evaluated TEWL and lag time after application of a vasoactive compound (methyl nicotinate) before and after removal of the stratum corneum by tape stripping. Before tape stripping, TEWL was 1.3 times greater in Blacks and Asians compared to Caucasians. No difference was found between Blacks and Asians, whereas after stripping, they found a significantly higher TEWL in Blacks and Asians than in Whites. In particular, after stripping Asians showed the highest TEWL (Asians 1.7 times greater than Caucasians). They concluded that, similar to previous studies [15, 16], skin permeability measured by TEWL is higher in Blacks than in Caucasians. They also concluded that Asian skin has the highest permeability among the groups studied. However, these findings have not yet been confirmed by other groups. In fact, Sugino et al. [12] also included Asians in their study but found that baseline TEWL was, in decreasing order, Blacks > Caucasians $\geq$ Hispanics $\geq$ Asians. Another study [17] looking at Asian skin has compared TEWL in Asians and Caucasians and found no statistically significant differences at baseline or after stripping; however, no vasoactive substance was applied.

Reed et al. [18] found differences in the recovery of the barrier between subjects with skin type II/III compared to skin type V/VI, but no differences between Caucasians in general and Asians. Darker skin recovered faster after barrier damage induced by tape stripping.

Biophysical Parameters

Transepidermal water loss (TEWL), skin conductance, and skin mechanical properties have been measured under basal conditions in Whites, Hispanics, and Blacks to assess whether skin color (melanin content) could induce changes in skin biophysical properties [19]. TEWL is defined as the amount of water vapor lost through the skin and appendages under non-sweating conditions. It is the most studied biophysical property when elucidating skin type variations. Differences appear in skin conductance are more evident in biomechanical features such as skin extensibility, skin elastic modulus, and skin recovery. They differ in dorsal and ventral sites according to races and highlight the influence of solar irradiation on skin and the role of melanin in maintaining it unaltered.

Wilson et al. [15] demonstrated higher in vitro TEWL values in Black compared to White skin taken from cadavers. They also found differences in Black and White skin physiology; in fact, the TEWL increased with skin temperature. In their own study, they concluded that Black skin would have a greater rise to achieve the same temperature and therefore a higher TEWL. Since TEWL depends on passive water vapor loss that is theoretically directly related to the ambient relative humidity and temperature [20], then, the increased TEWL in Black skin could be associated with an increase in temperature because it is well established that a difference in Black and Caucasian temperature exists.

Most studies using the forearm, back, and inner thigh [12–16, 21, 22] show a greater TEWL in Blacks compared to Whites; however, Warrier et al. [23] have demonstrated, studying a larger sample size, that TEWL is lower in Blacks than Whites when measuring on the cheeks and legs. No racial differences in TEWL exist either on the volar or dorsal forearms. However, water content is increased in Hispanics on the volar forearm and decreased in Whites (compared only to Blacks) on the dorsal forearm. These findings partially confirm previous observations [16, 24]. Skin lipids may play a role in modulating the relation between stratum corneum water content and TEWL resulting in higher conductance values in Blacks and Hispanics.

Racial differences in skin conductance are difficult to interpret in terms of stratum corneum water content, because other physical factors, such as the skin surface or the presence of hair, can modify the quality of the skin–electrode contact. In all races, significant differences exist between the volar and dorsal forearms [19]. These results are in apparent contrast with TEWL recordings. Indeed, increased stratum corneum water content, correlates with a higher TEWL [25]. These data may be explained on the basis of a different intercellular cohesion or lipid composition. A greater cell cohesion with a normal TEWL could result in increased skin water content.

Racial variability should be considered in terms of different skin responses to topical and environmental agents. Race provides a useful tool to investigate and compare the effects of lifetime sun exposure and ambient relative humidity. Evolution provided over 100 thousand years of genetic advantage to survive for those races living in a specific area with specific climatic conditions. Surviving in harmful environments requires an optimal adaptation of the outermost layers of our body, the skin on a structural, biochemical, and molecular level. For example, it is evident that melanin protection decreases sun damage; and furthermore, differences between sun-exposed and sun-protected areas are not detectable in races with dark skin.

However, transepidermal water loss studies are characterized by a large inter-individual variability and biased by environmental effects and eccrine sweating. To bypass these influences, an in vitro technique for measuring TEWL was used to compare TEWL in two racial groups (Blacks and Whites) [15]. Black skin had a significantly higher mean TEWL than White skin. In both groups a significant correlation between skin temperature and increased TEWL was found. The data confirm differences between races found in in vivo studies [16, 24]. The TEWL measurements with regards to Asian skin may be deemed inconclusive as baseline measurements have found Asian skin to have TEWL values that are equal to Black skin and greater than Caucasian skin [14], less than other ethnic groups [12], and no different than other ethnic groups [17]. Overall, data does not provide consistent, reproducible conclusions which may be attributed to anatomic site variation and/or disparate measurement parameters.

Irritation

Irritation, as measured by TEWL, [16, 24] revealed a different pattern of reaction in Whites after chemical exposure to sodium lauryl sulfate. Blacks and Hispanics developed stronger irritant reactions after exposure. We applied 0.5 and 2.0% sodium lauryl sulfate (SLS), to untreated, pre-occluded, and pre-delipidized Black and Caucasian skin and quantified the resulting level of irritation using water content (WC), TEWL, and laser Doppler velocimetry (LDV) of the stratum corneum [16]. There were only a statistical difference in irritation measuring TEWL after 0.5% SLS application to the pre-occluded area between the two groups. In fact, Blacks had 2.7 times higher TEWL levels than Caucasians, suggesting that Blacks in the pre-occluded state are more susceptible to irritation than Caucasians. In another study, we compared differences in irritation between Hispanic and Caucasian skin [16]. We found higher values of TEWL for Hispanics compared to Whites after SLS-induced irritation. However, these values were not statistically significant. The reaction of Hispanic skin to SLS resembles Black skin when irritated with the same substance. Therefore, these data oppose the traditional clinical view, based on observing erythema, that darker are less reactive to irritants than Whites.

Skin Aging

Skin aging is also associated with progressive atrophy of the dermis and changes in the architectural organization leading to folds and wrinkles [26].

Asian and Black skin has thicker and more compact dermis than White skin, with the thickness being proportional to the degree of pigmentation [27].

This likely contributes to the lower incidence of facial rhytides in Asians and Blacks. In addition, darker skin types are thought to have more cornified cell layers and greater lipid content compared to White stratum corneum [12, 19]. The major cell type of the dermis is the fibroblast, which synthesizes the main structural elements of the dermis. Black skin has been found to have more numerous, larger, and more nucleated fibroblasts, smaller collagen fiber bundles, and more macrophages than White skin [28]. Chronological aging reduces the life span of fibroblasts; their potential for division being lower in the elderly. Fibroblast functionality and reactivity likely contribute to both the aging phenomena and abnormal scarring. Individuals with darker skin are overall thought to have firmer and smoother skin than individuals with lighter skin of the same age; however, aging does occur in regards to mottled pigmentation, wrinkles, and skin laxity. Disorders of pigmentation associated with aging seem to occur earlier in Asians as compared to Caucasians, even though wrinkling appears years later [29, 30]. A complete knowledge of the structural and functional principles of mature ethnic skin is helpful to properly care for the aging skin of color population [31].

Conclusion

Ethnic differences in skin physiology have been minimally investigated. The current experimental human model for skin is largely based upon physical and biochemical properties known about Caucasian skin. Thus, anatomical or physiological properties in skin of different races that may alter a disease process or a treatment of that disease are not being accounted for. Therefore, we still cannot answer the question "how resistant is black skin compared to white?". There exists reasonable evidence to support that Black skin has a higher TEWL compared to White skin by means of objective measurements. Although some deductions have been made about Asian and Hispanic skin, the results are contradictory and further evaluation needs to be done. Perhaps more specificity about the origin of their heritage should also be included since "Asian" and "Hispanic" encompasses a broad spectrum of people. Regardless, we remain optimistic that further knowledge will lead to redefine claim support and more appropriated formulation for race-based skin care.

References

1. Shriver MD. Ethnic variation as a key to the biology of human disease. Ann Intern Med. 1997;127:401–3.
2. Freeman RG, Cockerell EG, Armstrong J, et al. Sunlight as a factor influencing the thickness of epidermis. J Invest Dermatol. 1962;39:295–7.
3. Thomson ML. Relative efficiency of pigment and horny layer thickness in protecting the skin of European and Africans against solar ultraviolet radiation. J Physiol (Lond). 1955;127:236.

4. Lock-Andersen J, Therkildsen P, de Fine Olivarius F et al. Epidermal thickness, skin pigmentation and constitutive photosensitivity. Photodermatol Photoimmunol Photomed. (1997) Aug;13(4):153–8.

5. La Ruche G, Cesarini JP. Histology and physiology of black skin Ann Dermatol Venereol. 1992;119(8):567–74.

6. Weigand DA, Haygood C, Gaylor JR. Cell layers and density of Negro and Caucasians stratum corneum. J invest Dermatol. 1974;62:563–5.

7. Kompaore F, Tsuruta H. In vivo differences between Asian, black and white in the stratum corneum barrier function. Int Arch Occup Environ Health. 1993;65(1 Suppl):S223–5.

8. Coderch L, Lopez O, De La Maza A, Parra JLV. Ceramides and skin function. Am J Clin Dermatol. 2003;4(2):107–29.

9. Rienertson RP, Wheatley VR. Studies on the chemical composition of human epidermal lipids. J Invest Dermatol. 1959;32:49–51.

10. Johnson LC, Corah NL. Racial differences in skin resistance. Science. 1963;139:766–9.

11. Corcuff P, Lotte C, Rougier A, Maibach H. Racial differences in corneocytes. Acta Derm Venereol (Stockh). 1991;71:146–8.

12. Sugino K, Imokawa G, Maibach H. Ethnic difference of stratum corneum lipid in relation to stratum corneum function. J Invest Dermatol. 1993;100:597.

13. Meguro S, Arai Y, Masukawa Y, Uie K, Tokimitsu I. Relationship between covalently bound ceramides and transepidermal water loss (TEWL). Arch Dermatol Res. 2000;292(9):463–8.

14. Kompaore F, Marty JP, Dupont Ch. In vivo evaluation of the stratum corneum barrier function in Blacks, Caucasians and Asians with two noninvasive methods. Skin Pharmacol. 1993;6:200–7.

15. Wilson D, Berardesca E, Maibach HI. In vitro transepidermal water loss: differences between black and white human skin. Brit J Dermatol. 1988;199:647–52.

16. Berardesca E, Maibach HI. Racial differences in sodium lauryl sulphate induced cutaneous irritation: black and white. Contact Dermatitis. 1988;18:136–40.

17. Yosipovitch G, Theng CTS. Asian skin: its architecture, function, and differences from caucasian skin. Cosmet Toiletr. 2002;117(9):57–62.

18. Reed JT, Ghadially R, Elias PM. Effect of race, gender and skin type on epidermal permeability barrier function. J Invest Dermatol. 1994;102:537.

19. Berardesca E, de Rigal J, Leveque JL, Maibach HI. In vivo biophysical characterization of skin physiological differences in races. Dermatologica. 1991;182:89–93.

20. Baker H. The skin as a barrier (1986). In: Rook A, editors. Textbook of dermatology. Blackwell Scientific, Oxford, 355.

21. Reed JT, Ghadially R, Elias PM. Skin type, but neither race nor gender, influence epidermal permeability function. Arch Dermatol. 1995;131(10):1134–8.

22. Berardesca E, Pirot F, Singh M, Maibach HI. Differences in stratum corneum pH gradient when comparino white caucasian and black african-american skin. Brit J Dermatol. 1998;139:855–7.

23. Warrier AG, Kligman AM, Harper RA, Bowman J, Wickett RR. A comparison of black and white skin using noninvasive methods. J Soc Cosmet Chem. 1996;47:229–40.

24. Berardesca E, Maibach HI. Racial differences in sodium lauryl sulphate induced cutaneous irritation: black and white. Contact Dermatitis. 1988;18:65–70.

25. Rietschel RL. A method to evaluate skin moisturizers in vivo. J Invest Dermatol. 1978;70:152–5.

26. Lapiere CM. The ageing dermis: the main cause for the appearance of "old" skin. Br J Dermatol. 1990;122(Suppl 35):5–11.

27. Montagna W, Prota G, Kenney J. The structure of black skin. In: Montagna W, Prota G, Kenney J, editors. Black skin structure and function. USA: Gulf Professional Publishing; 1993.

28. Montagna W, Carlisle K. The architecture of black and white facial skin. J Am Acad Dermatol. 1991;24(6 Pt 1):929–37.

29. Nouveau-Richard S, Yang Z, Mac-Mary S, et al. Skin aging: a comparison between Chinese and European populations. A pilot study. J Dermatol Sci. 2005;40(3):187–93.
30. Morizot F, Guehenneux S, Dheurle S, et al. Do features of aging differ between Asian and Caucasian women. J Invest Dermatol. 2004;123:A67.
31. Vashi NA, de Castro Maymone MB, Kundu RV. Aging differences in ethnic skin. J Clin Aesthetic Dermatol. 2016;9(1):31–8.

Chapter 4
Differences in Skin Structure and Function in Ethnic Populations

Lauren E. Wiznia and Nada Elbuluk

Skin structure and function have been studied in various populations. Knowledge of these structural and functional differences aids the dermatologist in understanding clinical cutaneous differences between skin types. Furthermore, understanding of these differences has additional implications on treatment considerations. Unfortunately, an overall lack of literature exists in the skin of color population. This chapter summarizes current data on differences in the layers and components of the skin in various skin types and how this can affect skin structure and function.

Epidermis

The epidermis, the outermost skin layer, serves as a protective barrier between one's internal organs and the external environment. The epidermis shields the body from fluid loss as well as from infections and pollutants in the external environment. The predominant cell types in the epidermis are keratinocytes, melanocytes, Langerhans cells, and Merkel cells. Keratinocytes are expressed throughout the epidermis, and are mitotically active in the basal layer [1]. As they progress through their development and move externally toward the stratum corneum, the keratins they express change as the keratinocytes withdraw from the cell cycle [2]. Eventually, keratinocytes differentiate into corneocytes that are ultimately shed from the skin into the environment. Keratinocytes and the melanocyte with which they are associated form a complex termed the epidermal melanin unit [3]. Each melanocyte in the epidermal melanin unit is associated with 30–40 keratinocytes, and melanocytes transfer melanosomes to the keratinocytes within their unit [4].

L.E. Wiznia · N. Elbuluk (✉)
The Ronald O. Perelman Department of Dermatology, NYU School of Medicine, 240 East 38th Street, 11th Floor, New York, NY 10016, USA
e-mail: Nada.elbuluk@nyumc.org

© Springer International Publishing AG 2017
N.A. Vashi and H.I. Maibach (eds.), *Dermatoanthropology of Ethnic Skin and Hair*, DOI 10.1007/978-3-319-53961-4_4

Two other cell types, Langerhans cells and Merkel cells, are less predominant in the epidermis but nonetheless serve important functions. Langerhans cells are dendritic cells confined to the epidermis that functions as antigen presenting cells within the adaptive immune system [1]. Their density decreases with age and in chronically UV-exposed skin [2]. Merkel cells are neuroendocrine cells in the basal layer of the epidermis. They are associated with nerve fibers and appendages and are involved with mechanoreception. [1]

The epidermis has several layers, which include the stratum basale, the stratum spinosum, stratum granulosum, and the stratum corneum (SC), which is the most external layer [5]. The stratum basale is the innermost layer of the epidermis and is composed of mitotically active keratinocytes attached to the basement membrane. The spinous layer, within the midepidermis, contains "spine-like" cells which are desmosomes that promote adhesion to surrounding cells [2]. As the keratinocytes differentiate and move toward the stratum corneum, they flatten and develop lamellar granules that deliver SC lipid precursors into the intercellular space [1]. The granular layer is named for the keratohyalin granules prominent in this layer. As keratinocytes continue to differentiate, they destroy most of their cellular contents. The SC, the outermost layer, is composed of anucleate cornified cells.

Stratum Corneum

The barrier formed by the stratum corneum is composed of two compartments, lipid-poor corneocytes and an extracellular lipid matrix. The lipid-rich membrane includes ceramides, cholesterol, and long-chain saturated fatty acids [1]. The SC prevents evaporative water loss from interior skin cell layers. Several studies have found differences in the SC between skin types (Table 4.1) [6, 7]. Weigand et al. studied Black and White skin by performing skin biopsies and "flooding" the samples with sodium hydroxide and methylene blue to count SC cell layers under magnification. The authors reported that a greater number of tape strippings was required to remove the SC in Black compared to White subjects. Since Black skin had more SC layers than White but there was no significant difference in SC thickness, the SC of Black skin was determined to be more cohesive and compact [6, 7].

Spontaneous desquamation of the SC, which is a reflection of epidermal cell proliferation, has also been reported as increased in Blacks compared to that of White and Chinese individuals [8]. Corcuff et al. [8] who reported this finding noted that the finding was not consistent with prior existing literature. In contrast, Warrier et al. reported a greater desquamation index in White subjects compared to Black [9]. There remains no clear consensus in the literature with regard to which skin type has greater SC desquamation.

The lipid composition of the SC has also been studied among various skin types. These differences are evaluated through transepidermal water loss (TEWL), which is the amount of water vapor lost through the skin and appendages under normal conditions [10]. Rates of TEWL increase when the SC barrier is compromised which

Table 4.1 Epidermal differences between black and white skin [6, 8, 16–20, 22, 25, 75]

Epidermal features	Black	White
Stratum corneum thickness	Same	Same
Number of stratum corneum layers	More layers	Fewer layers
Transepidermal water loss	Slightly higher to no significant difference[a]	Slightly lower to no significant difference[a]
Ceramide levels	Lower	Higher (same to lower than Asians [19, 20])
pH	Lower more superficially, same at deeper levels	Higher more superficially, same at deeper levels

[a]No clear consensus in the literature

can occur in various dermatologic conditions or after physical or chemical insults to the skin. Differences in TEWL, however, are difficult to interpret due to additional influencing factors including humidity, temperature, season, and the skin's baseline hydration level [10–12]. Data from prior studies lead to inconsistent conclusions. Kompaore et al. [10, 12] studied TEWL in Black, Asian, and Caucasian subjects after treatment with methyl nicotinate, an agent used to induce vasodilatation. Subsequently, TEWL was evaluated using noninvasive techniques including tape stripping and the use of an Evaporimeter. Higher TEWL values were reported in Blacks and Asians compared to Caucasians. Berardesca et al. also investigated TEWL and water content in Blacks, Hispanics, and Whites [13]. They found no significant baseline difference in either of these variables among the three groups.

Studies have also investigated TEWL at different anatomic sites in different skin types. In an in vitro study evaluating inner thigh skin using an evaporation chamber, Wilson et al. reported a TEWL 1.1 times greater in black as compared to white skin [13]. However, Warrier et al. reported TEWL in blacks to be lower on the cheeks and lower extremities compared with those of Whites [9]. The authors concluded that their findings of decreased TEWL in Blacks signified that black skin had superior barrier function in comparison to white skin.

Skin irritancy has also been assessed among various racial groups. Early research into skin irritancy was based on perceptible erythema induced by various irritants. These studies initially concluded that black skin was less likely to experience skin irritation as compared to white skin [14]. More current researches have used objective measurements including the aforementioned TEWL and water content to assess skin irritancy between skin types. Goh and Chia [15] found no significant difference in skin water vapor loss between fair-skinned Chinese, Malaysian, and Indian subjects. Berardesca et al. assessed skin irritation with the application of sodium lauryl sulfate to pre-occluded skin in two separate studies, one comparing Whites and Hispanics and the other comparing blacks and whites. To do so, the authors assessed nonvisual detection and quantification of erythema, vasodilation, and skin damage after exposure to irritants through the use of laser Doppler velocimetry and measurements of both transepidermal water loss and water content [16]. In the first study, Hispanics were found to have greater skin sensitivity, while in the second study Blacks had higher TEWL in pre-occluded skin signifying greater skin irriration [16–19]. The authors assert that the difference found in TEWL may be relevant in cases of occupational dermatitis and in the formulation of topical medications and cosmetics.

Ceramides, which also contribute to the SC's lipid-rich membrane, have an inverse relationship with TEWL. Hellemans et al. evaluated ceramides in several ethnic groups through tape strippings from subjects' forearms [3]. The ceramide levels from the strippings were then quantified and analyzed after hydrolysis. The authors reported a lower ceramide to protein ratio in African Americans than in Caucasians but similar levels in Asians and Caucasians [19]. Sugino et al. evaluated ceramides using an Evaporimeter and Impedance meter and reported the lowest ceramide levels in Black subjects, but higher ceramide levels in Whites, Hispanics, and Asians, in increasing order [20]. Muizzuddin et al. [21] evaluated transepidermal water loss through tape strippings in African American, Caucasian, and East Asian skin. East Asian and Caucasian skin was found to have low maturation and a weak skin barrier, while African American skin was found to have low ceramide levels. These results were felt to correlate clinically with increased sensitivity in East Asian skin and increased xerosis in African-American skin. Harding et al. studied intercellular lipid content in individuals with and without dandruff living in Thailand and the United Kingdom [11]. Dandruff was associated with a decrease in free lipids including ceramides, fatty acids, and cholesterol. Lower free lipids were felt to result in a decreased skin barrier, which could contribute to increased susceptibility to microbial activity on scalp skin. No consistent differences in intercellular lipid content were found between the two populations [11].

Water content, a measure of skin hydration, has also been studied in different ethnicities. It is measured as a factor of capacitance, conductance, impedance, and skin resistance using skin electrodes [22, 23]. Fotoh et al. studied water content in skin samples from the forehead and volar forearm of women categorized in one of three groups: (1) sub-Saharan African Blacks or Caribbean Blacks, (2) African or Caribbean Mixed races (from intermarriage between Black African or Black Caribbean and White European Caucasian), and (3) European Caucasians [22]. They found no significant difference in water content among these groups. A study in a Chinese population found that measurements from the forehead and forearm using a physiologic skin monitor showed SC hydration changes with anatomic site, age, and gender [23]. These studies collectively show that various anatomic and demographic factors may lead to differences in water content.

Skin pH, another skin characteristic studied in various skin types, is thought to play a role in epidermal permeability [24]. Berardesca et al. [25] studied the skin of African American and Caucasian women by removing SC layers using cellophane tape stripping and measuring TEWL and pH with every three strippings. They reported a lower pH in African American compared to Caucasian women on the midvolar forearm after three tape strippings. They found that further strippings led to no further significant pH differences and concluded that skin pH is similar within deeper skin layers of both groups.

Melanocytes, Melanosomes, and Melanin

Variability in the quantity and type of melanin, melanocyte activity, and melanosome number, size, type, and arrangement within melanocytes all contribute to differences in skin pigmentation (Table 4.2) [1, 2]. Melanocytes are located in the basal layer of the epidermis and in the matrix of hair bulbs [4]. Each melanocyte in the basal layer is associated with 30–40 keratinocytes located in the malphigian layer, forming the aforementioned epidermal melanin unit. The metabolic unit of the melanocyte, the melanosome, is the location of melanin synthesis. There are two types of melanin, produced within melanocytes, eumelanin and pheomelanin. Tyrosinase, the rate-limiting enzyme in this process, is formed within the Golgi apparatus of melanocytes and is transferred to the melanosome early in its development. As melanocytes develop, melanin content increases. In later stages of development, melanosomes are transferred from the melanocyte into the keratinocyte as either single or aggregated particles [26]. Differences in this melanosome packaging have been noted among skin types, with more singly dispersed melanosomes being more characteristic of darkly pigmented skin [27, 28].

While epidermal melanocyte number is the same among all skin types, melanocyte density can vary by anatomic location. For example, within an individual, melanocyte density is greater in the genital region as compared to the back [1]. The amount of melanin, type of melanin (ratio of eumelanin to pheomelanin), and

Table 4.2 Differences in melanocytes, melanosomes, melanin, and response to ultraviolet light in black and white skin [23, 27, 37, 38, 44, 45]

	Black	White
Melanocyte density	Same	Same
Rate of melanin production	Higher	Lower
Melanosomes	Larger, non-aggregated melanosomes throughout the epidermis	Smaller, aggregated melanosomes confined to basal layer of epidermis
Melanin	Greater melanin content	Lower melanin content
Eumelanin to pheomelanin ratio	Higher	Lower
Response to UV insult	Greater increase in melanin content	Lower increase in melanin content, diffuse keratinocyte activation, increased neutrophils, and activated proteolytic enzymes
Vitamin D production	Less efficient	More efficient
Photodamage	Decreased susceptibility	Increased susceptibility
Photocarcinogenesis	Lower rates of melanoma and non-melanoma skin cancer	Higher rates of melanoma and non-melanoma skin cancer

intracellular distribution and location of melanin within the skin all contribute to perceived skin color [27, 29]. Melanocytes cultured from Black skin have been reported to produce more melanin than White skin [30]. The rate of melanogenesis by melanocytes may also be affected by various factors, including intracellular pH of melanocytes [30, 31]. Smit et al. measured melanin content spectrophotometrically in neonatal foreskin in skin phototypes I, II, and VI and reported that melanocytes in patients with skin phototype VI contained approximately five times more melanin than those of patients with Fitzpatrick skin type I [27, 29]. These studies support the understanding that darker skin types have a greater rate of melanogenesis and melanin content.

Melanosomes are the organelles unique to melanocytes in which melanin is synthesized, transported, and deposited. Size, packaging, distribution, and degradation of melanosomes can differ among skin types. Melanosomes have been reported as more numerous in several ethnic groups including Africans, African-Americans, and Australian aborigines [32]. Lighter skin types have smaller, aggregated melanosomes as compared to the larger, non-aggregated melanosomes found in darker skin types [27, 28]. Melanosome size and aggregation differ even within individual ethnic groups; dark-skinned Africans have larger non-aggregated melanosomes compared to the smaller, aggregated melanosomes of lighter skinned Africans [28]. Caucasians have mainly clustered melanosomes, with groups of 2–10 melanosomes distributed within the lysosomes of keratinocytes, while African Americans have predominantly individual melanosomes, and Asians have a combination of individual and clustered melanosomes [28]. Melanosome size has been reported to increase progressively in size from Europeans to Chinese, Mexicans, Indians, and Africans with the latter having the largest melanosomes [29, 33]. Melanosome distribution within the epidermis also varies across ethnic groups [21, 34, 35]. Melanosomes in White skin are confined to the basal layer of the epidermis and are absent in the upper layers compared to melanosomes in Black skin that are found throughout the epidermis, including the SC [36]. This latter finding has been attributed to a slower rate of melanosome degradation in Black skin [21, 34, 35].

In addition to contributing to skin pigmentation, melanin also plays a role in the absorption and deflection of ultraviolet (UV) rays. The larger, non-aggregated melanosomes in Black skin have a higher melanin content and absorb more UV light than their counterparts in White skin, helping protect darker skin from UV light's damaging effects [37, 38]. The sun protection offered by Black skin has been reported as equal to a sun protective factor (SPF) of 13.4 compared to that in White skin in which the SPF has been reported as 3.4 [38]. A Japanese study by Abe et al. supported this finding by showing that skin with a lower melanin content is more photosensitive as measured by minimal erythema dose (MED) [39]. Kaidbey et al. reported that on average, five times as much UV light reaches the upper dermis of Caucasians as that of Blacks. The authors hypothesized that this difference in UV filtration may account for the decreased frequency with which Black individuals experience phototoxic drug reactions and actinic damage [38]. The photoprotective role of melanin may also account for the significantly lower rates of skin cancer reported in patients with skin of color. Specifically, rates of non-melanoma and melanoma skin cancers are 50 and 13 times greater in White than in Black skin, respectively [40, 41]. Furthermore, the annual incidence of melanoma has been reported as 1 per 100,000 in Blacks, 4 per 100,00 in Hispanics, and 25 per 100,000 in non-Hispanic Whites [42].

Rates of melanogenesis after UV exposure also vary among racial groups. Tadokoro et al. established the MED in Latino, Black or African American, Asian, and White patients by performing biopsies in patients' skin 7 min, 1 day, and 1 week after UV exposure [43]. Patients classified as Latino and Black/African American demonstrated a greater increase in melanin content after UV exposure than those classified as having Asian or White skin. This study reported that increasing melanin content inversely correlated with the extent of DNA damage [43]. Additional studies have shown increased p53 immunoreactivity in the epidermis of dark-skinned individuals after UV exposure, suggesting that Black skin has a more efficient UV damage repair system than White skin [44]. Rijken et al. [45] also studied Black and White skin's response to solar simulating radiation. The authors compared skin of volunteers with Fitzpatrick skin types I–III with skin of volunteers with Fitzpatrick skin type VI before and after UV exposure. They found that only for the former group, skin showed diffuse keratinocyte activation, increased neutrophils, and active proteolytic enzymes. The authors posit that these findings may help explain darker skin's decreased susceptibility to photoaging, sunburns, and skin carcinogenesis [45].

In addition to its role in photoprotection, changes in melanin can also result in pigmentary disorders. These disorders, such as postinflammatory pigment alteration and melasma can occur in all skin types but are more common in those with skin of color [1, 46]. Various factors such as melanin content, UV irradiation, melanocyte lability, and skin phototype can all influence the development and progression of pigmentary disorders [47].

Increased melanin may also affect vitamin D production among different skin types. The endogenous production of vitamin D relies on the conversion of 7-dehydrocholesterol to provitamin D_3 after skin is exposed to UVB radiation [1]. Although dietary intake can affect vitamin D levels, the lower levels of vitamin D in darker skin are also related to greater skin pigmentation that reduces UVB penetration and vitamin D photosynthesis [48]. This leads to less efficient vitamin D production in darker skin compared to lighter skin, which can consequently lead to vitamin D deficiency. Vitamin D deficiency is more common in Blacks than in Whites, with 53–76% of non-Hispanic Blacks having vitamin D levels below 50 nmol/l, as compared to 8–33% of non-Hispanic Whites [39, 48–50].

Dermal–Epidermal Junction

The dermal–epidermal junction (DEJ), also known as the basement membrane, represents the boundary between the epidermis and dermis. It is composed of two layers known as the lamina lucida and lamina densa. The DEJ provides resistance against external shearing forces and connects the epidermis and dermis [2]. Three networks form the DEJ, including anchoring fibrils which extend from the lamina densa into the papillary dermis, the basement membrane, and the hemidesmosome anchoring filament complex [2]. Projections of the papillary dermis, termed rete ridges, occur beneath the lamina densa. The DEJ, therefore, represents an important junction over which both nutrients and waste products are exchanged. Additionally, disruption of the DEJ which can occur from external trauma or various dermato-logic conditions can lead to pigment incontinence and subsequent pigmentary alteration. This can present clinically as post-inflammatory hyperpigmentation or hypopigmentation, both of which occur more commonly in the skin of color population [2]. Significant differences in the DEJ of different skin types have not been well elucidated. Studies have found conflicting results, with Girardeau et al. finding the DEJ to be thicker in African-Americans compared to Caucasians [51], while Querleux et al. reported the opposite [52].

Dermis

The dermis provides connective tissue support to the overlying epidermis and is composed of a fibrous matrix made of collagen, elastin, and fiber fragments, along with vascular structures, mast cells, and nerves [1]. The dermis also contains cutaneous appendages [5]. The dermis has two layers, the papillary dermis, which is more superficial, and the reticular dermis, which lies deeper. The fibroblast is the major cell type, producing collagen. The papillary dermis is primarily composed of a loose connective tissue including elastic fibers, extracellular matrix, and collagen fibers, whereas the reticular dermis contains tightly woven large-diameter collagen fibrils with surrounding branching elastic fibers [2].

Dermal differences including dermal thickness and number of dermal papillae have been studied in different skin types (Table 4.3). Querleux et al. [52] reported no significant difference in papillary dermis thickness amongst African-American, Mexican, Caucasian, and Chinese subjects. Another study by Sugiyama-Nakagiri et al. found dermal thickness to be the same across ethnic groups, but more dermal papillae in Hispanics and African-Americans than in Asians and Caucasians [53]. The clinical significance of this latter finding is uncertain.

Collagen, elastin, and fiber fragments in the dermis comprise the fibrous matrix and contribute to skin elasticity and laxity. Montagna et al. reported more closely stacked collagen bundles and numerous fiber fragments composed of collagen fibrils, glycoproteins, fibroblasts, and macrophages in Black compared to White subjects [34]. The authors hypothesize that these differences may account for the firmness or turgor of Black skin, although they did not comment on this finding's clinical implications.

Mast cells, another important component of the dermis, may differ between races. Sueki et al. evaluated ultrastructural differences in mast cell granules between Black and White skin and found that mast cells in Black skin had larger granules

Table 4.3 Dermal differences in black and white skin [6, 14, 34, 52]

Dermal Features	Black	White
Dermal thickness	Same	Same
Collagen fibers	More closely stacked	Less closely stacked
Fibroblasts	More numerous	Less numerous
Mast cells	Larger granules, greater levels of tryptase	Smaller granules, lower levels of tryptase

and greater levels of tryptase than White skin [54]. This finding may help account for the greater occurrence of keloids in Blacks, as mast cells have been speculated as playing a role in the aberrant fibrosis process that contributes to hypertrophic scar and keloid formation [55, 56]. In addition, these differences in tryptase may account for the greater pruritus experienced in Black versus White skin [54].

The subcutis, also known as the hypodermis, is formed predominantly of adipocytes [57, 58]. Lobules of adipocytes separated by septa of fibrous connective tissue are also accompanied by nerves, vessels, and lymphatics. The hypodermis provides insulation and protection to the skin, as well as serves as a reserve for energy supply [1]. Defects in the subcutis can be found in various dermatologic diseases including lipodystrophies [2]. No studies have been done examining differences in the subcutis in different skin types.

Cutaneous Appendages

Eccrine and Apocrine Glands

Eccrine glands are located throughout the skin, with the highest density on the palms and soles followed by the forehead and axillae [1, 5]. They are sweat glands which allow for evaporative heat loss, electrolyte balance, and maintenance of moisture in the stratum corneum [1]. There appears to be no significant racial difference in eccrine gland structure, although differences in function have been reported [34, 59]. McCance et al. reported White subjects to have higher sweating rates by cholinergic stimulation than Black subjects [60, 61].

Apocrine glands are confined to the axillae, areolae, nipples, vermilion lip, anogenital and periumbilical regions [1]. Apoeccrine glands have been reported only in adult axillae [62, 63]. Montagna et al. qualitatively reported a greater number of apoeccrine glands in Black compared to White skin [34]. The authors noted that they could not conclude if this difference was of any evolutionary significance.

Sebaceous Glands

Sebaceous glands produce sebum via holocrine secretion and are under androgenic influence [1]. Most sebaceous glands are associated with hair follicles although their overall distribution can vary. They are well developed on the upper back, chest, scalp, and face. Sebaceous glands contain androgen receptors that bind to dihydrotestosterone (DHT), which is a major contributor to gland development and sebum production [1]. Decreased sebum production can be associated with dry skin, whereas excessive production can result in seborrhea. Sebaceous gland activity is thought to play a role in certain dermatologic conditions such as acne vulgaris and rosacea.

Variations in sebaceous gland activity can also influence selection of dermatologic treatments and vehicles used for topical treatments. Studies have found inconsistent results in the differences in sebaceous glands and sebum production among skin types [22, 51, 64–66]. In some studies, Blacks have been reported to have larger sebaceous glands than Whites [14, 65]. With regard to sebum production, Kligman and Shelley reported an increase in sebum production in Blacks; [64] however, other studies have reported no differences among racial groups [67]. Grimes et al. [68] performed a study on sebum production of forehead skin of African American and White women using a sebumeter and found no statistically significant differences. A similar study evaluating sebum production with a sebumeter reported no significant differences in sebum production among African Americans, Whites, and Asians [67].

Hair Follicles

Hair follicle morphology as well as hair density and diameter have also been studied across different skin types [14, 34, 69, 70]. Melanosomes have been reported as being present in the outer root sheath and bulb of vellus hairs in Black but not White individuals [34]. Black hair has also been reported as being more heavily pigmented than White hair due to having larger melanin granules in their melanosomes [5, 18]. Hair density and the number of terminal hair follicles have also been reported as significantly lower in African Americans compared to Whites [69]. Mangelsdorf et al. and Otberg et al. both reported increased hair density of the forehead region of Caucasians [71, 72]. Mangelsdorf et al. also reported increased follicular infundibulum volumes in Caucasians as compared to Africans and Asians [71].

Hair shape and hair shaft diameters also differ among racial groups. Larger vellus hair shaft diameters have been reported in African subjects in the calf region as compared to Caucasians [71, 73]. In cross section, hair is elliptical and can vary from a more flattened ellipse with a major axis twice as long as its minor axis to a nearly circular ellipse with nearly equal major and minor axes [70]. Cross-sectional analyses of hair from different ethnic groups reported Black subjects to demonstrate more elliptical shapes, having the longest major axis compared to Chinese, Asian

Indians, and Western Europeans [70]. The same study compared cross-sectional areas of the hair shaft in men, and found it to be the largest in Chinese followed by Asian Indians and Blacks, and then smallest in Western Europeans [70]. Fewer elastic fibers have also been found to anchor hair follicles to the dermis in Black subjects [34]. These differences are thought to have implications for variants of alopecia including traction alopecia, which is more frequently reported in skin of color [34].

Conclusion

While there are certain similarities in skin structure and function among skin types, many differences have been found as well. Similarities have been reported in several skin components including stratum corneum thickness, melanocyte number, dermal thickness, and sebaceous gland number and function [1, 6, 7, 22, 51, 64–66]. Differences have been reported in other components of the epidermis and dermis as well as in melanogenesis after UV exposure, vitamin D production, photocarcinogenesis, and hair follicle density and diameter [6, 8–14, 16–21, 28, 34, 35, 39, 43, 48–50, 74]. Studies across different skin types, races, and ethnicities to evaluate skin structure and function still remain limited. More research is needed to draw more definitive conclusions not only about the differences that exist, but also to understand the clinical implications of these differences. Furthermore, studies need to objectively define skin types and study parameters in order to draw more accurate comparisons and conclusions between studies. As the global population continues to diversify with an increase in the skin of color population, future research will hopefully shed greater light on the differences and similarities in skin structure and function and their clinical implications across varied skin types.

References

1. Bolognia J, Jorizzo JL, Schaffer JV. Dermatology. 3rd ed. Philadelphia: Elsevier Saunders; 2012.
2. Goldsmith LA, Fitzpatrick TB. Fitzpatrick's dermatology in general medicine. 8th ed. New York: McGraw-Hill Medical; 2012.
3. Jimbow K, Quevedo WC, Fitzpatrick TB, Szabo G. Some aspects of melanin biology: 1950–1975. J Invest Dermatol. 1976;67:72–89.
4. Tobin DJ, Bystryn JC. Different populations of melanocytes are present in hair follicles and epidermis. Pigment Cell Res. 1996;9:304–10.
5. Badresha-Bansal S PMaTSTsafosIKA, Taylor SC, eds. Dermatology for Skin of Color. 2nd ed. New York, NY: McGraw-Hill; 2016.
6. Weigand DA, Haygood C, Gaylor JR. Cell layers and density of Negro and Caucasian stratum corneum. J Invest Dermatol. 1974;62:563–8.
7. Thomson ML. Relative efficiency of pigment and horny layer thickness in protecting the skin of Europeans and Africans against solar ultraviolet radiation. J Physiol. 1955;127:236–46.

8. Corcuff P, Lotte C, Rougier A, Maibach HI. Racial differences in corneocytes. A comparison between black, white and oriental skin. Acta Derm Venereol. 1991;71:146–8.

9. Warrier AGKA, Harper RA, Bowman J, Wickett RR. A comparison of Black and White skin using noninvasive methods. J Soc Cosmetic Chem. 1996;47:229–40.

10. Kompaore F, Dupont C, Marty JP. In vivo evaluation in man by two noninvasive methods of the stratum corneum barrier function after physical and chemical modifications. Int J Cosmet Sci. 1991;13:293–302.

11. Harding CR, Moore AE, Rogers JS, Meldrum H, Scott AE, McGlone FP. Dandruff: a condition characterized by decreased levels of intercellular lipids in scalp stratum corneum and impaired barrier function. Arch Dermatol Res. 2002;294:221–30.

12. Kompaore F, Marty JP, Dupont C. In vivo evaluation of the stratum corneum barrier function in blacks, Caucasians and Asians with two noninvasive methods. Skin Pharmacol. 1993;6:200–7.

13. Wilson D, Berardesca E, Maibach HI. In vitro transepidermal water loss: differences between black and white human skin. Br J Dermatol. 1988;119:647–52.

14. Taylor SC. Skin of color: biology, structure, function, and implications for dermatologic disease. J Am Acad Dermatol. 2002;46:S41–62.

15. Goh CL, Chia SE. Skin irritability to sodium lauryl sulphate–as measured by skin water vapour loss-by sex and race. Clin Exp Dermatol. 1988;13:16–9.

16. Berardesca E, Maibach HI. Racial differences in sodium lauryl sulphate induced cutaneous irritation: black and white. Contact Dermatitis. 1988;18:65–70.

17. Berardesca E, Maibach HI. Sodium-lauryl-sulphate-induced cutaneous irritation. Comparison of white and Hispanic subjects. Contact Dermatitis. 1988;19:136–40.

18. Berardesca E. Racial differences in skin function. Acta Derm Venereol Suppl (Stockh). 1994;185:44–6.

19. Hellemans L eaCoscpihsfadgbJID, 124:371.

20. Sugino KIG, Maibach HI. Ethnic difference of stratum corneum lipid in relation to stratum corneum function. J Invest Dermatol. 1993;100:59.

21. Muizzuddin N, Hellemans L, Van Overloop L, Corstjens H, Declercq L, Maes D. Structural and functional differences in barrier properties of African American, Caucasian and East Asian skin. J Dermatol Sci. 2010;59:123–8.

22. Fotoh C, Elkhyat A, Mac S, Sainthillier JM, Humbert P. Cutaneous differences between Black, African or Caribbean Mixed-race and Caucasian women: biometrological approach of the hydrolipidic film. Skin Res Technol. 2008;14:327–35.

23. Man MQ, Xin SJ, Song SP, et al. Variation of skin surface pH, sebum content and stratum corneum hydration with age and gender in a large Chinese population. Skin Pharmacol Physiol. 2009;22:190–9.

24. Hachem JP, Crumrine D, Fluhr J, Brown BE, Feingold KR, Elias PM. pH directly regulates epidermal permeability barrier homeostasis, and stratum corneum integrity/cohesion. J Invest Dermatol. 2003;121:345–53.

25. Berardesca E, Pirot F, Singh M, Maibach H. Differences in stratum corneum pH gradient when comparing white Caucasian and black African-American skin. Br J Dermatol. 1998;139:855–7.

26. Bolognia JL, Cooper DL, Glusac EJ. Toxic erythema of chemotherapy: a useful clinical term. J Am Acad Dermatol. 2008;59:524–9.

27. Smit NP, Kolb RM, Lentjes EG, et al. Variations in melanin formation by cultured melanocytes from different skin types. Arch Dermatol Res. 1998;290:342–9.

28. Thong HY, Jee SH, Sun CC, Boissy RE. The patterns of melanosome distribution in keratinocytes of human skin as one determining factor of skin colour. Br J Dermatol. 2003;149:498–505.

29. Alaluf S, Heath A, Carter N, et al. Variation in melanin content and composition in type V and VI photoexposed and photoprotected human skin: the dominant role of DHI. Pigment Cell Res. 2001;14:337–47.

30. Yohn JJ, Lyons MB, Norris DA. Cultured human melanocytes from black and white donors have different sunlight and ultraviolet A radiation sensitivities. J Invest Dermatol. 1992;99:454–9.

31. Ancans J, Tobin DJ, Hoogduijn MJ, Smit NP, Wakamatsu K, Thody AJ. Melanosomal pH controls rate of melanogenesis, eumelanin/phaeomelanin ratio and melanosome maturation in melanocytes and melanoma cells. Exp Cell Res. 2001;268:26–35.

32. Mitchell RE. The skin of the Australian Aborigine; a light and electronmicroscopical study. Australas J Dermatol. 1968;9:314–28.

33. Alaluf S, Atkins D, Barrett K, Blount M, Carter N, Heath A. Ethnic variation in melanin content and composition in photoexposed and photoprotected human skin. Pigment Cell Res. 2002;15:112–8.

34. Montagna W, Carlisle K. The architecture of black and white facial skin. J Am Acad Dermatol. 1991;24:929–37.

35. Herzberg AJ, Dinehart SM. Chronologic aging in black skin. Am J Dermatopathol. 1989;11:319–28.

36. Halder RMNP. Ethnic skin disorders overview. J Am Acad Dermatol. 2003;48(6 Suppl): S143–8.

37. Szabó G, Gerald AB, Pathak MA, Fitzpatrick TB. Racial differences in the fate of melanosomes in human epidermis. Nature. 1969;222:1081–2.

38. Kaidbey KH, Agin PP, Sayre RM, Kligman AM. Photoprotection by melanin–a comparison of black and Caucasian skin. J Am Acad Dermatol. 1979;1:249–60.

39. Abe T, Arai S, Mimura K, Hayakawa R. Studies of physiological factors affecting skin susceptibility to ultraviolet light irradiation and irritants. J Dermatol. 1983;10:531–7.

40. Halder RM, Bridgeman-Shah S. Skin cancer in African Americans. Cancer. 1995;75:667–73.

41. English DR, Armstrong BK, Kricker A, Fleming C. Sunlight and cancer. Cancer Causes Control. 1997;8:271–83.

42. American Cancer Society. Cancer Facts and Figures 2015. http://www.cancer.org/acs/groups/content/@editorial/documents/document/acspc-044552.pdf. Accessed Oct 15.

43. Tadokoro T, Kobayashi N, Zmudzka BZ, et al. UV-induced DNA damage and melanin content in human skin differing in racial/ethnic origin. FASEB J. 2003;17:1177–9.

44. de Winter S, Vink AA, Roza L, Pavel S. Solar-simulated skin adaptation and its effect on subsequent UV-induced epidermal DNA damage. J Invest Dermatol. 2001;117:678–82.

45. Rijken F, Bruijnzeel PL, van Weelden H, Kiekens RC. Responses of black and white skin to solar-simulating radiation: differences in DNA photodamage, infiltrating neutrophils, proteolytic enzymes induced, keratinocyte activation, and IL-10 expression. J Invest Dermatol. 2004;122:1448–55.

46. Grimes PE, Hunt SG. Considerations for cosmetic surgery in the black population. Clin Plast Surg. 1993;20:27–34.

47. Grimes PE. Management of hyperpigmentation in darker racial ethnic groups. Semin Cutan Med Surg. 2009;28:77–85.

48. Harris SS. Vitamin D and African Americans. J Nutr. 2006;136:1126–9.

49. Looker AC, Dawson-Hughes B, Calvo MS, Gunter EW, Sahyoun NR. Serum 25-hydroxyvitamin D status of adolescents and adults in two seasonal subpopulations from NHANES III. Bone. 2002;30:771–7.

50. Cornish DA, Maluleke V, Mhlanga T. An investigation into a possible relationship between vitamin D, parathyroid hormone, calcium and magnesium in a normally pigmented and an albino rural black population in the Northern Province of South Africa. BioFactors. 2000;11:35–8.

51. Girardeau S, Mine S, Pageon H, Asselineau D. The Caucasian and African skin types differ morphologically and functionally in their dermal component. Exp Dermatol. 2009;18:704–11.

52. Querleux B, Baldeweck T, Diridollou S, et al. Skin from various ethnic origins and aging: an in vivo cross-sectional multimodality imaging study. Skin Res Technol. 2009;15:306–13.

53. Sugiyama-Nakagiri Y, Sugata K, Hachiya A, Osanai O, Ohuchi A, Kitahara T. Ethnic differences in the structural properties of facial skin. J Dermatol Sci. 2009;53:135–9.

54. Sueki H, Whitaker-Menezes D, Kligman AM. Structural diversity of mast cell granules in black and white skin. Br J Dermatol. 2001;144:85–93.
55. Ketchum LD, Cohen IK, Masters FW. Hypertrophic scars and keloids. A collective review. Plast Reconstr Surg. 1974;53:140–54.
56. Kischer CW, Bunce H, Shetlah MR. Mast cell analyses in hypertrophic scars, hypertrophic scars treated with pressure and mature scars. J Invest Dermatol. 1978;70:355–7.
57. Avram AS, Avram MM, James WD. Subcutaneous fat in normal and diseased states: 2. Anatomy and physiology of white and brown adipose tissue. J Am Acad Dermatol. 2005;53:671–83.
58. Avram MM, Avram AS, James WD. Subcutaneous fat in normal and diseased states 3. Adipogenesis: from stem cell to fat cell. J Am Acad Dermatol. 2007;56:472–92.
59. Johnson LC, Landon MM. Eccrine sweat gland activity and racial differences in resting skin conductance. Psychophysiology. 1965;1:322–9.
60. McCance RA, Rutishauser IH, Knight HC. Response of sweat glands to pilocarpine in the Bantu of Uganda. Lancet. 1968;1:663–5.
61. McCance RA, Purohit G. Ethnic differences in the response of the sweat glands to pilocarpine. Nature. 1969;221:378–9.
62. Beer GM, Baumüller S, Zech N, et al. Immunohistochemical differentiation and localization analysis of sweat glands in the adult human axilla. Plast Reconstr Surg. 2006;117:2043–9.
63. Bovell DL, Corbett AD, Holmes S, Macdonald A, Harker M. The absence of apoeccrine glands in the human axilla has disease pathogenetic implications, including axillary hyperhidrosis. Br J Dermatol. 2007;156:1278–86.
64. Kligman AM, Shelley WB. An investigation of the biology of the human sebaceous gland. J Invest Dermatol. 1958;30:99–125.
65. Pochi PE, Strauss JS. Sebaceous gland activity in black skin. Dermatol Clin. 1988;6:349–51.
66. Yamamoto A, Serizawa S, Ito M, Sato Y. Effect of aging on sebaceous gland activity and on the fatty acid composition of wax esters. J Invest Dermatol. 1987;89:507–12.
67. Grimes PE. Aesthetics and cosmetic surgery for darker skin types. Philadelphia: Wolters Kluwer Health/Lippincott Williams & Wilkins; 2008.
68. Grimes P, Edison BL, Green BA, Wildnauer RH. Evaluation of inherent differences between African American and white skin surface properties using subjective and objective measures. Cutis. 2004;73:392–6.
69. Sperling LC. Hair density in African Americans. Arch Dermatol. 1999;135:656–8.
70. Vernall DG. A study of the size and shape of cross sections of hair from four races of men. Am J Phys Anthropol. 1961;19:345–50.
71. Mangelsdorf S, Otberg N, Maibach HI, Sinkgraven R, Sterry W, Lademann J. Ethnic variation in vellus hair follicle size and distribution. Skin Pharmacol Physiol. 2006;19:159–67.
72. Otberg N, Richter H, Schaefer H, Blume-Peytavi U, Sterry W, Lademann J. Variations of hair follicle size and distribution in different body sites. J Invest Dermatol. 2004;122:14–9.
73. Luther N, Darvin ME, Sterry W, Lademann J, Patzelt A. Ethnic differences in skin physiology, hair follicle morphology and follicular penetration. Skin Pharmacol Physiol. 2012;25:182–91.
74. Tadokoro T, Yamaguchi Y, Batzer J, et al. Mechanisms of skin tanning in different racial/ethnic groups in response to ultraviolet radiation. J Invest Dermatol. 2005;124:1326–32.
75. Berardesca E, Maibach H. Racial differences in skin pathophysiology. J Am Acad Dermatol. 1996;34:667–72.

Chapter 5
Photosensitivity and Photoreactivity in Ethnic Skin

Umer A. Ansari, Stephanie T. Le and Valerie M. Harvey

The Electromagnetic Spectrum—UVA, UVB, and Visible Light

Solar radiation comprises a continuum of wavelengths including ultraviolet radiation (UVR; 280–400 nm), visible light (VL; 400–760 nm), and infrared radiation (IR; 760 nm–1 mm) [1]. UVR is further categorized, and although several definitions exist, the classification scheme most widely employed in photodermatology separates UVB (290–320 nm) and UVA (320–400 nm) [2]. UVA is further divided into UVA1 (340–400 nm) and UVA2 (320–340 nm) (Fig. 5.1). Because the majority of wavelengths are absorbed by the ozone layer, only a fraction reaches the earth's surface. UV radiation accounts for only 3% of the radiation present on the earth's surface [3]. UVB reaches the earth's surface in relatively low amounts, accounting for only 0.5% of the solar spectrum at ground level [4]. In contrast, UVA is 20 times more abundant than UVB, as its longer wavelengths more efficiently penetrate through the ozone layer [4]. VL accounts for 44% of solar radiation at ground level, with IR accounting for the remaining portion [3, 5].

U.A. Ansari · S.T. Le
Eastern Virginia Medical School,
825 Fairfax Ave, Norfolk, VA 23507, USA

V.M. Harvey (✉)
Department of Dermatology, Eastern Virginia Medical School,
Norfolk, VA, USA
e-mail: Harveyvm@evms.edu

V.M. Harvey
Hampton University Skin of Color Research Institute, Hampton, VA, USA

© Springer International Publishing AG 2017
N.A. Vashi and H.I. Maibach (eds.), *Dermatoanthropology of Ethnic Skin and Hair*, DOI 10.1007/978-3-319-53961-4_5

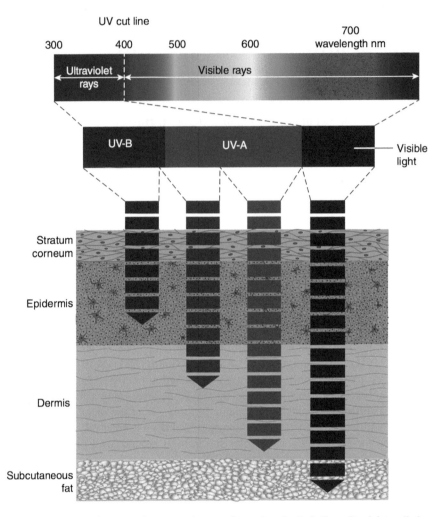

Fig. 5.1 Solar radiation comprises a continuum of wavelengths including ultraviolet radiation (UVR; 280–400 nm), visible light (VL; 400–760 nm), and infrared radiation (IR; 760 nm–1 mm)

The Biological Effects of Ultraviolet Radiation

UVA

The cellular and molecular impact of UVR on cutaneous structures is well documented. UVA's long wavelengths facilitate its penetration through the epidermis and into the dermis [6]; 20–50% of UVA reaches the depth of melanocytes, and approximately 30% of UVA is capable of infiltrating the dermis [4, 7].

One major mechanism by which UVA provokes epidermal and dermal injury is via generation of free radicals and reactive oxygen species (ROS) [4, 8]. UVA is absorbed by cutaneous chromophores including melanin, DNA, RNA, and aromatic amino acids, triggering photochemical reactions which produce the ROS [1, 9]. In vitro and in vivo studies have shown that, following UVA exposure, keratinocytes and fibroblasts increase their expression of biomarkers related to oxidative damage such as ferritin, lysozyme, matrix metalloproteinase-1 (MMP-1), heme oxygenase-1, and superoxide dismutase-2 [4, 10]. A recent study using human skin constructs showed that UVA exposure modulated the expression of genes implicated in oxidative stress and extracellular matrix modeling. Sixty of 74 genes were expressed after minimal amounts of sun exposure, suggesting that the threshold for UVA-induced change is quite low [10].

At the cellular level, ROS illicit a number of detrimental effects, including mitochondrial and cellular membrane injury, and apoptosis [7, 11, 12]. Structural sequelae of UVA-induced ROS are evident by the destruction of dermal elastin and collagen, and the effacement of the dermal–epidermal junction [4, 9, 10, 13]. ROS also mediate the release of cytokines and inflammatory mediators such as histamine, prostaglandins, and kinins [14] which cause dilatation of the vasculature in the subpapillary plexus [14, 15].

UVA causes direct damage to DNA through the formation of pyrimidine dimers [12]. Recent data suggests that UVA-induced dimers may be more mutagenic than those caused by UVB [12]. Runger et al. showed that UVA-irradiated primary human fibroblasts possess less-effective DNA repair and cell cycle arrest mechanisms compared to human fibroblasts exposed to equimutagenic doses of UVB [12].

Biological Effects of UVA in Darker Skin Types

There is evidence to suggest that melanin and its intermediaries exacerbate UVA-mediated damage. Eniko et al. demonstrated that cultured human type VI melanocytes exposed to UVA experience higher levels of DNA single-strand breaks compared to type I melanocytes, presumably secondary to the higher melanin content of the former [16]. Marrot et al. also found a correlation between DNA damage and cellular melanin content; breakage was more intense within melanocytes than in fibroblasts, and in cells with high versus low melanin content following melanogenic stimulation [17]. Together, these findings suggest that individuals with darker skin are in fact susceptible to UVA-induced phototoxicity, and strengthen the rationale for ethnic-specific sun protection.

UVB

UVB less effectively penetrates the epidermis than UVA; 9–15% of UVB reaches the melanocytes, while only 10% of UVB contacts the dermis [4, 7]. Because the plurality of UVB rays is absorbed by residents of the epidermis, much of its biological sequelae occur there. The relatively short wavelength of this light spectrum renders it more potent, imparting its deleterious effects at much lower doses [1]. UVB directly injures DNA, eventuating in the formation of cyclobutane–pyrimidine and pyrimidine–pyrimidine dimers within keratinocytes and melanocytes [1]. As mutagenesis progresses, cells gain the ability to evade the regulatory mechanisms of apoptosis [18]. Subsequent clonal expansion of genomically modified cells ultimately leads to carcinogenesis with the development of squamous cell carcinomas, basal cell carcinomas, or melanomas [18].

DNA dimer formation is associated with upregulation of melanogenic genes [6]. After UVB exposure, keratinocytes increase the expression of the p53 protein, which in turn activates transcription of proopiomelanocortin (POMC). POMC is processed into several different biologically active hormones, including alpha melanocyte stimulating hormone (alpha-MSH). Alpha-MSH then binds to Melanocortin-1 receptors on melanocytes and activates melanin redistribution, melanocyte proliferation, and de novo melanin synthesis [19]. This cascade of events is accompanied by elevated levels of tyrosinase mRNA [20]. Newly produced melanin is transferred to the superficial layers of the epidermis [7, 19, 20]. UVB-generated melanogenesis, in combination with epidermal acanthosis, provides broad spectrum coverage against subsequent UVA, UVB, and VL exposure [1, 12].

UVB is also integral to Vitamin D3 production (cholecalciferol). UVB converts dehydrocholesterol (provitamin D) to previtamin D3 in the basal and spinous layers of the epidermis [9]. Previtamin D3 is then heat converted to vitamin D3. Due to the increased absorbance of UVB by epidermal melanocytes, darker skinned individuals are less-efficient producers of Vitamin D and therefore more susceptible to vitamin D deficiency [21]. A detailed discussion on the formation and function of Vitamin D is provided in a review by Goring and Koshuchowa [22].

Biological Effects of UVB in Darker Skin

A number of factors provide darker skin with relative protection against the harmful effects of UVB. Melanin, an avid absorber and deflector of UVB [23, 24], serves as a physical shield for UVB exposed cells [12, 23], effectively diminishing the proportion of keratinocytes, melanocytes, and dermal fibroblasts exposed to UVB radiation [23, 24]. Furthermore, wavelengths less than 310 nm are preferentially absorbed by the stratum corneum (SC). Studies have shown that the SC of black skin has a greater number of layers [25, 26]. Although the SC of black and white skin are of equal thickness, an increase in its layers makes black skin more compact and cohesive, conferring increased relative protection to UVB. Together, these factors may account for the lower levels of UVB-propagated DNA damage observed in darker skin compared to lighter skin [27, 28].

Visible Light

Visible Light (VL) has recently been identified as a potential contributor to cutaneous carcinogenesis and photodamage. Like UVR, VL is absorbed by an array of chromophores including melanin, B-carotene, and protoporphyrin [15]. Similar to UVA, VL triggers free radical damage, inflammatory reactions, and the activation of matrix metalloproteinases, leading to subsequent dermal damage [15, 29]. A recent study by Chiarelli-Neto [28] showed that VL-generated singlet oxygen-free radicals via interaction with melanin [28]. Cells expressing higher melanin levels suffered the greatest amount of necro-apoptosis, suggesting that VL-induced phototoxicity may be more severe among darker skin types. The effects of VL are significant, since the majority of currently available proprietary sunscreens are ineffective against this spectrum of light [29].

Skin Classification Systems

The Fitzpatrick skin phototype system (SPS), based on a self-reported tendency to sunburn and ability to tan, was initially developed as a method to assess one's tolerance to UVR exposure [1]. It was originally created to classify skin phototype in Caucasians, (classes I to IV), with higher gradation correlating to darker skin. Skin types V and VI were later incorporated to expand the SPS to include individuals with brown and black skin, respectively. Although widely employed by dermatologists, the SPS has many shortcomings [27]. First, several studies have shown poor correlation between skin phototype, constitutive pigmentation and minimum erythema dose (MED) [30, 31]. Second, burning and tanning are subjective assessments with inter-individual differences in connotation [32]. Third, the classification is particularly unreliable in classifying black skin, and clinical trials have not shown a consistent correlation between skin phototype classification and sun sensitivity [33–35]. Finally, although people of color are commonly categorized into types IV–VI based on ethnicity, ethnic skin spans the entire spectrum of skin color [36].

Bino et al. proposed an alternate classification to the Fitzpatrick-SPS system, based on the Individual Typology Angle (ITA), as determined by colorimetric properties of skin L* (luminance) and b* (yellow/blue component) [27]. Bino et al. created six groups of skin color in which the ITA corresponded to relative melanin concentration, with lower ITA values signifying darker skin [27]. They were able validate the ITA measurements in ex vivo skin samples and showed consistent correlations between ITA measurements and constitutive pigmentation [27]. Furthermore, ITA correlated with the dose needed for skin to burn, with lower ITAs requiring higher doses to burn. While the ITA values were fairly consistent in white and African subjects across geographic regions, values ranged widely among Hispanics and Asians [27]. The ITA may provide a more accurate and objective measurement of constitutive pigmentation than the Fitzpatrick system and may prove to be more predictive of the physiological sequelae of UV exposure [27].

The Clinical Effects of UVR and Visible Light

UVA and Erythema

UVA radiation is 1000 times less potent in causing erythema than UVB [4, 37]. UVA-mediated erythema follows a biphasic pattern [1, 14]. An immediate erythematous reaction, typically only present in lighter skin types I/II, occurs within seconds to minutes of exposure [1, 14]. Delayed erythema, which occurs within minutes to hours, may or may not follow and is experienced irrespective of skin type [1, 14, 38]. However, the dose required to induce UVA-delayed erythema increases with baseline pigmentation, suggesting a protective role for melanin [7, 14].

UVA and Pigmentation

The pigmentary effects of UVR are classified based on the timing of onset and duration [39]. Immediate pigment darkening (IPD) occurs immediately after light exposure, is gray in color, and fades within minutes to hours [14, 40]. Persistent pigment darkening (PPD) is brown and can persist for as long as one day. Both IPD and PPD result from oxidation and redistribution of pre-existing melanin [1, 15]. Numerous studies have shown UVA to be more melanogenic than erythemogenic [15, 38]. UVA causes IPD within hours; with increased or repetitive exposure, UVA can also produce PPD. Both IPD and PPD are more pronounced in dark-skinned individuals than in those with fair skin [7].

UVA and Photoaging

Up to 95% of the visible signs of aging can be attributed to lifelong sun exposure [36]. Photoaging is characterized by patchy/mottled pigmentation, rhytid formation, laxity, sagging, and xerosis. Histologically, there is altered dermal collagen and elastin, epidermal atrophy, and pigmentary changes [4, 41, 42]. These changes occur less frequently and with less severity among darker skin types [43–45]. Photoaging manifests uniquely in different skin types. A growing body of evidence demonstrates the critical role of UVA in the pathogenesis of photoaging in ethnic skin. UVA has been suspected to exacerbate the prominent pigmentary component of aging ethnic skin, due to its melanogenic properties [15, 38, 46]. Multiple studies have shown that photoaging in Asians and African Americans is first evidenced as pigmentary changes including lentigines, dyschromias, and keratoses [47–49]. Compared to white counterparts, Chinese subjects show a 10-year delay in the development of rhytides [50, 51].

UV-mediated pigmentary lesions are markedly diminished when sunscreen contents are altered such that the ratio UVA protection factor (UVAPF) to Sun Protection Factor (SPF) (which provides UVB coverage) is increased [46]. Products with a UVAPF to SPF ratio greater than three are most effective in preventing pigmented lesions caused by exposure to sunlight [46]. In vitro studies show that sunscreens meeting this ratio provide better protection against dermal damage, produce fewer photoaging related biomarkers, and result in fewer clinically apparent pigmentary lesions [4, 52, 53].

UVB and Erythema

Sunburn, the most well-known consequence of excessive sun exposure is largely attributed to UVB injury, which triggers the release of cytokines and inflammatory mediators causing local inflammatory responses [6] leading to capillary dilation within the superficial dermis [15]. UVB is more erythemogenic than melanogenic, with a minimal erythema dose (MED) much lower than its minimal melanogenic dose (MMD) [38]. UVB produces erythema as its first cutaneous effect at relatively low quantities [1]. The MED increases linearly with the level of pigmentation [32]. Both constitutive pigmentation and delayed tanning (DT) pigmentation from prior UVB exposure protect against erythema and DNA damage from all forms of UV radiation [14, 54]. Immediate erythema, which preferentially occurs in lighter skin types, typically manifests 6–24 h post-exposure [14]. Darkly pigmented individuals are relatively protected in regards to the intensity and duration of UVB erythema. The time frame for subsequent fading and desquamation depends on baseline pigmentation. It may last for 1–2 weeks in lighter skin types (Fitzpatrick I/II), while in darker skinned individuals erythema often resolves within 72 h [14, 54].

UVB and Pigmentation

DT occurs 3–5 days after UVB exposure and is associated with newly synthesized melanin [54]. UVB-induced pigmentation is always preceded by erythema in lighter skin types, but this process is less common in darker skin [14]. The dose needed to cause DT is dependent on constitutive skin pigmentation, with darker skin types possessing higher MMDs [55]. The absolute pigmentary increase is independent of constitutive skin pigmentation but increases linearly with UVB dosage [56]. Thus, once the MMD dose of UVB is achieved, further increases in pigmentation depend only on UVB dosage, irrespective of pre-existing skin color.

The Impact of Visible Light on Erythema and Pigmentation

At very high doses, VL is capable of causing erythema [7]. In vivo studies have shown that exposure to increasing amounts of visible light results in increasing degrees of erythema associated with IPD in darker skin types [15]. Because VL penetrates to the deep dermis, the VL-mediated erythema is thought to occur by a similar mechanism to that of UVA [15]. It has been hypothesized that, in darker skin types, VL causes heat, the generation of which lead to vasodilation with subsequent erythema [57].

Recent studies have confirmed that VL, in the absence of UVR, can induce IPD, PPD, and DT [58, 59]. The IPD and PPD secondary to VL reveal a similar photometric action spectrum to UVA, and are thought to arise from the oxidization and redistribution pf pre-existing melanin [57, 60]. IPD and PPD are frequently only present in darker skin [15, 59]. VL is also able to initiate melanogenesis via mechanisms analogous to UVB [13]. After repeated exposure, VL is able to produce DT in all skin types [5]. Skin samples that have undergone DT showed increased transcription of tyrosinase and a redistribution of melanin to the upper strata of the epidermis [5]. It has been concluded that, in order for melanogenesis to occur, the skin may require priming via multiple VL exposures [57]. Therefore, depending on the circumstances of exposure, VL may generate pigmentation via mechanisms analogous to either UVA or UVB.

Photodermatoses

The photodermatoses are a group of disorders which are either caused or exacerbated by exposure to sunlight. A clue to their presence lies in their distribution, with confinement of symptoms to photoexposed body sites. Photodermatoses are broadly classified into four major categories: (1) idiopathic or immunologically mediated; (2) drug-induced photodermatoses (Table 5.1); (3) photo aggravation of pre-existing cutaneous conditions (Table 5.2); and (4) disorders of defective DNA repair disorders. Phytophotodermatitis is an additional subset of photodermatosis that deserves brief mention. This self-limited phototoxic inflammatory eruption is caused by ultraviolet A activation of furocoumarins, present in particular foods such as lemons, limes, parsley, and celery [61, 62]. The characteristic "streaky" linear rash can present with erythema, vesicle formation, and blistering localized to affected

Table 5.1 Causes of drug-induced photosensitivity reactions

Phototoxic agents	Photoallergic agents
• Amiodarone	• Amantadine
• Antineoplastic agents: 5-FU, dacarbazine, vinblastine	• Antimalarials: chloroquine, hydroxychloroquine, quinidine, quinine
• Antimalarials: chloroquine, hydroxychloroquine, quinidine, quinine	• Antimicrobials: chloramphenicol, pyrimethamine, quinolones
• Antimicrobials: ceftazidime, griseofulvin, ketoconazole, quinolones, tetracyclines, trimethoprim	• Benzodiazepines: chlordiazepoxide
	• Dapsone
• Atorvastatin	• Diphenhydramine
• Calcium channel blockers: Diltiazem	• Flu amide
• Nonsteroidal anti-inflammatory drugs (NSAIDS)	• Griseofulvin
– Oral: proprionic acid derivatives	• Nonsteroidal anti-inflammatory drugs (NSAIDS)
• Chlorpromazine	– Oral:
• Porphyrins	Piroxicam
• Psoralens	Celecoxib
• Retinoids: isotretinoin, etretinate	– Topical:
• Sulfur-containing medications: hydrochlorothiazide, furosemide, sulfonamides, sulfonylureas	Oxicams
	Proprionic acid derivatives
	• Phenothiazine
	• Pilocarpine
	• Pyridoxine
	• Ranitidine
	• Sulfur-containing medications: hydrochlorothiazide, furosemide, sulfonamides, sulfonylureas
	• Tricyclic antidepressants

Table 5.2 Common photoaggravated dermatoses

• Atopic dermatitis
• Chronic cutaneous lupus erythematosus
• Darier disease (synonyms: Darier-white disease, dyskeratosis follicularis, keratosis follicularis)
• Dermatomyositis
• Pellagra
• Pemphigus erythematosus

sites within the first 24–48 h of exposure. Patients can subsequently develop hyperpigmentation that may take months to resolve. Notably, the inflammatory stage may go unnoticed and patients may present only after pigmentary changes develop.

The approach to the patient suspected of suffering from photodermatoses includes a thorough history and physical exam, as well as phototesting. Additional laboratory testing may be necessary based on the clinical findings, and may include skin biopsies, screening for antinuclear antibodies, porphyrins, a comprehensive metabolic panel, and a urine analysis. While the medical treatment of these conditions may vary, meticulous photoprotective measures—including minimizing sun exposure, the use of broad-spectrum sunscreens, and wearing protective clothing are mandatory.

Sun Protection

The SPF measures how well a product protects against UVB radiation. The Food and Drug Administration defines SPF as the ratio of MED with an applied product to the MED unprotected [63]. For example, skin applied with a sunscreen of SPF 30 will sustain thirty times more sunlight before burning compared to unprotected skin. Sunscreens with an SPF 30 prevent 97% of the sun's rays from penetrating the skin. There is no data to indicate significant additional benefit from applying sunscreen with a SPF of greater than 50 [63]. SPF does not provide information on a products' efficacy in protection from UVA or visible light [64].

Chemical sunscreens are composed of organic compounds that work by absorbing UV radiation. Commonly used organic ingredients are include avobenzone, oxybenzone, ensulizole, octinoxate, and octisalate [64]. Depending on the compound, the degree and spectrum of UVA and UVB protection varies [64]. These compounds are also vulnerable to photodegradation and may be prone to generating free radicals [64]. They can subsequently cause photosensitizing or photoirritating reactions in susceptible individuals [64]. Newer ingredients such as ecamsule, bemotrizinol, and bisoctrizole have been added to formulations as they protect against both UVB and UVA and function as photostabilizers when paired with avobenzone [64].

Physical sunscreens are composed of inorganic compounds and protect skin by absorbing, deflecting, and scattering solar radiation [64]. They are composed of inorganic compounds such as iron oxide (FeO), titanium dioxide (TiO_2), and zinc oxide (ZnO) [64]. Their spectrum of action covers UVB, UVA, and visible light. Iron oxide specifically has been shown to be more effective than the other inorganic compounds in preventing the erythema and irritation caused by visible light [65]. Iron oxide inorganic compounds are generally safe for use and are favorable by consumers due to their tinted formulations and, therefore, increased transparency upon application [66].

The American Academy of Dermatology (AAD) recommends that all individuals apply sunscreen prior to outdoor exposure regardless of age, gender, or race [67]. The AAD recommends water-resistant sunscreens with an SPF of 30 or higher [67]. Sunscreens should be applied 15 min prior to going outdoors, and reapplied approximately every two hours, or after swimming or sweating [67]. Guidelines also recommend usage of protective clothing such as long-sleeved shirts, pants, and a wide brimmed hat.

Conclusion

Human skin experiences both immediate and delayed effects as a consequence of exposure to UVR and visible light. These effects vary in magnitude and degree across skin types. Although higher levels of melanin confers darker skin with some protection against UVB-induced erythema, studies show that darker skin may be more susceptible to the cellular toxicity and subsequent photoaging caused by UVA. Emerging data also shows that the toxic effects of visible light may be more pronounced in darker skin types. Additional studies characterizing the effects of UV and visible light on photodermatoses and photoaging are warranted in order to optimize the treatment and management of all patients.

References

1. Sklar LR, Almutawa F, Lim HW, Hamzavi I. Effects of ultraviolet radiation, visible light, and infrared radiation on erythema and pigmentation: a review. Photochem Photobiol Sci. 2013;12(1):54–64. doi:10.1039/c2pp25152c.
2. Diffey B. What is light? Photodermatol Photoimmunol Photomed. 2002;18(2):68–74.
3. Qiang F. Radiation (Solar). In: Holton JR, editor. Encyclopedia of atmospheric Sciences. 5th ed.; 2003, p. 1859–63.
4. Battie C, Jitsukawa S, Bernerd F, Del Bino S, Marionnet C, Verschoore M. New insights in photoaging, UVA induced damage and skin types. Exp Dermatol. 2014;23(Suppl 1):7–12. doi:10.1111/exd.12388.
5. Randhawa M, Seo I, Liebel F, Southall MD, Kollias N, Ruvolo E. Visible light induces melanogenesis in human skin through a photoadaptive response. PLoS ONE. 2015;10(6): e0130949. doi:10.1371/journal.pone.0130949.
6. Marrot L, Meunier JR. Skin DNA photodamage and its biological consequences. J Am Acad Dermatol. 2008;58(5 Suppl 2):139–48. doi:10.1016/j.jaad.2007.12.007.
7. Maddodi N, Jayanthy A, Setaluri V. Shining light on skin pigmentation: the darker and the brighter side of effects of UV radiation. Photochem Photobiol. 2012;88(5):1075–82. doi:10. 1111/j.1751-1097.2012.01138.x.
8. Ou-Yang H, Stmatas G, Saliou C, Kollias N. A chemiluminescence study of UVA-induced oxidative stress in human skin in vivo. J Invest Dermatol. 2004;122(4):1020–9.
9. Romanhole RC, Ataide JA, Moriel P, Mazzola PG. Update on ultraviolet A and B radiation generated by the sun and artificial lamps and their effects on skin. Int J Cosmet Sci. 2015:366–70. doi:10.1111/ics.12219.
10. Marionnet C, Pierrard C, Lekuene F, Bernerd F. Modulations of gene expression induced by daily ultraviolet light can be prevented by a broad spectrum sunscreen. Photochem Photobiol Sci. 2012;116:37–47.
11. Agar N, Young AR. Melanogenesis: a photoprotective response to DNA damage? Mutat Res—Fundam Mol Mech Mutagen. 2005;571(1-2 SPEC. ISS.):121–32. doi:10.1016/j.mrfmmm. 2004.11.016.
12. Rünger TM, Farahvash B, Hatvani Z, Rees A. Comparison of DNA damage responses following equimutagenic doses of UVA and UVB: a less effective cell cycle arrest with UVA may render UVA-induced pyrimidine dimers more mutagenic than UVB-induced ones. Photochem Photobiol Sci. 2012;11(1):207. doi:10.1039/c1pp05232b.
13. Bernerd F, Asselineau D. UVA exposure of human skin reconstructed in vitro induces apoptosis of dermal fibroblasts: subsequent connective tissue repair and implications in photoaging. Differ Cell Death. 1998;5(9):792–802.
14. Hönigsmann H. Erythema and pigmentation. Photodermatol Photoimmunol Photomed. 2002;18:75–81. doi:10.1034/j.1600-0781.2002.180204.x.
15. Mahmoud BH, Hexsel CL, Hamzavi IH, Lim HW. Effects of visible light on the skin. Photochem Photobiol. 2008;84(2):450–62. doi:10.1111/j.1751-1097.2007.00286.x.

16. Wenczl E, Van Der Schans GP, Roza L, et al. (Pheo)melanin photosensitizes UVA-induced DNA damage in cultured human melanocytes. J Invest Dermatol. 1998;111(4):678–82. doi:10.1046/j.1523-1747.1998.00357.x.

17. Marrot L, Belaidi JP, Meunier JR, Perez P, Agapakis-Causse C. The human melanocyte as a particular target for UVA radiation and an endpoint for photoprotection assessment. Photochem Photobiol. 1999;69(6):686–93.

18. Brash DE. Roles of the transcription factor p53 in keratinocyte carcinomas. Br J Dermatol. 2006;154(Suppl):8–10. doi:10.1111/j.1365-2133.2006.07230.x.

19. Cui R, Widlund HR, Feige E, et al. Central role of p53 in the suntan response and pathologic hyperpigmentation. Cell. 2007;128(5):853–64. doi:10.1016/j.cell.2006.12.045.

20. D'Orazio J, Jarrett S, Amaro-Ortiz A, Scott T. UV radiation and the skin. Int J Mol Sci. 2013;14(6):12222–48. doi:10.3390/ijms140612222.

21. Jablonski NG. The evolution of human skin colouration and its relevance to health in the modern world. J R Coll Physicians Edinb. 2012;42(1):58–63.

22. Göring H, Koshuchowa S. Vitamin D. The sun hormone. Life in environmental mismatch. Biochem Biokhimiiā. 2015;80(1):8–20. doi:10.1134/S0006297915010022.

23. Antoniou C, Lademann J, Schanzer S, et al. Do different ethnic groups need different sun protection? Skin Res Technol. 2009;15(3):323–9. doi:10.1111/j.1600-0846.2009.00366.x.

24. Kaidbey KH, Agin PH, Sayre RM, Kligman AM. Photoprotection by melanin–a comparison of black and Caucasian skin. J Am Acad Dermatol. 1979;1:249–60.

25. Thomson M. Relative efficiency of pigment and horny layer thickness in protecting the skin of Europeans and Africans against solar ultraviolet radiation. J Physiol. 1955;127:236–46.

26. Weigand D, Haygood C, Gaylor J. Cell layers and density of Negro and Caucasian stratum corneum. J Invest Dermatol. 1974;62(6):563–8.

27. Del Bino S, Bernerd F. Variations in skin colour and the biological consequences of ultraviolet radiation exposure. Br J Dermatol. 2013;169 Suppl (3):33–40. doi:10.1111/bjd.12529.

28. Chiarelli-Neto O, Ferreira AS, Martins WK, et al. Melanin photosensitization and the effect of visible light on epithelial cells. PLoS ONE. 2014;9(11):1–9. doi:10.1371/journal.pone.0113266.

29. Liebel F, Kaur S, Ruvolo E, Kollias N, Southall MD. Irradiation of skin with visible light induces reactive oxygen species and matrix-degrading enzymes. J Invest Dermatol. 2012;132 (7):1901–7. doi:10.1038/jid.2011.476.

30. Youn J, Oh J, Kim B, et al. Relationship between skin phototype and MED in Korean, brown skin. Photodermatol Photoimmunol Photomed. 1997;13(5–6):208–11.

31. Leenutaphong V. Relationship between skin and cutaneous response to UV radiation in Thai. Photodermatol Photoimmuno. 1995;11:198–203.

32. Eilers S, Bach DQ, Gaber R, et al. Accuracy of self-report in assessing Fitzpatrick skin phototypes I through VI. JAMA Dermatology. 2016;60611(11):1289–94. doi:10.1001/jamadermatol.2013.6101.

33. Pichon L, Landrine H, Corral I, Hao Y, Mayer J, Hoerster K. Measuring skin cancer risk in African Americans: is the Fitzpatrick Skin Type Classification Scale culturally sensitive? Ethn Dis. 2010;20(2):174–9.

34. Kelser E, Linos E, Kanzler M, Lee W, Sainani K, Tang J. Reliability and prevalence of digital image skin types in the United States: results from National Health and Nutrition Examination Survey 2003–2004. J Am Acad Dermatol. 2012;66(1):163–5.

35. Sanclemente G, Zapata JF, García JJ, Gaviria Á, Gómez LF, Barrera M. Lack of correlation between minimal erythema dose and skin phototype in a colombian scholar population. Skin Res Technol. 2008;14(4):403–9. doi:10.1111/j.1600-0846.2008.00306.x.

36. Agbai ON, Buster K, Sanchez M, et al. Skin cancer and photoprotection in people of color: a review and recommendations for physicians and the public. J Am Acad Dermatol. 2014;70 (4):748–62. doi:10.1016/j.jaad.2013.11.038.

37. Ravnbak MH, Philipsen PA, Wiegell SR, Wulf HC. Skin pigmentation kinetics after exposure to ultraviolet A. Acta Derm Venereol. 2009;89(4):357–63. doi:10.2340/00015555-0635.

38. Kollias N, et al. Erythema and melanogenesis action spectra in heavily pigmented individuals as compared to fair-skinned Caucasians. Photodermatol Photoimmunol Photomed. 1996;12:183–8. doi:10.1111/j.1600-0781.1996.tb00197.x.
39. Wolber R, Schlenz K, Wakamatsu K, et al. Pigmentation effects of solar simulated radiation as compared with UVA and UVB radiation. Pigment Cell Melanoma Res. 2008;21(4):487–91. doi:10.1111/j.1755-148X.2008.00470.x.Pigmentation.
40. Roh K, Kim D, Ha S, Ro Y, Kim J, Lee H. Pigmentation in Koreans: study of the differences from caucasians in age, gender and seasonal variations. Br J Dermatol. 2001;144(1):94–9.
41. Kotrakaras R, Kligman A. The effect of topical tretinoin on photodamaged facial skin: the Thai experience. Br J Dermatol. 1993;129:302–9.
42. Beradesca E, Leveqe J-L, Maibach H. Ethnic Skin and Hair. 2006.
43. Halder R, Ara C. Skin cancer and photoaging in ethnic skin. Dermatol Clin. 2003;21(4): 725–32.
44. Taylor S. Enhancing the care and treatment of skin of color, Part 2: understanding skin physiology. Cutis. 2005;76(5):302–6.
45. Zastrow L, Ferrero L, Herrling T, Groth N. Sun protection under asian light. Asian soc Cosm Sci. 2007;4:62–8.
46. Fourtanier A, Moyal D, Seite S. UVA filters in sun-protection products: regulatory and biological aspect. Photochem Photobiol Sci. 2012;11:81–9.
47. Griffiths C, Wang T, Hamilton T, Voorhees J, Ellis C. A photonumeric scale for the assessment of cutaneous photodamage. Dermatology, Arch. 1992;128(3):347–51.
48. Larnier C, Ortonne J, Venot A, et al. Evaluation of cutaneous photodamage using photographic scale. Br J Dermatol. 1994;130(2):167–73.
49. Vierkotter A, Krutmann J. Environmental influences on skin aging and ethnic-specific manifestations. Dermatoendocrinol. 2012;4(3):227–31.
50. Nouveau-Richard S, Yang Z, Mac-Mary S, et al. Skin ageing: a comparison between Chinese and European populations: a pilot study. J Dermatol Sci. 2005;40(3):187–93. doi:10.1016/j.jdermsci.2005.06.006.
51. Chan H, Jackson B. Laser treatment on ethnic skin. In: Lim HW, Hoenigsmann H, Hawk JLM, editors. Photodermatol New York Inf Healthc. 2007.
52. Lejeune F, Christiaens F, Bernerd F. Evaluation of sunscreen products using a reconstructed skin model exposed to simulated daily ultraviolet radiation: relevance of filtration profile and SPF value for daily photoprotection. Photodermatol Photoimmunol Photomed. 2008;24 (5):249–55.
53. Marionnet C, Grether-Beck S, Seite S, et al. A broad-spectrum sunscreen prevents UVA radiation-induced gene expression in reconstructed skin in vitro and in human skin in vivo. Exp Dermatol. 2011;20(6):466–82.
54. Miyamura Y, Coelho SG, Schlenz K, et al. The deceptive nature of UVA tanning versus the modest protective effects of UVB tanning on human skin. Pigment Cell Melanoma Res. 2011;24(1):136–47. doi:10.1111/j.1755-148X.2010.00764.x.
55. Ravnbak MH, Wulf HC. Pigmentation after single and multiple UV-exposures depending on UV-spectrum. Arch Dermatol Res. 2007;299(1):25–32. doi:10.1007/s00403-006-0728-3.
56. Ravnbak MH, Philipsen PA, Wiegell SR, Wulf HC. Skin pigmentation kinetics after UVB exposure. Acta Derm Venereol. 2008;88(3):223–8. doi:10.2340/00015555-0431.
57. Mahmoud BH, Ruvolo E, Hexsel CL, et al. Impact of long-wavelength UVA and visible light on melanocompetent skin. J Invest Dermatol. 2010;130(8):2092–7. doi:10.1038/jid.2010.95.
58. Kollias N, Baqer A. An experimental study of th changes in pigmentation in human skin in vivo with visible and near infrared light. Photochem Photobiol. 1984;39(5):651–9.
59. Rosen CF, Jacques SL, Stuart ME, Gange RW. Immediate pigment darkening: visual and reflectance spectrophotometric analysis of action spectrum. Photochem Photobiol. 1990;51 (5):583–8. doi:10.1111/j.1751-1097.1990.tb01969.x.
60. Ramasubramaniam R, Roy A, Sharma B, Nagalakshmi S. Are there mechanistic differences between ultraviolet and visible radiation induced skin pigmentation? Photochem Photobiol Sci. 2011;10(12):1887–93. doi:10.1039/c1pp05202k.

61. Marcos LA, Kahler R, Quaak MS, et al. Phytophotodermatitis. Int J Infect Dis. 2015;38:7–8. doi:10.1016/j.ijid.2015.07.004.
62. Raam R, DeClerck B, Jhun P, et al. Phytophotodermatitis: the other "lime" disease. Ann Emerg Med. 2016;67(4):554–6. doi:10.1016/j.annemergmed.2016.02.023.
63. Al-Jamal MS, Griffith JL, Lim HW. Photoprotection in ethnic skin. Dermatol Sin. 2014;32 (4):217–24. doi:10.1016/j.dsi.2014.09.001.
64. Morabito K, Shapley NC, Steeley KG, Tripathi A. Review of sunscreen and the emergence of non-conventional absorbers and their applications in ultraviolet protection. Int J Cosmet Sci. 2011;33(5):385–90. doi:10.1111/j.1468-2494.2011.00654.x.
65. Bissonnette R, Nigen S, Bolduc C, Méry S, Nocera T. Protection afforded by sunscreens containing inorganic sunscreening agents against blue light sensitivity induced by aminole-vulinic acid. Dermatol Surg. 2008;34(11):1469–74. doi:10.1111/j.1524-4725.2008.34311.x.
66. Nohynek G. Nanotechnology, cosmetics and the skin: is there a health risk? Skin Pharmacol Physiol. 2008;21(3):136–49.
67. American Academy of Dermatology—Sunscreen FAQs. 2016. Website https://www.aad.org/media/stats/prevention-and-care/sunscreen-faqs. Accessed 5 May 2016.

Chapter 6
Stratum Corneum Lipids and Water-Holding Capacity

Dimitrios Rigopoulos and Ekaterini Tiligada

The Epidermis

The skin is the largest organ of the body that covers its entire surface and provides a protective mechanical, biochemical and immunological barrier against the outside world. The epidermis (Greek *epi*, on top; *derma*, skin) is the outermost stratified epithelial compartment that is separated from the dermis by a stabilizing and dynamic interface provided by the basal membrane [1, 2].

The epidermis lacks blood vessels and is composed of four main layers of unique architecture: the superficial stratum corneum (SC) or horny layer, the stratum granulosum (SG), the stratum spinosum (SS) or squamous cell layer and the innermost stratum basale (SB). In thick skin, a small number of parallel arrays of dead keratinocytes containing keratohyalin form the stratum lucidum (SL) between the SG and the SC. The SG, SS and SB form the 50–100 μm thick viable epidermis, whereas the SC forms the 10–30 μm thick non-viable epidermis [1, 3–5].

The epidermis protects the organism by preventing excessive trans-epidermal water loss (TEWL), the passive outward water diffusion process of the water-saturated viable epidermis and by stopping environmental insults to harm the body [6, 7]. It is characterized by the dynamic continuous self-renewal attributed to the keratinocytes that undergo programmed differentiation during their migration from the SB toward the SC [8, 9]. The communication of keratinocytes through

D. Rigopoulos (✉)
2nd Department of Dermatology and Venereology, Medical School, 'Attikon' General University Hospital, National and Kapodistrian University of Athens, Rimini 1, 12462 Haidari, Greece
e-mail: drigop@hol.gr

E. Tiligada
Department of Pharmacology, Medical School, National and Kapodistrian University of Athens, M. Asias 75, 11527 Athens, Greece
e-mail: aityliga@med.uoa.gr

© Springer International Publishing AG 2017
N.A. Vashi and H.I. Maibach (eds.), *Dermatoanthropology of Ethnic Skin and Hair*, DOI 10.1007/978-3-319-53961-4_6

different signaling pathways with the melanin-producing melanocytes [10], Merkel cells [11] and the Langerhans cells (dendritic cells), the first line immune defense players [12], contributes to the complex skin homeostatic network (Fig. 6.1). In the SC, the keratinocytes shed approximately every two weeks as corneocytes proceed through the desquamation process [9]. In the healthy epidermis, the balance between cell proliferation in the lower layers and desquamation in the SC results in a complete renewal approximately every four weeks [8].

Keratinocytes and Corneocytes

The keratinocyte is the predominant epidermal cell type that is formed in the SB and proliferates through to the SG. During their maturation toward the final transformation into the non-viable corneocytes, keratinocytes express a range of lipids and proteins, including keratins. Keratins are epithelial proteins that form heterodimeric intermediate filaments anchoring skin cells to the extracellular matrix through desmosomes involved in cell–cell adhesion [13–15]. Keratin intermediate filaments provide structural support and integrity to the epithelium and regulate cellular growth, proliferation, migration and apoptosis via interactions with diverse cellular proteins [14]. Furthermore, keratinocytes at the lower epidermal layers synthesize precursor lipids that are assembled in lamellar bodies (LBs) in the upper layers and secreted into the extracellular space by exocytosis in the interface between the SG and SC [1, 16].

In late differentiated stages, keratinocytes are transformed into the flattened anucleated corneocytes. They become filled with water-retaining filaggrin-linked keratin intermediate filaments and secrete lipids into the extracellular space [17–19]. Corneocytes, also referred to as squames, are remnants of the differentiated keratinocytes that are devoid of cytoplasmic organelles and provide the skin with structural integrity and elasticity. They contribute to the barrier properties of the SC together with the surrounding densely cross-linked protein layers of the cornified cell envelope and the attached lipid monolayer that forms the cornified lipid envelope [1, 20]. Thus, keratinocyte differentiation is an important process that establishes and maintains the SC. At the terminal differentiation stage after 4–6 weeks, they are converted by cornification into the building blocks of the epidermal barrier, the dead corneocytes [5, 9].

Architecture of the Stratum Corneum

The SC is composed of a multilayer of corneocytes and gives the skin its characteristic look, feel and health. At the interface with the external environment, it provides a water-resistant protective barrier to the inner structures by retaining water and offering protection against dehydration and environmental damage from

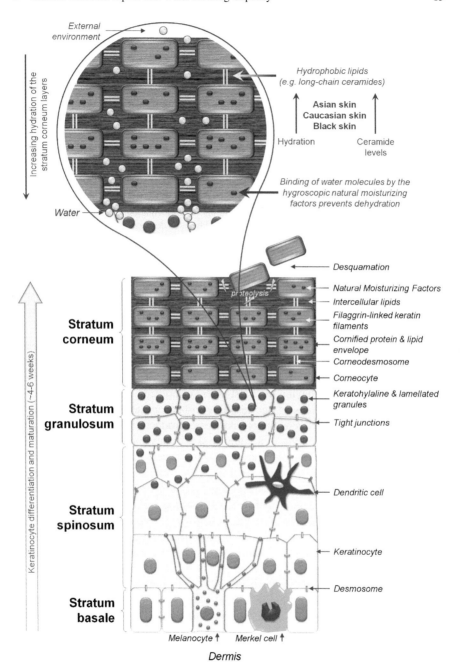

◄**Fig. 6.1** Schematic representation of the main epidermal layers. The epidermis is a keratinized stratified squamous epithelium consisting primarily of keratin-producing keratinocytes bridged by intercellular desmosomes and constantly differentiating and migrating from the deeper epidermal layers toward the skin surface. The innermost stratum basale lies adjacent to the dermis and consists of a single layer of proliferating keratinocytes. Multiple layers of nondividing keratinocytes form the stratum spinosum. Keratinocytes communicate with melanin-producing melanocytes, tactile (Merkel) cells and dendritic (Langerhans) cells that are pivotal to the dermal immune response. The stratum granulosum consists of 3–5 layers of flat keratinocytes with deteriorating organelles and accumulation of keratohylaline and lamellar granules containing glycoproteins that are released to the extracellular space to reduce water loss. At the interface between stratum granulosum and stratum corneum, the keratinocytes secrete the lipid contents of the lamellar bodies to the intercellular space. They are terminally differentiated into the dead, keratin-filled corneocytes that are surrounded by a cornified envelope composed of cross-linked proteins and lipids. Corneocytes eventually shed when the interconnecting corneodesmosomes are degraded by proteolytic extracellular enzymes resulting in desquamation. The stratum corneum is compared to 'bricks and mortar' consisting of 20–30 layers of dead corneocytes (bricks) that are embedded in lipid lamellar structures (mortar). The spatial corneocytes arrangement and the hydrophobic lamellar lipids prevent the loss of water from the body to the drier external environment. In parallel, the hygroscopic natural moisturizing factors selectively retain free water and keep the outermost layers hydrated. In general, deeper stratum corneum layers are more hydrated than the upper layers, while variations in hydration and ceramide levels seem to be implicated in the racial differences in barrier function

xenobiotics and pathogen invasion [5, 6, 20, 21]. Moreover, it is considered to be a rate-limiting barrier for the intra-cutaneous penetration of various agents, including drugs and cosmetics [5, 7]. SC thickness largely varies with the anatomical location, with the palms and soles having the most layers of corneocytes. Generally, the SC becomes thicker with increasing age resulting in barrier alterations and loss of its protective capacity [22]. Interestingly, skin care products have been reported to decrease SC thickness resulting in a younger skin appearance [23].

The interest in SC morphology, physiology and biochemistry dates back to the late nineteenth and early twentieth centuries [24]. Yet, the recent technological advances in visualization options and biochemical tools allowed a more detailed dissection of its vital structural and functional homeostatic properties, with significant implications in dermatology, pharmacology, toxicology, and cosmetology [20, 25]. The SC is often referred to as a 'brick and mortar' structure based on a two-phase model described in an effort to investigate some of the pharmacokinetic properties of topically applied drugs on the skin [26]. It is composed of 15–20 layers of lipid-depleted corneocytes that are oriented almost in parallel to the skin surface and embedded as 'bricks' in the extracellular matrix that mainly contains the lipids secreted by the differentiated keratinocytes and compared to 'mortar' (Fig. 6.1). Despite this common simplistic description, the structural and functional complexity of the SC is remarkably high considering its metabolic adaptation and constant renewal [5, 20, 21]. About 5–10 highly ordered and densely packed lipid-enriched lamellar membranous sheets that consist of some 13 species of complex ceramides, cholesterol, and free fatty acids (FFAs) constitute the skin permeability barrier and maintain its integrity. The SC also contains corneodesmosomes interconnecting the corneocytes primarily via the proteins loricrin and involucrin, their degradation leading to exfoliation; intracellular and extracellular natural moisturizing factor (NMF) formed by filaggrin proteolysis into small hygroscopic molecules including amino acids; lipid-processing lipolytic enzymes; proteolytic enzymes catalyzing the degradation of corneodesmosomes; and secreted contents of LBs at the interface between the SC and the SG [6, 20, 27–29].

The Stratum Corneum as a Homeostatic Biochemical Barrier

The biochemical skin barrier consists of water, lipids, acids, hydrolytic enzymes, and antimicrobial peptides. Secretory LBs are crucial to the homeostasis and the barrier function of the SC [30, 31]. LBs are produced in the keratinocytes of the SS and contain lysosomal enzymes such as cathepsin D and vacuolar H^+-ATPase. Their secretion products at the interface between SG and SC include lipids, such as glucosylceramides, sphingomyelin and cholesterol; lipid-processing enzymes, including β-glucocerebrosidase, acid sphingomyelinase, and secretory phospholipase A_2; structural proteins like corneodesmosin implicated in corneocyte cohesion; proteases, such as kallikreins and cathepsins; protease inhibitors involved in the control of desquamation; and antimicrobial peptides such as defensins and cathelicidins [18].

The Lipid Milieu

Despite being composed of dead corneocytes, the SC is characterized by a high lipid metabolic activity that largely defines the permeability and barrier properties of the skin. Notably, the cornified lipid envelope contains ω-hydroxy-ceramides that covalently bind mainly to the cornified envelope protein involucrin to bridge the hydrophilic corneocytes and the surrounding lipophilic multi-lamellar lipid sheets [32]. On a dry-weight basis, the SC contains 5–15% lipids, 75–80% proteins, and 5–10% other materials [33].

Although the exact spatial arrangement of the SC lipids is not completely elucidated and described in various structural models [20, 34], the lipid matrix is unanimously accepted to display a highly ordered intercellular organization that directs the permeability and barrier integrity of the SC [20, 34]. The intercellular lipids of the SC are organized in layers forming *S*hort (SPP; repeat distance 6 nm) and *L*ong (LPP; repeat distance 13 nm) *P*eriodicity lamellar *P*hases. Within the lamellae, lipids are laterally packed in a very dense, ordered orthorhombic arrangement, a less dense, ordered hexagonal, or a disordered liquid organization [35]. The lamellae play a vital role in the selective permeability of the skin, including the intradermal penetration of topically applied drugs [1, 31, 33].

The composition of the SC lipid lamellae is unique as common membrane phospholipids are virtually absent. The lamellar polar glycosphingolipids, sterols, and phospholipids released in the interface between SG and SC serve as precursors of the enzymatically derived nonpolar lipids in the SC that are assembled into lamellar structures surrounding the corneocytes [20]. The constituents of the SC lipid lamellae are mainly complex ceramides (40–50%), cholesterol (20–30%) and mostly long-chain saturated FFAs ($\sim 10\%$), as well as cholesterol-3-sulfate and cholesteryl esters [20, 30, 33]. In particular, ceramides are composed of a sphingoid base linked through an amide bond to a fatty acid moiety with variable chain length and exhibit a remarkable biodiversity [16, 35]. Linoleic acid and protein-esterified ceramides are crucial for structuring and maintaining barrier integrity. A plethora of metabolic enzymes and regulatory factors mediate the production and the organization of epidermal lipids, including ceramides that are essential for proper SC function and barrier homeostasis [16].

Additional surface lipids include triglycerides ($\sim 16\%$), wax/sterol esters ($\sim 26\%$), squalene ($\sim 12\%$), hexadecenoic acid and other FFAs ($\sim 33\%$) that are secreted by sebaceous glands and elicit a number of actions and antimicrobial effects [20, 34, 36]. Interestingly, the actual lipid composition of the SC exhibits interindividual and racial variability and seasonal variations [37, 38], as well as differences related to the anatomical location, skin depth, age, sex, dermal dysfunctions, and pathological conditions [3, 23, 36].

Water-Holding Capacity

The specialized biochemical modifications that promote the migration of keratinocytes from the lower SB toward the outer SC lead to the cornification process that marks their terminal differentiation to corneocytes and thereby the beginning of the SC maturation and the formation of a highly efficient barrier against water loss [7, 9, 17, 38]. The resulting structure provides the natural physical and water-retaining barrier of the skin, being able to absorb three times its weight in water.

The SC is a biochemically active structure in which continuous anabolic and catabolic reactions support its maturation and facilitate its normal intrinsic hydration, the maintenance of tissue cohesion, integrity, and thickness and the loss of corneocytes upon completion of the maturation process during desquamation [9, 21, 39]. Under normal conditions, the water content of the SC is vital for maintaining tissue flexibility and for facilitating the biochemical activity that is critical for optimal tissue functioning and maturation, whereas when the water content is less than 10% the SC cracks [27]. For instance, free water is essential for effective corneodesmolysis, the degradation of corneodesmosomes by serine proteases in the intercellular space resulting in desquamation [21, 27, 39].

The hydration of SC exhibits considerable differences depending on the body location, with the scalp, eyelids, nasal tip, anterior neck, antecubital, and popliteal fossae and the areola mammae being highly hydrated [7]. Moreover, water is not uniformly distributed in the SC, deeper SC layers being progressively more hydrated than the uppermost SC layers [7]. At least three components have been implicated in the water-holding capacity of the SC. These are related to the spatial arrangement of corneocytes, the organization of the intercellular lamellar lipids and the presence of NMFs [17, 21, 27, 39].

Corneocyte Arrangement

Corneocyte packing, lectins, and desmosomes in the SC increase the path length of traversing water molecules and enhance the structural cohesiveness of the tissue [17]. Water seems to be unevenly distributed in the SC, its content being related to the penetration and binding capacities of the different corneocyte layers [40, 41]. Differences in the hydration levels have been observed at water content of 57–87% (w/w), corneocytes in central SC parts being more swollen that their superficial and deeper counterparts, whereas extracellular water pools have been reported at hydration levels >300% (w/w) [40, 41]. Studies in patients with dry skin revealed that premature expression of the corneocyte cross-linking protein involucrin also contributes to the reduced water-binding capacity of the skin [38].

Intercellular Lipids

The effectiveness of the SC barrier highly depends on the content of the different intercellular lipids. During SC maturation, enzymatic lipid modifications decrease their polarity. In addition to the composition that influences the passage of water through the SC, lipid lateral packing also affects the barrier function. Altered ratios of fatty acids esterified to ceramides have been reported to increase skin moisture loss, without excluding the involvement of altered expression of various keratins, exemplified by decreased keratins K1 and K10 and increased basal keratins K5 and K14 [38]. Moreover, the dense orthorhombic laterally packed lipids of the solid crystalline state reduce the rate of water flux through the tissue and contribute to the more efficient barrier in the lower SC, compared to the gel state of the hexagonally packed lipids that weaken the barrier in the outer SC [17, 39, 42].

The differences in lipid lateral arrangements are attributed to the role played by the fatty acids. In contrast, cholesterol and ceramides seem to be decisive for the lamellar conformations [39]. Further information on the role of ceramides in the SC barrier function comes from more recent studies on lesional and non-lesional skin from patients with atopic dermatitis. These reports associate TEWL increases with decreasing ceramide chain length and skin barrier dysfunction with increased levels of short-chain ceramides [35, 43]. Notably, ceramide chain length rather than the ratio of lipid subclasses appears to play a critical role in TEWL, skin permeability, and barrier function [35, 42].

Additional evidence on the role of ceramides in the water-retaining capacity of the SC is provided by observations on the racial differences in dermal properties that influence the ability of the skin to retain water. Lower skin hydration and higher TEWL has been reported in African American compared to Caucasian skin, whereas Asian skin demonstrated higher levels of hydration, yet the poorest barrier function upon mechanical challenge [38, 44]. Similarly, ceramide levels in the SC have been found to be highest in Asian skin, followed by Caucasian and Black skin [38].

Natural Moisturizing Factor

The hygroscopic NMF components act as humectants that play a central role in the selective free water retention of the SC by binding water molecules and preventing dehydration of the outermost layers [17]. NMF consists of small water-soluble molecules, including mostly amino acids or their derivatives, such as pyrrolidone carboxylic and urocanic acid, as well as sweat-derived lactic acid, urea, citrate, and sugars that create an effective moisture barrier [17]. NMF is a degradation product of filaggrin and it is present in high concentrations within healthy corneocytes [17, 27]. Interestingly, NMF levels decrease with age as well as by bathing or ultraviolet light [27].

Factors Influencing the Stratum Corneum Water-Holding Capacity

The extent of environmental humidity influences the hydration of the SC and promotes an adaptive response in the barrier function, in part by modifying the relative levels of epidermal ceramide species [17]. Moreover, low humidity may change the moisture content of the SC and induce or exacerbate various seasonal cutaneous pathologies characterized by accumulation of corneocytes on the skin surface as a result of impaired corneodesmosomal degradation, altered ceramide biochemistry and structure, and reduced NMF levels [17, 27, 45]. Other exogenous factors that are linked to the ability of the skin to maintain moisture include dry climates, cold, excessive showering or bathing, and exposure to alkali and detergents [46]. In addition to exogenous factors, ambient, lifestyle, and endogenous components that have been associated with loss of skin moisture include malnutrition, renal insufficiency, aging, racial differences, and hereditary disorders, such as ichthyosis vulgaris and atopy [37, 38].

Conclusion

The vital role of the epidermis in maintaining skin integrity and flexibility largely relies on the structural and biochemical properties of the SC, the outer epidermal layer that guards the interface between the organism and the external environment. The water-holding capacity of the SC contributes to the natural physical barrier of the skin. The spatial arrangement of corneocytes, the organization of the intercellular lamellar lipids, and the presence of natural moisturizing factors are decisive parameters for the ability of the skin to retain water. Among the pivotal elements that have been associated with SC hydration and the barrier homeostasis, are the relative levels of epidermal ceramide species, which exhibit racial variability and can be modified by both exogenous factors and endogenous components.

References

1. Bouwstra JA, Ponec M. The skin barrier in healthy and diseased state. Biochim Biophys Acta. 2006;1758:2080–95.
2. Baroni A, Buommino E, De Gregorio V, Ruocco E, Ruocco V, Wolf R. Structure and function of the epidermis related to barrier properties. Clin Dermatol. 2012;30:257–62.
3. Ya-Xian Z, Suetake T, Tagami H. Number of cell layers of the stratum corneum in normal skin—relationship to the anatomical location on the body, age, sex and physical parameters. Arch Dermatol Res. 1999;291:555–9.
4. Simpson CL, Patel DM, Green KJ. Deconstructing the skin: cytoarchitectural determinants of epidermal morphogenesis. Nat Rev Mol Cell Biol. 2011;12:565–80.
5. Böhling A, Bielfeldt S, Himmelmann A, Keskin M, Wilhelm KP. Comparison of the stratum corneum thickness measured in vivo with confocal Raman spectroscopy and confocal reflectance microscopy. Skin Res Technol. 2014;20:50–7.
6. Menon GK, Cleary GW, Lane ME. The structure and function of the stratum corneum. Int J Pharm. 2012;435:3–9.
7. Tagami H. Electrical measurement of the hydration state of the skin surface in vivo. Br J Dermatol. 2014;171(S3):29–33.
8. Webb A, Li A, Kaur P. Location and phenotype of human adult keratinocyte stem cells of the skin. Differentiation. 2004;72:387–95.
9. Eckhart L, Lippens S, Tschachler E, Declercq W. Cell death by cornification. Biochim Biophys Acta. 2013;1833:3471–80.
10. Cichorek M, Wachulska M, Stasiewicz A, Tymińska A. Skin melanocytes: biology and development. Postepy Dermatol Alergol. 2013;30:30–41.
11. Irmak MK. Multifunctional Merkel cells: their roles in electromagnetic reception, finger-print formation, Reiki, epigenetic inheritance and hair form. Med Hypotheses. 2010;75:162–8.
12. Matsui T, Amagai M. Dissecting the formation, structure and barrier function of the stratum corneum. IntImmunol. 2015;27:269–80.
13. Windoffer R, Beil M, Magin TM, Leube RE. Cytoskeleton in motion: the dynamics of keratin intermediate filaments in epithelia. J Cell Biol. 2011;194:669–78.
14. Pan X, Hobbs RP, Coulombe PA. The expanding significance of keratin intermediate filaments in normal and diseased epithelia. Curr Opin Cell Biol. 2013;25:47–56.
15. Loschke F, Seltmann K, Bouameur JE, Magin TM. Regulation of keratin network organization. CurrOpin Cell Biol. 2015;32:56–64.

16. Rabionet M, Gorgas K, Sandhoff R. Ceramide synthesis in the epidermis. Biochim Biophys Acta. 2014;1841:422–34.
17. Rawlings AV, Harding CR. Moisturization and skin barrier function. Dermatol Ther. 2004;17:43–8.
18. Raymond AA, Gonzalez de Peredo A, Stella A, Ishida-Yamamoto A, Bouyssie D, Serre G, Monsarrat B, Simon M. Lamellar bodies of human epidermis: proteomics characterization by high throughput mass spectrometry and possible involvement of CLIP-170 in their trafficking/secretion. Mol Cell Proteomics. 2008;7:2151–75.
19. Kezic S, Jakasa I. Filaggrin and skin barrier function. Curr Probl Dermatol. 2016;49:1–7.
20. Sahle FF, Gebre-Mariam T, Dobner B, Wohlrab J, Neubert RH. Skin diseases associated with the depletion of stratum corneum lipids and stratum corneum lipid substitution therapy. Skin Pharmacol Physiol. 2015;28:42–55.
21. Rawlings AV. Molecular basis for stratum corneum maturation and moisturization. Br J Dermatol. 2014;171(Suppl 3):19–28.
22. Bielfeldt S, Böhling A, Wilhelm K-P. Bioengineering methods to assess aging parameters in the depth of the skin. SOFW. 2011;J137:2–9.
23. Imbert I, Guerif-Ferreira Y, Oberto G, Berghi A, Mouser P, Cucumel K, Domloge N. In vivo study of age-related skin changes using in vivo confocal microscopy. IFSCC1. 2012:15–21.
24. Rein H. Die Gleichstromleitereigenschaften und elektromotorischen Kräfte der menschlichen Haut unddihre Auswertungzur Untersuchung von Funktionszuständen des Organes I-IV. Ztschr f Biol. 1926;85:195–247.
25. Machado M, Salgado TM, Hadgraft J, Lane ME. The relationship between transepidermal water loss and skin permeability. Int J Pharm. 2010;384:73–7.
26. Michaels AS, Chandrasekaran SK, Shaw JE. Drug permeation through human skin: theory and in vitro experimental measurement. AIChE J. 1975;21:985–96.
27. Harding CR, Watkinson A, Rawlings AV, Scott IR. Dry skin, moisturization and corneodesmolysis. Int J Cosmet Sci. 2000;22:21–52.
28. Robinson M, Visscher M, Laruffa A, Wickett R. Natural moisturizing factors (NMF) in the stratum corneum (SC). I. Effects of lipid extraction and soaking. J Cosmet Sci. 2010;61:13–22.
29. Feingold K, Elias P. The important role of lipids in the epidermis and their role in the formation and maintenance of the cutaneous barrier. Biochim Biophys Acta. 2014;1841:279.
30. Elias PM. Epidermal barrier function: intercellular lamellar lipid structures, origin, composition and metabolism. J Control Release. 1991;15:199–208.
31. van Smeden J, Janssens M, Gooris GS, Bouwstra JA. The important role of stratum corneum lipids for the cutaneous barrier function. Biochim Biophys Acta. 2014;1841:295–313.
32. Mizutani Y, Mitsutake S, Tsuji K, Kihara A, Igarashi Y. Ceramide biosynthesis in keratinocyte and its role in skin function. Biochimie. 2009;91:784–90.
33. Hatfield RM, Fung LW. Molecular properties of a stratum corneum model lipid system: large unilamellar vesicles. Biophys J. 1995;68:196–207.
34. Takigawa H, Nakagawa H, Kuzukawa M, Mori H, Imokawa G. Deficient production of hexadecanoic acid in the skin is associated in part with the vulnerability of atopic dermatitis patients to colonization by Staphylococcus aureus. Dermatology. 2005;211:240–8.
35. Janssens M, van Smeden J, Gooris GS, Bras W, Portale G, Caspers PJ, Vreeken RJ, Hankemeier T, Kezic S, Wolterbeek R, Lavrijsen AP, Bouwstra JA. Increase in short-chain ceramides correlates with an altered lipid organization and decreased barrier function in atopic eczema patients. J Lipid Res. 2012;53:2755–66.
36. Giacomoni PU, Mammone T, Teri M. Gender-linked differences in human skin. J Dermatol Sci. 2009;55:144–9.
37. Darlenski R, Fluhr JW. Influence of skin type, race, sex, and anatomic location on epidermal barrier function. Clin Dermatol. 2012;30:269–73.
38. Wan DC, Wong VW, Longaker MT, Yang GP, Wei FC. Moisturizing different racial skin types. J Clin Aesthet Dermatol. 2014;7:25–32.

39. Rawlings AV, Matts PJ. Stratum corneum moisturization at the molecular level: an update in relation to the dry skin cycle. J Invest Dermatol. 2005;124:1099–110.
40. Bouwstra JA, de Graaff A, Gooris GS, Nijsse J, Wiechers JW, van Aelst AC. Water distribution and related morphology in human stratum corneum at different hydration levels. J Invest Dermatol. 2003;120:750–8.
41. Richter T, Peuckert C, Sattler M, Koenig K, Riemann I, Hintze U, Wittern KP, Wiesendanger R, Wepf R. Dead but highly dynamic-the stratum corneum is divided into three hydration zones. Skin Pharmacol Physiol. 2004;17:246–57.
42. Groen D, Poole DS, Gooris GS, Bouwstra JA. Is an orthorhombic lateral packing and a proper lamellar organization important for the skin barrier function? Biochim Biophys Acta. 2011;1808:1529–37.
43. Ishikawa J, Narita H, Kondo N, Hotta M, Takagi Y, Masukawa Y, Kitahara T, Takema Y, Koyano S, Yamazaki S, Hatamochi A. Changes in the ceramide profile of atopic dermatitis patients. J Invest Dermatol. 2010;130:2511–4.
44. Berardesca E, Maibach HI. Racial differences in sodium lauryl sulphate induced cutaneous irritation: black and white. Contact Dermatitis. 1988;18:65–70.
45. Denda M, Sato J, Masuda Y, Tsuchiya T, Koyama J, Kuramoto M, Elias PM, Feingold KR. Exposure to a dry environment enhances epidermal permeability barrier function. J Invest Dermatol. 1998;111:858–63.
46. Guenther L, Lynde CW, Andriessen A, Barankin B, Goldstein E, Skotnicki SP, Gupta SN, Choi KL, Rosen N, Shapiro L, Sloan K. Pathway to dry skin prevention and treatment. J Cutan Med Surg. 2012;16:23–31.

Chapter 7
Physiologic Pigmentation

Catherine M. Higham and Neelam A. Vashi

Skin color is determined by melanocyte activity. Physiologic pigmentation refers to nonpathologic variations in intensity of pigmentation that, by definition, fall within the spectrum of what is considered normal pigmentation. For example, across all skin types, but more apparent in skin of color, skin over dorsal surfaces is typically more pigmented than skin over ventral surfaces [1]. There are a number of specific categories that fall under the general umbrella of physiologic pigmentation, which are elaborated in the following sections. In general, physiologic pigmentation is more prevalent in skin of color. It typically develops during the first two decades of life but may not be noticed until later. The unifying histologic feature found in all of these entities is an increase in melanin deposition in the affected skin. This is due to increased melanocytic activity rather than an increased number of melanocytes, which is similar across all skin types, ethnicities, and races.

Pigmentation of the Newborn

Newborn skin tends to be relatively less pigmented than adult skin. It is thought that pigmentation rapidly increases from birth to around 6 months of age, at which point it has reached adult levels [2]. Additionally, it is not uncommon for newborns to

C.M. Higham
Boston University Medical Center, 609 Albany Street, J-205,
Boston, MA 02118, USA
e-mail: catherine.higham@bmc.org

N.A. Vashi (✉)
Department of Dermatology, Center for Ethnic Skin,
Boston University, Boston, MA, USA
e-mail: nvashi419@gmail.com

N.A. Vashi
Boston University School of Medicine, Boston Medical Center,
Boston, MA, USA

© Springer International Publishing AG 2017
N.A. Vashi and H.I. Maibach (eds.), *Dermatoanthropology of Ethnic Skin and Hair*, DOI 10.1007/978-3-319-53961-4_7

have varied degrees of pigmentation by body site. Most noticeably, a number of studies have demonstrated that the forehead is most commonly the most intensely pigmented site in neonates [3, 4]

Pigmentary Demarcation Lines

Clinical Presentation

Pigmentary demarcation lines (PDLs) reflect variations in the degree of pigmentation between adjacent segments of skin [5, 6]. They appear clinically as well-demarcated patches of varying intensities of pigmentation and are typically symmetric [5, 7, 8]. The entity was first described by Motzumoto [9] in 1913 and has since been further characterized by a number of case reports and cross-sectional studies. There are currently eight recognized types of PDLs, types A-H, based on anatomic location [5].

Type A   Lateral area of upper anterior arm, extending across to pectoral region
Type B   Posterior medial leg
Type C   Vertical hypopigmented patches in pre- and para-sternal skin
Type D   Skin surrounding posterior medial spine
Type E   Lateral chest, extending from mid-third of clavicle to periareolar area
Type F   V-shaped hyperpigmented patch extending from malar prominence to temple
Type G   W-shaped hyperpigmented patch extending from malar prominence to temple
Type H   Hyperpigmented patches extending from angle of mouth to lateral chin

Epidemiology

PDLs are present in all skin types but are significantly more common in patients with darker skin [6]. One study found that among black participants, 79% of females and 75% of males had at least one PDL [6]. They are thought to most commonly arise during early childhood [6], although there are also reports of cases with the initial presentation occurring during adulthood [10]. It is not entirely clear if there were underlying subtle changes that were present previously but only became more noticeable after a specific trigger, such as pregnancy, puberty, or viral infections [10]. There are numerous reports of PDLs appearing during pregnancy, in particular type B [7, 8, 11].

Etiology

PDLs represent variations in the activity of melanocytes in adjacent areas of skin. The underlying developmental events that result in such differences remain unclear. Some have postulated that PDLs follow the distribution of cutaneous nerves and are related to variation in neural stimulation [8, 12, 13], while others hypothesize that they follow the lines of Blaschko [14].

Pigmentary demarcation lines must be distinguished from other patterns of pigmentary mosaicism that may warrant additional workup. There are a number of patterns of pigmentary mosaicism—variation in pigmentation that typically follow lines of Blaschko—that can be associated with systemic pathology, including hypomelanosis of Ito, linear and whorled nevoid hypermelanosis, and systematized epidermal nevus. Typically, the risk of systemic abnormalities is greatest in patients with widespread cutaneous involvement. As such, patients with large areas of cutaneous involvement should typically be worked up for systemic pathology [15].

Clinical Course/Treatment

Typically, PDLs are persistent but do not change significantly in size or intensity [5]. The exception is PDLs that arise during pregnancy and often will resolve spontaneously following pregnancy [7, 16]. Treatment is not medically necessary, as PDLs are within the spectrum of normal pigment variation. If desired for cosmetic reasons, the q-switched lasers have been shown to be an effective option [17].

Periorbital Hyperpigmentation

Definition/Clinical Presentation

Periorbital hyperpigmentation refers to darkening of the periorbital skin. It is known by a variety of names, including periorbital melanosis, dark circles, infraorbital darkening, or idiopathic cutaneous hyperchromia of the orbital region [18, 19]. It has a varied appearance, ranging from light brown to dark black round or semi-circular discoloration of the periorbital skin [18, 20]. It can extend as inferiorly as the malar prominence and midway down the nasal sidewall [19]. As discussed below, etiology for most cases of periorbital hyperpigmentation involves multiple etiologic forces; however, a component of this is physiologic based on underlying skin pigmentation.

Etiology

Data remain inconclusive regarding the underlying etiology of periorbital hyperpigmentation. Moreover, periorbital hyperpigmentation can be the end result of a number of different processes including dermal melanosis, excessive vascularity of the area, venous stasis, periorbital edema, thinness of the periorbital skin, and skin laxity and tear tough formation associated with aging [18, 20–23]. Additionally, there are forms of periorbital hyperpigmentation that are associated with other pigmentary disease processes, including post-inflammatory hyperpigmentation that must be distinguished clinically. It also must be distinguished from various systemic illnesses (including Addison's disease, thyroid disease, hemochromatosis, liver cirrhosis, Cushing's syndrome, chronic kidney disease) that are associated with periorbital darkening [24, 25].

There have been observational reports suggesting possible genetic associations [26], although Verschoore et al. [19] did not find any familial associations in their 2012 study. Sun exposure is thought to worsen periorbital hyperpigmentation [19]. There has been thought to lesions being exacerbated during periods of stress, illness, or fatigue, possibly due to increased vascular congestion and/or dermal edema [19, 22–24], although data behind this hypothesis are lacking.

Dermal melanosis is thought to play a major role in the constitutional or physiologic form of periorbital hyperpigmentation. A 2012 study by Verschoore et al. [19] used spectrophotometric intracutaneous analysis (SIA) to noninvasively assess the presence of melanin and hemoglobin in affected skin. They found the concentrations of total melanin, dermal melanin, and hemoglobin to be greater in affected skin compared to normal skin. Watanabe et al. [22] also found dermal melanosis to be present on histologic examination of biopsies of the affected skin in 12 out of 12 patients with bilateral homogenous periorbital hyperpigmentation. There is some thought that perhaps—at least in some cases—periorbital hyperpigmentation is a clinical variant of type F pigmentary demarcation lines [10].

Treatment

Treatment should be tailored to the underlying etiology. Hydroquinone, tretinoin, chemical peels, topical vitamin C, laser and light therapy, autologous fat transplantations, and fillers have all been shown to have some effect in the treatment of periorbital hyperpigmentation, depending on the specific etiology. [18, 20, 27–30]. In terms of laser and light therapy, the carbon dioxide resurfacing laser [23], Q-switched (QS) ruby laser [22, 31], QS alexandrite [32], QS Nd; YAG [33], and intense pulsed light [24] have all demonstrated some degree of effectiveness. Sunscreen and other means of photoprotection should be encouraged [21].

Acquired Idiopathic Pattern Facial Pigmentation

Acquired idiopathic pattern facial pigmentation (AIPFP) is an entity recently characterized by Sarma et al. [34] based on evidence from a survey of 187 patients. AIPFP presents most commonly as symmetric, uniform grayish-colored hyperpigmentation over periorbital, zygomatic, malar upper nasal, perioral, and mandibular regions. It appears to worsen over time, possibly due to chronic UV exposure. Based on this study, it also seems to arise most commonly in adulthood, although the study cannot prove this based on its retrospective design. These authors do not distinguish periorbital hyperpigmentation as a separate entity but rather a subtype of AIPFP. Moreover, they suggest that AIPFP perhaps is a more overarching diagnosis that includes both periorbital hyperpigmentation and pigmentary demarcation lines of the face. They hypothesize that these variations in pigmentation represent a form of pigmentary mosaicism that follow lines of Blaschko.

Oral Mucosal Hyperpigmentation

Gingival and mucosal pigmentation tends to roughly correlate with that of skin. Importantly, there can be significant color variation of normal, healthy mucosa [35]. Oral mucosal hyperpigmentation is common, particularly in darker skin patients [35]. It can be diffuse (mucosal melanosis) or focal (oral melanotic macules) [36]. Melanotic macules can also be seen in the genital mucosa as well.

Mucosal Melanosis

Also commonly known as "black gums," mucosal melanosis most commonly affects the gingiva [35, 37]. This is followed by the buccal mucosa, lips, palate, and tongue [35]. Gingival involvement most commonly presents as symmetric, well-demarcated dark brown bands [35, 37]. Notably, it usually spares the marginal gingiva, which can help distinguish it from hyperpigmentation related to Addison's disease. Mucosal melanosis involving the palate and buccal mucosa usually consists of poorly demarcated and irregularly shaped patches [35].

It is important to note that there are a number of systemic conditions associated with hyperpigmentation of the oral mucosa, and these should be ruled out clinically before a diagnosis of physiologic mucosal melanosis is made. These diseases include Addison's disease, Peutz-Jeghers disease, hemochromatosis, and HIV infection [35, 36]. There are also a number of other secondary causes of oral mucosal hyperpigmentation including dental amalgam tattoo and other foreign body reactions [35, 38], smoker's melanosis [39], drug-induced hyperpigmentation

[35], and post-inflammatory hyperpigmentation that should be considered in the patient with darkening of oral mucosal surfaces [36].

Mucosal melanosis most commonly presents in infancy but will typically darken further with age [35, 40]. It is more common in patients with darker skin types [41, 42]. One study reported a prevalence of 5% in Caucasians and 38% in darker skinned patients [40]. Histopathologic examination shows an increase in melanin without an increase in number of melanocytes [36].

Oral Melanotic Macules

Oral melanotic macules are also relatively common. They typically present as brown, blue, or black homogenously pigmented macules, either as solitary lesions or multiple within a single patient [35, 38, 43]. The vermillion border is the most commonly affected site, followed by the gingiva [38, 43, 44]. It is more common in women and, unlike diffuse mucosal melanosis, is more likely to first present in adulthood [43, 44]. Like diffuse mucosal melanosis, lesions typically result from increased melanocyte activity as opposed to increased melanocyte number, although the precise etiology of this entity remains unclear [36, 45]. It has been suggested that lesions may be related to post-inflammatory hyperpigmentation [35]. Importantly, oral melanotic macules must be differentiated from oral melanomas. It has been recommended that any lesion be biopsied if it is of new onset, changing, or associated with irregular features [36]. The palate is the most common site of oral melanoma, so any pigmented lesion in that location should be treated with particular caution [36, 43, 46].

Treatment of Oral Hyperpigmentation

Although no treatment is necessary, cryotherapy and lasers have both shown some degree of success in treating physiologic oral hyperpigmentation [47, 48]. A 2012 case report showed resolution of oral hyperpigmentation with liquid nitrogen cryotherapy with no evidence of recurrence at 12 months of follow-up [48].

Melanotic Macules of the Genitals

Melanotic macules that are histologically identical to oral melanotic macules can also be seen on the genital mucosa in both men and women. One small study found that these lesions most commonly arise during adulthood. They range in color from tan to dark brown to black. They appear to not change significantly in clinical appearance over time [49]. Biopsy to rule out melanoma should be performed if a lesion is changing, atypical, symptomatic or if the lesion has irregular color, symmetry, or border [49].

Palmar/Plantar Melanotic Macules

Melanotic macules of the volar surfaces are more common in darker skinned individuals, although they can be seen in light-skinned patients as well [50]. They most commonly present as light brown to medium-dark brown macules on the palms and soles [50, 51]. Like mucosal melanotic macules, palmar/plantar melanotic macules histologically have an increase in the amount of melanin without an increase in the number of melanocytes [52]. Similarly, the etiology is also still unclear. Post-inflammatory hyperpigmentation has been raised as a possibility [51]. The differential diagnosis of volar melanotic macules includes lentigines, melanocytic nevi, melanoma, drug-induced lesions (most classically 5-fluorouracil), Peutz-Jeghers syndrome, tinea nigra, and post-inflammatory hyperpigmentation [51, 53].

Physiologic Longitudinal Melanonychia

Longitudinal melanonychia is brown-black hyperpigmentation that extends longitudinally from the proximal nail fold to the free edge of the nail plate [54]. Physiologic longitudinal melanonychia—sometimes also referred to as racial melanonychia—is the most common type of longitudinal melanonychia seen in Hispanic, African American, and Japanese patients [54]. Differential diagnosis for longitudinal melanonychia is broad, however, and includes melanoma, non-melanoma skin cancers (rare), benign melanocytic hyperplasia, benign nevus, lentigo, hemorrhage, bacterial or fungal infection, systemic disease such as Addison's disease, and drug-induced hyperpigmentation [54–56].

The classic presentation of physiologic longitudinal melanonychia consists of 1–3 mm wide light-to-dark brown longitudinal bands. It commonly affects more than one nail. It can sometimes also be associated with mucosal melanosis [54]. Under dermoscopy, the characteristic finding of physiologic longitudinal melanonychia is a gray band consisting of homogenous gray lines [55, 56]. Histopathologically, there is an increase in melanin deposition with no increase in number of melanocytes [54].

It is of critical importance to differentiate physiologic longitudinal melanonychia from subungual melanoma, and, unfortunately, this is often quite challenging [57–59]. There are no clear consensus-based guidelines to aid in the workup of longitudinal melanonychia. Some authors recommend nail matrix biopsy if the entire nail plate is affected, if there is significant color variegation, if the patient reports any significant change in color or width of the band, or if the patient presents with new-onset melanonychia even if there is more than one nail affected [54]. Other authors biopsy any new longitudinal melanonychia in adults [58]. Longitudinal melanonychia affecting more than one nail is more likely to represent a benign process; however, there are cases of subungual melanoma arising in patients with melanonychia of more than one nail [54]. Other features that make melanoma more likely include brown background coloration with irregular longitudinal lines under dermoscopy, single affected nail, any abrupt development of pigment change, pigmentation of the proximal and/or lateral nailfold, associated nail dystrophy, blurring or darkening of pigment near the nail matrix, and melanonychia of the thumb, index finger, or great toe in particular [55, 56, 58, 60]. There is less consensus about width of the band, but in general, a band >3–5 mm is more concerning [58].

Conclusion

Physiologic pigmentation lies within the spectrum of normal. Practicing clinicians should be aware of normal variation patterns as patients may come to clinic with a chief complaint related to one of the entities discussed in this chapter. Physiologic alteration of pigment is more common in skin of color but is seen to some extent in all skin types. As it falls within the realm of normal pigmentation, the above variations do not require medical treatment. If desired for cosmetic reasons, a variety of lasers and surgical techniques have been employed (tailored to the particular etiology) with varying success. As emphasized above, it is of paramount importance to rule out other secondary causes of pigmentation variation before settling on a diagnosis of physiologic pigmentation, as this affects management and prognosis.

References

1. Vrieling H, Duhl DMJ, Millar SE, Miller KA, Barsh GS. Differences in dorsal and ventral pigmentation result from regional expression of the mouse agouti gene. Proc National Academy Sci. 1994;91:5667–71.
2. Walsh RJ. Variation in the melanin content of the skin of New Guinea natives at different ages. J Invest Dermatolo. 1964;42(3):261–5.
3. Park JH, Lee MH. A study of skin color by melanin index according to site, gestational age, birth weight and season of birth in Korean neonates. J Korean Med Sci. 2005;20(1):105–8.
4. Post PW, Krauss AN, Walcman S, Auld PA. Skin reflectance of newborn infants from 25 to 44 weeks gestational age. Hum Biol. 1976;48(3):541–57.
5. Zhang R, Zhu W. Coexistence of pigmentary demarcation lines types C and E in one subject. Int J Dermatol. 2011;50(7):863–5.
6. James WD, Carter JM, Rodman OG. Pigmentary demarcation lines: a population survey. J Am Acad Dermatol. 1987;16(3):584–90.
7. Kumari R, Laxmisha C, Thappa DM. Pigmentary demarcation lines associated with pregnancy. J Cosmetic Dermatolo. 2006;5(2):169–70.
8. Chandran V, Kurien G, Mohan V. Pigmentary demarcation lines in pregnancy. Indian J Dermatol. 2016;61(1):127.

9. Matzumoto SH. Über eine eigentümliche Pigmentverteilung an den Voigtschen Linien. (Beitrag zur Kenntnis der Voigtschen Grenzen). Archiv für Dermatologie und Syphilis. 1913;118(1):157–64.

10. Malakar S, Lahiri K, Banerjee U, Mondal S, Sarangi S. Periorbital melanosis is an extension of pigmentary demarcation line-F on face. Indian J Dermatol Venereol Leprol. 2007;73 (5):323–5.

11. James WD, Meltzer MS, Guill MA, Berger TG, Rodman OG. Pigmentary demarcation lines associated with pregnancy. J Am Acad Dermatol. 1984;11(3):438–40.

12. Miura O. On the demarcation lines of pigmentation observed among the Japanese, on inner sides of their extremities and on anterior and posterior sides of their medial regions. Tohoku J Exp Med. 1951;54(2):135–40.

13. Maleville J, Taieb A. Pigmentary demarcation lines as markers of neural development. Arch Dermatol. 1997;133(11):1459.

14. Krivo JM. How common is pigmentary mosaicism? Arch Dermatol. 1997;133(4):527–8.

15. Treat J. Patterned pigmentation in children. Pediatric Clin. 2010;57(5):1121–9.

16. Peck J, Cusack C. Futcher lines: a case report in pregnancy and literature review. Cutis. 2013;92(2):100–1.

17. Bukhari IA. Effective treatment of Futcher's lines with q-switched Alexandrite laser. J Cosmetic Dermatol. 2005;4(1):27–8.

18. Sarkar R, Ranjan R, Garg S, Garg VK, Sonthalia S, Bansal S. Periorbital hyperpigmentation: a comprehensive review. J Clin Aesthetic Dermatol. 2016;9(1):49–55.

19. Verschoore M, Gupta S, Sharma VK, Ortonne J-P. Determination of melanin and haemoglobin in the skin of idiopathic cutaneous hyperchromia of the orbital region (ICHOR): a study of Indian patients. J Cutaneous Aesthetic Surg. 2012;5(3):176–82.

20. Roh MR, Chung KR. Infraorbital dark circles: definition, causes, and treatment options. Dermatol Surg. 2009;35(8):1163–71.

21. Ranu H, Thng S, Goh BK, Burger A, Goh CL. Periorbital hyperpigmentation in Asians: an epidemiologic study and a proposed classification. Dermatol Surg. 2011;37(9):1297–303.

22. Watanabe S, Nakai K, Ohnishi T. Condition known as "dark rings under the eyes" in the Japanese population is a kind of dermal melanocytosis which can be successfully treated by Q-switched ruby laser. Dermatol Surg. 2006;32(6):785–9.

23. West TB, Alster TS. Improvement of infraorbital hyperpigmentation following carbon dioxide laser resurfacing. Dermatol Surg. 1998;24(6):615–6.

24. Cymbalista NC. Oliveira ZNPd. Treatment of idiopathic cutaneous hyperchromia of the orbital region (ICHOR) with intense pulsed light. Dermatol Surg. 2006;32(6):773–83.

25. Sarkar R. Idiopathic cutaneous hyperchromia at the orbital region or periorbital hyperpigmentation. JCutaneous Aesthetic Sur. 2012;5(3):183–4.

26. Goodman RM, Belcher RW. Periorbital hyperpigmentation: an overlooked genetic disorder of pigmentation. Arch Dermatol. 1969;100(2):169–74.

27. Ranjan R, Sarkar R, Garg VK, Gupta T. A comparative study of two modalities, 4% hydroquinone versus 30% salicylic acid in periorbital hyperpigmentation and assessment of quality of life before and after treatment. Indian J Dermatol. 2016;61(4):413–7.

28. Bosniak S, Sadick NS, Cantisano-Zilkha M, Glavas IP, Roy D. The hyaluronic acid push technique for the nasojugal groove. Dermatol Surg. 2008;34(1):127–31.

29. Roh MR, Kim TK, Chung KY. Treatment of infraorbital dark circles by autologous fat transplantation: a pilot study. Br J Dermatol. 2009;160(5):1022–5.

30. Ohshima H, Mizukoshi K, Oyobikawa M, Matsumoto K, Takiwaki H, Kanto H, et al. Effects of vitamin C on dark circles of the lower eyelids: quantitative evaluation using image analysis and echogram. Skin Res Technol. 2009;15(2):214–7.

31. Lowe NJ, Wieder JM, Shorr N, Boxrud C, Saucer D, Chalet M. Infraorbital pigmented skin. Preliminary observations of laser therapy. Dermatol Surg. 1995;21(9):767–70.

32. Manuskiatti W, Fitzpatrick RE, Goldman MP. Treatment of facial skin using combinations of CO_2 Q-switched alexandrite, flashlamp-pumped pulsed dye, and Er: YAG lasers in the same treatment session. Dermatol Sur. 2000;26(2):114–20.

33. Cisneros JL. RIo R, Palou J. The Q-switched neodymium (Nd):YAG laser with quadruple frequency. Clinical histological evaluation of facial resurfacing using different wavelengths. Dermatol Surg. 1998;24(3):345–50.

34. Sarma N, Chakraborty S, Bhattacharya SR. Acquired, idiopathic, patterned facial pigmentation (AIPFP) including periorbital pigmentation and pigmentary demarcation lines on face follows the lines of Blaschko on face. Indian J Dermatol. 2014;59(1):41–8.

35. Eisen D. Disorders of pigmentation in the oral cavity. Clin Dermatol. 2000;18(5):579–87.

36. Muller S. Melanin-associated pigmented lesions of the oral mucosa: presentation, differential diagnosis, and treatment. Dermatol Ther. 2010;23(3):220–9.

37. Chandra S, Keluskar V, Bagewadi A, Sah K. Extensive physiologic melanin pigmentation on the tongue: an unusual clinical presentation. Contemp Clin Dent. 2010;1(3):204–6.

38. Buchner A, Hansen LS. Amalgam pigmentation (amalgam tattoo) of the oral mucosa. A clinicopathologic study of 268 cases. Oral Sur Oral Med Oral Pathol. 1980;49(2):139–47.

39. Hedin CA, Axell T. Oral melanin pigmentation in 467 Thai and Malaysian people with special emphasis on smoker's melanosis. J Oral Pathol Med. 1991;20(1):8–12.

40. Fry L, Almeyda JR. The incidence of buccal pigmentation in caucasoids and negroids in Britain. Br J Dermatol. 1968;80(4):244–7.

41. Lenane P, Powell FC. Oral pigmentation. J Eur Acad Dermatol Venereol. 2000;14(6):448–65.

42. Amir E, Gorsky M, Buchner A, Sarnat H, Gat H. Physiologic pigmentation of the oral mucosa in Israeli children. Oral Sur Oral Med Oral Pathol. 1991;71(3):396–8.

43. Buchner A, Merrell PW, Carpenter WM. Relative frequency of solitary melanocytic lesions of the oral mucosa. J Oral Pathol Med. 2004;33(9):550–7.

44. Kaugars GE, Heise AP, Riley WT, Abbey LM, Svirsky JA. Oral melanotic macules. A review of 353 cases. Oral Sur Oral Med Oral Pathol. 1993;76(1):59–61.

45. Meleti M, Vescovi P, Mooi WJ, van der Waal I. Pigmented lesions of the oral mucosa and perioral tissues: a flow-chart for the diagnosis and some recommendations for the management. Oral Sur Oral Med Oral Pathol Oral Radiol Endodontol. 2008;105(5):606–16.

46. Hicks MJ, Flaitz CM. Oral mucosal melanoma: epidemiology and pathobiology. Oral Oncol. 2000;36(2):152–69.

47. Lin YH, Tu YK, Lu CT, Chung WC, Huang CF, Huang MS, et al. Systematic review of treatment modalities for gingival depigmentation: a random-effects poisson regression analysis. J Esthetic Restorative Dent. 2014;26(3):162–78.

48. Talebi M, Farmanbar N, Abolfazli S, Shirazi AS. Management of physiological hyperpigmentation of oral mucosa by cryosurgical treatment: a case report. J Dental Res Dental Clin Dental Prospects. 2012;6(4):148–51.

49. Lenane P, Keane CO, Connell BO, Loughlin SO, Powell FC. Genital melanotic macules: clinical, histological, immunohistochemical, and ultrastructural features. J Am Acad Dermatol. 2000;42(4):640–4.

50. Blossom J, Altmayer S, Jones DM, Slominski A, Carlson JA. Volar melanotic macules in a gardener: a case report and review of the literature. Am J Dermatopathol. 2008;30(6):612–9.

51. Kiyohara T, Kumakiri M, Kouraba S, Lao LM, Sawai T. Volar melanotic macules in a Japanese man with histopathological postinflammatory pigmentation: the volar counterpart of mucosal melanotic macules. J Cutan Pathol. 2001;28(6):303–6.

52. Chapel TA, Taylor RM, Pinkus H. Volar melanotic macules. Int J Dermatol. 1979;18(3):222–5.

53. Cho KH, Chung JH, Lee AY, Lee YS, Kim NK, Kim CW. Pigmented macules in patients treated with systemic 5-fluorouracil. J Dermatol. 1988;15(4):342–6.

54. Dominguez-Cherit J, Roldan-Marin R, Pichardo-Velazquez P, Valente C, Fonte-Avalos V, Vega-Memije ME, et al. Melanonychia, melanocytic hyperplasia, and nail melanoma in a Hispanic population. J Am Acad Dermatol. 2008;59(5):785–91.

55. Ronger S, Touzet S, Ligeron C, Balme B, Viallard AM, Barrut D, et al. Dermoscopic examination of nail pigmentation. Arch Dermatol. 2002;138(10):1327–33.

56. Braun RP, Baran R, Gal FAL, Dalle S, Ronger S, Pandolfi R, et al. Diagnosis and management of nail pigmentations. J Am Acad Dermatol. 2007;56(5):835–47.

57. Molina D, Sanchez JL. Pigmented longitudinal bands of the nail. A clinicopathologic study. Am J Dermatopathol. 1995;17(6):539–41.
58. Haneke E, Baran R. Longitudinal melanonychia. Dermatol Surg. 2001;27(6):580–4.
59. Husain S, Scher RK, Silvers DN, Ackerman AB. Melanotic macule of nail unit and its clinicopathologic spectrum. J Am Acad Dermatol. 2006;54(4):664–7.
60. Baran R, Kechijian P. Longitudinal melanonychia (melanonychia striata): diagnosis and management. J Am Acad Dermatol. 1989;21(6):1165–75.

Chapter 8
Mucosal Lesions in Skin of Color

Mayra B.C. Maymone and Allison R. Larson

Physiologic Variation in Mucosal Areas

The mucosal surfaces of the body are areas where keratinized epithelium, of ectodermal origin, adjoin nonkeratinized epithelium, of endodermal origin [1]. Both keratinized and nonkeratinized mucosal surfaces have unique features. The epithelium is thick in these areas, and muscle present more superficially [2]. The nonkeratinized stratified squamous epithelium is highly glycogenated [1, 2]. Specialized structures such as salivary glands, taste buds, terminal hairs, eccrine glands, and sebaceous glands are seen, depending on the location [1, 2].

Similar to other cutaneous surfaces, melanocytes reside within the basal layer of the epithelium. They are regularly spaced among basal keratinocytes. Mucosal epithelia contain roughly the same numbers of melanocytes from person to person; however, there is considerable color variation between people. Genetic determinates affect melanin synthesis and melanosome characteristics [3]. Typically, mucosal pigmentation is related to overall skin tone. The darker one's skin, the more color is manifest in the mucosal areas. Physiologic pigmentation is frequently not one uniform color throughout the mucosa and is due to greater activity of melanocytes rather than an increase in melanocyte number. Pigment differs based on the degree of keratinization, melanocytic activity, vascularization, and the type of submucosal tissue (muscle, bone) present in a particular site [4].

Within the oral cavity, the gingiva and buccal mucosa tend to have the darkest pigmentation but physiologic pigmentation can also be seen on the lips, palate, and tongue [4]. Physiologic pigmentation generally develops within the first two decades of life. However, patients may not notice this difference until years later. Even within

M.B.C. Maymone · A.R. Larson (✉)
Department of Dermatology, Boston Medical Center,
609 Albany St. J-202, Boston, MA 02118, USA
e-mail: arlarson@bu.edu

© Springer International Publishing AG 2017
N.A. Vashi and H.I. Maibach (eds.), *Dermatoanthropology of Ethnic Skin and Hair*, DOI 10.1007/978-3-319-53961-4_8

87

a given area, there are often patchy differences in color. Within the oral mucosa, there has been found to be some increase in numbers of melanocytes with age [4].

Oral Pigmented Lesions

Oral Melanotic Macules and Lentigines

Oral melanotic macules are benign foci of hyperpigmentation. The most common site of occurrence is on the lower lip (33%) (Fig. 8.1), followed by the gingiva, buccal mucosa, and palate [5]. Labial melanotic macules occur in about 3% of the population, most commonly in young women [6]. They are generally solitary lesions. The color change is primarily a result of increased melanin production and deposition, though an increase in the number of melanocytes and dermal melanophages can also contribute [6, 7]. Despite the lower lip predominance, they are not related to sun exposure [6]. There is a 2:1 female predominance. They are most common in women over 30 years of age with greatest incidence in the fifth decade [7]. All skin types are susceptible to macules, however, black patients develop more lesions on the buccal mucosa [6]. Intraoral lesions are typically larger than those on the lips. On dermoscopy, there is diffuse structureless pigmentation, typically evenly distributed [4]. On histology, these lesions lack both the rete ridge elongation as well as melanocytic hyperplasia seen in lentigines [4, 7].

Lentigines present similarly as sharply demarcated brown macules, typically on the vermillion border of the lips or perioral skin [4]. When multiple oral lentigines are present, especially in a child, this brings up the possibility of a syndrome such

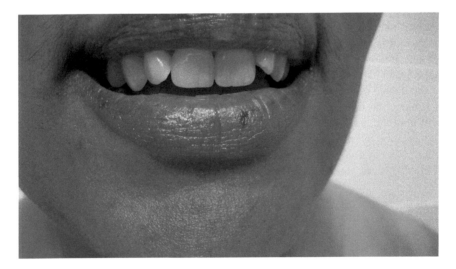

Fig. 8.1 Labial melanotic macules

as Peutz–Jeghers, Laugier–Hunziker, Cronkhite–Canada, LEOPARD (lentigines, electrocardiographic conduction defects, ocular hypertelorism, pulmonary stenosis, abnormalities of the genitals, retarded growth resulting in short stature, sensorineural deafness), LAMB (lentigines, atrial myxomas, mucocutaneous myxomas, blue nevi), or others [6]. On histology, lentigines exhibit elongation of the rete ridges and melanocytic hyperplasia [7]. Treatment of oral melanotic macules and lentigines is not necessary.

Melanoacanthosis

Oral melanoacanthosis (OM), alternatively termed melanoacanthoma, is a rare benign mucosal lesion, considered to be the oral equivalent of cutaneous melanoacanthoma [8]. Most often reported in darker-skinned women between their third and fourth decades, few reports exist of melanoacanthosis during the first two decades of life [9].

Clinically, OM presents as an asymptomatic, pigmented and rapidly growing lesion. It can spontaneously regress. Lesions are usually solitary, but multifocal lesions have also been described [10]. The most frequently involved locations are the buccal mucosa, lips, palate, and gingiva. Although the etiology has not been fully elucidated, it is thought to be a reactive process related to masticatory and frictional trauma [8]. The differential diagnosis is broad and includes a spectrum of pigmented and vascular lesions [9]. A biopsy may be warranted to exclude malignant melanoma [10]. On histology, OM exhibits numerous benign-appearing dendritic melanocytes within areas of epithelial acanthosis. Mild spongiosis, melanophages, and variable chronic inflammation within the lamina propria can be seen [2]. No treatment is necessary.

Smoker's Melanosis

Smoker's melanosis (SM) is a benign diffuse melanocytic pigmentation occurring in tobacco smokers. It is the most frequent oral lesion among smokers in Chennai, India [11]. Another study from Turkey found that gingival hyperpigmentation was present in 27.5% of smokers and only in 8.6% of nonsmokers [12]. Women appear to be more frequently affected than men, raising the possibility of a hormonal factor [5].

The characteristic diffuse, asymmetric brown-black pigmentation is usually noted on the anterior mandibular gingiva, but other sites such as the buccal mucosa, lips, and hard palate can also be affected [13]. The observed increase in melanin is thought to be due to the stimulating effect of tobacco on oral melanocytes. Diagnosis is made based on clinical presentation and a history of smoking. The diagnosis may be especially challenging in darker skin types, due to similarities with physiologic hyperpigmentation [14]. Histologically, the features are the same as post-inflammatory hyperpigmentation, with increased basilar melanin, no or mild melanocytic hyperplasia, pigment incontinence, melanophages, and variable chronic inflammation within the lamina propria [2]. Treatment is not necessary. Discontinuing smoking may improve the condition [15].

Amalgam Tattoo

Amalgam tattoo is an iatrogenic, nonmelanocytic lesion that results from traumatic inlay of dental amalgam into the soft tissue. It usually presents as a single, asymptomatic, gray-black to blue macule located near the amalgam-filled tooth [16]. The most commonly affected sites are the gingiva, buccal and alveolar mucosa, palate, and tongue [17]. The mandibular area is more frequently affected than the maxilla.

Although this a benign condition, a biopsy may be needed to exclude malignancy. Histology reveals brown granules scattered along collagen bundles as well as around blood vessels and nerves. A scar may also be present, and larger particles may incite formation of foreign-body granulomas [2, 16]. Surgical or laser treatment can be performed for cosmetic reasons.

Melanocytic Nevi

Oral melanocytic nevi (OMN) are uncommon foci of oral pigmentation that may be congenital or, more commonly, acquired. Most are noted in the third to fourth decade of life. Compared to cutaneous nevi, the incidence of OMN is low. A study from the Netherlands found that OMN occurred at a rate of 4.35 cases per 10 million people [18]. In a retrospective study conducted in Texas, OMN comprised 0.067% of biopsies sent to an oral pathology service [19]. There is a 1.6:1 female predominance.

Usually single, small, well-defined brown-gray to blue-black macules or papules. The most common site of involvement is the hard palate, followed by the buccal mucosa, vermillion lip, and gingiva. Rarely, they are seen on the tongue or floor of the mouth [18]. There are six histological subtypes of OMN: junctional, compound, intramucosal, blue (common or cellular), combined, and dysplastic. The most common subtype is intramucosal, in which lesions are often nonpigmented. The second most common subtype is blue. OMN cannot be differentiated from melanoma based on clinical presentation, therefore, biopsy is recommend in any new or otherwise suspicious oral pigmented lesion [19]. Histology varies based on the lesion's subtype [2].

Oral Mucosal Melanoma

Oral mucosal melanoma is a very rare, highly aggressive malignancy. It accounts for 0.2–8% [20] of all melanomas. A 2005 article on melanomas in the United States (US) reported that mucosal melanomas (from any mucosal site) make up 1.4% of all melanomas [21]. In Hispanics, oral mucosal melanomas amount to 14.4% of reported melanomas, compared to 12.2% in Blacks, 11.3% in Asian/Pacific Islander, and 8.2% in whites [22]. Higher rates of oral mucosal melanoma are observed in Africa, India, and Japan [23]. Most studies suggest a male predominance of 2:1 [20, 23]; however, a recent study by Altieri et al. [22] reported oral cavity melanomas to be more common among women of Hispanic and Asian ethnicity. Oral mucosal melanoma (OMM) is usually diagnosed between the fourth and seventh decades. It is exceedingly rare among younger individuals. The most common sites of involvement are the palate and maxillary anterior gingiva (80%) [23].

To date, there are no known risk factors or precursor lesions related to the development of oral mucosal melanoma. Various tumor suppressor genes and oncogenes have been linked to OMM, with c-kit being the most frequently associated [24]. The clinical appearance is variable. Lesions are usually asymptomatic, irregularly shaped, black-blue to brown macules, papules, or nodules. Pain, ulceration, bleeding, bone destruction, and paresthesia may be present in later stages. Up to one third of oral mucosal melanomas can be amelanotic [25]. Based on clinical features, OMM can be classified into five subtypes: pigmented nodular, nonpigmented nodular, pigmented macular, pigmented mixed, and nonpigmented mixed type [20].

Histology of mucosal melanoma in situ reveals spindled or epithelioid melanocytes arranged in a lentiginous array or exhibiting pagetoid spread within the epithelium. Sheets or nests of cells that extend into the lamina propria or below are classified as invasive disease [2, 25]. In amelanotic variants, immunohistochemical staining for melanocytic markers is helping in making the diagnosis. Breslow depth and Clark level do not apply to the oral mucosa.

Wide local excision with clear margins is the cornerstone of therapy. Depending on the clinical stage, further treatment may involve lymph node dissection and chemotherapy [20]. Careful oral examination is imperative as OMM has an extremely poor prognosis. Early diagnosis is a key factor in maximizing survival.

Drug-Induced Hyperpigmentation

Numerous medications can cause symmetric ill-defined brown, blue, or gray hyperpigmentation in the oral mucosa as a side effect. Common culprits include oral contraceptives, minocycline (Fig. 8.2), antimalarials, clofazimine, nicotine, zidovudine, ketoconazole, and some chemotherapeutics [2, 4]. This occurs via local accumulation following systemic absorption of particles that chelate with iron or melanin or by direct stimulation of melanin production [2].

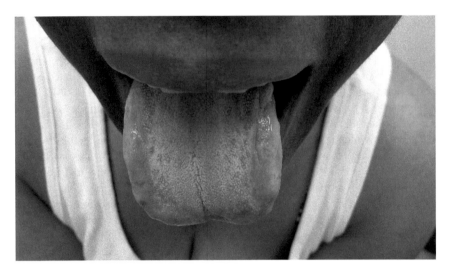

Fig. 8.2 Minocycline tongue hyperpigmentation

Post-Inflammatory Hyperpigmentation

In the setting of chronic inflammation, melanocytes will often react with increased melanin production and hyperpigmentation. The mucosa is no exception to this phenomenon. Oral post-inflammatory hyperpigmentation may be diffuse or localized depending on the inflammatory pattern. Potential triggers include dermatitis such as lichen planus, or externally induced phenomena such as radiation therapy [2]. Mild nonspecific inflammation can also cause hyperpigmentation. This increased pigment fades over months [2].

Nonpigmented Oral Lesions

Leukoedema

Oral leukoedema is a benign thickening of the oral mucosal epithelium due to fluid accumulation. It is the most common benign oral condition in patients with skin of color. It presents as an asymptomatic, symmetrical white-gray mucosal alteration located most often on the buccal mucosa, but it is also seen on floor of the mouth and palatopharyngeal tissues [26].

The prevalence is higher among dark-skinned people, especially African Americans and Hispanics. Reports in the United States estimate that this condition affects 70–90% of African American adults and 50% of African American children [27]. A study conducted in Mexico found leukoedema to be the most common oral lesion in this population [28]. Although a common condition, the etiology is unknown. Given its high prevalence, some consider leukoedema a normal variation rather than a pathologic condition. Stretching of the affected area leads to temporary reversal of the white-gray appearance, facilitating the diagnosis. Leukoedema is not associated with an increased risk of malignancy [26]. No treatment is necessary.

Submucous Fibrosis

Oral submucous fibrosis is a potentially malignant disorder associated with chewing of betel quid, a mixture of betel leaves, areca nuts, slaked lime, and spices. This chronic condition is characterized by mucosal paleness, a burning sensation, mouth dryness, ulceration, and fibrosis of the oral mucosa. The abnormal accumulation of collagen in subepithelial layers may extend to the underlying musculature forming fibrous bands that lead to stiffness of the involved tissues [29]. Oral submucous fibrosis evolves in stages. The first stage, stomatitis, is characterized by mouth soreness, intolerance to spicy foods, and vesicles that later ulcerate. These heal with fibrosis, the second stage. The third and final stage presents with pain during palpation of the fibrous bands and trismus due to fibrosis of pterygomandibular raphea. It may result in deafness caused by fibrosis of the Eustachian tubes and dysphagia to solids if fibrous bands extend to oropharynx [30]. The buccal mucosa has a pale leathery texture, and petechiae have been observed in 22% of patients without any history of blood dyscrasias [29].

Submucous fibrosis affects predominantly people from India, Asia, South Africa, and the United Kingdom, who chew betel. There is a slight male predominance, yet it can affect both sexes. The reported rates of malignant transformation range from 2.3 to 7.6% [31]. The pathogenesis is not fully understood and thought to be multifactorial. The exposure to areca nuts and their constituent alkaloids (mostly arecoline and arecaidine), flavonoids, copper, and tannins seems to interfere with deposition and degradation of extracellular matrix molecules in susceptible individuals [32]. Alkaloids stimulate fibroblast proliferation and collagen formation. Flavonoids are implicated in reduced breakdown of collagen. Increased copper observed in the mucosa of affected patients plays a potential role as a fibrosis mediator [32]. Localized mucosal inflammation due to betel quid promotes secretion of inflammatory cytokines and growth factors (transforming growth factor beta) and inhibits enzymes responsible for collagen degradation. Patients need frequent monitoring for malignant transformation and may require surgical intervention to release fibrotic bands.

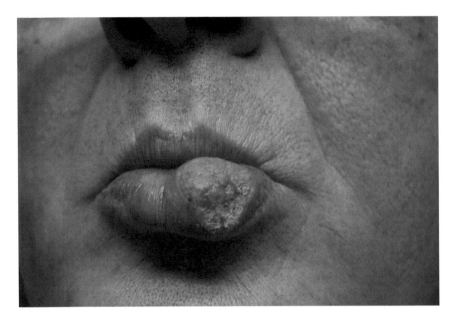

Fig. 8.3 Lip SCC in a Mediterranean man

Squamous Cell Carcinoma

Oral squamous cell carcinomas make up >90% of oral cavity malignancies in virtually all populations. The presentation is varied. Such lesions can present as either as a white patch (leukoplakia), red patch (erythroplakia), a mass (Fig. 8.3), or nonhealing ulcer [2]. Risk of metastasis and recurrence increases with increasing tumor thickness [2]. The incidence of oral squamous cell carcinoma varies not only among countries and regions within countries but also between ethnic groups living in the same region. This variation speaks to the truly multifactorial etiology of oral squamous cell carcinoma (SCC). Factors that play a large role in its development include tobacco, alcohol, areca nut chewing, human papilloma virus (HPV) infection, prolonged immunosuppression, age, and personal or family history of cancer [2]. HPV-related SCCs and verrucous carcinomas, well-differentiated variants of SCC, have a better prognosis.

In the United States, men tend to develop oral cancer more often than women, with a ratio of about 2.2:1 [33], however, this is not true in all countries [34]. In the United States, oral cancer is the 11th most common malignancy [2]. In some locations, it is the most common cancer overall [10]. Regional variations within ethnic groups are often explained by use of tobacco, alcohol, or other carcinogenic exposures [34, 35]. In a recent US study, whites and in particular white men, had a higher incidence of oral and oropharyngeal cancer than all other ethnic groups [33]. This has not always been the case. Between 1987 and 1991, African Americans experienced a higher incidence of oropharyngeal cancer than their white counterparts [36]. A separate US study on tongue cancer in women, of which the vast majority were SCC, found that while the incidence was similar among different ethnic groups, African American women had lower survival rates at 1, 5, and 10 years though this trend was not significant (33% vs 54% 10-year survival) [37]. Similarly for men, the annual mortality rate among African Americans was found to be 1.5 times that of whites [38]. Emphasis should be placed on early detection and lifestyle modifications that will aid in preventing oral SCC. Any persistent oral lesion should be biopsied, particularly given the relatively high rate of metastasis from oral SCCs. A second primary lesion of the aerodigestive tract is found in up to one quarter of patients with oral SCCs [39]. Aggressive surgical intervention is the mainstay of treatment. This may include lymph node sampling and/or neck dissection [40]. External beam radiotherapy is also used when lymph nodes are involved, and adjuvant chemotherapy may be needed in cases of recurrent or metastatic disease [39].

Kaposi's Sarcoma

Kaposi's sarcoma (KS) presents with violaceous or red-brown vascular plaques, caused by human herpesvirus-8 (HHV-8). There are multiple forms of KS, including that associated with acquired immune deficiency syndrome (AIDS), the African endemic form, the iatrogenic form resulting from immunosuppression, and the classic type, which is most commonly seen in elderly men from Eastern Europe and the Mediterranean [41]. AIDS-associated KS represents the majority of the disease, and this form often involves the oral mucosa [41]. Oral KS typically involves the hard and soft palate, gingiva, and dorsal tongue in either a solitary or multifocal pattern. In AIDS-associated oral KS, 71% of patients have concurrent cutaneous and visceral disease [42]. Among those with KS affected by AIDS, women are more likely to have oral lesions [41].

The rate of HHV-8 seropositivity is especially high in regions of Africa, around 40–50% [41]. The prevalence of KS is higher in many African countries compared to other regions given the combination of high HHV-8 seropositivity and high rates of human immunodeficiency virus (HIV) infection. Since the advent of antiretroviral therapy, the incidence of KS has decreased significantly. However, KS has been found to flare with initial immune reconstitution [42]. In transplant patients, higher incidences of KS have been found among African Blacks, Mediterranean, and Caribbean patients, likely related to frequencies of HHV-8 seropositivity in these populations [42].

Histological examination reveals proliferations of spindle cells, extravasated erythrocytes, hemosiderin, eosinophilic globules, and possibly mitotically active cells [2]. Treatment is largely determined by the stage and extent of disease. Thorough investigations of the dermatologic, otolaryngeal, ophthalmologic, lymphatic, gastrointestinal, and pulmonary systems should be undertaken [42]. HIV status should be checked. Local therapeutic measures for focal disease include excision, sclerotherapy, intralesional injection with vinca alkaloids, photodynamic therapy, radiotherapy, and cryotherapy [42]. Systemic therapies for more wide-spread disease include antiretroviral therapy for those with HIV and systemic chemotherapeutics [43].

Actinic Prurigo

Actinic prurigo is a chronic photosensitive disorder more frequently observed in mestizos (a Latin American term typically referring to a person of combined European and Native American descent) and native Latin Americans living in altitudes over 1000 m above sea level. The usual age of onset is during childhood, but it may appear later in early adult life [44]. It affects predominantly women at a ratio of 2:1–4:1; however, in Asians, the less common adult-onset presentation seems to have a male predilection.

Actinic prurigo presents as symmetric, intensely pruritic erythematous macules, papules, and nodules that are often excoriated on sun-exposed areas of the skin, lips, and conjunctiva. Lip involvement was observed in 82.7% of patients. The vermilion borders are erythematous, swollen, and crusted, and fissures can be covered by serohemorrhagic scales, referred to as actinic prurigo cheilitis. This is the only manifestation of actinic prurigo in 27.6% of patients. The vermillion border location can be distinguished from angular cheilitis, a disease of fissuring and maceration at the corners of the mouth, often caused by Candida species, and seen especially in denture-wearers or the immunocompromised. Often times, anterior gingival hyperplasia can be observed, possibly due to secondary mouth breathing from painful lesions on the lower lip [45]. Conjunctival involvement appears to be a late manifestation that affects about 45% of patients. It presents with hyperemia, photophobia, increased tearing, and pseudopterygium formation [46].

A genetic susceptibility characterized by a strong association with human leukocyte antigen (HLA) subtype DRB1*0407 is present in 60–80% [44, 46] of patients, and HLA DRB1*0401 is the second most common subtype found in up to 20% of those afflicted [47]. Although the exact pathogenesis remains elusive, exposure to solar radiation, especially ultraviolet A, B, and visible light, appears to result in a form of abnormal immune response.

On histology, actinic prurigo cheilitis is characterized by acanthosis, spongiosis, and dense lymphocytic inflammation with intermixed eosinophils. Treatment includes photoprotection, topical steroids, and/or thalidomide [45].

Oral Ulcers

Recurrent Aphthous Stomatitis

Recurrent aphthous stomatitis (RAS) is the most common of oral mucosal diseases, presenting as well defined, oval to round shallow ulcerations with erythematous borders and yellow-gray fibromembranous bases [48]. Prevalence varies from 2 to 50% [49] of the general population and may be higher in woman, as well as children whose parents have RAS [50]. Lesions are frequently observed in childhood and adolescence, and they tend to diminish in frequency and severity with time. Although the pathogenesis is not well-known, proposed predisposing factors include trauma, stress, various nutritional deficiencies (iron, zinc, vitamins B1, B2, B6, and B12), allergies, infectious conditions, gluten sensitivity, and genetic susceptibility [48, 49]. Associated systemic conditions include Behçet's disease, celiac disease, HIV, inflammatory bowel disease, *Heliobacter pylori* infection, MAGIC syndrome (mouth and genital ulcers with inflamed cartilage), PFAPA syndrome (periodic fever, aphthosis, pharyngitis, and adenitis), and systemic lupus [49, 50].

Lesions are painful and typically involve nonkeratinized mucosa. RAS can be classified based on clinical severity or morphology. Based on clinical severity, RAS is divided into a milder type known as simple aphthosis and a more severe type known as complex aphthosis. Based on morphology (size, number, and location of lesions), RAS is classified as minor aphthous ulcers (MiAU), major aphthous ulcers (MjAU), or herpetiform ulcers (HU). MiAU is the most common type with few, quick healing, small ulcers localized on the anterior mucosa. MjAU are larger, slower-healing, more painful ulcers that can occur on either the anterior or posterior mucosa. HU is the least common type, presenting as grouped small ulcers on both the anterior or posterior mucosa [49].

Although RAS heals spontaneously, symptomatic relief it is often required. MjAU often heal with scarring. Treatment options include topical medications (amlexanox, antibiotics, calcineurin inhibitors, corticosteroids in dental/oral paste, sulcralfate, chlorhexidine gluconate mouthwash) or systemic therapy, which can be specific to an underlying etiology (i.e., vitamin B12) or nonspecific (corticosteroids, colchicine, tetracycline antibiotics, and thalidomide) [49].

Pemphigus Vulgaris

Pemphigus vulgaris, the most common pemphigus variant, is an autoimmune disorder characterized by flaccid and easily ruptured bullae on skin and mucous membranes. It affects men and women equally [51] and is more commonly seen in the fourth to sixth decades of life. Oral lesions are the first site of involvement in 50–70% of patients [52] and, in some cases, are the sole disease manifestation [53]. Pemphigus vulgaris presents as vesicles and bullae that quickly rupture resulting in painful erosions and ulcerations affecting the buccal mucosa, palate, tongue, and labial mucosa [54]. Desquamative or erosive gingivitis and involvement of other mucosal sites such as ocular, esophageal, and anogenital can occur, causing significant morbidity [52].

Pemphigus vulgaris result from autoantibodies (IgG) directed against intracellular cadherins, specifically desmogleins in desmosomes within stratified squamous epithelia. Both anti-desmogleins 1 and 3 are found in the serum of patients with mucocutaneous pemphigus vulgaris. Anti-desmoglein 3 alone is associated with the mucosal-limited variant [51]. On histology, pemphigus vulgaris has suprabasilar clefting and acantholysis with variable lymphocytic inflammation in the lamina propria [2]. Direct immunofluorescence studies reveal intercellular IgG and sometimes intercellular IgA within the epithelium [2].

The incidence of pemphigus vulgaris is higher among those of Mediterranean or Jewish descent [54]. It is the most common autoimmune blistering disease (80%) in India, China, Malaysia, and the Middle East [53]. There is a strong association with HLA class II, specifically HLA-DR4 (DRB1*0402) in Ashkenazi Jews, DRw14 (DRB1*1041) and DQB1*0503 in Europeans and Asians [51].

Corticosteroids are the mainstay of therapy. Other anti-inflammatory and steroid-sparing agents are used to minimize adverse effects including azathioprine, methotrexate, dapsone, cyclophosphamide, mycophenolate mofetil, plasmapheresis, intravenous immunoglobulin, rituximab, and tumor necrosis factor alpha (TNF-α) antagonists [52, 54].

Behçet's Disease

Behçet's disease is a chronic inflammatory multisystem disease defined by the International Study Group as a combination of recurrent oral aphthous ulcers plus two of the following: recurrent genital aphthous ulcers, eye lesions (anterior uveitis, posterior uveitis, vitreal cells, or retinal vasculitis), skin lesions (erythema nodosum, pseudofolliculitis, papulopustular or acneiform lesions), or a positive pathergy test. The oral ulcers are painful, typically last for weeks, and heal with scarring. Behçet's disease usually presents around the third or fourth decade of life [55]. It is more common in males and believed to be precipitated by an unknown trigger in genetically susceptible individuals [56]. HLA-B51 is strongly associated with this disease; presence of this variant confers an almost sixfold increased odds of developing Behçet's disease [55].

Sometimes referred to as the 'Silk Route' disease, it most frequently affects people in the Mediterranean and Middle East, especially Turkey, and also Japan. While some have reported phenotypic variation in different populations, a 2007 study found only slight differences in the disease manifestations in different ethnic groups either within or between countries [57].

Oral ulcers, one of the defining features of the disease, are also one of the most frequently occurring disease features. The most common locations for these are the mucosal surfaces of the lips, buccal mucosa, tongue, and soft palate. The lesions start as red papules or vesicles and quickly become oval to round ulcers with an erythematous rim, rolled borders, and a gray or yellow base. They are indistinguishable from non-Behçet's-associated aphthae. They can be induced by trauma and take weeks to resolve [55].

Behçet's disease is classified as a form of vasculitis. It can affect any size or type of vessel. Vasculitis is seen commonly on biopsies of mucocutaneous lesions in this condition [55].

Treatment options include topical agents such as antimicrobials, corticosteroids, and pimecrolimus. Systemic therapies are also frequently employed including colchicine with or without penicillin, corticosteroids, azathioprine, thalidomide, and TNF-α antagonists [55].

Conclusion

Examination of the oral mucosa is an important part of a complete skin exam. As the population of the United States continues to become more ethnically and racially diverse, it is imperative to recognize both normal and pathologic features of oral mucosal conditions. Pigmented, nonpigmented, inflammatory, and ulcerative conditions may present with unique characteristics and at different frequencies in those with richly pigmented skin. It is essential to understand how presentations, triggers, prognoses, and treatment options vary in this patient population.

References

1. Hoang MPSM. Vulvar Pathology. In: Hoang MP, Selim MA, editors. New York: Springer; 2015.
2. Woo S-B. Oral Pathology. 1st ed. Philadephia: Elsevier; 2012.
3. Feller L, Masilana A, Khammissa RA, Altini M, Jadwat Y, Lemmer J. Melanin: the biophysiology of oral melanocytes and physiological oral pigmentation. Head Face Med. 2014;10(8):8.
4. Meleti M, Vescovi P, Mooi WJ, van der Waal I. Pigmented lesions of the oral mucosa and perioral tissues: a flow-chart for the diagnosis and some recommendations for the management. Oral Sur Oral Med Oral Pathol Oral Radiol Endodontol. 2008;105(5):606–16.
5. Müller S. Melanin-associated pigmented lesions of the oral mucosa: presentation, differential diagnosis, and treatment. Dermatol Therapy. 2010;23(3):220–9.
6. Lenane P, Powell FC. Oral pigmentation. J Eur Acad Dermatol Venereol. 2000;14(6):448–65.
7. Weedon D. Weedon's skin pathology. Elsevier; 2010.
8. Contreras E, Carlos R. Oral melanoacanthosis (melanoachantoma): report of a case and review of the literature. Med oral Patolo Oral Cir Bucal. 2004;10(1):11–2.

9. Brooks JK, Sindler AJ, Scheper MA. Oral Melanoacanthoma in an Adolescent. Pediatr Dermatol. 2010;27(4):384–7.
10. Cantudo-Sanagustín E, Gutiérrez-Corrales A, Vigo-Martínez M, Serrera-Figallo MÁ, Torres-Lagares D, Gutiérrez-Pérez JL. Pathogenesis and clinicohistopathological caractheristics of melanoacanthoma: a systematic review. J Clin Exp Dentistry. 2016;8(3):e327.
11. Behura SS. Oral mucosal lesions associated with smokers and chewers–a case-control study in chennai population. J Clin Diagnostic Res: JCDR. 2015;9(7):ZC17–22.
12. Marakoglu K, Gursoy UK, Toker HC, Demirer S, Sezer RE, Marakoglu I. Smoking status and smoke-related gingival melanin pigmentation in army recruitments. Mil Med. 2007;172 (1):110–3.
13. Bellew SG, Alster TS. Treatment of exogenous ochronosis with a Q-switched alexandrite (755 nm) laser. Dermatol Sur. 2004;30(4):555–8.
14. Hassona Y, Sawair F, Al-karadsheh O, Scully C. Prevalence and clinical features of pigmented oral lesions. Int J Dermatol. 2016;55(9):1005–13.
15. Hedin CA, Pindborg JJ, Axell T. Disappearance of smoker's melanosis after reducing smoking. J Oral Pathol Med. 1993;22(5):228–30.
16. Amano H, Tamura A, Yasuda M, et al. Amalgam tattoo of the oral mucosa mimics malignant melanoma. J Dermatol. 2011;38(1):101–3.
17. Ricart J, Martin JM. Acquired amalgam tattoo. A possible diagnostic pitfall. J Cosmet Dermatol. 2011;10(1):70–1.
18. Meleti M, Mooi WJ, Casparie MK, van der Waal I. Melanocytic nevi of the oral mucosa—no evidence of increased risk for oral malignant melanoma: an analysis of 119 cases. Oral Oncol. 2007;43(10):976–81.
19. Ferreira L, Jham B, Assi R, Readinger A, Kessler HP. Oral melanocytic nevi: a clinicopathologic study of 100 cases. Oral Surg Oral Med Oral Pathol Oral Radiol. 2015;120(3):358–67.
20. Mohan M, Sukhadia VY, Pai D, Bhat S. Oral malignant melanoma: systematic review of literature and report of two cases. Oral Surg Oral Med Oral Pathol Oral Radiol. 2013;116(4): e247–54.
21. McLaughlin CC, Wu XC, Jemal A, Martin HJ, Roche LM, Chen VW. Incidence of noncutaneous melanomas in the U.S. Cancer. 2005;103(5):1000–7.
22. Altieri L, Wong MK, Peng DH, Cockburn M. Mucosal melanomas in the racially diverse population of California. J Am Acad Dermatol. 2017;76(2):250–7.
23. Ulusal BG, Karatas O, Yildiz AC, Oztan Y. Primary malignant melanoma of the maxillary gingiva. *Dermatol Surg*. 2003;29(3):304–307. http://www.ncbi.nlm.nih.gov/pubmed/ 12614430.
24. Chatzistefanou I, Kolokythas A, Vahtsevanos K, Antoniades K. Primary mucosal melanoma of the oral cavity: current therapy and future directions. Oral Surg Oral Med Oral Pathol Oral Radiol. 2016;122(1):17–27.
25. Lamichhane NS, An J, Liu Q, Zhang W. Primary malignant mucosal melanoma of the upper lip: a case report and review of the literature. BMC Res Notes. 2015;8(1):499.
26. Madani FM, Kuperstein AS. Normal variations of oral anatomy and common oral soft tissue lesions. Med Clin North Am. 2014;98(6):1281–98.
27. Martin JL. Leukoedema: an epidemiological study in white and African Americans. *J Tenn Dent Assoc*. 1997;77(1):18-21. http://www.ncbi.nlm.nih.gov/pubmed/9520752.
28. Castellanos JL, Díaz-Guzmán L. Lesions of the oral mucosa: an epidemiological study of 23785 Mexican patients. Oral Surg Oral Med Oral Pathol Oral Radiol Endod. 2008;105 (1):79–85.
29. Arakeri G, Brennan PA. Oral submucous fibrosis: an overview of the aetiology, pathogenesis, classification, and principles of management. Br J Oral Maxillofac Surg. 2013;51(7):587–93.
30. Aziz SR. Oral submucous fibrosis: case report and review of diagnosis and treatment. J Oral Maxillofac Surg. 2008;66(11):2386–9.
31. Angadi PV, Rao SS. Areca nut in pathogenesis of oral submucous fibrosis: Revisited. Oral Maxillofac Surg. 2011;15(1):1–9.

32. Tilakaratne WM, Klinikowski MF, Saku T, Peters TJ, Warnakulasuriya S. Oral submucous fibrosis: review on aetiology and pathogenesis. Oral Oncol. 2006;42(6):561–8.
33. Weatherspoon DJ, Chattopadhyay A, Boroumand S, Garcia I. Oral cavity and oropharyngeal cancer incidence trends and disparities in the United States: 2000-2010. Cancer Epidemiol. 2015;39(4):497–504.
34. . Idris A, Vani N, Saleh S, et al. Relative Frequency of Oral Malignancies and Oral Precancer in the Biopsy Service of Jazan Province, 2009-2014. *Asian Pac J Cancer Prev*. 2016;17 (2):519–525. http://www.ncbi.nlm.nih.gov/pubmed/26925637.
35. Lewin F, Norell SE, Johansson H, et al. Smoking tobacco, oral snuff, and alcohol in the etiology of squamous cell carcinoma of the head and neck: a population-based case-referent study in Sweden. Cancer. 1998;82(7):1367–75.
36. Walker B, Figgs LW, Zahm SH. Differences in cancer incidence, mortality, and survival between African Americans and whites. Environ Health Perspect. 1995;103:275–81.
37. Joseph LJ, Goodman M, Higgins K, et al. Racial disparities in squamous cell carcinoma of the oral tongue among women: a SEER data analysis. Oral Oncol. 2015;51(6):586–92.
38. Siegel RL, Miller KD, Jemal A. Cancer statistics, 2015. CA Cancer J Clin. 2015;65(1):5–29.
39. Sciubba JJ. Oral cancer. The importance of early diagnosis and treatment. *Am J Clin Dermatol*. 2001;2(4):239–251. http://www.ncbi.nlm.nih.gov/pubmed/11705251.
40. Abu-Ghanem S, Yehuda M, Carmel NN, Leshno M, Abergel A, Gutfeld O, Fliss DM. Elective neck dissection vs observation in early-stage squamous cell carcinoma of the oral tongue with no clinically apparent lymph node metastasis in the neck: a systematic review and meta-analysis. JAMA Otolaryngol-Head Neck Sur. 2016;142(9):857–65.
41. Koski L, Ngoma T, Mwaiselage J, Le L, Soliman AS. Changes in the pattern of kaposi's sarcoma at ocean road cancer institute in Tanzania (2006–2011). Int J STD AIDS. 2015;26 (7):470–8.
42. Fatahzadeh M, Schwartz RA. Oral Kaposi's sarcoma: a review and update. Int J Dermatol. 2013;52(6):666–72.
43. Organization WH. No Title. 2014; http://www.ncbi.nlm.nih.gov/pubmed/26203484.
44. Suárez A, Valbuena MC, Rey M, Porras de Quintana L. Association of HLA subtype DRB1*0407 in Colombian patients with actinic prurigo. Photodermatol Photoimmunol Photomed. 2006;22(2):55–8.
45. Vega-Memije ME, Mosqueda-Taylor A, Irigoyen-Camacho ME, Hojyo-Tomoka MT, Domínguez-Soto L. Actinic prurigo cheilitis: Clinicopathologic analysis and therapeutic results in 116 cases. Oral Surg Oral Med Oral Pathol Oral Radiol Endod. 2002;94(1):83–91.
46. Vera Izaguirre DS, Zuloaga Salcedo S, González Sánchez PC, et al. Actinic prurigo: a case-control study of risk factors. Int J Dermatol. 2014;53(9):1080–5.
47. Ross G, Foley P, Baker C. Actinic prurigo. Photodermatol Photoimmunol Photomed. 2008;24 (5):272–5.
48. Akintoye SO, Greenberg MS. Recurrent aphthous stomatitis. Dent Clin North Am. 2014;58 (2):281–97.
49. Cui RZ, Bruce AJ, Rogers RS. Recurrent aphthous stomatitis. Clin Dermatol. 2016;34 (4):475–81.
50. Chattopadhyay A, Shetty KV. Recurrent aphthous stomatitis. Otolaryngol Clin North Am. 2011;44(1):79–88.
51. Scully C, Mignogna M. Oral mucosal disease: pemphigus. Br J Oral Maxillofac Sur. 2008;46 (4):272–7.
52. Scully C, Paes De Almeida O, Porter SR, de Gilkes JJH. Pemphigus vulgaris: the manifestations and long-term management of 55 patients with oral lesions. Br J Dermatol. 1999;140(1):84–9.
53. Venugopal SS, Murrell DF. Diagnosis and clinical features of pemphigus vulgaris. Immunol Allergy Clin North Am. 2012;32(2):233–43.
54. Taylor J, McMillan R, Shephard M, et al. World workshop on oral medicine VI: a systematic review of the treatment of mucous membrane pemphigoid. Oral Sur Oral Med Oral Pathol Oral Radiol. 2015;120(2):161–71.

55. Alpsoy E. Behçet's disease: A comprehensive review with a focus on epidemiology, etiology and clinical features, and management of mucocutaneous lesions. J Dermatol. 2016;43 (6):620–32.
56. Kalayciyan A, Zouboulis CC. An update on Behçet's disease. J Eur Acad Dermatol Venereol. 2007;21(1):1–10.
57. Lewis KA, Graham EM, Stanford MR. Systematic review of ethnic variation in the phenotype of Behcet's disease. Scandinavian J Rheumatol. 2007;36(1):1–6.

Chapter 9
Acne and Rosacea

Christina N. Lawson and Valerie D. Callender

Acne Vulgaris

Acne vulgaris is one of the most commonly encountered dermatologic conditions in the United States across all racial groups. A recent analysis of nationally representative data from dermatology practice surveys found that acne was the leading dermatologic disorder among African Americans, Asian or Pacific Islanders, and Hispanic or Latino populations [1]. Notably, in this same analysis, dyschromia was listed as a leading condition among African Americans and Hispanic populations [1]. Although acne is found predominantly during adolescence, it is a common problem among adults, especially females with skin of color [2]. One photographic study consisting of 2895 females of all racial groups found that clinical acne was more prevalent in African-American and Hispanic women (37 and 32% respectively) than in Continental Indian, Caucasian, and Asian women (23, 24, and 30% respectively) [3]. Hyperpigmentation was more prevalent in African-American and Hispanic women (65 and 48% respectively) than in Asian, Continental Indian, and Caucasian women (18, 10, and 25% respectively) [3]. These findings are in congruence with previous surveys, which reported that dyschromia or pigmentary disorders (other than vitiligo) were the second [4] and third [5] most commonly diagnosed conditions seen in dermatology practices composed of predominantly African-American patients.

C.N. Lawson (✉)
Dermatology Associates of Lancaster, 1650 Crooked Oak Drive,
Suite 200, Lancaster, PA 17601, USA
e-mail: clawson2011@gmail.com

V.D. Callender
Callender Dermatology and Cosmetic Center,
12200 Annapolis Rd, Suite 315, Glenn Dale, MD 20769, USA
e-mail: drcallender@callenderskin.com

© Springer International Publishing AG 2017
N.A. Vashi and H.I. Maibach (eds.), *Dermatoanthropology of Ethnic Skin and Hair*, DOI 10.1007/978-3-319-53961-4_9

The pathogenesis of acne in skin of color is thought to involve the four same mechanisms as in Caucasian skin: follicular hyperkeratinization leading to plugging of the follicle, excess sebum production from increased androgenic stimulation, *Propionibacterium acnes* (*P. acnes*) overgrowth, and inflammation [6]. One study of 60 women reported a trend toward a greater overall density of *P. acnes* in 30 African-American women as compared with 30 Caucasian women [7]. A few studies have found differences with respect to sebaceous gland size and activity between African-American and Caucasian subjects [8, 9]. However, because these studies included small patient populations, generalized conclusions cannot be made [6].

New research indicates that inflammation plays a crucial role in the pathogenesis of acne and has been shown in studies to occur prior to and concurrently with follicular hyperkeratinization and microcomedone formation [10]. This novel finding is in agreement with Halder et al. [11] who reported significant histological differences between acne in African Americans compared to Caucasian skin. Notably, the authors reported that biopsy specimens of facial comedonal, papular, and pustular lesions from 30 African-American females demonstrated marked inflammation in all acne lesions, including comedones that lacked inflammation based on clinical appearance. The study suggested that this baseline-enhanced inflammation on histology might explain the tendency for darker -skinned individuals to develop post-inflammatory hyperpigmentation (PIH).

Acne in skin of color affects heavily populated sebaceous areas of the skin similar to Caucasians, such as the face, upper chest, and back. Papules, pustules, comedones, and hyperpigmented macules are the most common lesions seen in patients with skin of color [12]. Although nodulocystic acne is less commonly seen in the African-American population, one study revealed that cystic lesions occurred in 25.5% of Hispanics, 18% of African Americans, and 10.5% of Asians [6]. Adult female acne in skin of color characteristically presents with acneiform lesions or hyperpigmented macules or papules distributed along the lower one-third of the face, particularly the jawline and chin, which is considered to be a hormonal distribution (Fig. 9.1) [2].

PIH is a frequent, prominent feature of acne in darker skinned individuals and commonly may be of greater distress to the patient than the actual acneiform lesions themselves [12, 13]. In the co-author's 20-year private practice experience in treating patients from diverse ethnic backgrounds, PIH is often the presenting reason for a visit to the dermatologist and many of these patients will have already attempted the use of over-the-counter (OTC) 1–2% hydroquinone preparations or topical corticosteroids with the intent to fade these blemishes [13]. Hypertrophic scarring and keloid formation are additional unfortunate sequelae of acne in skin of color.

A few studies have highlighted important racial differences regarding the clinical characteristics, behaviors, expectations, and treatment patterns among patients with skin of color compared to Caucasians with acne. A cross-sectional, Web-based survey of 208 subjects with adult female acne reported that non-Caucasian women experienced more PIH than Caucasian women ($P < 0.0001$) [14]. Furthermore, lesion clearance was the most important aspect of acne clearing to Caucasian

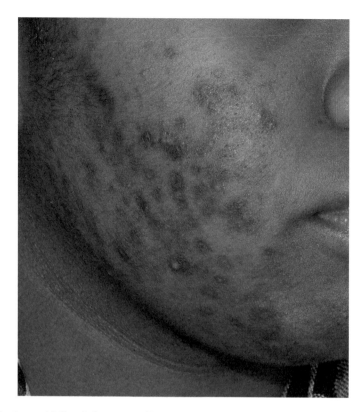

Fig. 9.1 Acne with Post-inflammatory Hyperpigmentation (Courtesy of Valerie Callender, MD; Callender Dermatology & Cosmetic Center, Glenn Dale, MD)

women (57.9% vs. non-Caucasian 31.7%, $P < 0.001$) whereas PIH clearing was most important for many non-Caucasian females (41.6% vs. Caucasian 8.4%, $P < 0.001$) [14]. Another cross-sectional, Web-based observational survey of 313 subjects was conducted to support this initial pivotal study [15]. The authors found that African Americans reported recent use of PIH treatments more often than did other racial groups (African American 40.6%; Hispanic 25.5%; Asian/other 27.8%; Caucasian 23.4%; $P = 0.07$) [15]. Among those patients using PIH treatments, a higher proportion of African-American (64.1%) and Hispanic subjects (78.6%) reported using a skin-lightening agent in the past three months compared with Asian/other (46.7%) and Caucasian (40%) subjects ($P = 0.07$) [15]. Therefore, this data further emphasizes the observation that patients with skin of color are more likely to present with pigmentary changes as a result of their acne, which warrants early prevention and treatment.

Pomade acne is commonly seen in African Americans and clinically manifests as comedones, papules, and/or pustules noted on the forehead, temples, and anterior hairline. It occurs due to the frequent application of oil-based hair products, which are comedogenic hair moisturizers commonly used to style and manage dry, fragile hair and to aid in the treatment of inflammatory conditions such as seborrheic dermatitis [13]. A survey by Taylor [6] reported that nearly half (46.2%) of acne subjects with skin of color reported hair oil or pomade use; of these subjects, 70.3% manifested with forehead acne. Treatment of pomade acne includes minimizing use of pomades, educating patients to apply the product only to the scalp hair (1 inch behind the hairline) and avoiding contact with facial skin [16]. For patients who desire a light hair moisturizer, clinicians should recommend silicone-based styling products instead of oil-based products [17]. Standard treatments for acne (e.g., topical antimicrobials or retinoids) may be used in persistent cases. Steroid acne is also not uncommon in skin of color as some racial groups may frequently use topical corticosteroid-containing fade creams in an attempt to treat underlying PIH. In such cases, discontinuation of the corticosteroid will resolve the acne [16].

Treatment of acne in ethnic skin should focus on three major objectives: (1) early and aggressive initiation of treatment for active inflammatory lesions, (2) prevention and management of PIH, and (3) minimizing skin irritation. Because PIH and scarring are more prevalent in skin of color, the clinician must plan a treatment regimen that carefully balances diminishing the acneiform lesions with avoiding potentially irritating, drying agents that could exacerbate preexisting PIH. In patients with skin of color, more severe forms of acne (especially truncal) can lead to the development of keloids and permanent scarring [18]. Treatment options for acne in skin of color are similar to Caucasians and include topical comedolytic agents, topical and oral antibiotics, topical and systemic retinoids, oral contraceptive agents, and procedural therapies. However, a major concern with the use of topical agents in skin of color is the potential for irritant contact dermatitis (ICD) [6, 13]. An appropriate individualized selection of topical acne medications is essential for patients with skin of color as these agents may lead to worsening PIH in those with dry, sensitive skin. Table 9.1 summarizes selected clinical trials evaluating the safety and efficacy of various treatments for acne in skin of color.

Topical retinoids are generally considered a first-line treatment for mild to moderate acne in skin of color [19]. Retinoids have several advantages in skin of color patients with acne as they improve hyperkeratosis, decrease comedogenesis, possess anti-inflammatory effects [20], and help alleviate PIH by causing melanin granule dispersion and removal [21]. In an 8-week, double-blind, vehicle-controlled study with tretinoin cream, Halder [22] demonstrated a decrease in papules and pustules and in hyperpigmented macules in 83% of 12 African-American patients treated with tretinoin 0.025% cream compared with 13% of 15 patients treated with vehicle cream only (unpublished data). More recent clinical trials have demonstrated the efficacy and safety of all three topical retinoids (adapalene, tretinoin, and tazarotene) for acne in skin of color patients (Table 9.1).

Topical retinoids in pigmented skin can produce irritation known as "retinoid dermatitis," however, there are many useful strategies available to lessen this potential risk [23]. The first is selecting an appropriate retinoid based on the patient's skin type (dry/oily/combination). Adapalene gel appears to be well tolerated across all skin types [6]. Second, initiating therapy with lower concentrations in a cream or

Table 9.1 Summary of selected studies of acne in skin of color

Agent(s)	Author(s)	Study design	Demographics	Summary of results
Topical retinoids	Jacyk et al. [45]	Two-center, open-label, noncomparative study	N = 65 64 African, 1 Indian	Statistically significant reductions from baseline in total acne lesion counts were seen after 4 weeks' treatment with once-daily adapalene 0.1% gel ($P < 0.01$). Adapalene 0.1% gel demonstrated statistically significant improvements in the degree of PIH at weeks 4, 8, and 12 versus baseline ($P < 0.01$). Less than 5% of patients reported moderate to severe skin irritation during the study
	Tu et al. [46]	Multicenter, randomized study	N = 150 1 FST I, 8 FST II, 89 FST III, 52 FST IV (all Chinese)	By week 8, adapalene 0.1% gel and tretinoin 0.025% gel (each applied once daily) were essentially equivalent, both producing 70% reductions in the total number of noninflammatory lesions from baseline. By the end of the treatment course, adapalene had produced a 74.8% reduction in inflammatory lesions as compared with 72.2% for tretinoin. In general, irritation was mild, but was more common and more severe in the tretinoin group versus the adapalene group (45.7% tretinoin vs. 32.4% adapalene)
	Goh et al. [47]	Single-center, randomized, investigator-masked and intra-individual comparison	N = 73 19 Chinese, 20 Malay, 20 Indian, 14 Caucasian	The irritation potential of adapalene gel 0.1% was significantly lower than that of tretinoin gel 0.025% in all tolerability assessments, irrespective of the volunteers' ethnic origins. The differences between the two treatments were statistically significant in all cases ($P < 0.03$), suggesting that adapalene gel 0.1% had a much lower irritancy potential than tretinoin gel 0.025%

(continued)

Table 9.1 (continued)

Agent(s)	Author(s)	Study design	Demographics	Summary of results
	Tirado-Sanchez et al. [48]	Single-center, randomized, double-blinded placebo-controlled study	N = 171 (all Mexican, including FST III and IV)	At 90 days of treatment, the efficacy rates of tretinoin 0.05% gel, adapalene 0.3% gel, and adapalene 0.1% gel were 80, 70, and 59% respectively. Tolerance was better with adapalene 0.1% gel than with adapalene 0.3% and tretinoin 0.05% gel ($P = 0.001$)
	Grimes, PE, Callender, VD [49]	Randomized, double-blinded, vehicle-controlled study	N = 74 69 African American, 1 Hispanic, 1 Asian, 2 Other	Once-daily tazarotene 0.1% cream was significantly more effective than vehicle in lessening PIH overall ($P = 0.010$) and in reducing the intensity ($P = 0.044$) and area of hyperpigmented lesions ($P = 0.026$) within 18 weeks
	Alexis et al. [50]	Multicenter, randomized, double-blinded, placebo-controlled study	N = 238 2 FST II, 4 FST III, 25 FST IV, 95 FST V, 112 FST VI	After 12 weeks, significant reductions in median total, inflammatory, and noninflammatory lesion counts were observed with adapalene 0.1%/BPO 2.5% gel than vehicle
Topical antibiotics	Callender VD [51]	Multicenter, randomized, double-blinded, vehicle-controlled study	N = 797 419 FST I-III, 378 FST IV-VI	Treatment success and median reductions in inflammatory, noninflammatory, and total lesions with clindamycin phosphate 1.2%/BPO 2.5% gel were comparable between FST I-III and FST IV-VI at week 12. Patients with FST IV-VI were not found to be more susceptible to irritation from the combination treatment as compared to patients with FST I-III
	Callender et al. [52]	Multicenter, randomized, double-blinded, placebo-controlled study	N = 33 32 African American, 1 African American/Caucasian	Clindamycin phosphate 1.2%/tretinoin 0.025% gel-treated patients had a greater decrease in inflammatory lesion counts from baseline than vehicle group at week 12 ($P = 0.05$)

(continued)

Table 9.1 (continued)

Agent(s)	Author(s)	Study design	Demographics	Summary of results
Azelaic acid	Kircik LH [53]	Single-center, open-label pilot study	N = 20 (all African American)	At week 16, azelaic acid 15% gel applied twice-daily resulted in 92% of subjects with at least a one-point improvement in IGA for acne and 100% of subjects had at least a 2-point improvement in IGA for PIH. Tolerability was rated as good throughout the treatment period with no serious adverse events reported
Topical dapsone	Piette et al. [54]	Randomized, double-blinded, vehicle-controlled crossover study	N = 64 56 African American, 4 Asian, 1 Hispanic, 3 other	Subjects with glucose-6-phosphate dehydrogenase deficiency (G6PD) treated with dapsone 5% gel had only a 0.32 g/dL decrease in hemoglobin levels from baseline to 2 weeks; however, no changes were noted in reticulocytes, haptoglobin, bilirubin or lactate dehydrogenase levels
	Alexis et al. [55]	Multicenter, open-label, single-group study	N = 68 (all females, FST IV–VI)	Twice-daily monotherapy with topical dapsone 5% gel resulted in significantly decreased Global Acne Assessment Score (GAAS) from baseline to week 12 ($P < 0.001$; 39% improvement). Subjects experienced significant reductions in mean total lesions (52% decrease), inflammatory lesions (65%), and comedone counts (41%; all $P < 0.001$)
Oral antibiotics	Thiboutot et al. [56]	Multicenter, randomized, investigator-blinded, vehicle-controlled, parallel-group study	N = 467 291 Caucasian, 62 Black, 13 Asian, 96 Hispanic, 5 other	At week 12, the combination of adapalene 0.1% gel + doxycycline 100 mg capsule was significantly superior to doxycycline 100 mg capsule alone for change from baseline in total ($P < 0.001$), inflammatory ($P = 0.02$), and noninflammatory ($P < 0.001$) lesions

(continued)

Table 9.1 (continued)

Agent(s)	Author(s)	Study design	Demographics	Summary of results
	Fleischer et al. [57]	Multicenter, randomized, double-blinded, placebo-controlled study	N = 1038 767 Caucasian, 107 African American, 126 Hispanic, 3 American Indian, 19 Asian/Pacific Islander, 16 other	Treatment with extended-release minocycline (1 mg/kg) significantly reduced ($P < 0.001$) the number of inflammatory lesions and significantly improved ($P < 0.001$) their Evaluator's Global Severity Assessment (EGSA) scores (phase 3 studies)
	Ullah et al. [58]	Single-center, randomized controlled study	N = 386 (study conducted in Pakistan)	Azithromycin 500 mg daily before meals for 4 consecutive days monthly for 3 months resulted in an excellent response in 3.1% and a good response in 22.8%. Doxycycline 100 mg daily after meals for 3 months resulted in an excellent response in 11.4% and a good response in 55.4% of subjects. The authors concluded that doxycycline is the better treatment option for acne
	Tan et al. [59]	Multicenter, randomized, controlled, noninferiority, investigator-blinded study	N = 266 16 FST I, 80 FST II, 112 FST III, 46 FST IV, 8 FST V, 4 FST VI	After 20 weeks, doxycycline 200 mg plus adapalene 0.1%/benzoyl peroxide 2.5% gel showed a favorable composite efficacy/safety profile compared with oral isotretinoin, indicating that this combination can be an option for severe nodular acne
Oral retinoids	Kelly AP, Sampson DD [37]	Case series	N = 10 (all African American)	Treatment with isotretinoin resulted in an early onset flare of nodulocystic lesions at sites initially devoid of acne lesions at weeks 2–4 (notably the temporal and submandibular areas). At completion of the study, an improvement in PIH was noted. Between weeks 2–8, most subjects developed a reversible ashen or grayish facial hue (due to the drying and desquamative effects of isotretinoin)

(continued)

Table 9.1 (continued)

Agent(s)	Author(s)	Study design	Demographics	Summary of results
Procedural therapies	Karnik et al. [43]	Multicenter, randomized, double-blinded, controlled study	N = 147 (>20% subjects with FST V and VI)	Polymethylmethacrylate (PMMA)-collagen injections resulted in statistically significant improvements in atrophic acne scars (64%) compared with saline injections (33%) (P = 0.0005). The treatment showed excellent safety with generally mild, reversible adverse events
	Fabbrocini et al. [60]	Prospective, non-blinded study	N = 60 10 FST I-II, 45 FST III to V, 5 FST VI	After 3 monthly treatments with percutaneous collagen induction, a statistically significant improvement in atrophic acne scars was achieved. Transient posttreatment erythema occurred most prominently in patients with FST I-III. No reports of dyschromia were noted in any group at 1 year after final treatment
	Alexis et al. [61]	Investigator-initiated, randomized, blinded, split-face comparative study	N = 12 (FST IV–VI)	Treatment with the fractional 1550-nm nonablative laser resulted in significantly improved quantitative global scarring grading system (QGSGS) scores from baseline to 16 and 24 weeks (P = 0.0277). Five of seven and three of seven patients in the higher and lower density treatment group, respectively, experienced mild or moderate hyperpigmentation

Abbreviations: *BPO* benzoyl peroxide; *PIH* post-inflammatory hyperpigmentation; *FST* Fitzpatrick skin type; *IGA* investigator global assessment lotion vehicle (rather than gel) in patients with dry/sensitive skin or a history of prior irritation from topical acne medications may also help reduce irritation [13]. Third, educating patients to use alternate-day dosing for the first two weeks of therapy with a gradual transition to nightly application thereafter will further help reduce the potential for irritation. Finally, the use of a moisturizer prior to the application of the retinoid may help alleviate dryness, peeling, and erythema [24]. If the initial lower concentration retinoid is well tolerated, it can be slowly titrated to a higher strength after four to six weeks of treatment if necessary [13]. Patients should also be instructed to discontinue any harsh soaps, astringents, toners or exfoliating cleansers as these may potentiate cutaneous side effects of topical retinoids.

Topical antimicrobials are often used in combination for the treatment of mild to moderate acne. Benzoyl peroxide (BPO) has bactericidal, keratolytic, and anti-inflammatory properties. BPO may be utilized as monotherapy or in combination with other topical antibiotics or retinoids and has been studied in skin of color (Table 9.1). A lower concentration of BPO is recommended initially in treating skin of color patients in order to minimize skin irritation and dryness. In one study involving 153 patients, 2.5% BPO gel was found to be equivalent in efficacy to the 5 and 10% concentrations in reducing the number of papules and pustules, and to have less cutaneous adverse effects (desquamation, erythema, and burning) than the 10% preparation [25]. Topical clindamycin and erythromycin work by reducing *P. acnes* counts in the pilosebaceous units and also possess anti-inflammatory properties. These agents are less effective monotherapy; however, when combined with BPO, the potential for antibiotic resistance is reduced [26].

Azelaic acid is a naturally occurring, saturated, dicarboxyclic acid, which serves as an excellent non-retinoid alternative for patients with skin of color, mainly due to its effect on treating pigmentary disorders. Due to its ability to reversibly inhibit tyrosinase, azelaic acid may be a useful option in patients who exhibit PIH from acne but may have had prior hypersensitivity to topical retinoids or other skin-lightening agents [19]. Azelaic acid's mechanism of action in treating acne involves anti-inflammatory effects, stabilization of differentiation of keratinocytes in the follicular infundibulum, and antimicrobial effects on *P. acnes* and *Staphylococcus epidermidis* [27]. It is often used concomitantly with other topical antimicrobials or retinoids for increased efficacy [19]. Azelaic acid has been safely studied in skin of color patients and demonstrates a low irritation potential.

Topical dapsone is an effective alternative for acne due to its anti-inflammatory and antimicrobial properties [28]. One major concern with the use of oral dapsone in skin of color patients is the risk for hemolytic anemia in those with glucose-6-phosphate dehydrogenase (G6PD) deficiency, a common condition found among patients of African, South Asian, Middle Eastern, and Mediterranean descent [19]. However, the efficacy and safety of topical dapsone gel has been demonstrated in patients with skin of color, indicating it is safe (Table 9.1). Recently, a higher concentration of topical dapsone gel (7.5%) became FDA-approved for the treatment of acne vulgaris [29]. Patients should be counseled that the use of concomitant BPO with topical dapsone can cause a temporary yellow to orange discoloration at sites of application.

The most commonly used oral antibiotics for moderate to severe inflammatory acne in skin of color are the tetracycline antibiotics (e.g., doxycycline and minocycline). These agents reduce *P. acnes* counts and possess anti-inflammatory properties, which are critical in preventing PIH from acne in skin of color [12]. A lower threshold for initiation of oral antibiotics may be considered in skin of color patients to reduce inflammation at an earlier stage, thus decreasing the risk of PIH and scarring [18]. Doxycycline and minocycline have been associated with gastrointestinal side effects, photosensitivity, and photo-onycholysis [30]. Three distinct types of cutaneous minocycline-induced pigmentation have been described [31], with a frequency ranging between 2.4 and 14.8% in several longitudinal studies [32]. In particular, minocycline has been associated with an increased rate of a lupus-like syndrome compared to the other tetracyclines in young healthy acne patients [33]. It remains unclear if any specific ethnic group is more likely to develop this drug-induced condition [12]. Minocycline may also cause a drug hypersensitivity syndrome (DHS), and this severe drug reaction has been studied in ethnic populations [34].

Female patients with skin of color who develop adult-onset acne should be evaluated for possible underlying endocrine disorders, especially in the setting of hirsutism, irregular menses, and other signs of hyperandrogenism. Those patients who are thought to exhibit primarily hormonal acne will likely benefit from hormonal therapies, such as oral contraceptives and androgen-receptor blockers (e.g., spironolactone), even in the setting of normal laboratory findings [35]. Using hormonal therapies for acne in skin of color do not appear to require modifications based on skin type, however, more studies are needed [13].

Isotretinoin (13-cis-retinoid acid) is an oral retinoid FDA-approved for the treatment of severe inflammatory acne in patients who have failed conventional acne therapies. It should be considered early in the course of nodulocystic or severe forms of acne in skin of color to reduce the risk for permanent scarring [36]. The efficacy and safety of isotretinoin has been studied in patients of various ethnic groups [37–40]. Patient education and extensive counseling is crucial prior to initiation of isotretinoin as the drug is associated with several mucocutaneous and serious systemic toxicities including teratogenicity, dyslipidemia, hepatotoxicity, pancreatitis, pseudotumor cerebri, psychiatric disorders, and gastrointestinal adverse effects [19].

The importance in addressing PIH secondary to acne cannot be emphasized enough since PIH is often the driving force for acne patients with skin of color to pursue a dermatologic evaluation [36]. The gold standard therapy for treating hyperpigmentation from acne includes the use of hydroquinone, which is a phenolic product that inhibits conversion of tyrosine to melanin and alters several normal activities of the melanosome [13]. Hydroquinone is available OTC in strengths of 1–2%, whereas the prescription strength is usually between 3 and 4%. Given the small risk of allergic contact dermatitis to hydroquinone, it is recommended to initially limit the product only to a small test area for a few days, and if well tolerated, then apply the product on the remaining hyperpigmented areas [17]. Hydroquinone should be applied carefully with a Q-tip as temporary hypopigmentation or depigmentation of the surrounding normal skin ("the halo effect") may result from improper use [13]. Caution should be used as prolonged treatment with hydroquinone may lead to exogenous ochronosis, which may develop even with lower concentration OTC strengths and is difficult to treat [41]. Topical retinoids and azelaic acid are excellent alternative therapies for skin of color patients as they simultaneously treat the acneiform lesions and address PIH by various mechanisms on melanocyte biology [42].

Acne scarring is a potential sequela in skin of color patients, and treatment requires a careful, stepwise approach [18]. Treatments for acne scarring in skin of color may include chemical peels, microdermabrasion, injectables, microneedling, and lasers (Table 9.1). Patients with skin of color with acne and PIH typically benefit from superficial chemical peels, such as glycolic acid or salicylic acid [17]. Bellafill® (Suneva Medical, Inc.), a polymethylmethacrylate (PMMA)-collagen dermal filler, is FDA-approved for the treatment of atrophic facial acne scars and has demonstrated safety and efficacy in skin of color patients [43]. Microneedling is an evolving technique that may offer a more favorable safety profile compared to conventional resurfacing procedures and has been shown to be effective in treating acne and acne scarring in skin of color patients [44]. Any procedural therapy in skin of color patients needs to be undertaken with caution and experience as aggressive treatment may lead to worsening PIH and scarring.

In summary, the treatment of acne vulgaris is similar across various racial/ethnic groups; however, the increased risk of PIH and scarring in ethnic patients mandates a higher level of attention on addressing these particular sequelae. It is important to design a treatment regimen that balances early aggressive treatment of the inflammatory process with methods to reduce PIH, while still minimizing the risk of medication-induced irritation for the skin of color patient.

Rosacea

Rosacea is a chronic inflammatory disorder that affects the vasculature and pilosebaceous units of facial skin. While rosacea is less common in skin of color, it is not rare [62]. The prevalence of rosacea in different racial groups is not well described because the condition may be underestimated [63]. Some data suggest that approximately 4% of rosacea patients are of African, Latino, or Asian descent [12]. In a study analyzing data from the National Ambulatory Medical Care Survey (NAMCS) in 2010, results showed that of all patients diagnosed with rosacea, 2.0% were African American, 2.3% were Asian or Pacific Islander, and 3.9% were Hispanic or Latino [63]. In a 5-year longitudinal cohort study of 2587 rosacea patients enrolled in North Carolina Medicaid and prescribed at least 1 topical prescription for rosacea, the authors found that 16.27% of the patients were African American and 10.98% were of "other race" indicating that this disorder may be more common in skin of color than once previously believed [64].

Although the pathogenesis of rosacea remains to be fully elucidated, it is hypothesized that recurrent vascular dilatation, inflammation, and microorganisms play a role. It has been shown that increased expression of the cathelicidin antimicrobial peptide gene (CAMP), kallikrein 5 (KLK5), and Toll-like receptor 2 (TLR2) have been identified in facial skin of rosacea patients [65]. It is hypothesized that these biomarkers augment the innate immune response in rosacea and contribute to the pathophysiology of the disease. Sun exposure may also play a role in the disorder. A study of 168 Korean patients with Fitzpatrick skin types (FST) II through V reported that the degree of sun exposure had significant correlation with the development and severity of the erythematotelangiectatic subtype ($P < 0.05$), however, no such correlation was observed for the papulopustular, ocular, and phymatous subtypes [66]. Triggers of rosacea may include emotional stress, environmental temperature extremes, hot and spicy foods, red wine or alcohol, and topical irritants or allergens found in common cosmetic products [67].

The four major subtypes of rosacea are erythematotelangiectatic rosacea, papulopustular rosacea, phymatous rosacea, and ocular rosacea. Although rhinophyma is more commonly identified in Caucasian men, there are case reports in the literature describing this condition in ethnic groups [68, 69].

Data on the clinical manifestations of rosacea in patients with ethnic skin is limited [70]. Lesions in ethnic populations typically develop in the same zones of the face as in Caucasian skin (notably the glabella, nose, cheeks, and chin), however, because of the constitutive skin pigmentation in darker skinned patients, they may not appear as erythematous and telangiectasias may not be as easily appreciated [12, 62, 71]. One study found that patients of color less frequently received a diagnosis of rosacea despite exhibiting the same reasons for visit that often prompted a diagnosis of rosacea in Caucasian patients [63]. Patients with skin of color may report sensitivity, burning or stinging to various skin care products and episodic facial warmth (without visible flushing) in response to usual rosacea triggers [62]. In addition, facial flushing, ocular symptoms, or acneiform eruptions lacking comedones in patients of color should prompt the physician to consider rosacea as a possible diagnosis [63].

Extrafacial sites, although rarely reported in the literature, can also be affected and may serve as clues to the diagnosis in ethnic skin. In one study consisting of 50 female patients with rosacea from Saudi Arabia (FST IV through VI), extrafacial lesions affecting the ears, neck, upper chest, and back were identified in 7 (14%) patients [70]. The authors concluded that because extrafacial sites of rosacea are more likely to be involved, performing a clinical examination of these sites is essential [70]. Interestingly, the same authors also found that post-inflammatory pigmentary changes were not reported during their clinical study in patients with darker skin. This result is in accord with the clinical observation by Alexis [62], who commented that PIH secondary to rosacea is rare compared to acne vulgaris in skin of color. It has been hypothesized that this finding may be due to differences in the inflammatory mediators implicated in the specific disorders [62]. Furthermore, it is possible that the inflammation from rosacea in patients with skin of color may

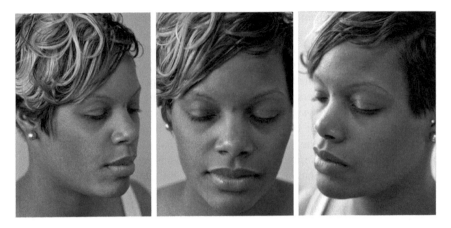

Fig. 9.2 Rosacea with post-inflammatory hypopigmentation (Courtesy of Valerie Callender, MD; Callender Dermatology & Cosmetic Center, Glenn Dale, MD)

resolve with post-inflammatory erythema that can be difficult to differentiate from the background erythema intrinsic to the disorder [70]. Future studies are needed to investigate these hypotheses.

In the co-author's private practice experience, treating many patients with skin of color, central facial erythema associated with hypopigmentation surrounding the borders of the erythematous regions can also point to the diagnosis of rosacea (Fig. 9.2). It is important to consider the differential diagnosis of rosacea in skin of color patients, which includes lupus erythematosus, sarcoidosis, seborrheic dermatitis, and other photodermatoses. In such patients, obtaining an antinuclear antibody (ANA) test should be considered.

The manifestations of ocular rosacea may include chalazion, blepharitis, meibomianitis, conjunctival hyperemia, corneal vascularization, corneal thinning and perforation, episcleritis, and iritis [71, 72]. In a case report of three African-American men with varying degrees of severity of ocular rosacea, the diagnosis was not initially suspected because the pathognomonic skin changes of rosacea were obscured by the skin hyperpigmentation [72]. Therefore, because the erythema may be slightly more difficult to appreciate in darker skinned individuals, it is important for the clinician to closely examine patients presenting with such eye complaints [12].

Granulomatous rosacea is considered a variant seen mostly in African Americans and Afro Caribbeans [12]. Clinically, it presents with firm, yellowish-brown papules and nodules in the malar, perioral, and periocular regions of the face. Both clinically and histologically, granulomatous rosacea can resemble sarcoidosis or cutaneous tuberculosis. In a case series of three African-American males with rosacea, biopsies revealed that two of the three patients were found to have the granulomatous form of the disease [71]. Future larger studies are needed to determine why patients with skin of color may be more susceptible to this variant.

FACE syndrome (*f*acial *A*fro-Caribbean *c*hildhood *e*ruption) is a subtype of granulomatous rosacea reported in the literature exclusively seen in African-American and Afro-Caribbean children [73]. Children with this condition typically present with monomorphic flesh-colored or hypopigmented papules particularly around the mouth, eyelids, ears, and nose [74]. The condition occurs at an earlier age than acne, and the etiology is poorly understood. The lesions persist for several months before resolving spontaneously without scarring [73].

General facial skin care recommendations for rosacea patients should include the use of a daily gentle cleanser or mild hypoallergenic syndet bar. Patients should avoid certain irritants such as astringents, exfoliators, toners, and potentially allergenic cosmetics. A daily sunscreen with both ultraviolet A (UV-A) and UV-B properties with an SPF >30 is beneficial. The physical blockers, titanium dioxide, and zinc oxide, are tolerated best by most rosacea patients [75]. The use of green-tinted makeup may help provide coverage of the erythematous areas in lighter skinned patients (FST III–V). Clinicians should emphasize to the patient that the goal in treatment is control of the disease, rather than cure, as rosacea is a chronic condition.

Food and Drug Administration (FDA)-approved topical agents for the treatment of mild rosacea include metronidazole, azelaic acid, ivermectin, sodium sulfacetamide/sulfur, and brimonidine. Alternative topical agents such as BPO, clindamycin, erythromycin, retinoids, and calcineurin inhibitors are considered off-label, but may be prescribed in select cases. For mild-moderate disease, oral antibiotics in the tetracycline family of antibiotics remain the most effective and are often combined with topical agents for maintenance. In severe and recalcitrant cases, low-dose isotretinoin may be considered, but recurrence upon discontinuation is commonplace.

While many published clinical trials exist comparing the various topical and oral therapeutic agents for rosacea, these trials generally include smaller numbers of patients with skin of color [62]. Therefore, there is a lack of data with respect to comparing the efficacy of certain treatments based on different FST. To our knowledge, no published clinical studies have been conducted exclusively in rosacea patients with skin of color. While the following sections describe the FDA-approved therapies for rosacea, it is important to note that these clinical trials contain a very small number of subjects with ethnic skin (Table 9.2).

Topical metronidazole (available in 0.75% cream, lotion or gel; 1% cream or gel) was the first topical agent approved for the treatment of rosacea. Nielsen first reported the efficacy of 1% metronidazole cream over placebo for rosacea in the early 1980s [76]. The mechanism of action of metronidazole in rosacea may include inhibition of neutrophil-generated reactive oxygen species and immunomodulator activity [64]. At least 10 randomized, placebo-controlled trials consisting of greater than 500 actively treated subjects have demonstrated the efficacy and tolerability of topical metronidazole in the treatment of rosacea [77]. Metronidazole may be used in a variety of FST due to its excellent safety, efficacy, and tolerability profile [64].

Azelaic acid 15% gel was approved by the FDA in 2002 for the treatment of mild to moderate papulopustular rosacea [78]. A newer formulation, 15% azelaic

Table 9.2 Summary of selected studies of rosacea in skin of color

Agent(s)	Author(s)	Study design	Demographics	Summary of results
Topical metronidazole versus azelaic acid	Elewski et al. [89]	Multicenter, double-blinded, randomized, parallel-group study	N = 251 93.5% Caucasian, 2.5% African American, 3.5% Hispanic, 0.5% Asian, 0.5% other	Twice-daily 15% azelaic acid gel was superior to twice-daily 0.75% metronidazole gel in reduction of mean nominal lesion count ($P = 0.003$) and mean percent decrease in inflammatory lesions ($P < 0.001$). An improvement in erythema severity was observed in 56% of azelaic acid gel-treated patients versus 42% of metronidazole gel-treated patients ($P = 0.02$)
	Wolf et al. [90]	Randomized, investigator-blinded, active-controlled, parallel-group study	N = 160 86.15% Caucasian, 1.25% African American, 11.3% Hispanic, 1.25% other	Once-daily metronidazole 1% gel was compared to twice-daily azelaic acid 15% gel for moderate rosacea. Both treatment groups showed similar reductions in inflammatory lesion counts at week 15 (77% for metronidazole gel and 80% for azelaic acid gel) and reduction in erythema (42.7% for metronidazole and 42.3% for azelaic acid)
	Colon et al. [91]	Single-center, investigator-blinded study	N = 32 87.5% Caucasian, 3.1% African American, 6.3% Hispanic	This study demonstrated a significantly greater potential for irritation from azelaic acid 15% gel compared with 0.75% metronidazole gel ($P < 0.0001$), which had significantly greater potential for irritation compared with 1% metronidazole gel ($P = 0.0054$)

(continued)

Table 9.2 (continued)

Agent(s)	Author(s)	Study design	Demographics	Summary of results
Azelaic acid	Thiboutot et al. [92]	Two multicenter, randomized, double-blinded, parallel-group, vehicle-controlled studies	N = 664 92.5% Caucasian, 0.75% African American, 5.75% Hispanic, 0.25% Asian, 0.75% other	Twice-daily azelaic acid 15% gel yielded statistically significantly higher reductions in mean inflammatory lesion count compared to vehicle gel within 12 weeks of treatment. Significantly higher proportions of subjects treated with azelaic acid gel experienced improvement in facial erythema compared with vehicle gel
Topical ivermectin	Stein et al. [93]	Two identically designed, multicenter, randomized, double-blinded, parallel-group, vehicle-controlled studies	N = 1371 95.6% Caucasian, 1.4% African American, 1.6% Asian, 1.3% other	A greater proportion of subjects in the ivermectin group achieved treatment success (IGA "clear" or "almost clear") at week 12 (38.4 and 40.1% for ivermectin compared to 11.6 and 18.8% for vehicle, both $p < 0.001$). Ivermectin was superior to vehicle with respect to reduction from baseline in inflammatory lesion counts (76.0 and 75.0% for ivermectin compared to 50.0% for both vehicle groups, $P < 0.001$)
Topical brimonidine	Fowler et al. [94]	Two multicenter, randomized and vehicle-controlled studies	N = 122 7 FST I, 72 FST II, 39 FST III, 3 FST IV, 1 FST V	Once-daily brimonidine tartrate gel 0.5% is well tolerated and provides statistically significantly greater efficacy than vehicle gel for the

(continued)

Table 9.2 (continued)

Agent(s)	Author(s)	Study design	Demographics	Summary of results
				treatment of moderate to severe erythema of rosacea ($P < 0.001$)
	Holmes et al. [95]	Two multicenter, randomized, double-blinded, parallel-group, vehicle-controlled Phase 3 studies; one multicenter, open-label, long-term safety study	N = 1002 86 FST I, 490 FST II, 328 FST III, 87 FST IV, 10 FST V, 1 FST VI	The most commonly reported adverse events from use of topical brimonidine 0.33% gel were flushing and erythema, occurring in 5.4% of subjects in the Phase 3 studies and 15.4% of subjects in the long-term study. These adverse events occurred early in the course of treatment, were short-lived, and mild or moderate in severity
Topical calcineurin inhibitors	Lee et al. [96]	Open-label, investigator-blinded, split-face study	N = 15 (Asian subjects, FST IV included)	Twice-daily pimecrolimus 1% cream demonstrated safety and efficacy in the treatment of steroid-induced rosacea over 8 weeks
Doxycycline monotherapy	Del Rosso et al. [97]	Two phase III, parallel-group, multicenter, randomized, double-blinded, placebo-controlled studies	N = 537 (91% Caucasian, other specifics of patient demographics not mentioned)	Monotherapy with once-daily anti-inflammatory dose of doxycycline (40 mg) demonstrated statistically significant greater reductions from baseline in total inflammatory lesion counts at week 16 compared to placebo ($P < 0.001$)
	Alexis et al. [98]	Open-label, multicenter, community-based study	N = 826 768 Caucasian, 6 African American, 11 Asian, 1 American Indian/Alaska Native, 3 Native	Subjects received doxycycline 40 mg capsules (30 mg immediate release and 10 mg delayed-release beads) once daily as monotherapy for 12 weeks. Treatment success, defined

(continued)

Table 9.2 (continued)

Agent(s)	Author(s)	Study design	Demographics	Summary of results
			Hawaiian/Pacific Islander, 37 other/mixed	as an IGA score of 0 ("clear") or 1 ("near clear") was achieved in 74.6 and 74.3% of patients with FST I-III and FST IV-VI, respectively at week 12 ($P < 0.001$)
Doxycycline + topical metronidazole	Sanchez et al. [99]	Randomized, double-blinded, placebo-controlled study	N = 40 11 Caucasian, 28 Hispanic, 1 African American	Adjunctive use of doxycycline hyclate 20 mg twice daily significantly reduced the clinical signs of rosacea in comparison with monotherapy with topical metronidazole
Doxycycline + azelaic acid	Thiboutot et al. [100]	One initial open-label, non-randomized study followed by a multicenter, double-blinded, randomized, vehicle-controlled, parallel-group study	N = 308 284 Caucasian, 12 Hispanic, 3 African American, 1 Asian, 8 other	By week 12 of the open-label phase (azelaic acid 15% gel + doxycycline 100 mg both twice daily), 81.4% of subjects had reached a 75% or greater reduction in inflammatory lesion count. During the second study (maintenance phase), azelaic acid 15% gel provided better maintenance response than vehicle

Abbreviations: *FST* Fitzpatrick skin type; *IGA* investigator global assessment acid foam, was recently approved in 2015 for the treatment of mild to moderate papulopustular rosacea. Azelaic acid is a naturally occurring dicarboxylic acid with several proposed mechanisms of action, including antimicrobial, anti-inflammatory/antioxidant, and keratinolytic properties [79]. Azelaic acid 15% gel has also been shown to directly inhibit KLK5 in cultured keratinocytes and gene expression of KLK5, Toll-like receptor-2 and cathelicidin in mouse skin, mediators that are upregulated in rosacea-affected skin [65]. Azelaic acid can provide a twofold benefit in the treatment of rosacea and hyperpigmentation in skin of color given its ability to inhibit tyrosinase.

There has been increasing interest in the use of agents that possess anti-parasitic activity in the treatment of rosacea. Many studies have demonstrated commensal *Demodex* mite overgrowth in some patients with rosacea, which is thought to exacerbate inflammation in rosacea [80]. One study reported that *Demodex folliculorum* was found in 20 of 25 rosacea patients but in only 2 of 20 control subjects, suggesting the presence of this mite in rosaceous skin could contribute to the pathophysiology of the disease [81]. Ivermectin is a semi-synthetic macrocyclic lactone derivative of the avermectin family [80]. Ivermectin inhibits lipopolysaccharide-induced production of certain inflammatory cytokines, such as TNF-α and IL-1β, and increases the anti-inflammatory cytokine IL-10 [82]. The drug's anti-inflammatory and broad-spectrum anti-parasitic properties are thought to account for its efficacy in treating rosacea [80]. A topical formulation of the drug (available in 1% cream) was FDA-approved in 2014 as a once-daily application for the treatment of papulopustular rosacea.

Brimonidine gel is a highly selective alpha-2 adrenergic receptor agonist with vasoconstrictive properties, which are thought to play a role in reducing the facial erythema in patients with rosacea. In 2013, once-daily brimonidine 0.33% gel was approved by the FDA as the first agent available for the topical treatment of persistent (nontransient) facial erythema linked to rosacea [83]. The efficacy and safety of brimonidine tartrate in the treatment of moderate to severe facial erythema has been demonstrated in multiple Phase II and III clinical trials [84].

There are case reports of an exaggerated or "rebound" erythema occurring after brimonidine tartrate use. One case series describes three female patients (1 Latino and 2 Caucasian) who experienced a reduction in erythema followed by severe rebound erythema (worse from baseline) and burning in the areas of application over the next 12 h and lasting roughly 12 h [85]. This self-limited reaction is thought to be due to a rebound dilation of capillaries caused by down-regulation of alpha-2 adrenergic receptors after use of the drug. Therefore, the clinician should advise patients to apply a small amount of the drug, select a test area, and limit use to special occasions. Educating patients about the potential for temporary worsening of erythema is critical.

Topical calcineurin inhibitors (tacrolimus and pimecrolimus) may be useful in certain situations, particularly steroid-induced rosacea. A preliminary report demonstrated the efficacy of tacrolimus ointment for the treatment of steroid-induced rosacea [86]. However, the use of topical calcineurin inhibitors for rosacea has been debated, as other case reports have described rosacea-like eruptions developing after use of tacrolimus [87] or pimecrolimus [88] for facial dermatitis.

Among the oral pharmacologic agents, the tetracycline family of antibiotics has remained the basis of systemic therapy for the treatment of moderate to severe rosacea. Several clinical trials have demonstrated the efficacy of doxycycline in the treatment of papulopustular rosacea (Table 9.2). A sub-antimicrobial dose of doxycycline is beneficial in treating rosacea as it provides anti-inflammatory effects without the potential threat of emergence of antibiotic-resistant bacteria. Other antibiotics such as oral metronidazole, dapsone, erythromycin, and penicillin have demonstrated variable success in selected rosacea patients [71].

In summary, topical and oral anti-inflammatory agents remain the standard of care for papulopustular rosacea and are often used in combination for increased efficacy. The oral antibiotic of choice is typically administered over several weeks with a gradual taper, while long-term therapy with a topical agent such as metronidazole or azelaic acid is used to maintain remission [77]. For moderate to severe cases of ocular rosacea, the tetracycline group of antibiotics has been shown to be as effective in the management of ocular rosacea in ethnic skin as previously described in Caucasian patients [72]. In recalcitrant, severe cases of rosacea, oral administration of isotretinoin (13-cis-retinoid acid) is beneficial and has been studied in African-American patients [71]. Unfortunately, relapses may occur after discontinuation of therapy. Treatment of rhinophyma is largely via surgical approaches, including carbon dioxide laser, electrosurgery, or surgical excision. Light-based therapy with the intense pulsed light and pulsed dye laser have shown efficacy in decreasing the erythema and telangiectasias, however, due to the risk of dyschromia and scarring in patients with darker skin types, there is limited data regarding such procedures in skin of color patients with rosacea.

Conclusion

Acne remains the leading dermatologic condition among patients with skin of color in this nation. Rosacea, an entity previously assumed to be rare among ethnic racial groups, is often underrecognized but should be considered among the differential diagnoses of facial erythema in skin of color patients. In general, the pathogenesis and treatments for acne and rosacea are similar to Caucasian skin; however, special attention should be aimed at minimizing potential outcomes that are increasingly more frequent in skin of color, such as post-inflammatory pigmentary alterations and scarring. PIH associated with acne is a critical concern among skin of color patients; therefore, early recognition and treatment of PIH in a balanced, effective manner is key to improving patient outcomes. It is the authors' hope that this comprehensive chapter provides the clinician with a detailed approach to the diagnosis and treatment of acne and rosacea in skin of color.

References

1. Davis SA, Narahari S, Feldman SR, Huang W, Pichardo-Geisinger RO, McMichael AJ. Top dermatologic conditions in patients of color: an analysis of nationally representative data. J Drugs Dermatol. 2012;11:466–73.
2. Lawson C, Hollinger J, Sethi S, Rodney I, Sarkar R, Dlova N, Callender V. Updates in the understanding and treatments of skin & hair disorders in women of color. Int J Womens Dermatol. 2015;1(2):59–75.
3. Perkins AC, Cheng CE, Hillebrand GG, Miyamoto K, Kimball AB. Comparison of the epidemiology of acne vulgaris among Caucasians, Asian, Continental Indian and African American women. J Eur Acad Dermatol Venerol. 2011;25:1054–60.
4. Alexis AF, Sergay AB, Taylor SC. Common dermatologic disorders in skin of color: a comparative practice survey. Cutis. 2007;80:387–94.
5. Halder RM, Grimes PE, McLaurin CI, Kress MA, Kenney JA. Incidence of common dermatoses in a predominantly black dermatologic practice. Cutis. 1983;32:388–90.
6. Taylor SC, Cook-Bolden F, Rahman Z, Strachan D. Acne vulgaris in skin of color. J Am Acad Dermatol. 2002;46(suppl 2):S98–106.
7. Warrier AG, Kligman AM, Harper RA, Bowman J, Wickett RR. A comparison of black and white skin using non-invasive methods. J Soc Cosmet Chem. 1996;47:229–40.
8. Nicolaides N, Rothman S. Studies on the chemical composition of human hair fat. II, The overall composition with regard to age, sex and race. J Invest Dermatol. 1952;21:90.
9. Kligman AM, Shelley WB. An investigation of the biology of the sebaceous gland. J Invest Dermatol. 1958;30:99–125.
10. Kircik N. Advances in the understanding of the pathogenesis of inflammatory acne. J Drugs Dermatol. 2016;15(1 Suppl 1):s7–10.
11. Halder RM, Holmes YC, Bridgeman-Shah S, Kligman AM. A clinicohistopathologic study of acne vulgaris in black females. J Invest Dermatol. 1996;106:888.
12. Halder RM, Brooks HL, Callender VD. Acne in ethnic skin. Dermatol Clin. 2003;21(4):609–15, vii.
13. Callender VD. Acne in ethnic skin: special considerations for therapy. Dermatol Ther. 2004;17:184–95.
14. Callender VD, Alexis AF, Daniels SR, Kawata AK, Burk CT, Wilcox TK, Taylor SC. Racial differences in clinical characteristics, perceptions and behaviors, and psychosocial impact of adult female acne. J Clin Aesthet Dermatol. 2014;7(7):19–31.
15. Rendon MI, Rodriguez DA, Kawata AK, Degboe AN, Wilcox TK, Burk CT, Daniels SR, Roberts WE. Acne treatment patterns, expectations, and satisfaction among adult females of different races/ethnicities. Clin Cosmet Investig Dermatol. 2015;2(8):231–8.
16. Taylor S, Badreshia-Bansal S, Callender V, Gathers R, Rodriguez D. Treatments for skin of color. Edinburgh: Saunders; 2011.
17. Spann CT. Ten tips for treating acne vulgaris in Fitzpatrick skin types IV-VI. J Drugs Dermatol. 2011;10(6):654–7.
18. Shah SK, Alexis AF. Acne in skin of color: practical approaches to treatment. J Dermatol Treat. 2010;21:206–11.
19. Davis EC, Callender VD. A review of acne in ethnic skin: pathogenesis, clinical manifestations, and management strategies. J Clin Aesthet Dermatol. 2010;3:24–38.
20. Wolf JE Jr. Potential anti-inflammatory effects of topical retinoids and retinoid analogues. Adv Ther. 2002;19(3):109–18.
21. Ortonne JP, Passeron T. Melanin pigmentary disorders: treatment update. Dermatol Clin. 2005;23(2):209–26.
22. Halder RM. The role of retinoids in the management of cutaneous conditions in blacks. J Am Acad Dermatol. 1998;39(2 Pt 3):S98–103.
23. Geria AN, Lawson CN, Halder RM. Topical retinoids for pigmented skin. J Drugs Dermatol. 2011;10(5):483–9.

24. Zeichner J. Strategies to minimize irritation and potential iatrogenic post-inflammatory pigmentation when treating acne patients with skin of color. J Drugs Dermatol. 2011;10(12 Suppl):s25–6.
25. Mills OH Jr, Kligman AM, Pochi P, Comite H. Comparing 2.5%, 5%, and 10% benzoyl peroxide on inflammatory acne vulgaris. Int J Dermatol. 1986;25(10):664–7.
26. Leyden J, Levy S. The development of antibiotic resistance in Propionibacterium acnes. Cutis. 2001;67(2 Suppl):21–4.
27. Vargas-Diez E, Hofmann MA, Bravo B, Malgazhdarova G, Katkhanova OA, Yutskovskaya Y. Azelaic acid in the treatment of acne in adult females: case reports. Skin Pharmacol Physiol. 2014;27(Suppl 1):18–25.
28. Draelos ZD, Carter E, Maloney JM, Elewski B, Poulin Y, Lynde C, Garrett S; United States/Canada Dapsone Gel Study Group. Two randomized studies demonstrate the efficacy and safety of dapsone gel, 5% for the treatment of acne vulgaris. J Am Acad Dermatol. 2007;56:439.e1–10.
29. Fellner C. Pharmaceutical approval update. P T. 2016;41(4):220–1.
30. Kircik LH. Doxycycline and minocycline for the management of acne: a review of efficacy and safety with emphasis on clinical implications. J Drugs Dermatol. 2010;9:1407–11.
31. Mouton RW, Jordaan HF, Schneider JW. A new type of minocycline-induced cutaneous hyperpigmentation. Clin Exp Dermatol. 2004;29:8–14.
32. Soung J, Cohen J, Phelps R, Cohen S. Case reports: minocycline-induced hyperpigmentation resolves during oral isotretinoin therapy. J Drugs Dermatol. 2007;6:1232–6.
33. Sturkenboom MC, Meier CR, Jick H, Stricker BH. Minocycline and lupuslike syndrome in acne patients. Arch Intern Med. 1999;159(5):493–7.
34. Muller P, Dubreil P, Mahé A, Lamaury I, Salzer B, Deloumeaux J, Strobel M. Drug hypersensitivity syndrome in a West-Indian population. Eur J Dermatol. 2003;13(5):478–81.
35. Zeichner JA. Evaluating and treating the adult female patient with acne. J Drugs Dermatol. 2013;12:1418–27.
36. Alexis AF. Acne vulgaris in skin of color: understanding nuances and optimizing treatment outcomes. J Drugs Dermatol. 2014;13(6):s61–5.
37. Kelly AP, Sampson DD. Recalcitrant nodulocystic acne in black Americans: treatment with isotretinoin. J Natl Med Assoc. 1987;79:1266–70.
38. Ghaffarpour G, Mazloomi S, Soltani-Arabshahi R, Seyed KS. Oral isotretinoin for acne, adjusting treatment according to patient's response. J Drugs Dermatol. 2006;5(9):878–82.
39. Ng PP, Goh CL. Treatment outcome of acne vulgaris with oral isotretinoin in 89 patients. Int J Dermatol. 1999;38(3):213–6.
40. Dhir R, Gehi NP, Agarwal R, More YE. Oral isotretinoin is as effective as a combination of oral isotretinoin and topical anti-acne agents in nodulocystic acne. Indian J Dermatol Venereol Leprol. 2008;74(2):187.
41. Levin CY, Maibach H. Exogenous ochronosis. An update on clinical features, causative agents and treatment options. Am J Clin Dermatol. 2001;2(4):213–7.
42. Woolery-Lloyd HC, Keri J, Doig S. Retinoids and azelaic acid to treat acne and hyperpigmentation in skin of color. J Drugs Dermatol. 2013;12(4):434–7.
43. Karnik J, Baumann L, Bruce S, Callender V, Cohen S, Grimes P, Joseph J, Shamban A, Spencer J, Teldaldi R, Werschler W, Smith S. A double-blind, randomized, multicenter, controlled trial of suspended polymethylmethacrylate microspheres for the correction of atrophic facial acne scars. J Am Acad Dermatol. 2014;71:77–83.
44. Cohen BE, Elbuluk N. Microneedling in skin of color: a review of uses and efficacy. J Am Acad Dermatol. 2016;74(2):348–55.
45. Jacyk WK, Mpofu P. Adapalene gel 0.1% for topical treatment of acne vulgaris in African patients. Cutis. 2001;68(4 Suppl):48–54.
46. Tu P, Li GQ, Zhu XJ, et al. A comparison of adapalene gel 0.1% vs. tretinoin gel 0.025% in the treatment of acne vulgaris in China. J Eur Acad Dermatol Venereol. 2001;15(Suppl 3):31–6.

47. Goh CL, Tang MB, Briantais P, Kaoukhov A, Soto P. Adapalene gel 0.1% is better tolerated than tretinoin gel 0.025% among healthy volunteers of various ethnic origins. J Dermatolog Treat. 2009;20(5):282–8.
48. Tirado-Sanchez A, Espindola YS, Ponce-Olivera RM, Bonifaz A. Efficacy and safety of adapalene gel 0.1% and 0.3% and tretinoin gel 0.05% for acne vulgaris: results of a single-center, randomized, double-blinded, placebo-controlled clinical trial on Mexican patients (skin type III-IV). J Cosmet Dermatol. 2013;12:103–7.
49. Grimes PE, Callender VD. Tazarotene cream for postinflammatory hyperpigmentation and acne vulgaris in darker skin: a double-blind, randomized, vehicle-controlled study. Cutis. 2006;77:45–50.
50. Alexis AF, Johnson LA, Kerrouche N, Callender VD. A subgroup analysis to evaluate the efficacy and safety of adapalene-benzoyl peroxide topical gel in black subjects with moderate acne. J Drugs Dermatol. 2014;13:170–4.
51. Callender VD. Fitzpatrick skin types and clindamycin phosphate 1.2%/benzoyl peroxide gel: efficacy & tolerability of treatment in moderate to severe acne. J Drugs Dermatol. 2012;11:643–8.
52. Callender VD, Young CM, Kindred C, Taylor SC. Efficacy and safety of clindamycin phosphate 1.2% and tretinoin 0.025% gel for the treatment of acne and acne-induced post-inflammatory hyperpigmentation in patients with skin of color. J Clin Aesthet Dermatol. 2012;5:25–32.
53. Kircik LH. Efficacy and safety of azelaic acid (AzA) gel 15% in the treatment of post-inflammatory hyperpigmentation and acne: a 16-week, baseline-controlled study. J Drugs Dermatol. 2011;10:586–90.
54. Piette WW, Taylor S, Pariser D, Jarratt M, Sheth P, Wilson D. Hematologic safety of dapsone gel, 5%, for topical treatment of acne vulgaris. Arch Dermatol. 2008;144:1564–70.
55. Alexis AF, Burgess C, Callender VD, Herzog JL, Roberts WE, Schweiger ES, Stockton TC, Gallagher CJ. The efficacy and safety of topical dapsone gel, 5% for the treatment of acne vulgaris in adult females with skin of color. J Drugs Dermatol. 2016;15(2):197–204.
56. Thiboutot DM, Shalita AR, Yamauchi PS, Dawson C, Arsonnaud S, Kang S; Differin Study Group. Combination therapy with adapalene gel 0.1% and doxycycline for severe acne vulgaris: a multicenter, investigator-blind, randomized, controlled study. Skinmed. 2005;4 (3):138–46.
57. Fleischer AB Jr, Dinehart S, Stough D, Plott RT; Solodyn Phase 2 Study Group; Solodyn Phase 3 Study Group. Safety and efficacy of a new extended-release formulation of minocycline. Cutis. 2006;78:21–31.
58. Ullah G, Noor SM, Bhatti Z, Ahmad M, Bangash AR. Comparison of oral azithromycin with oral doxycycline in the treatment of acne vulgaris. Br J Dermatol. 2014;171:1508–16.
59. Tan J, Humphrey S, Vender R, Barankin B, Gooderham M, Kerrouche N, Audibert F, Lynde C; POWER study group. A treatment for severe nodular acne: a randomized investigator-blinded, controlled, noninferiority trial comparing fixed-dose adapalene/benzoyl peroxide plus doxycycline vs. oral isotretinoin. Br J Dermatol. 2014;171:1508–16.
60. Fabbrocini G, De Vita V, Monfrecola A, De Padova MP, Brazzini B, Teixeira F, Chu A. Percutaneous collagen induction: an effective and safe treatment for post-acne scarring in different skin phototypes. J Dermatolog Treat. 2014;25(2):147–52.
61. Alexis AF, Coley MK, Nijhawan RI, Luke JD, Shah SK, Argobi YA, Nodzenski M, Veledar E, Alam M. Nonablative fractional laser resurfacing for acne scarring in patients with Fitzpatrick skin phototypes IV–VI. Dermatol Surg. 2016;42(3):392–402.
62. Alexis AF. Rosacea in patients with skin of color: uncommon but not rare. Cutis. 2010;86 (2):60–2.
63. Al-Dabagh A, Davis SA, McMichael AJ, Feldman SR. Rosacea in skin of color: not a rare diagnosis. Dermatol Online J. 2014;20(10).

64. Jayawant SS, Feldman SR, Camacho FT, Yentzer B, Balkrishnan R. Prescription refills and healthcare costs associated with topical metronidazole in Medicaid enrolled patients with rosacea. J Dermatolog Treat. 2008;19(5):267–73.
65. Coda AB, Hata T, Miller J, Audish D, Kotol P, Two A, Shafiq F, Yamasaki K, Harper JC, Del Rosso JQ, Gallo RL. Cathelicidin, kallikrein 5, and serine protease activity is inhibited during treatment of rosacea with azelaic acid 15% gel. J Am Acad Dermatol. 2013;69 (4):570–7.
66. Bae YI, Yun SJ, Lee JB, Kim SJ, Won YH, Lee SC. Clinical evaluation of 168 Korean patients with rosacea: the sun exposure correlates with the erythematotelangiectatic subtype. Ann Dermatol. 2009;21(3):243–9.
67. Culp B, Scheinfeld N. Rosacea: a review. P T. 2009;34(1):38–45.
68. Khoo CT, Saad MN. Rhinophyma in a negro: case report. Br J Plast Surg. 1980;33(2): 161–3.
69. Furukawa M, Kanetou K, Hamada T. Rhinophyma in Japan. Int J Dermatol. 1994;33(1): 35–7.
70. Al Balbeesi AO, Halawani MR. Unusual features of rosacea in saudi females with dark skin. Ochsner J. 2014;14(3):321–7.
71. Rosen T, Stone MS. Acne rosacea in blacks. J Am Acad Dermatol. 1987;17(1):70–3.
72. Browning DJ, Rosenwasser G, Lugo M. Ocular rosacea in blacks. Am J Ophthalmol. 1986;101(4):441–4.
73. Williams HC, Ashworth J, Pembroke AC, Breathnach SM. FACE–facial Afro-Caribbean childhood eruption. Clin Exp Dermatol. 1990;15(3):163–6.
74. Child FJ, Fuller LC, Higgins EM, Du Vivier AW. A study of the spectrum of skin disease occurring in a black population in south-east London. Br J Dermatol. 1999;141(3):512–7.
75. Pelle MT, Crawford GH, James WD. Rosacea: II. Therapy. J Am Acad Dermatol. 2004;51 (4):499–512; quiz 513–4.
76. Nielsen PG. Treatment of rosacea with 1% metronidazole cream. A double-blind study. Br J Dermatol. 1983;108(3):327–32.
77. Wolf JE Jr. The role of topical metronidazole in the treatment of rosacea. Cutis. 2004;73(1 Suppl):19–28.
78. Del Rosso JQ, Kircik LH. Update on the management of rosacea: a status report on the current role and new horizons with topical azelaic acid. J Drugs Dermatol. 2014;13(12): s101–7.
79. Del Rosso JQ, Baum EW, Draelos ZD, Elewski BE, Fleischer AB Jr, Kakita LS, Thiboutot D. Azelaic acid gel 15%: clinical versatility in the treatment of rosacea. Cutis. 2006;78(5 Suppl):6–19.
80. Deeks ED. Ivermectin: a review in Rosacea. Am J Clin Dermatol. 2015;16(5):447–52.
81. Sibenge S, Gawkrodger DJ. Rosacea: a study of clinical patterns, blood flow, and the role of Demodex folliculorum. J Am Acad Dermatol. 1992;26(4):590–3.
82. Scheinfeld N. 1% Ivermectin cream (Soolantra) for the treatment of Rosacea. Skinmed. 2015;13(3):222–4.
83. Johnson AW, Johnson SM. The role of topical brimonidine tartrate gel as a novel therapeutic option for persistent facial erythema associated with Rosacea. Dermatol Ther (Heidelb). 2015;5(3):171–81.
84. Jackson JM, Knuckles M, Minni JP, Johnson SM, Belasco KT. The role of brimonidine tartrate gel in the treatment of rosacea. Clin Cosmet Investig Dermatol. 2015;23(8):529–38.
85. Routt ET, Levitt JO. Rebound erythema and burning sensation from a new topical brimonidine tartrate gel 0.33%. J Am Acad Dermatol. 2014;70(2):e37–8.
86. Goldman D. Tacrolimus ointment for the treatment of steroid-induced rosacea: a preliminary report. J Am Acad Dermatol. 2001;44:995–8.
87. Fujiwara S, Okubo Y, Irisawa R, Tsuboi R. Rosaceiform dermatitis associated with topical tacrolimus treatment. J Am Acad Dermatol. 2010;62(6):1050–2.
88. El-Heis S, Buckley DA. Rosacea-like eruption due to topical pimecrolimus. Dermatol Online J. 2015;18;21(5).

89. Elewski BE, Fleischer AB Jr, Pariser DM. A comparison of 15% azelaic acid gel and 0.75% metronidazole gel in the topical treatment of papulopustular Rosacea: results of a randomized trial. Arch Dermatol. 2003;139(11):1444–50.

90. Wolf JE Jr, Kerrouche N, Arsonnaud S. Efficacy and safety of once-daily metronidazole 1% gel compared with twice-daily azelaic acid 15% gel in the treatment of rosacea. Cutis. 2006;77(4 Suppl):3–11.

91. Colón LE, Johnson LA, Gottschalk RW. Cumulative irritation potential among metronidazole gel 1%, metronidazole gel 0.75%, and azelaic acid gel 15%. Cutis. 2007;79(4):317–21.

92. Thiboutot D, Thieroff-Ekerdt R, Graupe K. Efficacy and safety of azelaic acid (15%) gel as a new treatment for papulopustular Rosacea: results from two vehicle-controlled, randomized phase III studies. J Am Acad Dermatol. 2003;48(6):836–45.

93. Stein L, Kircik L, Fowler J, Tan J, Draelos Z, Fleischer A, Appell M, Steinhoff M, Lynde C, Liu H, Jacovella J. Efficacy and safety of ivermectin 1% cream in treatment of papulopustular Rosacea: results of two randomized, double-blind, vehicle-controlled pivotal studies. J Drugs Dermatol. 2014;13(3):316–23.

94. Fowler J, Jarratt M, Moore A, Meadows K, Pollack A, Steinhoff M, Liu Y, Leoni M on behalf of the Brimonidine Phase II Study Group. Once-daily topical brimonidine tartrate gel 0.5% is a novel treatment for moderate to severe facial erythema of rosacea: results of two multicentre, randomized and vehicle-controlled studies. Br J Dermatol. 2012; 166(3): 633–641.

95. Holmes AD, Waite KA, Chen MC, Palaniswamy K, Wiser TH, Draelos ZD, Rafal ES, Werschler WP, Harvey AE. Dermatological adverse events associated with topical brimonidine gel 0.33% in subjects with erythema of Rosacea: a retrospective review of clinical studies. J Clin Aesthet Dermatol. 2015;8(8):29–35.

96. Lee DH, Li K, Suh DH. Pimecrolimus 1% cream for the treatment of steroid-induced rosacea: an 8-week split-face clinical trial. Br J Dermatol. 2008;158(5):1069–76.

97. Del Rosso JQ, Webster GF, Jackson M, Rendon M, Rich P, Torok H, Bradshaw M. Two randomized phase III clinical trials evaluating anti-inflammatory dose doxycycline (40-mg doxycycline, USP capsules) administered once daily for treatment of Rosacea. J Am Acad Dermatol. 2007;56(5):791–802.

98. Alexis AF, Webster G, Preston NJ, Caveney SW, Gottschalk RW. Effectiveness and safety of once-daily doxycycline capsules as monotherapy in patients with Rosacea: an analysis by Fitzpatrick skin type. J Drugs Dermatol. 2012;11(10):1219–22.

99. Sanchez J, Somolinos AL, Almodóvar PI, Webster G, Bradshaw M, Powala C. A randomized, double-blind, placebo-controlled trial of the combined effect of doxycycline hyclate 20-mg tablets and metronidazole 0.75% topical lotion in the treatment of Rosacea. J Am Acad Dermatol. 2005;53(5):791–7.

100. Thiboutot DM, Fleischer AB, Del Rosso JQ, Rich P. A multicenter study of topical azelaic acid 15% gel in combination with oral doxycycline as initial therapy and azelaic acid 15% gel as maintenance monotherapy. J Drugs Dermatol. 2009;8(7):639–48.

Chapter 10
Inflammatory Disorders

Porcia Bradford Love

Atopic Dermatitis

Atopic dermatitis, also known as eczema, is a common inflammatory skin disease characterized by pruritic, erythematous scaly patches. Patients have a chronic, relapsing course, and many have an "atopic tendency," meaning they may develop any combination of atopic dermatitis, asthma, and allergic rhinitis.

Epidemiology

Atopic dermatitis is the most common inflammatory skin condition and has an estimated prevalence of 17% in the United States [1]. Atopic dermatitis is more common in industrialized nations and urban areas. Immigrants from developing countries living in developed countries have a higher incidence of atopic dermatitis than the indigenous population [2]. Atopic dermatitis affects all ages; however, the majority of cases occur before age 5. The disease may have periods of complete remission, particularly in adolescence, and may then recur in early adult life. Atopic dermatitis occurs in all races and ethnicities; however, it disproportionately affects patients with skin of color [3]. There is an increased incidence in patients of African and Asian descent [4, 5], and a 1993–2009 National Ambulatory Medical Care Survey showed that atopic dermatitis was in the top ten diagnoses for African Americans and Asians, but not Caucasians [6]. African-American children are more

P.B. Love (✉)
River region Dermatology and Laser, University of Alabama School of Medicine,
2060 Berryhill Road, Montgomery, AL 36117, USA
e-mail: porcialove@gmail.com

© Springer International Publishing AG 2017
N.A. Vashi and H.I. Maibach (eds.), *Dermatoanthropology of Ethnic Skin and Hair*, DOI 10.1007/978-3-319-53961-4_10

likely than Caucasian children to have severe atopic dermatitis [7], potentially due to poor access to care or delayed diagnosis. However, there is a lack of research studies.

Pathophysiology

The pathophysiology of atopic dermatitis remains poorly defined. The predominant theory is that there is alteration of the epithelial barrier, possibly leading to the entry of antigens, as well as immune dysregulation resulting in the production of inflammatory cytokines [8]. Mutations in the gene encoding filaggrin, a key epidermal barrier protein, cause ichthyosis vulgaris and are the strongest known genetic risk factors for the development of AD [9]. Filaggrin mutations are associated with early-onset atopic dermatitis and with airway disease in the setting of atopic dermatitis [10]. Although filaggrin is strongly linked to atopic dermatitis, mutations are only found in 30% of European patients, begging the question of whether other genetic variants may also be responsible for some of the findings in the pathogenesis of atopic dermatitis [11]. Given the fact that filaggrin is critical for epithelial integrity, it is now thought that loss of filaggrin function leads to increased transepidermal penetration of environmental allergens, increasing inflammation and sensitivity and potentially leading to the atopic march [12].

Clinical Presentation

Atopic dermatitis is characterized by pruritus, erythema, lichenification, and scale (Fig. 10.1a, b). Erythema is often difficult to appreciate in dark skin. Instead, edema, warmth of skin, and scaling in particular distributions are clues to the diagnosis of atopic dermatitis in darker skin tones [13]. The SCORAD (SCORing Atopic Dermatitis), a clinical tool used to assess the extent and severity of atopic dermatitis, is often worse in African Americans [14].

Atopic dermatitis can present differently in different age groups. In infants, pruritic, erythematous patches and plaques are common on the forehead, cheeks, trunk, and extensor surfaces. There is often secondary edema, fissuring, and crusting. Severe pruritus often disturbs sleeping patterns [1]. Children ages 2–13 often display lichenified plaques on the hands, antecubital and popliteal fossa, and feet [1]. In adults, atopic dermatitis is often found on the face, neck, and upper arms.

In skin of color, especially darker skin, a follicular subset of atopic dermatitis is often found. It is characterized by monomorphic follicular papules coalescing into plaques on the trunk and extensors (Fig. 10.1c) [7, 13]. Patients with atopic dermatitis also have an increased risk of secondary infections, including staphyloccus aureus, herpes simplex, molluscum contagiosum, and warts [1]. Palmar hyperlinearity, periorbital involvement, perifollicular accentuation, keratosis pilaris, and

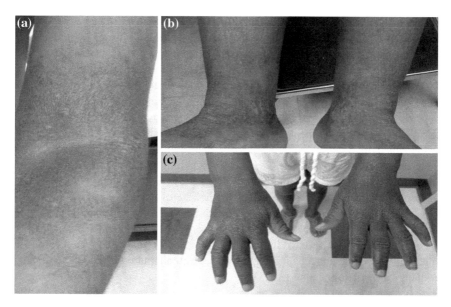

Fig. 10.1 Atopic dermatitis. Erythematous, eczematous patches are noted on the antecubital fossa (**a**) and feet (**b**). The follicular variant of atopic dermatitis is noted on the hands (**c**)

ichthyosis vulgaris [13] are also seen. One-third of atopic dermatitis patients also have asthma or allergic rhinitis.

Histopathology

Atopic dermatitis is typically diagnosed clinically. Classic histopathologic findings will show an acute, subacute, or chronic spongiotic dermatitis.

Treatment

The treatment of atopic dermatitis is the same among ethnic groups. Topical corticosteroids reduce inflammation and pruritus. It is important to give an adequate amount to cover the affected area [15]. Fluticasone is a topical steroid that can be used in infants as young as 3 months [16]. The side effects of topical steroids should be discussed with patients and include striae, telangiectasias, skin thinning, perioral dermatitis, acneiform eruptions, hypothalamic–pituitary–adrenal (HPA) axis suppression, and hypopigmentation [15]. Topical calcineurin inhibitors like tacrolimus and pimecrolimus are steroid sparing agents that inhibit transcription of inflammatory cytokines.

Patients with extensive involvement or who are unresponsive to topical treatments need systemic therapy. Options include systemic corticosteroids, methotrexate, azathioprine, mycophenolate mofetil, and cyclosporine. Of note, African Americans may need higher doses of cyclosporine to maintain therapeutic concentrations, due to its lower bioavailability compared to Caucasians [15]. African Americans are also at risk for azathioprine toxicity due to thiopurine methyltransferase (TPMT) enzyme deficiencies since azathioprine is partially metabolized by the TMPT enzyme [7]. Narrowband UVB phototherapy may also be used to treat atopic dermatitis.

Patients with atopic dermatitis have a compromised epidermal barrier, with enhanced transepidermal water loss. Therefore, skin hydration and moisturizers are important. Bleach baths are thought to decrease the risk of secondary infection [16]. African Americans have lower ceramide to cholesterol ratios, thus an increased risk of xerosis; therefore, higher potency steroids in ointment formulation are often needed [15]. Family education and a plan for flares and maintenance must be stressed. The patient should also avoid irritants and food allergies. It is also important to ask patients about complementary and alternative medicine treatment, as many can irritate the skin [17].

Psoriasis

Psoriasis vulgaris is a chronic, multifactorial, hyperproliferative skin disease. Skin disease may be associated with arthritis.

Epidemiology

Psoriasis appears to be most prevalent in northern European populations and is thought to be observed less frequently in patients with skin of color; however, there is a lack of consensus on the issue. In one study, patients with psoriasis constituted approximately only 0.8% of dermatology cases in Northern Nigeria over five years [18]. However, a population based study in the United States from 2005 showed that although psoriasis is less common in African Americans than in Caucasians, it is not rare and carries a substantial burden in both groups. The prevalence of psoriasis was 2.5% in Caucasians and 1.3% in African Americans. African Americans had an approximately 52% reduction in the prevalence of psoriasis compared with Caucasians [19]. In a cross-sectional study using National Health and Nutrition Examination Survey data from 2009 to 2010, the psoriasis prevalence was highest in Caucasians at 3.6%, followed by African Americans (1.9%), Hispanics (1.6%), and others (1.4%) [20]. The psoriasis prevalence is estimated to be approximately 0.3% in Asians (18). Psoriasis, even severe psoriasis, may occur in the pediatric age group, with a prevalence of 0.5–2% of children [21].

Pathophysiology

The pathogenesis of psoriasis is not completely understood; however, it is thought that genetic and immune-mediated factors lead to immune dysregulation and hyperproliferation of epidermal keratinocytes with increased epidermal cell turnover. Numerous agents have been found to trigger psoriasis, including an infectious episode (staphylococcus, streptococcus, HIV), traumatic insult (i.e., surgery), alcohol, or medications (beta blockers, steroid withdrawal, lithium, antimalarials) [22]. Once triggered, there appears to be substantial leukocyte recruitment to the dermis and epidermis resulting in the characteristic psoriatic plaques [23]. Extensive research in recent decades has shown that the major inflammatory cells are T-cells which, once activated, induce changes in keratinocytes, vascular endothelial cells, and other inflammatory cells. Patients with psoriasis have a genetic predisposition for the disease, with the HLA-Cw6 antigen having the strongest association with psoriasis. The presence of HLA-Cw6 correlates with early age at onset and a positive family history [24]. HLA-Cw6 is found in approximately 50–80% of Caucasian psoriatic patients [25]. However, in Asian studies, 17–18% of Chinese [26] and Taiwanese [27] psoriatic patients, respectively, were found to have the HLA Cw6 allele. Obesity is another factor associated with psoriasis. The onset or worsening of psoriasis with weight gain and/or improvement with weight loss is observed [28].

Clinical Manifestations

Psoriasis presents similarly across skin types. Psoriasis is characterized by erythematous, well-demarcated plaques with silvery scale (Fig. 10.2a, b). Lesions are most commonly found on the elbows, knees, scalp, umbilicus, and intergluteal folds. The palms and soles may contain sterile pustules and thick scale. External trauma (rubbing, scratching, surgery) may lead to the koebner phenomenon [23]. In darker skin, the distribution is similar; however, plaques are violaceous with gray scale, and erythema is sometimes difficult to identify (Fig. 10.2c). Nonpustular psoriasis has two peak age ranges; early onset occurs in the second decade and late onset peaks between the ages of 50 and 60 [29].

Guttate psoriasis is characterized by the rapid onset of red, salmon-colored papules and plaques that may be covered with fine silvery scale. In darker skin, violaceous and gray colors predominate. Guttate psoriasis most commonly occurs in young patients and is often associated with viral or streptococcal pharyngitis. Pustular psoriasis is characterized by groups of sterile pustules at the periphery of stable plaques. Pustular psoriasis may occur as a primary manifestation of palmoplantar psoriasis and can be confused with dyshidrotic eczema. Generalized psoriasis, a potentially fatal disorder, is characterized by large sheets of pustules on a fiery red base. It is seen in patients with extensive psoriasis who have been treated with systemic or intensive and prolonged topical corticosteroids. Patients often have systemic symptoms (fever, chills, or peripheral leukocytosis). Erythrodermic

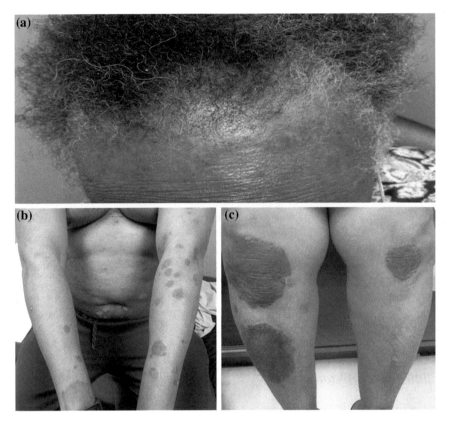

Fig. 10.2 Psoriasis. Erythematous, well-demarcated plaques with silvery scale are noted on the scalp (**a**) and arms (**b**). In *darker* skin, the distribution is similar; however, plaques are often *brown* or violaceous, and erythema is sometimes difficult to appreciate (**c**)

psoriasis is characterized by generalized redness, scaling, and warmth of the skin. Body temperature is often erratic, and patients are severely ill, secondary to sudden withdrawal of long-term steroids [29].

Psoriasiform nail changes have no relationship to severity of disease. Nail findings include nail pitting (most common finding), leukonychia, longitudinal grooves and ridges, the oil drop sign, and subungual hyperkeratosis. Psoriatic arthritis affects approximately 10–30% of those with skin disease. It produces stiffness, pain, and progressive joint damage, usually in the hands and feet [29].

Recent studies show an association between psoriasis and an adverse cardiometabolic profile. Outcome-based studies often suggest that patients with more severe psoriasis have an increased risk of major cardiovascular events independent of traditional risk factors [30].

Histopathology

Psoriasis is typically diagnosed clinically; however, some cases may be difficult to recognize. In difficult cases and to rule out alternative diagnoses, biopsy of the skin can be undertaken. Classic histopathologic findings include parakeratosis, basal cell hyperplasia, proliferation of subepidermal vasculature, and absence of normal cell maturation. In addition, polymorphonuclear leukocytes and lymphocytes are seen to infiltrate the dermis and epidermis.

Treatment

Treatment for psoriasis is similar across ethnicities. Mild to moderate psoriasis is treated with topical corticosteroids, vitamin D derivatives, topical calcineurin inhibitors, retinoids, anthralin, and tar-based formulations. For psoriasis that is nonresponsive to topical treatments and for moderate to severe psoriasis, systemic treatment is often needed. Options include systemic retinoids, methotrexate, cyclosporine, and apremilast [31]. Many of the systemic therapies for psoriasis manipulate the function of the immune system and expose the patient to the risk of severe infections while blunting the body's response. In these patients, findings suggestive of minor infections must be taken seriously, and the risk versus the benefit of continuing the drug in the face of the infection must be weighed [31].

Biologic immune modifying agents have revolutionized psoriasis therapy. Several are now available and block TNF-alpha, IL 12/23, and IL 17, all inflammatory cytokines involved in psoriasis pathogenesis. The risks of these biologic agents include infections, tuberculosis reactivation, and hematologic malignancies [32]. Therefore, the benefit of using these medications must be weighed against the side effects while selecting appropriate patients for treatment. Phototherapy may also be used to treat moderate to severe plaque psoriasis. There is a risk of increased pigmentation (tanning) and post-inflammatory hyperpigmentation in skin of color. Various ultraviolet (UV) light treatments are used, with UVB being the most common, although psoralen + UVB (PUVA) is still used. [33]. It is also important to control cardiometabolic factors and to counsel patients that stress can exacerbate the condition.

Lichen Planus

Lichen planus is an autoimmune inflammatory mucocutaneous condition that can affect the scalp, oral mucosa, skin, and nails.

Epidemiology

Lichen planus can be found in approximately 1% of adults. There is no overt racial predisposition, and women develop the condition more than men. Two-thirds develop the disease between 30 and 60 years old; however, lichen planus can occur at any age [34, 35]. Oral lichen planus is found in 50–70% of cutaneous lichen planus, and cutaneous lichen planus is found in 10–20% of oral lichen planus. One-fourth has solely mucosal involvement [35]. More than two-thirds of lichen planus patients are aged 30–60 years;

Pathogenesis

Lichen planus is a T-cell-mediated autoimmune process against basal keratinocytes. Caspase 3 is often elevated in cutaneous and oral lesions, and it is suspected that apoptosis of basal keratinocytes as mediated by cytotoxic T-cells is involved [36]. Five percent of hepatitis C patients have lichen planus. Medications that may cause lichen planus include beta blockers, ACE inhibitors, NSAIDs, antimalarials, quinidine, hydrochlorothiazide, gold, and penicillamine. Autoimmune liver disease, myasthenia gravis, and ulcerative colitis may also be associated with lichen planus [35]. There is a higher prevalence of serum autoantibodies in Chinese patients with oral lichen planus [37], and a strong correlation between the presence of hepatitis C and lichen planus in the Japanese. In one study, longstanding hepatitis C virus infection, hypoalbuminemia, and smoking were significant risk factors for the presence of oral lichen planus in patients [38]. In oral lichen planus, prolonged exposure to amalgam fillings has been implicated. Many have regression of disease with removal of the metal [39].

Clinical Features

Cutaneous lichen planus is characterized by small, polygonal, violaceous, flat-topped papules that coalesce into plaques (Fig. 10.3). The surface is often shiny with a network of fine lines, also known as Wickham's striae. The koebner phenomenon is commonly seen. Lesions often involve the flexor surfaces of the wrists and forearms, the dorsal surfaces of the hands, and the anterior aspect of the lower legs. In skin of color, the classic purple color may be black, gray, brown, or violaceous. If exacerbation occurs, it usually takes 2–16 weeks for maximal spread to occur. Lesions are intensely pruritic, often out of proportion to the amount of disease [35]. There are numerous variants of lichen planus (Table 10.1).

Lichen planus actinicus, also known as actinic lichen planus, is a photo distributed variant of lichen planus more common in darker skinned individuals from

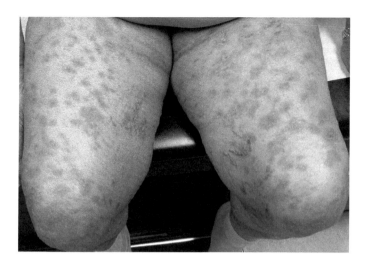

Fig. 10.3 Lichen planus. Polygonal, violaceous, flat-topped papules that coalesce into plaques with Wickham's striae are noted on the thighs

Table 10.1 Variants of lichen planus (Adapted from [35])

Variants	Characteristics	Notes
Acute lichen planus	Eruptive lesions that occur most often on the trunk	
Annular lichen planus	Lesions with central inactivity or involution	Occurs in about 10% of patients
Atrophic lichen planus	Resolving lesions that are classically found on the lower leg	
Bullous lichen planus	Lesions that exhibit blisters within long-standing plaques	
Hypertrophic lichen planus	Lesions that present with thick hyperkeratotic plaques	Risk of squamous cell carcinoma, more common in blacks
Lichen nitidus	Presents as tiny skin colored or hypopigmented papules involving the trunk or extremities	Most common in children
Lichen planopilaris	Follicular variant that can result in scarring alopecia of the scalp	
Lichen planus pemphigoides	Manifests as bullae in previously uninvolved skin of patients with LP	Circulating IgG autoantibodies against BPAG2 (type XVII collagen)
Linear lichen planus	Linear lesions that occur spontaneously along the lines of Blaschko	

(continued)

Table 10.1 (continued)

Variants	Characteristics	Notes
Lichen planus-lupus erythematosus overlap syndrome	Patients with characteristics of both lichen planus and lupus erythematosus	
Nail lichen planus	Nail thinning, ridging, fissuring, pterygium formation	
Oral lichen planus	White, reticular lacy patches on the buccal mucosa	More common in women; occurs in ~50–75% of patients; risk of squamous cell carcinoma
Ulcerative lichen planus	Consists of bullae and permanent loss of toenails	

Adapted from Bridges K. Lichen planus. In: Kelly AP TS, editor. Dermatology for Skin of Color. New York: McGraw Hill; 2009. p. 152–7, with permission

subtropical climates and individuals of Middle Eastern, African, and Asian descent [35, 40]. Sun exposure is a triggering factor. The lateral aspect of the forehead is the most common involved area. It has an earlier age of onset and a longer course. There is a female predominance. Pruritus, scaling, nail involvement, and the koebner phenomenon are often present [35, 41]. Lichen planus pigmentosus is another variant that is more common in Latin Americans and darker skin. Asymptomatic dark brown macules or patches in sun exposed areas and flexural folds are found (Fig. 10.4).

Histopathology

A skin biopsy can be undertaken to assist in the diagnosis of lichen planus. Distinguishing histopathologic features include irregular acanthosis, colloid bodies in the epidermis with degeneration of the basal layer, and a band-like infiltrate of

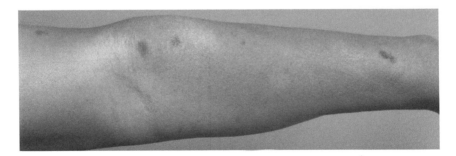

Fig. 10.4 Lichen planus pigmentosus. *Dark brown* macules and patches found on the arms

lymphocytes and histiocytes in the upper dermis obscuring the dermoepidermal junction. Characteristically, there is an irregular epidermal hyperplasia, forming a "saw-tooth" appearance with wedge-shaped hypergranulosis.

Treatment

Lichen planus is often self-limiting with most patients remitting in 1 year; however, treatment is often indicated to prevent post-inflammatory hyperpigmentation. Topical corticosteroids are first-line treatment. For lesions refractory to topical treatment or lesions that are more hyperkeratotic, intralesional or systemic corticosteroids may be indicated. Additional therapy for lesions that are refractory to topical treatment and are steroid sparing include acitretin, dapsone, methotrexate, hydroxychloroquine, cyclosporine, thalidomide, low molecular weight heparin, mycophenolate mofetil, and metronidazole. Narrow band UVB phototherapy may also be used [42]. It is important to check for exacerbating factors (for example, medications and infections). Treatment of oral lichen planus is often more difficult. Treatments include topical, intralesional, or systemic steroids, topical immunomodulators, retinoids, cyclosporine, griseofulvin, antimalarials, and methotrexate [39]. Removal of a contact allergen is also often indicated.

Conclusion

Inflammatory skin conditions, including atopic dermatitis, psoriasis, and lichen planus, are very common in patients with skin of color. However, these conditions can have varied presentations in different skin tones, and erythema is often difficult to appreciate. Edema, warmth of skin, and scaling in particular distributions are clues to the diagnosis of atopic dermatitis in patients with skin of color. Additionally, a follicular subset of atopic dermatitis is often found in patients with darker skin tones. Psoriasis plaques are often violaceous with gray scale in patients with skin of color. In lichen planus, the classic purple color may be black, gray, brown, or violaceous. If untreated, inflammatory conditions in patients with skin of color can lead to post-inflammatory hyperpigmentation, which can be very difficult to treat.

References

1. Spergel JM, Paller AS. Atopic dermatitis and the atopic march. J Allergy Clin Immunol. 2003;112(6 Suppl):S118–27.
2. Rottem M, Geller-Bernstein C, Shoenfeld Y. Atopy and asthma in migrants: the function of parasites. Int Arch Allergy Immunol. 2015;167(1):41–6.

3. Desai NAA. Atopic dermatitis and other eczemas. In: Kelly ATS, editor. Dermatology for skin of color. China: McGraw Hill; 2009. p. 163–6.
4. Williams HC, Pembroke AC, Forsdyke H, Boodoo G, Hay RJ, Burney PG. London-born black Caribbean children are at increased risk of atopic dermatitis. J Am Acad Dermatol. 1995;32(2 Pt 1):212–7.
5. Mar A, Tam M, Jolley D, Marks R. The cumulative incidence of atopic dermatitis in the first 12 months among Chinese, Vietnamese, and Caucasian infants born in Melbourne, Australia. J Am Acad Dermatol. 1999;40(4):597–602.
6. Davis SA, Narahari S, Feldman SR, Huang W, Pichardo-Geisinger RO, McMichael AJ. Top dermatologic conditions in patients of color: an analysis of nationally representative data. J Drugs Dermatol JDD. 2012;11(4):466–73.
7. Vachiramon V, Tey HL, Thompson AE, Yosipovitch G. Atopic dermatitis in African American children: addressing unmet needs of a common disease. Pediatr Dermatol. 2012;29 (4):395–402.
8. Agrawal R, Woodfolk JA. Skin barrier defects in atopic dermatitis. Curr Allergy Asthma Rep. 2014;14(5):433.
9. Osawa R, Akiyama M, Shimizu H. Filaggrin gene defects and the risk of developing allergic disorders. Allergol Int. 2011;60(1):1–9.
10. Palmer CN, Irvine AD, Terron-Kwiatkowski A, Zhao Y, Liao H, Lee SP, et al. Common loss-of-function variants of the epidermal barrier protein filaggrin are a major predisposing factor for atopic dermatitis. Nat Genet. 2006;38(4):441–6.
11. Margolis DJ, Kim B, Apter AJ, Gupta J, Hoffstad O, Papadopoulos M, et al. Thymic stromal lymphopoietin variation, filaggrin loss of function, and the persistence of atopic dermatitis. JAMA Dermatol. 2014;150(3):254–9.
12. Kubo A, Nagao K, Amagai M. Epidermal barrier dysfunction and cutaneous sensitization in atopic diseases. J Clin Invest. 2012;122(2):440–7.
13. Jackson-Richard DPA. Dermatology atlas for skin of color. New York: Springer; 2014.
14. Ben-Gashir MA, Hay RJ. Reliance on erythema scores may mask severe atopic dermatitis in black children compared with their white counterparts. Br J Dermatol. 2002;147(5):920–5.
15. Kathuria PKR. Atopic Dermatitis. In: Love PBKR, editor. Clinical cases in skin of color. Switzerland: Springer; 2016. p. 63–72.
16. Boguniewicz M, Eichenfield LF, Hultsch T. Current management of atopic dermatitis and interruption of the atopic march. J Allergy Clin Immunol. 2003;112(6 Suppl):S140–50.
17. Silverberg JI, Lee-Wong M, Silverberg NB. Complementary and alternative medicines and childhood eczema: a US population-based study. Dermatitis. 2014;25(5):246–54.
18. Jacyk WK. Psoriasis in Nigerians. Trop Geogr Med. 1981;33(2):139–42.
19. Gelfand JM, Stern RS, Nijsten T, Feldman SR, Thomas J, Kist J, et al. The prevalence of psoriasis in African Americans: results from a population-based study. J Am Acad Dermatol. 2005;52(1):23–6.
20. Rachakonda TD, Schupp CW, Armstrong AW. Psoriasis prevalence among adults in the United States. J Am Acad Dermatol. 2014;70(3):512–6.
21. Bronckers IM, Paller AS, van Geel MJ, van de Kerkhof PC, Seyger MM. Psoriasis in children and adolescents: diagnosis, management and comorbidities. Paediatr Drugs. 2015;17(5):373–84.
22. Krueger JG, Bowcock A. Psoriasis pathophysiology: current concepts of pathogenesis. Ann Rheum Dis. 2005;64 Suppl 2:ii30–6.
23. Shah NJKR. Psoriasis. In: Love PBKR, editor. Clinical cases in skin of color. Switzerland: Springer; 2016. p. 73–80.
24. Ikaheimo I, Tiilikainen A, Karvonen J, Silvennoinen-Kassinen S. HLA risk haplotype Cw6, DR7, DQA1*0201 and HLA-Cw6 with reference to the clinical picture of psoriasis vulgaris. Arch Dermatol Res. 1996;288(7):363–5.
25. Wuepper KD, Coulter SN, Haberman A. Psoriasis vulgaris: a genetic approach. J Invest Dermatol. 1990;95(5 Suppl):2S–4S.

26. Cao K, Song FJ, Li HG, Xu SY, Liu ZH, Su XH, et al. Association between HLA antigens and families with psoriasis vulgaris. Chin Med J (Engl). 1993;106(2):132–5.
27. Tsai TF, Hu CY, Tsai WL, Chu CY, Lin SJ, Liaw SH, et al. HLA-Cw6 specificity and polymorphic residues are associated with susceptibility among Chinese psoriatics in Taiwan. Arch Dermatol Res. 2002;294(5):214–20.
28. Correia B, Torres T. Obesity: a key component of psoriasis. Acta Biomed. 2015;86(2):121–9.
29. Geng AMJ, Zeikus PS, McDonald CJ. Psoriasis. In: Kelly APTS, editor. Dermatology for skin of color. China: McGraw-Hill; 2009. p. 139–46.
30. Parisi R, Rutter MK, Lunt M, Young HS, Symmons DP, Griffiths CE, et al. Psoriasis and the risk of major cardiovascular events: cohort study using the clinical practice research datalink. J Invest Dermatol. 2015;135(9):2189–97.
31. Menter A, Korman NJ, Elmets CA, Feldman SR, Gelfand JM, Gordon KB, et al. Guidelines of care for the management of psoriasis and psoriatic arthritis: section 4. Guidelines of care for the management and treatment of psoriasis with traditional systemic agents. J Am Acad Dermatol. 2009;61(3):451–85.
32. Menter A, Gottlieb A, Feldman SR, Van Voorhees AS, Leonardi CL, Gordon KB, et al. Guidelines of care for the management of psoriasis and psoriatic arthritis: Section 1. Overview of psoriasis and guidelines of care for the treatment of psoriasis with biologics. J Am Acad Dermatol. 2008;58(5):826–50.
33. Menter A, Korman NJ, Elmets CA, Feldman SR, Gelfand JM, Gordon KB, et al. Guidelines of care for the management of psoriasis and psoriatic arthritis: Section 5. Guidelines of care for the treatment of psoriasis with phototherapy and photochemotherapy. J Am Acad Dermatol. 2010;62(1):114–35.
34. Balasubramaniam P, Ogboli M, Moss C. Lichen planus in children: review of 26 cases. Clin Exp Dermatol. 2008;33(4):457–9.
35. Bridges K. Lichen planus. In: Kelly APTS, editor. Dermatology for skin of color. New York: McGraw Hill; 2009. p. 152–7.
36. Abdel-Latif AM, Abuel-Ela HA, El-Shourbagy SH. Increased caspase-3 and altered expression of apoptosis-associated proteins, Bcl-2 and Bax in lichen planus. Clin Exp Dermatol. 2009;34(3):390–5.
37. Chang JY, Chiang CP, Hsiao CK, Sun A. Significantly higher frequencies of presence of serum autoantibodies in Chinese patients with oral lichen planus. J Oral Pathol Med. 2009;38(1):48–54.
38. Nagao Y, Sata M. A retrospective case-control study of hepatitis C virus infection and oral lichen planus in Japan: association study with mutations in the core and NS5A region of hepatitis C virus. BMC Gastroenterol. 2012;12:31.
39. Goyal AKR. Lichen planus. In: Love PBKR, editor. Clinical cases in skin of color. Switzerland: Springer; 2016. p. 91–101.
40. Sharma VK, Sahni K, Wadhwani AR. Photodermatoses in pigmented skin. Photochem Photobiol Sci. 2013;12(1):65–77.
41. Meads SB, Kunishige J, Ramos-Caro FA, Hassanein AM. Lichen planus actinicus. Cutis. 2003;72(5):377–81.
42. Taylor S. Treatments for skin of color. St. Louis: Saunders/Elsevier; 2011.

Chapter 11
Tinea Versicolor and Tinea Capitis

Stavonnie Patterson and Lisa Akintilo

Infections with viruses, bacteria, parasites, fungi, and yeast are ubiquitous. However, some infections are particularly notable in skin of color. Some infections are predisposed in skin of color and other infections present uniquely or have special considerations in this population. For example, tinea capitis (TC) occurs much more commonly in skin of color. Tinea versicolor (TV) presents with hypopigmented and hyperpigmented macules and patches in persons of color and can result in much more prominent and long-lasting dyschromia. Tinea nigra is important to note because the differential diagnosis of this entity includes acral nevi and acral lentiginous melanoma. In this chapter, we will review infectious disorders with unique clinical features and considerations in skin of color.

Tinea Capitis

Tinea capitis (TC) is a fungal infection of the scalp and hair that most commonly affects children. It is caused by dermatophytes of two genera, *Trichophyton* and *Microsporum*. The most common etiologic agent varies by region and has evolved over time. In the United States, the most common cause of infection is *Trichophyton tonsurans*. The clinical presentation has tremendous variation ranging from diffuse scale on the scalp to inflammatory pustules and scarring alopecia. TC is a common cause of alopecia in school-aged children and is highly contagious. Thus, adequate treatment is paramount in preventing transmission. The infection is

S. Patterson (✉) · L. Akintilo
Department of Dermatology, Northwestern University Feinberg School of Medicine,
676 N. St. Clair St. Suite 1600, Chicago, IL 60611, USA
e-mail: spatters@nm.org

© Springer International Publishing AG 2017
N.A. Vashi and H.I. Maibach (eds.), *Dermatoanthropology of Ethnic Skin and Hair*, DOI 10.1007/978-3-319-53961-4_11

spread by person-to-person contact, animals, soil, and fomites. Asymptomatic carrier states exist in which persons have no symptoms of TC but may infect others. This likely contributes to the difficulty in eradicating TC from some communities. Oral antifungals are the standard treatment for TC.

Epidemiology

Tinea capitis is most prevalent among prepubertal children. Among this group, ages greater than 2 and less than 10 are most commonly affected [1]. This infection is less common in adults but does occur. The increased sebum production at the onset of puberty is thought to be protective as sebum has fungistatic properties. Among adults, the immunocompromised and postmenopausal women are more susceptible. With the onset of menopause, there is involution of sebaceous glands as a result of decreased estrogen levels resulting in increased susceptibility. One series noted that 80% of the adults with TC in their cohort were immunosuppressed in some way [2]. This included a history of diabetes mellitus, connective tissue disease, human immunodeficiency virus (HIV) infection, and long-term use of systemic steroids.

Among children with TC, a slightly higher incidence in boys has been found. However, in adult populations, women are most likely to be affected, and this finding has been attributed to the high rate of females as primary caregivers for children [3].

Black and Hispanic populations have higher rates of TC when compared to other ethnicities. In an urban population based study, the prevalence rates among white students was 1.1%, Hispanic students was 1.6%, and black students was 13% with rates as high as 18% in younger Black students [4]. This was similar to other population studies showing prevalence rates of 13% [5, 6]. Interestingly, in this large metropolitan population, the genetic diversity of the tonsurans species isolated suggested that this pathogen is endemic among black children and special efforts to prevent infection are needed [4]. A recent study in a low-income, rural, Ethiopian population showed a prevalence rate of 24.6% [7]. This was similar to rates reported in other low-income countries [8].

The reason for higher rates of TC in Blacks and Hispanics is unclear, but many reasons have been proposed. This includes hair care practices such as less frequent shampooing, which has some spore-removal benefits, and certain hair styles. Traction styling may lead to increased fungal access to the impaired hair shaft. However, recent case-control research has found no association between hair care practices and the acquisition of TC. The number of shampoos per month, hairstyles such as braids or ponytails, use of a comb, pick, brush, straightener, curler, oil, grease, and sharing of hair utensils were considered [9]. Among an Indian population, amla, cantharidine, and coconut oils used for routine hair care were found to be protective [10].

Pathogenesis

Tinea capitis is a dermatophytosis. This is a fungal infection caused by organisms with the ability to invade the keratinized tissue of the skin, hair, and nails. The pathogens feed on the keratin in the skin and hair. Dermatophytes are characterized as anthropophilic—carried by humans, zoophilic—transmitted by animals, or geophilic—carried in the soil.

Dermatophytes are further characterized by where they invade the hair. Ectothrix infections invade both the shaft and the outer hair. *Microsporum* species generally result in ectothrix infections. These infections can be identified by Wood's Lamp; they will fluoresce green. Endothrix infections are those where the pathogen solely invades the hair shaft. *Trichophyton* species cause endothrix infections. Favus is a severe, chronic hair infection that is most commonly caused by *Trichophyton schoenleinii*. Figure 11.1 outlines species that cause each type of infection.

For years, *Microsporum audouinii* was the most common cause of TC in the United States. *T. tonsurans* has now emerged as the most common cause. Across Europe, the predominant agent is *Microsporum canis*; however, in the United Kingdom, *Tricholosporum violaceum* accounts for over half of culture-proven TC.

Clinical Presentation

Clinical features of TC are variable. Lesions can be inflammatory or noninflammatory. Typically, there is a combination of scale and patchy alopecia that raises clinical suspicion and leads to the diagnosis. Some clinical features are associated

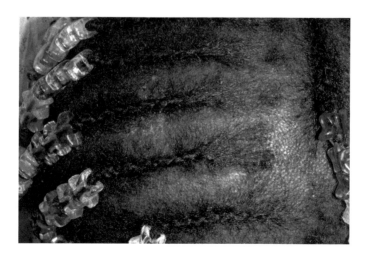

Fig. 11.1 Tinea capitis—isolated patch of hypekeratosis without alopecia. Courtesy of Anthony Mancini

with particular species. Below are descriptions of common clinical presentations [11].

1. Diffuse Scale—(1%) [12] Some patients present with a diffuse scale on the scalp without evidence of alopecia. This may be difficult to distinguish from seborrheic dermatitis clinically. However, seborrheic dermatitis is typically not seen in young, preadolescent children [13] and thus, this presentation should prompt evaluation for TC (Fig. 11.1).
2. Black Dot—(31%) [12] This refers to patches of fine scale with broken off hairs, resembling black dots. These hairs are infected with *Trichophyton*, an endothrix infection, resulting in breakage. The color of the dots will vary based on hair color, but is most commonly referred to as "Black Dot" due to the increased presence in children of color with dark hair.
3. Gray Patch—(35%) [12] This pattern consists of circular patches of alopecia with fine scale and a gray appearance. The gray color is a result of arthrospores coating the affected hairs and is most commonly seen with *Microsporum* infections.
4. Diffuse Pustular—(3%) [12] This is an inflammatory variant of TC with diffuse patchy alopecia and superimposed pustules (Fig. 11.2).
5. Kerion—(25%) [12] This is an extremely inflamed variant in which a boggy, pustular nodule is present. These lesions can be tender and often are crusted. This may result in permanent hair loss of the affected area.
6. Favus—(5%) [12] Favus is a chronic inflammatory dermatophyte infection characterized by scutula. Scutula are yellow, cup-shaped crusts that surround and pierce the hair. The most common cause is *T. schoenleinii* [14]. Other less common causes of favus include *T. violaceum*, *T. verrucosum*, zoophilic *T. mentagrophytes*, *M. canis*, and geophilic *M. gypseum* [15]. Favus most

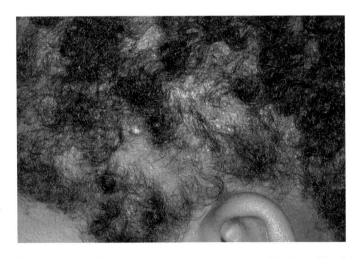

Fig. 11.2 Tinea capitis—patchy alopecia with pustules. Courtesy of Anthony Mancini

commonly represents a variant of TC but can also involve the skin and nails. There are air spaces between the hyphae in infected hair, and this represents autolysis of hyphae. This infection can persist for years and can be seen in long hair. The hair fluoresces green.

Inflammatory variants can be associated with cervical and postauricular lymphadenopathy. In addition, some infections may be accompanied by an id reaction. TC can result in scarring alopecia, thus recognition and appropriate management are critical.

Workup/Diagnosis

Microscopy

Evaluation of the hair shaft with light microscopy can aid in the diagnosis. Plucked hairs and scalp scrapings can be mounted in 10–30% potassium hydroxide. Hyphae or arthroconidia may be visualized with the light of fluorescence microscopy.

Wood's Lamp

With *Microsporum* and *T. schoenleinii* infections, there may be green fluorescence with Wood's lamp examination. *Trichophyton* species are generally non-fluorescing.

Culture

Culture is useful and recommended to allow for identification of the causative organism and to direct therapy. Generally, samples are plated on Sabouraud agar with cycloheximide to inhibit nondermatophyte mold growth and potentially chloramphenicol, an antibacterial agent. Mycosel is a dermatophyte test medium that contains all of the above and a phenol red pH indicator. Dermatophyte identification medium is similar but has a purple indicator.

There are several collection techniques. With the cotton swab technique, a moistened cotton swab is used to swab scalp sites with erythema, scale, and/or alopecia. The swab is then inoculated onto Mycosel medium [16]. A sterile cytobrush has also been utilized for sample collection and reported to result in increased culture sensitivity [17]. With the cytobrush technique, the affected area is rubbed with a commercial, sterile cytobrush, and placed into test tubes containing Sabouraud dextrose agar or Mycosel. The cytobrush method produces similar results to the cotton swab technique with the added advantage of commercial availability and sterile state. Alternatively, a scalpel can be used to scrape scale from the scalp and pluck affected hairs to plate in culture medium [16].

Cultures are generally followed for at least 4 weeks. Dermatophytes grown on dermatophyte test medium grow faster (within 10 days) than those grown on Saboraud's dextrose agar (up to 3 weeks) with equal efficacy. However, for species-level identification of growth on dermatophyte test medium, subculturing with Saboraud's dextrose agar is needed [18]. Both dermatophyte test medium and Saboraud's dextrose agar are slightly more effective than enriched dermatophyte medium, which contains soytone, carbohydrate, growth stimulants, cycloheximide, color indicator, and agar in distilled water. However, enriched dermatophyte medium is easier to use and has the shortest incubation period of 1–2 days [19].

Dermoscopy

Dermoscopy has become a useful tool in the diagnosis of hair and scalp conditions. Dermoscopic findings may aid in making a quick diagnosis while awaiting confirmation with a culture. This is particularly true in dark-skinned patients when erythema is not apparent. In one review, comma hairs and corkscrew hairs were consistent findings in six Black children with culture-proven TC. These findings were distinct from matched controls without TC [20]. Comma hairs are short bent hairs with uniform thickness. Corkscrew hairs are coiled hairs; they are most commonly seen with comma hairs in Black patients. Black dots, broken hairs, and hair casts are other dermoscopic findings.

Pathology

Biopsy is not necessary and typically not performed to make the diagnosis of TC. Histologic findings include arthroconidia and hyphae within and outside of the hair shafts to the level of Adamson's fringe (limit of the zone of keratinization) and hyphae in the stratum cornea [14, 21].

Differential Diagnosis

The differential diagnosis for noninflammatory TC includes alopecia areata, scalp psoriasis, atopic dermatitis, trichotillomania, and seborrheic dermatitis. Seborrheic dermatitis is uncommon in children aged 2–7 years old. Thus, a seborrheic dermatitis presentation should alert the provider to investigate for TC. Alopecia areata generally has no erythema or scale. The geographic pattern of hair loss would help to differentiate trichotillomania. The differential diagnosis for inflammatory variants of TC includes impetigo, dissecting cellulitis, folliculitis decalvans, and lupus erythematosus.

Treatment

After laboratory confirmation or strong clinical suspicion of TC, treatment should be started immediately to prevent spread of disease. Treatment options are identical for skin of color and non-skin of color patients. Topical therapies are ineffective against eradication of TC infections. Systemic therapy is required (Table 11.1). Factors influencing drug choice are the species isolated, cost, compliance, safety, and availability of liquid formulation. Griseofulvin, a fungistatic drug, has been used for over five decades in the eradication of TC. In children, griseofulvin micronized liquid suspension at a dosage of 20–25 mg/kg taken daily for six to eight weeks is a first-line treatment. Griseofulvin is also available in a tablet form in both the micronized and ultramicronized formulations. The bioavailability of the ultrami-cronized formulation is greater. Thus, it is generally dosed at 10 mg–15 mg/kg/day as compared to 20–25 mg/kg/day for the micronized form. Griseofulvin is also effective in treating adults with TC, but care must be taken due to the drug's contraindication in pregnancy and requirement for men to avoid fathering a child for 6 months post treatment [11]. Taking the medication with a fatty meal may increase absorption.

Terbinafine, a fungicidal medication, has recently been shown to be more effective than griseofulvin in children with *T. tonsurans* infections given increasing resistance to griseofulvin. Griseofulvin remains superior in treating *M. canis* infections [22, 23]. Oral terbinafine granules 5–8 mg/kg taken daily for 4 weeks is an effective treatment for TC [11, 24, 25].

Fungicidal and fungistatic itraconazole (5 mg/kg) taken daily for 2–6 weeks or fluconazole (6 mg/kg) taken for 2–6 weeks are viable second-line alternatives that can be used in the management of TC [11]. Studies have shown that these newer antifungal agents offer shorter durations of treatment than griseofulvin with similar efficacy and safety profiles [26]. These therapies can be used as alternatives in patients who do not demonstrate clearance with griseofulvin or when there is concern about compliance due to the long duration of therapy with griseofulvin.

Table 11.1 Oral Tinea capitis treatment

Drug	Dose	Duration
Griseofulvin (micronized)	20–25 mg/kg (child) 500 mg (adult)	Daily for 6–8 weeks
Griseofulvin (ultramicronized)	10–15 mg/kg (child) 300–375 mg (adult)	
Terbinafine	Child: 125 mg (<25 kg), 187.5 mg (25–35 kg) or 250 mg (>35 kg) 250 mg (adult)	Daily for 3–4 weeks
Itraconazole	5 mg/kg (child) 5 mg/kg (adult)	Daily for 3–6 weeks
Fluconazole	6 mg/kg (child) 6 mg/kg (adult)	Daily for 3–6 weeks

It is important to note that although topical therapy is not recommended for TC management, topical agents are helpful in reducing the transmission of spores. Shampooing twice a week with 2.5% selenium sulfide, povidone-iodine, or 2% ketoconazole can be effective in reducing viable fungal spores. As such, these topical therapies can be used as adjunctive therapy and prophylaxis for asymptomatic family members to reduce the carrier state [11, 25]. For asymptomatic carriers with a low spore load, topical therapy alone can eradicate the fungi [11]. Oral therapy should be considered for asymptomatic carriers with a high spore load.

Irrespective of therapy regimen, patient follow-up with repeat mycological sampling is recommended at the end of the treatment period and then monthly afterwards until total mycological clearance is documented.

It is important to take specific measures to prevent the spread of infection. Because viable spores have been sequestered from hairbrushes and combs, these fomites should be cleansed with disinfectants such as simple bleach. It is unnecessary for children to stay home from school or nursery if they are receiving appropriate therapy. They should be allowed to attend school or nursery without fear of transmission of infection to unaffected classmates [11]. Considering the endemic nature of *T. tonsurans* infection among black children in metropolitan areas, special efforts to prevent infection may be necessary in large urban areas [26].

Tinea Versicolor

Tinea versicolor (TV), also known as pityriasis versicolor, is the superficial overgrowth of fungi from the *Malassezia* genus [27]. It is one of the most common etiologies of pigmentation disorders across the globe [28] and is characterized by hypopigmented, hyperpigmented, and/or erythematous skin changes frequently found in seborrheic regions of the upper arms and upper trunk. Unlike other superficial fungal disorders using the term tinea (i.e., tinea pedis, tinea cruris, tinea capitis), TV is not a dermatophyte infection. TV is common in tropical climates, with prevalence rates up to 50% in tropical countries compared to 1% in Scandinavia [29]. It is seen more often during the summer months than the winter months. TV has a high prevalence in young adults, though other age groups may be affected. Treatment with topical and oral antifungals is very effective. However, there is a high rate of recurrence, with 60% of patients having recurrence within one year of initial diagnosis and 80% within two years [30].

Epidemiology

Many studies have looked at the variability of TV's occurrence between different racial populations. Some researchers have found that it is more prevalent in darker skin versus lighter skin [31, 32]. One review of clinic visits in a Black population in southeast London showed that 3.8% of all visits were for TV [32]. Similarly, Halder et al. [33] found that in the United States (US), 2.2% of all dermatologic visits among Black and Hispanic patients were for TV. Mellen et al. [34] noted that ambulatory visits in US clinics for TV were highest among African American and Native American patients. Others have discovered a tendency of TV to involve the face (especially the forehead) and neck of individuals of color as opposed to the torso being more commonly involved in fair skin types [35–37].

With regards to gender and age, some investigators found a higher rate of TV in males attributable to their increased sebaceous activity as compared to females [38, 39]. Similarly, there seems to be a higher predilection of TV for adolescents and young adults as compared to older adults. Malassezia requires oil to grow, and younger persons have increased sebaceous activity [40]. Some have suggested that TV infection in prepubertal children should prompt investigation of possible precocious puberty [41]. Sebum production decreases as adults age, thus correlating with low rates of TV in older populations.

Rarely, neonatal colonization by *Malassezia* occurs due to colonization of the mother or transmission via the hands of healthcare workers. One report describes TV like lesions in an dark-skinned ICU neonate with consistent microscopic findings. Colonization in susceptible neonates carries a risk of potentially severe fungemia [42].

Pathogenesis/Etiology

Malassezia globosa is the most common causative agent of TV. However, *M. furfur*, *M. restricta*, *M. sloffiae*, and *M. sympodialis* are other common species responsible for TV [43]. No difference in the causative species of TV has been documented in the literature between dark- and light-skinned patients. *Malassezia* yeasts are part of normal skin flora (especially *M. sympodialis* [14]). TV results when Malassezia transforms from saprophytic, round-celled, or yeast phases into the mycelial phase. This change may be prompted by high temperature and high humidity. Immunocompetent individuals are able to eliminate virulent *Malassezia* through a T-helper cell driven dendritic cell pathway [27]. However, predisposing factors impact patients' ability to effectively mount this protective response. Such factors include hyperhidrosis, malnutrition, immunosuppression, and use of oral contraceptives. Use of body oils and lubricants may also increase the growth of Malassezia.

Malassezia is present in all layers of the stratum corneum, especially the lower part of the horny layer. This lipophilic yeast invades keratinocytes and produces lipoxygenases that act on surface lipids and oxidize oleic acid to azelaic acid. Oxidation of oleic acid leads to the inhibition of tyrosinase, damage to melanocytes, and hypopigmented macules. Furthermore, the build-up of lipid-like material from *Malassezia* in the stratum corneum can block UV light and lead to the apparent lightening of skin. This hypopigmentation can be more apparent in skin of color patients. Hyperpigmented macules are caused by inflammation created directly by *Malassezia* overgrowth [27]. *Malassezia* may also modify melanosome size and distribution within melanocytes and keratinocytes. This can lead to hypopigmentation when the melanosomes are abnormally small and hyperpigmentation when the melanosomes are abnormally large [44].

Clinical Features

TV lesions are well-demarcated, round or oval macules, papules, patches, or plaques with mild scale. Generally, TV lesions are hypopigmented, hyperpigmented, or erythematous compared to normal skin. However, lesions vary in color (hence the name versicolor) and may appear white, pink, tan, gray, or brown. This dyschromia is more apparent in persons of color due to the stark contrast between the lesions and the patients' dark skin. While hypopigmented lesions are common in dark-skinned patients with TV, up to one-third of patients of color have hyperpigmented lesions [45]. In dark-skinned patients, hyperpigmented lesions are often gray-brown (Fig. 11.3).

Lesions are mostly a cosmetic concern for patients due to significant dyspigmentation, although mild pruritus has been reported in some patients [29]. Fine scale present on the lesions becomes more apparent when the skin is stretched or scraped; this is referred to as the evoked scale sign. Lesions are most commonly found on the upper trunk and upper arms in adults. In children, TV lesions have a predilection for the face, especially the forehead. Furthermore, facial involvement is more common in skin of color than in fair skin [40]. Such facial involvement is often secondary to infection of the trunk or upper arms. TV macules may also be

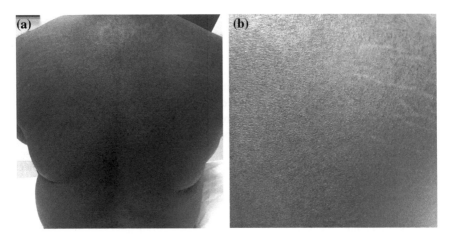

Fig. 11.3 **a** Tinea versicolor—gray-brown lesions common in skin of color. **b** Tinea versicolor—magnified view of *right upper back*

present on the proximal aspect of the lower extremities, such as the groin, penis, or popliteal fossa. TV macules may become confluent and coalesce into irregularly shaped patches. A phenomenon unique to the African American population is "acid skin", or the formation of coalescing hypopigmented plaques due to recurrent TV and/or other papulosquamous disorders. The term "acid skin" originated from the false belief that this condition is due to excess consumption of acidic foods such as carbonated beverages or foods high in protein. Treatment of the underlying condition typically leads to lesion resolution [27].

Diagnosis

Tinea versicolor is generally a clinical diagnosis. KOH preparation of skin scrapings or a Wood's light skin examination can be helpful. With a KOH preparation, the short, septate, non-branched pseudohyphae and spores, colloquially termed "spaghetti and meatballs", of the *Malassezia* fungi will become apparent, representing the yeast transforming to its mycelial form [29]. Examination of skin under a Wood's light (portal quartz lamp emitting filtered UV light with a peak of 365 nm held 4–5 in. from affected skin) will show yellow-green fluorescence if infected by *Malassezia*. However, it is important to note that a negative Wood's light examination does not exclude the diagnosis of TV, as not all *Malassezia* species fluoresce. Biopsy is typically not required, but if performed, demonstrates a thick basket weave stratum corneum with hyphae and spores.

Differential Diagnosis

The differential diagnosis of TV includes: melasma, confluent, and reticulated papillomatosis, pityriasis alba, pityriasis rosea, post-inflammatory hyperpigmentation (PIH) and hypopigmentation, progressive macular hypomelanosis, seborrheic dermatitis, secondary syphilis, tinea corporis, and vitiligo. Vitiligo, in particular, is often confused with hypopigmented lesions of TV in dark-skinned patients. Wood's lamp evaluation can differentiate between the depigmented vitiligo lesions illuminating with white fluorescence and hypopigmented TV lesions as described above.

Treatment

When choosing an effective treatment for a patient with TV, it is important to consider the extent and location of lesions, risks and benefits of particular therapies, patient age, patient compliance, and medication cost. Treatment of TV is the same regardless of skin color. However, some research has shown that treatment should be more aggressive in dark-skinned patients due to the increased likelihood of post-inflammatory dyspigmentation in this population [27]. Initial steps for mild infection include topical antifungal (fungistatic) and/or keratolytic shampoos, creams, and lotions to remove infected stratum corneum (Table 11.2). Nonspecific agents such as selenium sulfide are able to physically or chemically remove an infected stratum corneum. Treatment of the entire skin from the neck down to the knees has been shown to have high success rates. Preparations should be lathered onto affected areas and then left on the skin for 10–15 min before rinsing. For severe, extensive, and/or refractory lesions, oral medications can be used (Table 11.3).

It is important to note that current reports have demonstrated significant concerns about the safety of oral ketoconazole. This was the first broad spectrum antifungal medication and previously the first-line oral therapy option for TV. The most concerning side effect is hepatotoxicity, which can be life threatening. Other potential adverse effects are multiple drug interactions and endocrine dysregulation, primarily decreased testosterone production and consequent sequelae [46]. Oral ketoconazole was withdrawn from European and Australian markets in 2013. The US Food and Drug Administration (FDA) and Canada have updated product labeling with warnings regarding hepatotoxicity and drug interactions. Users are encouraged to restrict use of ketoconazole to severe fungal infections when alternatives are not available or tolerated. Increased liver function tests monitoring, avoidance in patients with liver disease, and heightened awareness of drug interactions is also recommended [47]. Topical ketoconazole is safe and remains first-line therapy for TV. In fact, although all azoles are effective, topical ketoconazole has the best minimum inhibitory concentration against *Malassezia*.

Table 11.2 Topical tinea versicolor treatment regimens

Drug	Duration
Ketoconazole shampoo (2%)	Twice weekly for 2–4 weeks
Selenium sulfide shampoo (2.5%)	Twice weekly for 2–4 weeks
Azole creams/lotions[a]	Once or twice-daily for 1–4 weeks
Zinc pyrithione shampoo (1 or 2%)	Twice weekly for 2–4 weeks
Ciclopirox 0.77% cream	Twice-daily for 2 weeks
Ciclopirox olamine 1% shampoo	Twice weekly for 2 weeks

[a]Topical azole antifungals include: clotrimazole 1%, econazole 1%, ketoconazole 2%, miconazole 2%, oxiconazole 1%, sulconazole 1%

Table 11.3 Oral tinea versicolor treatment regimens

Drug	Dose (mg)	Duration
Fluconazole	300	Once weekly for 2 weeks
Fluconazole	400	One-time dose
Itraconazole	200	Once-daily for 5–7 days
Itraconazole	400	One-time dose

Table 11.4 Prophylactic regimens for Tinea versicolor

Drug	Dose	Frequency
Ketoconazole shampoo 1 or 2%	Topical application	Once weekly to monthly
Zinc pyrithione shampoo	Topical application	Once weekly to monthly
Oral fluconazole	300 mg	Once a month
Oral itraconazole	400 mg	Once a month

Newer antifungal agents such as itraconazole and fluconazole have fewer drug interactions and are valid alternatives. If systemic oral therapy is necessitated, fluconazole is the preferred agent due to itraconazole's variable bioavailability and increased risk of gastrointestinal side effects and drug interactions [48, 49]. Furthermore, some evidence has shown fluconazole to be more effective in preventing TV recurrence than itraconazole [50].

Before initiating treatment, it is important to advise patients that changes in cutaneous pigment often persist even after successful treatment. Pigmentation can return after a period of weeks to months. Recurrence is common despite treatment choice. Immunocompromised patients are at heightened risk for TV recurrence. Effective prophylaxis can be attained with an intermittent prophylactic treatment regimen (Table 11.4).

As aforementioned, post-inflammatory dyspigmentation after an episode of TV is particularly common in skin of color. Treatment of this condition includes prevention with photoprotection and avoiding unnecessary trauma such as picking, rubbing, or scratching. Hydroquinone is the gold standard for PIH as it inhibits tyrosinase. Other possible treatments for PIH include topical retinoids, arbutin, kojic acid, licorice extract, N-acetyl glucosamine, and niacinamide [27, 51].

Tinea Nigra

Tinea nigra is a superficial phaeohyphomycosis affecting the palms, soles, neck, and trunk. It occurs primarily in tropical climates. The causative agent is *Hortaea werneckii* (*H. werneckii*), formerly known as *Exophiala werneckii* [52–54]. This agent is an environmental pathogen found in sewage, soil, decaying vegetation, and shower stalls [55]. Lesions of tinea nigra are irregular, sharply demarcated, asymptomatic, green to brown to black macules or patches that can present as single or multiple lesions. The macules enlarge centrifugally and often have accentuated pigment at the border. The lesions may appear velvety or have mild scale. The most common sites of involvement are the palms and soles. This entity is notable in skin of color because the lesions may resemble and be misdiagnosed as acral nevi and acral lentiginous melanoma. Palmar plantar macular hyperpigmentation, a common benign finding in skin of color, is also in the differential diagnosis [55, 56].

Diagnostic measures such as KOH preparation, culture, and dermoscopy help to differentiate tinea nigra from melanocytic lesions. KOH examination reveals septate, pigmented hyphae in the upper stratum corneum. Biopsy has similar findings. Dermoscopy shows the classic findings of superficial, fine, pigmented spicules without respect for dermatoglyphic lines [54]. The spicules form what resembles a reticulated patch. The pigmented hyphae do not follow the commonly noted dermoscopic patterns of acral nevi or acral melanomas. Dermoscopy is an efficient tool that can aid in prompt diagnosis, early treatment, and avoidance of unnecessary diagnostic tests.

Tinea nigra responds quickly to treatment with topical azoles or allylamine antifungal agents and keratolytics. Lesions typically resolve within two to three weeks of topical therapy. Treatment for several weeks may be considered to prevent recurrence. Systemic therapy is not required.

Conclusion

It is important to identify unique features of dermatologic conditions in skin of color. This includes infectious processes. Infections can have a higher prevalence, distinctive presentations, and require consideration of important differential diagnoses. TC is more common in persons of color. Appropriate management is important to prevent spread of disease and prevent scarring alopecia in those affected. TV is a common dermatosis affecting all ethnicities, but can result in notable dyschromia that is more prominent in dark skin. Lesions are often hypopigmented in skin of color and when they are hyperpigmented appear a gray brown to black color versus light brown in lighter skin. There are effective and safe therapies. Tinea nigra most often occurs on the palms and soles and may mimic acral nevi, palmar planter hyperpigmentation, and malignant melanoma. Proper identification is important to avoid unnecessary diagnostic procedures and treatment.

Key Points

1. Tinea Capitis

   a. The most common cause in the US is *T. tonsurans*
   b. High prevalence in Black and Hispanic children
   c. Requires systemic therapy
   d. Newer antifungal agents are effective and safe
   e. Asymptomatic carriers contribute to the endemic nature and should be treated

2. Special considerations for treating TV in skin of color include:

   a. Unique predilection for facial lesions
   b. Lesions can cause notable hypo- and/or hyperpigmentation
   c. May resemble other skin conditions common in this population such as vitiligo
   d. Potential need for more aggressive treatment due to heightened risk of post-inflammatory dyspigmentation
   e. Recurrence is common and can be prevented with preventative therapy

3. Tinea Nigra

   a. May resemble acral nevi and acral lentiginous melanoma
   b. Dermoscopy can be a helpful tool in differentiating this from melanocytic lesions
   c. Responds to topical antifungal agents.

References

1. Coley MK, et al. Scalp hyperkeratosis and alopecia in children of color. J Drugs Dermatol. 2011;10(5):511–6.
2. Khosravi AR, Shokri H, Vahedi G. Factors in etiology and predisposition of adult Tinea Capitis and review of published literature. Mycopathologia. 2016;181(5–6):371–8.
3. Silverberg NB, Weinberg JM, DeLeo VA. Tinea capitis: focus on African American women. J Am Acad Dermatol. 2002;46(2 Suppl Understanding):S120–4.
4. Abdel-Rahman SM, et al. The prevalence of infections with *Trichophyton tonsurans* in schoolchildren: the CAPITIS study. Pediatrics. 2010;125(5):966–73.
5. Williams JV, et al. Prevalence of scalp scaling in prepubertal children. Pediatrics. 2005;115(1):e1–6.
6. Ghannoum M, et al. Tinea capitis in Cleveland: survey of elementary school students. J Am Acad Dermatol. 2003;48(2):189–93.
7. Leiva-Salinas M, et al. Tinea capitis in schoolchildren in a rural area in southern Ethiopia. Int J Dermatol. 2015;54(7):800–5.
8. Hogewoning AA, et al. Prevalence and causative fungal species of tinea capitis among schoolchildren in Gabon. Mycoses. 2011;54(5):e354–9.
9. Sharma V, et al. Do hair care practices affect the acquisition of tinea capitis? A case-control study. Arch Pediatr Adolesc Med. 2001;155(7):818–21.
10. Garg AP, Muller J. Inhibition of growth of dermatophytes by Indian hair oils. Mycoses. 1992;35(11–12):363–9.
11. Fuller LC, et al. British Association of Dermatologists' guidelines for the management of tinea capitis 2014. Br J Dermatol. 2014;171(3):454–63.
12. Farooqi M, et al. Clinical types of tinea capitis and species identification in children: an experience from tertiary care centres of Karachi, Pakistan. J Pak Med Assoc. 2014;64(3):304–8.
13. Borda LJ, Wikramanayake TC. Seborrheic dermatitis and dandruff: a comprehensive review. J Clin Investig Dermatol. 2015;3(2).
14. Elewski BE. In: Bolognia JL, Jorizzo JL, Schaffer JV, editors. Dermatology. Elsevier Limited; 2012. p. 1251–84.
15. Ilkit M. Favus of the scalp: an overview and update. Mycopathologia. 2010;170(3):143–54.

16. Friedlander SF, et al. Use of the cotton swab method in diagnosing tinea capitis. Pediatrics. 1999;104(2 Pt 1):276–9.
17. Bonifaz A, et al. Cytobrush-culture method to diagnose tinea capitis. Mycopathologia. 2007;163(6):309–13.
18. Poluri LV, Indugula JP, Kondapaneni SL. Clinicomycological study of dermatophytosis in South India. J Lab Physicians. 2015;7(2):84–9.
19. Singh S, Beena PM. Comparative study of different microscopic techniques and culture media for the isolation of dermatophytes. Indian J Med Microbiol. 2003;21(1):21–4.
20. Hughes R, et al. Corkscrew hair: a new dermoscopic sign for diagnosis of tinea capitis in black children. Arch Dermatol. 2011;147(3):355–6.
21. Hinshaw MA, Longley BJ. In: Elder DE, editor. Lever's histopathology of the skin. Wolters Kluwer; 2014. p. 593–4.
22. Chen X, et al. Systemic antifungal therapy for tinea capitis in children. Cochrane Database Syst Rev. 2016;Cd004685 (5).
23. Elewski BE, et al. Terbinafine hydrochloride oral granules versus oral griseofulvin suspension in children with tinea capitis: results of two randomized, investigator-blinded, multicenter, international, controlled trials. J Am Acad Dermatol. 2008;59(1):41–54.
24. Bennasar A, Grimalt R. Management of tinea capitis in childhood. Clin Cosmetic Invest Dermatol. 2010;3:89–98.
25. Kakourou T, Uksal UA. Guidelines for the managemnent of tinea capitis in children. Pediatr Dermatol. 2010;27(3):226–8.
26. Bhanusali D, et al. Treatment outcomes for tinea capitis in a skin of color population. J Drugs Dermatol. 2012;11(7):852–6.
27. Kallini JR, Riaz F, Khachemoune A. Tinea versicolor in dark-skinned individuals. Int J Dermatol. 2014;53(2):137–41.
28. Park HJ, et al. Skin characteristics in patients with pityriasis versicolor using non-invasive method, MPA5. Ann Dermatol. 2012;24(4):444–52.
29. Gupta AK, Bluhm R, Summerbell R. Pityriasis versicolor. J Eur Acad Dermatol Venereol. 2002;16(1):19–33.
30. Kelly Ap, Taylor SC. Dermatology for skin of color. New York: McGraw Hill; 2016. p. 425–30 (Ch 59).
31. Berry M, Khachemoune A. Extensive tinea versicolor mimicking Pityriasis rubra pilaris. J Drugs Dermatol. 2009;8(5):490–1.
32. Child FJ, et al. A study of the spectrum of skin disease occurring in a black population in South-East London. Br J Dermatol. 1999;141(3):512–7.
33. Halder RM, Nootheti PK. Ethnic skin disorders overview. J Am Acad Dermatol. 2003;48(6 Suppl):S143–8.
34. Mellen LA, et al. Treatment of pityriasis versicolor in the United States. J Dermatolog Treat. 2004;15(3):189–92.
35. Halder RM, Nandedkar MA, Neal KW. Pigmentary disorders in ethnic skin. Dermatol Clin. 2003;21(4):617–28 (vii).
36. Pontasch MJ, Kyanko ME, Brodell RT. Tinea versicolor of the face in black children in a temperate region. Cutis. 1989;43(1):81–4.
37. Testa J, Belec L, Bouree P. Epidemiological survey of 126 cases of pityriasis versicolor in the Central African Republic. Ann Soc Belg Med Trop. 1991;71(2):153–4.
38. Rao GS, et al. Clinico-epidermiological studies on tinea versicolor. Indian J Dermatol Venereol Leprol. 2002;68(4):208–9.
39. Belec L, Testa J, Bouree P. Pityriasis versicolor in the Central African Republic: a randomized study of 144 cases. J Med Vet Mycol. 1991;29(5):323–9.
40. Nenoff P, et al. Mycology—an update part 2: dermatomycoses: clinical picture and diagnostics. J Dtsch Dermatol Ges. 2014;12(9):749–77.
41. Hawkins DM, Smidt AC. Superficial fungal infections in children. Pediatr Clin North Am. 2014;61(2):443–55.
42. Jubert E, et al. Neonatal pityriasis versicolor. Pediatr Infect Dis J. 2015;34(3):329–30.

43. Ibekwe PU, et al. The spectrum of Malassezia species isolated from students with pityriasis vesicolor in Nigeria. Mycoses. 2015;58(4):203–8.
44. Schwartz RA. Superficial fungal infections. Lancet. 2004;364(9440):1173–82.
45. Aljabre SH, et al. Pigmentary changes of tinea versicolor in dark-skinned patients. Int J Dermatol. 2001;40(4):273–5.
46. Gupta AK, Daigle D, Foley KA. Drug safety assessment of oral formulations of ketoconazole. Expert Opin Drug Saf. 2015;14(2):325–34.
47. Gupta AK, Lyons DC. The rise and fall of oral ketoconazole. J Cutan Med Surg. 2015;19(4): 352–7.
48. Hald M, et al. Evidence-based Danish guidelines for the treatment of Malassezia-related skin diseases. Acta Derm Venereol. 2015;95(1):12–9.
49. Hu SW, Bigby M. Pityriasis versicolor: a systematic review of interventions. Arch Dermatol. 2010;146(10):1132–40.
50. Pantazidou A, Tebruegge M. Recurrent tinea versicolor: treatment with itraconazole or fluconazole? Arch Dis Child. 2007;92(11):1040–2.
51. Davis EC, Callender VD. Postinflammatory hyperpigmentation: a review of the epidemiology, clinical features, and treatment options in skin of color. J Clin Aesthet Dermatol. 2010;3(7): 20–31.
52. Solak B, Unus Z. Tinea nigra on the fingers. BMJ Case Rep. 2015;2015.
53. Criado PR, Delgado L, Pereira GA. Dermoscopy revealing a case of tinea nigra. An Bras Dermatol. 2013;88(1):128–9.
54. Maia Abinader MV, et al. Tinea nigra dermoscopy: a useful assessment. J Am Acad Dermatol. 2016;74(6):e121–2.
55. Bolognia JL, Jorizzo JL, Schaffer JV. Dermatology chapter 77 fungal diseases. Philadelphhia, Saunders; 2012. p. 1251–55.
56. James WD, Berger T, editors. Andrews diseases of the skin: clinical dermatology. 12th ed. St. Louis: Elsevier; 2015. p. 302 (Ch 15).

Chapter 12
Autoimmune and Connective Tissue Disease in Skin of Color

Babu Singh, Scott Walter, Daniel J. Callaghan III., Jennifer Paek and Christina Lam

Systemic Lupus Erythematosus in Skin of Color

Systemic lupus erythematosus (SLE) is a disorder mediated by a complex interplay of genetic predisposition, alterations in immune functioning, environmental triggers, and socioeconomic factors. SLE can involve and cause irreversible damage to almost all organ systems, including the central nervous system, cutaneous, cardiovascular, musculoskeletal, renal and pulmonary systems. Cutaneous lupus erythematosus (CLE) manifests as a broad spectrum of skin lesions, some with a propensity for scarring and disfigurement. Importantly, the integument may be the first organ system involved and, when identified clinically, warrants careful evaluation for internal disease. Patients of different ethnicities may have important differences in disease presentation and evolution in both cutaneous and systemic lupus, including disease onset, predilection for particular organ involvement,

B. Singh · S. Walter · D.J. Callaghan III. · C. Lam (✉)
Department of Dermatology, Boston University Medical Center,
609 Albany Street, Boston, MA 02118, USA
e-mail: cslam@bu.edu

B. Singh
e-mail: singhba@bu.edu

D.J. Callaghan III.
e-mail: DanielJCallaghan3@gmail.com

J. Paek
Boston University School of Medicine, 609 Albany St., Boston, MA 02118, USA

© Springer International Publishing AG 2017
N.A. Vashi and H.I. Maibach (eds.), *Dermatoanthropology of Ethnic Skin and Hair*, DOI 10.1007/978-3-319-53961-4_12

disease severity and response to treatment. Furthermore, advances in genomic research have identified specific genetic markers with increased prevalence in certain ethnic groups that may provide prognostic information.

Epidemiology of Cutaneous Lupus Erythematosus

Population-based data by Durosaro et al. demonstrated an age- and sex-adjusted incidence of CLE to be 4.30 per 100,000; however, this population was predominantly Caucasian, limiting its generalizability to skin of color populations [1]. In terms of ethnic cohorts, data on the incidence of CLE is limited and is based on retrospective analyses. Osio-Salido et al. reported a 30–50 per 100,000 prevalence of CLE in a review of 24 countries in Asia [2]. A retrospective cohort study by Rees et al. investigated the epidemiology of lupus in the UK over the period 1999–2012 and found Black Caribbean patients to have the highest incidence (6.23/100,000 people) and prevalence (125.51/100,000 people) of CLE, which included cutaneous-only subtypes [3]. A similar trend was also found in their cohort of SLE patients. The malar rash and discoid lesions were identified in 36.4 and 33.1%, respectively, in a cohort of African Caribbean patients with SLE in Barbados [4]. In a retrospective epidemiological study of 888 Brazilian patients with SLE, 90.7% of patients presented with mucocutaneous manifestations, consisting of malar rash (83%) and photosensitivity (76.9%) [5]. Furthermore, the malar rash was observed more in female patients than male patients with SLE.

Pathogenesis

Gene Linkage and Genome-wide Association Studies in Skin of Color
Genome-wide association, microarray transcriptional and candidate gene studies have identified numerous susceptibility genes for SLE in different ethnic groups. Furthermore, genetic polymorphisms in certain genes have been identified to confer an increased risk for disease severity and prognostic information in certain ethnic groups. However, few studies have compared these polymorphisms between ethnic groups.
Genomic Studies in Hispanics
Gene linkage studies have identified human leukocyte antigen (HLA) specific to ethnic groups that predispose to LE. Castano-Rodriquez et al. determined that HLA-DR3 and HLA-DR2 occur in higher frequencies in Latin American patients with SLE, with the allele HLA-DRB1*0301 being the most strongly associated. Furthermore, HLA-DR5 appears to confer protection against developing SLE in these patients [6]. In another study, expression of HLA-DR1 (DRB1*01) and C4A*3 alleles were associated with increased disease severity in Hispanic and

African Americans [7]. A single nucleotide polymorphism (rs1143679) in the ITGAM (The Integrin AlphaM Protein) was associated with SLE in Hispanic American populations [8].

Genomic Studies in Asians

Genetic polymorphism of the genes FcγRIIA, FcγRIIB, FcγRIIIA, and FcγRIIB has been described in Asians with SLE [9–10]. The F158 allele of FcγRIIIA gene, which encodes the IgG receptor FcγRIIIA, has been found in a meta-analysis to be significantly associated with lupus nephritis among Asian patients, but not in Caucasian or Africans [11]. Furthermore, in a cohort of Malaysians, a specific single nucleotide polymorphism in STAT4 was associated with an increased risk for SLE. The authors of this study, however, found no significant association with polymorphisms in TNFAIP3 and IRF5, other genes involved in type I interferon pathways [12]. Katkam et al. identified a specific polymorphism in exon-1 of the CTLA-4 (Cytotoxic T Lymphocyte Associated protein) gene, an important negative regulator of T-cell activation, that was associated with increased serum levels of TNF-alpha in a cohort of South Indian patients with SLE. The authors concluded that this association may play a role in the risk of developing SLE [13]. Chua et al. identified an association between a specific gene polymorphism in PDCD1 (Programmed Cell Death 1) and SLE in Malaysian patients, which is an important gene in the negative regulation of autoreactive T and B lymphocytes [14].

Diagnosis of Systemic Lupus Erythematosus

The classification criteria by the American College of Rheumatology (ACR) is the most widely used in SLE [15]. Four of the items in the ACR criteria are cutaneous manifestations of SLE: malar rash, discoid rash, photosensitivity, and oral ulcers. Other criteria include non-erosive arthritis (affecting greater than or equal to two peripheral joints), neurologic disorders (including seizures or psychosis) serositis (i.e., pleuritic rub, pleural effusion, and pericarditis), renal dysfunction, hematologic abnormalities (i.e., hemolytic anemia, leukopenia, lymphopenia and thrombocytopenia), and finally, two positive immunologic markers (including autoantibodies to dsDNA, Smith, or antiphospholipid, and anti-nuclear antibody [ANA]). To classify a patient with SLE, a patient must satisfy four or more items.

Clinical Presentation

LE more frequently affects young females. CLE can be divided broadly into two categories consisting of LE-specific (or diagnostic) skin lesions versus LE-nonspecific (or associated) skin lesions. LE-specific skin lesions we discuss histology separately below consist of the following subcategories: chronic CLE (CCLE), subacute CLE (SCLE), and acute CLE (ACLE). LE-associated skin lesions are broad, some of which include vasculitis, Raynaud's phenomenon, livedoid vasculopathy, livedo reticularis, and alopecia. The 3 forms of specific CLE lesions present similarly among all ethnicities, however in darker skin types the initial lesions may be difficult to discern because erythema can be masked by normal skin tone. Photosensitivity may not be as prominent in darker skin types. Furthermore, scarring and pigmentation changes may be more prominent and disfiguring in skin of color patients because of the contrast between lesions and unaffected normal skin. Finally, CLE lesions may have minimal erythema and be mostly hyper- or hypopigmented, thus making the clinical diagnosis less obvious [16].

Acute Cutaneous Lupus Erythematosus

Acute Cutaneous Lupus Erythematosus (ACLE) classically presents as bilateral erythema of the malar prominences and bridge of the nose, otherwise known as the "butterfly rash", that typically resolves without scarring [17]. The rash characteristically spares the nasolabial folds (due to it being relatively photoprotected), which helps differentiate this from other facial dermatoses, such as erythemato-telangiectatic rosacea or dermatomyositis. Occasionally, the erythema may be palpable from associated edema. ACLE may also be more widespread and involve the extremities and torso. When ACLE affects the dorsal hands, there is characteristic sparing of the finger joints with involvement of the interphalangeal spaces. This subtype is strongly associated with SLE, and the eruption may occur with flairs of SLE causing long-term residual dyspigmentation [18].

Subacute Cutaneous Lupus Erythematosus

Subacute cutaneous lupus erythematosus (SCLE) typically affects the sun-exposed surfaces of the upper chest, upper back and extensor arms, with occasional involvement of the face and neck. Two variants of SCLE are usually seen: annular or papulosquamous/psoriasiform. Annular lesions present with raised erythematous to violaceous borders with central clearing. Papulosquamous or psoriasiform lesions appear as erythematous, scaly thin plaques. As opposed to DLE, lesions of SCLE do not scar, however significant dyspigmentation may result, particularly prominent in skin of color patients (Fig. 12.1a, b). The anti-Ro/SS-A antibody is strongly associated with SCLE and accounts for the significant photosensitivity seen with this eruption [19].

Chronic Cutaneous Lupus Erythematosus

The CCLE subset consists of discoid lupus erythematosus (DLE), tumid lupus, lupus panniculitis, and chilblain lupus. DLE lesions can be hypertrophic or mucosal and there may be a lichen planus/DLE overlap. DLE lesions are most frequently localized to the cheeks, extensor forearms, forehead, scalp, nose, and conchal bowls [20]. Uncommonly, lesions may present on mucosal surfaces, such as the lip, nasal mucosa, genitals and conjunctiva [21]. Red lunulae has been reported to be associated with LE [22]. Early lesions are inflammatory in nature and present as ill-defined violaceous to erythematous thin plaques, which can be missed clinically in darker skin types, as the erythema may be more difficult to appreciate (Fig. 12.2). As lesions progress, dyspigmentation, follicular plugging, and scaling occur;

(a)   **(b)**

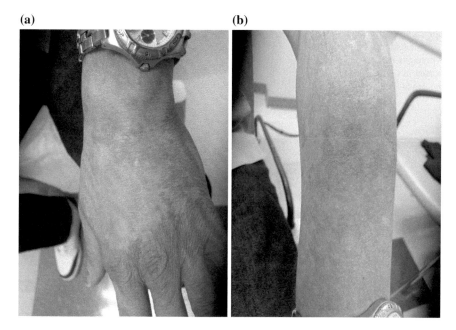

Fig. 12.1 Erythematous and scaly thin papules and plaques on photoexposed surfaces of the dorsal hand (**a**) and forearm (**b**). The depigmented vitiligo-like patches visualized under the erythema is a manifestation of the isotopic response that can occur following lupus lesions

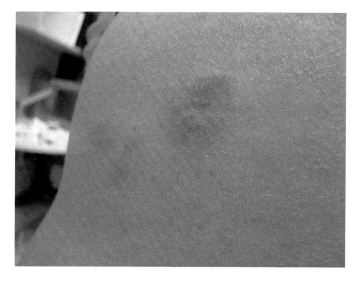

Fig. 12.2 Erythematous annular plaque with central hyperpigmentation occurring on the back representing an early discoid lupus lesion

Fig. 12.3 Classic discoid
lupus with central
depigmentation, peripheral
hyperpigmentation and scale
located in the conchal bowl
and pre-auricular area

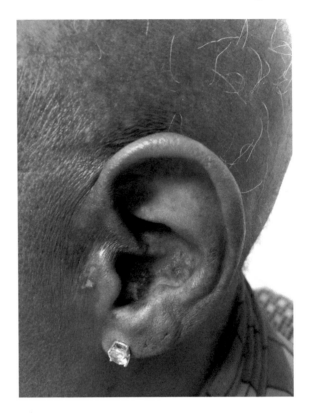

the former can be particularly pronounced in skin of color (Fig. 12.3). End stage
lesions typically have a hypopigmented, atrophied, and telangiectatic center with
hyperpigmented peripheral border. In skin of color patients, there may also be
striking vitiligo-like depigmentation centrally. Lesions, if left untreated, will
inevitably lead to pigmentary changes, scarring, loss of follicular orifices with
alopecia, and if severe, disfigurement of facial structures [23]. The striking contrast
between normal and lesional skin can be psychologically devastating to patients.
Furthermore, in long-standing untreated DLE lesions, squamous cell carcinoma
may develop, even in skin of color. Fernandes et al. reported that 0.98–3.4% of
patients from India developed SCC in long-standing DLE lesions [24]. The most
commonly reported site was the upper lip (28.57%), and the development of SCC
occurred approximately 10 years after the onset of DLE lesion. Keith et al. reported
two cases of SCC occurring in DLE lesions in African Americans, one of which
was on the lip [25]. DLE lesions that are localized to the head and neck region
confer a less than 5% risk of progression to SLE, while in patients with lesions that
are more diffuse and widespread, there is a 20% risk of progression to SLE [18].

Lupus erythematosus tumidus (or tumid lupus) presents as erythematous plaques most frequently distributed on photoexposed areas of the face and upper chest. The lesions have no appreciable follicular plugging, scarring, or atrophy as the process is predominantly dermal. The lesions appear and resolve intermittently, and therefore this entity is also known as intermittent CLE (ICLE).

Lupus panniculitis occurs when inflammation affects the subcutaneous tissue and commonly occurs at sites of abundant subcutaneous fat, such as the face, upper extremities, breasts, thighs, and buttocks. Initially, the lesions are characterized by intense inflammation presenting as indurated nodules that resolve with lipoatrophy, resulting in alterations in body contours. In the lupus profundus variant, there are changes of DLE overlying the panniculitis.

Chilblain lupus presents as red to dusky purple papules and plaques on the distal fingertips, toes, and nose. The lesions typically occur after exposure to cold temperatures [18].

Histology of Lupus Erythematosus

Histologic features of CLE include basal layer vacuolar degeneration, superficial, and deep perivascular lymphocytic infiltrate, basement membrane thickening and mucin deposition [26]. In DLE, the inflammation is predominantly periadnexal and follicular plugging may be seen. Lesions of LE tumidus have heavy dermal lymphocytic infiltrate with mucin leading to the indurated feel of the lesions with minimal epidermal changes [26]. Direct immunofluorescence (DIF) staining often reveals a homogeneous or granular band along the dermal-epidermal junction of IgG, IgM or complement, also known as the "lupus band test" [17]. This test has classically been reported as positive in uninvolved and involved skin of patients with SLE and in involved skin in patients with DLE [27].

Immunopathologic Features of Lupus Erythematosus

LE is characterized by an aberrant production of autoantibodies that can aid in diagnosis and may correspond with specific manifestations of disease activity. Anti-nuclear antibodies (ANAs) consist of a group of autoantibodies that react with the nucleus or nuclear associated antigens. ANA is present in >90% of patients with SLE, but has been found to be lower in patients with skin-limited cutaneous disease [28]. Higher titers of ANA (generally greater than 1:160) have been associated with a greater risk of developing SLE.

Epidemiology of Systemic Lupus Erythematosus in Skin of Color

Prevalence in Asia and Populations of Asian Descent

Osio-Salido et al. determined the prevalence of SLE in 24 Asian countries to be 30–50 per 100,000 population [2]. In this study, cutaneous (52–98%), musculoskeletal (36–95%), and renal involvement (greater than 50%) were the most common manifestations of SLE. Jakes et al. determined the prevalence of SLE in the Asia-Pacific region to be between 4 and 45 per 100,000 through a systematic literature search [29]. SLE in a Chinese population living in Oahu, Hawaii was estimated to be 24 per 100,000, which was higher than that estimated for white Europeans (6 per 100,000) [30]. Another study reported the overall prevalence rate for SLE in Asians (including people of Indian descent) to be 48.8 per 100,000, which was higher than for whites (20.3 per 100,000), but lower than that for people of Afro-Caribbean descent (207 per 100,000) [31]. Samanta et al. estimated prevalence of SLE in Leicester, England to be 0.4 per 1000 for Asians and 0.2 per 1000 for Caucasians [32].

Prevalence in Africa and Populations of African Descent

Deligny et al. performed a retrospective epidemiological study on 45 patients of African descent living with cutaneous lupus in French Guiana [33]. They found that the cutaneous manifestations of their cohort were similar to Caucasian patients living in the same area; however, those of African descent were younger at diagnosis. Flower et al. performed a retrospective study to characterize the epidemiology, clinical features, and outcomes of African Caribbean patients with SLE in Barbados using a national registry (Barbados National Lupus Registry) [4]. Over a 9-year period, they reported an annual incidence rate of 12.21 per 100,000 person-years for women and 0.84 per 100,000 person-years for men. The prevalence of SLE in Afro-Caribbean, West African, and European descent women living in southern London was reported to be 177, 110 and 35 per 100,000, respectively [34].

Overall, the prevalence of SLE appears greatest in populations of African descent, followed by Asian and lowest for Caucasian populations. Generally, women are more commonly affected by CLE, including DLE and SLE, than men [35].

Disease Severity in Skin of Color

Disease Severity in Asians

Asian patients with SLE have been found to have different clinical presentations compared to Caucasian or African patients. In a prospective study of patients of Chinese descent living in Canada, the age of diagnosis was lower for the Chinese cohort compared to the African Canadian and Caucasian patients [36]. Furthermore, renal involvement was more prevalent among the African and Chinese groups compared to Caucasians. In a retrospective study evaluating the Systemic Lupus International Collaborative Clinics/American College of Rheumatology (SLICC/ACR) Damage Index, Asian patients were found to have a significantly higher mean damage score at 5 and 10 years and a higher renal damage score at 10 years compared to scores for Afro-Caribbean and Caucasian populations [37]. Another study revealed a prevalence of biopsy-proven lupus nephritis in Chinese patients to be 110.3 cases per 100,000, compared to 99.2 per 100,000 for Afro-Caribbean patients and 5.6 per 100,000 for Caucasian patients [38]. Samanta et al. also determined a younger age on onset for Asian patients (age 24) compared to Caucasian subjects (age 31) [32]. Furthermore in this study, Asian patients were found to have higher prevalence of proteinuria, neuropsychiatric disease, muscle disease (as measured by increased serum muscle enzymes), and higher serum ANA levels compared to their Caucasian counterparts.

Disease Severity in Hispanics

In the LUMINA (Lupus in Minorities: Nature vs. nurture) study, patients were followed at multiple centers in the United States, including a center in Puerto Rico. Study cohorts included Hispanics from Texas, Hispanics from Puerto Rico, and African Americans from multiple medical centers. Caucasians were also included in this study as a comparison group. Skin of color patients were found to have worse outcomes including higher disease activity according to the Systemic Lupus Activity Measure (SLAM) and higher incidences of organ damage [7, 39]. Hispanics from Texas were found to have a higher rate of organ damage from SLE than African Americans and Caucasians, and the Hispanic ethnicity was a significant predictor of organ damage in a multivariate analysis. Positive anti-dsDNA antibodies were more frequent in Hispanics from Texas and African Americans, whereas anti-U1 RNP, anti-Smith and antiphospholipid antibodies were more frequent among African Americans [39]. Furthermore, the physician's global assessment of disease activity, as measured on a ten-point scale, was higher in Hispanic and African American groups. Hispanic and African American patients also had a higher number of ACR criteria at enrollment in the study compared to Caucasians.

The GLADEL study (Latin American Group for the Study of Lupus), another large prospective multicenter study of skin of color patients with SLE, included 1214 patients of Mestizo (combined European and Amerindian descent), Caucasian, and African Latin American ethnicity [40]. In this study, skin of color was associated with renal disease and higher number of ACR criteria met at inception compared to Caucasian group. Patients of the Mestizo cohort had higher rates of renal damage compared to the Caucasian group, after accounting for clinical and socio-demographic variables.

Disease Severity in Africans and African Americans

Evidence suggests that SLE severity is highest for the Afro-Caribbean patients compared to Asian and Caucasian populations. Tan et al. determined that African American men were more likely to have a history of smoking, proteinuria and renal involvement than African American women [41]. Furthermore, African American men were also more likely to have neuropsychiatric and cardiovascular damage and have higher mortality. Similar observations were made when comparing Caucasian men to women. When comparing African American men to Caucasian men, African American men were more likely to have discoid lesions, alopecia, proteinuria, renal insufficiency, and anti-Smith antibodies. Furthermore, African American men were more likely to have a higher mortality than Caucasian men. Another study found that black women with SLE were the youngest compared to other racial groups when analyzing cardiovascular disease complications of SLE [42].

Overall, the above studies suggest that African American, Asian and Hispanic populations have more severe disease compared to their Caucasian counterparts.

Survival and Mortality in Skin of Color with Lupus Erythematosus

Variations exist in the morbidity and mortality observed in SLE patients of different ethnicities. Wadee et al. performed a retrospective study to determine the long-term outcome and mortality patterns of patients with SLE at a tertiary center in Soweto, South Africa. Five-year survival of these patients was 57%, and the most common cause of death was infection (32.7%) and renal failure (16.4%). They found that nephritis, neuropsychiatric disease, and hypocomplementemia were associated with increased mortality [43]. Gomez-Puerta et al. [44] in a large cohort of Medicaid patients found the overall mortality rate per 1000 person-years to be highest for Native Americans (27.52), followed by African Americans (24.13), Caucasians (20.17), Hispanics (7.12), and Asians (5.18). Wang et al. performed a systematic retrospective review and identified over 4000 published cases of Chinese patients with SLE and determined a pooled survival rate for SLE of 94% at 5 years and 89% at 10 years. The major causes of death were infection (33.2%), renal involvement (18.7%), encephalopathy (13.8%), and cardiovascular disease (11.5%) [45]. Flower et al. performed a retrospective study to characterize the epidemiology, clinical features and outcomes of African Caribbean patients in Barbados using a national registry (Barbados National Lupus Registry) [4]. The overall 5-year survival rate for this cohort of 183 cases was 79.5%. Another study found that the African American race independently worsened the probability of survival [46]. According to the LUMINA cohort study, the 5-year survival rate for Hispanic Americans was 86.9%, compared to 89.8% for African Americans and 94% for Caucasians. African American and Asian patients were found to have high disease activity on renal biopsy and higher renal-related death compared to Caucasians [47]. A study analyzing data over a ten-year period from the National Center for Health Statistics found that Chinese, Japanese, and Filipino patients had higher adjusted annual rates of death compared to Caucasians [48]. These Asian subgroups were found to have an annual mortality rate of 6.8 per million population compared to 2.8 per million for Caucasians. Another study revealed that African American women with SLE were about 20 years younger than race and sex-matched controls at the time of cardiovascular-related death [42]. In summary, the above studies suggest that African Americans have greater mortality and higher disease activity compared to their Asian and Caucasian counterparts.

Treatment

The management of CLE follows an algorithmic approach and is similar in all patients independent of skin color. Many of these therapies are added rather than substituted as a multimodal approach will have synergistic effects. The first step always includes photoprotection, including diligent use of sunscreens, avoidance of sunlight during peak midday hours, and the use of sun-protective clothing. This can be particularly challenging for patients with darker skin types to adhere to as they do not burn as easily as fair-skinned patients do and are usually not as attentive to their photoprotective habits [49]. Sun avoidance is important for both cutaneous-limited and systemic disease, as sun exposure can precipitate flairs of both. For limited cutaneous disease, local therapies, including topical or intralesional corticosteroids and topical calcineurin inhibitors are used. For more severe disease or if lesions are recalcitrant to the previously outlined therapies, antimalarials are subsequently added to the regimen. The most commonly used agents include hydroxychloro-quine, chloroquine, and quinacrine [35]. Hydroxychloroquine is more frequently used in the US at a typical dose of 200 mg twice daily. Patients should be counseled that full efficacy may take up to two to three months and response to therapy is usually assessed after this time before starting a second-line agent [50]. The most concerning side effect of hydroxychloroquine is irreversible retinal toxicity (bull's eye maculopathy), which increases with higher doses and long-term use of the medication [51]. It is generally thought that the risk for retinal toxicity is highest for chloroquine and least for quinacrine [50]. A recent publication by the American Academy of Ophthalmology recommended that a baseline fundus exam be performed to evaluate for preexisting maculopathy and annual screening be performed after 5 years of use for patients on standard doses, as the risk of retinal toxicity increases substantially after that time. Weight-based dosing for hydroxychloroquine of 5 mg/kg/day of real body weight was recommended to decrease the risk of retinal toxicity [51].

Particular attention should be paid to patients who smoke, as cigarette smoking has been associated with increased disease severity in SLE and may decrease the efficacy of antimalarial drugs used. Second-line agents that can be used in combination with antimalarials or used alone include methotrexate (7.5–25 mg/week), mycophenolate mofetil (1000–3000 mg/day), thalidomide (25–100 mg/day), and dapsone (50–150 mg/day) [35].

In addition, it appears that ethnicity may play a role in patients' response to systemic therapies. In a retrospective study of a cohort with a large number of ethnic patients, immunosuppressive drugs (oral prednisone, chloroquine and intravenous cyclophosphamide) were found more frequently to be used in non-Caucasians compared with Caucasians [52]. Furthermore, in the Aspreva Lupus Management Study, African American and Hispanic patients who had induction treatment with mycophenolate mofetil (MMF) versus intravenous cyclophosphamide (IVC) for lupus nephritis had higher response rates to MMF compared to IVC, whereas the response rates to both agents were comparable in the Asian and Caucasian cohorts [53]. African Americans and Hispanics from Texas were found to more likely have received corticosteroids and cyclophosphamide compared to Caucasian patients [7]. Another study reported that immunosuppressive treatments were required more in Asian patients compared to Caucasian patients [32]. Interestingly, using antimalarial drugs for greater than 2 years in a skin of color population was associated with a lower mortality rate and a 38% delay in the occurrence of death [52].

SLE Key Points

The clinical presentation, course, and survival of patients with SLE appear to vary by ethnic group. Gene linkage studies have identified gene polymorphisms specific to ethnic groups that confer a risk of LE development and associated prognostic information. The prevalence of SLE is greatest in populations of African descent and this population appears to have more severe disease compared to their Caucasian counterparts. Furthermore, African Americans appear to have greater mortality and higher disease activity compared to their Asian and Caucasian counterparts.

Systemic Sclerosis in Skin of Color

Systemic sclerosis (SSc), or scleroderma, is an autoimmune connective tissue disorder that causes thickening of skin in association with internal organ involvement. In skin of color, scleroderma is noted for its distinct clinical presentation, clinical course, autoantibody profile, and prognosis. SSc can be broadly divided into two clinical subtypes based on distribution of skin lesions and pattern of systemic disease. The limited form of SSc is characterized by sclerotic changes (manifested clinically as skin hardening) of the distal extremities and face. This form of SSc can also involve internal organs, such as the lungs and gastrointestinal tract, but with usually different manifestations than the diffuse form. In the diffuse subtype of SSc, the skin thickening progresses from distal to proximal extremities as well as involving the trunk and face. In addition to more widespread skin and internal organ involvement, diffuse SSc has a higher associated mortality than the limited form of SSc.

Epidemiology of SSc in Skin of Color

SSc has a worldwide distribution and has been reported to affect all races. Women are affected more commonly than men in a 3–4:1 ratio. A positive family history of SSc confers up to a 15-fold higher risk of developing SSc than the general population [54]. The age of onset of SSc typically ranges from 40 to 50 years old. The authors in one study reported a 2.5-fold higher incidence in their African American cohort (20 per million per year), compared to their Caucasian cohort (8 per million per year) [55]. In a large epidemiological study of female patients with SSc from Michigan over a 10-year period, the annual incidence for African American women was estimated to be 22.5 per million population and was lower for Caucasian women at 12.8 per million [56]. In one large cohort study, African American patients presented at a younger age compared to Caucasian patients (mean age at first visit 44.8 vs. 50) [57]. Furthermore in a study over a 20-year period, the incidence of diffuse SSc was reported to be higher among African Americans compared to Caucasians, especially in the younger age range 15–24 [58]. In a smaller case-control study of 12 SSc cases, full-blooded Choctaws of Native American descent were found to have a higher prevalence (66/100,000) compared to the other Native Americans in Oklahoma (9.5/100,000), who had a similar prevalence to that reported for Caucasians [59].

Pathogenesis

The etiology for SSc is complex and only partially understood. The earliest pathophysiologic change in SSc is endothelial injury with altered response to vasoconstriction and vasodilation [60]. Eventually, vessel lumens decrease in diameter and become occluded, leading to localized hypoxia with production of profibrotic cytokines and fibroblastic activation [61]. The final pathway in SSc is fibrosis with proliferation of fibroblasts and deposition of collagen, fibronectin, proteoglycans, fibrillins, and various other molecules. An important growth factor that has been implicated in the pathogenesis of SSc is transforming growth factor $\beta1$ (TGF-$\beta1$), which is involved in fibrinogenesis and fibrosis. In dermal fibroblasts isolated from patients with SSc, receptors for TGF-$\beta1$ are increased with abnormal downstream signaling [60]. Caveolin-1 is a plasma membrane protein that is regulated by expression of TGF-$\beta1$ and thought to be involved in the predisposition of blacks to SSc [62].

Multiple alleles of the human leukocyte antigen have been associated with the risk of developing SSc in certain ethnic groups. Furthermore, frequencies of certain SSc-associated autoantibodies have been found to differ in various ethnic groups compared to Caucasians. In a cohort of Han Chinese patients, DRB1*11 was found to confer risk of developing SSc, which the authors note is consistent with studies of Hispanic and Spanish populations. Furthermore, DRB1*15 was associated with Han Chinese patients with SSc who were positive for anti-topoisomerase autoantibodies. This haplotype was also found in anti-topoisomerase positive Black South African and Korean patients with SSc [63]. In a case-control study of 52 Black South Africans, greater frequency of DRB1*0301 was observed in the limited SSc subset and DQB1*0301/4 in the diffuse subset. The authors of this study also found that pulmonary fibrosis was associated with DRB1*11. Topoisomerase I autoantibodies were associated with DPB1*1301 and DRB1*15 [64]. In a large cohort of 944 patients with SSc, HLA-DRB1*1104 and HLA-DQB1*0301 haplotypes were found to have higher frequencies in cohorts from Spain and Italy [65]. One study found that DRB1*0804, DQA1*0501, DQB1*0301 alleles are associated with black subjects with SSc [66].

Diagnosis of Systemic Sclerosis

The diagnosis of systemic sclerosis is based on a constellation of clinical manifestations and laboratory findings. The 2013 American College of Rheumatology/European League Against Rheumatism classification (ACR/EULAR) criteria for SSc includes weighted scores for various clinical features and scleroderma-related autoantibodies [67]. Clinical features with the highest weighted score(s) includes skin thickening of fingers of both hands extending proximal to the metacarpophalangeal joints (score of 9), skin thickening affecting an entire finger past the metacarpophalangeal joint (score of 4), puffy fingers (score of 2), digital tip ulcers (score of 2), and pitting scars (score of 3). Additional cutaneous features in the classification criteria include telangiectasias and abnormal nailfold capillary changes. Systemic features in the classification criteria include pulmonary arterial hypertension, interstitial lung disease, and Raynaud's phenomenon. Finally, the criteria include the most commonly detected autoantibodies in scleroderma, including anti-topoisomerase I (Scl-70), anti-centromere, and anti-RNA polymerase III (RNAP3). Patients with a score of 9 or greater are classified as having definite SSc.

Cutaneous and Systemic Features

Patients with SSc often experience an evolution in their skin disease over time, whereby there is an early edematous phase with erythema and edema of the skin, which is typically described as nonpitting [60]. This phase is followed by subsequent hardening with the appearance of shiny and tight overlying epidermis, which is known as the indurated phase. With progression, the overlying epidermis becomes thinner resulting in the atrophic phase [68]. With time and progressive disease, the digits may develop flexion contractures due to the thickened bound-down skin and ulcerations due to tissue hypoxia and trauma. Involvement of the face can cause tightening of the skin with loss of wrinkles, decrease in diameter of the oral aperture (microstomia), and beaked nose giving the face a characteristic appearance [69]. In skin of color patients, dyspigmentation can frequently be observed over sclerotic areas as well as unaffected areas. The classically described "salt and pepper" sign is most frequently distributed over the upper trunk and central face, and consists of focal areas of depigmentation with normal follicular pigmentation and a normal-appearing epidermis. Changes in pigmentation are a common finding in skin of color patients. In one study, 82% of African American patients had hyperpigmentation or hypopigmentation, compared to 51% in Caucasian patients [70]. The types of pigmentary changes described are variable, ranging from ill-defined hyper- or hypopigmented patches to vitiligo-like areas (such as the above-mentioned "salt and pepper" sign) to a mixture of both hyper- and hypopigmented areas [71]. Telangiectasias are more frequent in patients with limited SSc and may be harder to appreciate in skin of color. Telangiectasias are most frequently distributed on the face, lips, and palmar surfaces. On capillaroscopy of the proximal nailfolds, an alternating pattern of loss of capillary loops ("drop out") with dilated loops is characteristic of SSc and can be observed in up to 90% of patients [72]. CREST syndrome is a variant of limited SSc, consisting of Calcinosis, Raynaud's phenomenon, Esophageal dysmotility, Sclerodactyly, and Telangiectasias. This syndrome is most frequently observed in women and is associated with the anti-centromere antibody.

Additional cutaneous manifestations of SSc include dystrophic calcinosis, pruritus, alopecia, and Raynaud's phenomenon. SSc is one of the most common causes of Raynaud's phenomenon, a symmetric vasospasm of the digital arteries resulting in sequential discoloration (white to blue to red) of the distal fingers in response to cold. Digital ulcerations are commonly observed in patients with SSc. Ulcerations on the fingertips are usually due to ischemia and those over dorsal interphalangeal joints or pressure points are most likely caused by trauma. These ulcerations may be challenging to manage, may require specialty care, and can be a nidus for infection. In addition, severe cases of digital ischemia and ulcerations can result in osteolysis and digit shortening. The gastrointestinal tract (GIT) is commonly affected, particularly the upper GIT in up to 90% of patients with SSc [73]. When the esophagus is affected, patients typically present with dyspepsia and dysphagia. Pulmonary involvement may manifest as pulmonary arterial hypertension or interstitial lung disease and represents the leading cause of death in scleroderma [74]. The most dreaded complication from kidney involvement is the scleroderma renal crisis, which is the sudden onset of hypertension and/or acute renal failure and is associated with high mortality.

Histology

Histologic features of SSc depend on the stage of the lesion. Earlier lesions of SSc have a mixed inflammatory infiltrate (lymphocytes, histiocytes, and plasma cells) between collagen bundles and also around blood vessels. Thickening or hyalinization of collagen bundles has been noted to occur in the lower dermis and fibrous septa and then extend to the upper dermis. Eventually, the densely packed collagen bundles replace the dermis and subcutaneous fat. Adnexal structures such as eccrine glands and hair follicles can become "trapped" because of the increase in collagen deposition. Blood vessels also become hyalinized. These changes also occur in lesions of morphea and histologically the two cannot be distinguished [60].

Serologic Markers in Systemic Sclerosis

Several autoantibodies have been found in patients with scleroderma and are helpful in diagnosing and characterizing the associated clinical features of patients with this disease. In particular, anti-centromere antibody (ACA) has been associated with the limited subtype of SSc and pulmonary arterial hypertension, anti-topoisomerase I (topo I) antibody with the diffuse subtype of SSc and interstitial lung disease, and anti-RNA polymerase III (RNA pol III) antibody with the diffuse subtype and scleroderma renal crisis [57, 73]. It appears that ethnicity may also influence antibody profiles as certain authors found anti-U1RNP and anti-U3RNP (fibrillarin) in combination with topo I to be the most frequent in African Americans with SSc, whereas the most common in Caucasians appeared to be ACA, topo I, and RNA pol III [57]. There is also some evidence to suggest that this racial difference in antibody profiles may affect severity of clinical manifestations, as African Americans with anti-topo I and U1-RNP were found to have more severe pulmonary fibrosis than Caucasians with the same antibodies [57].

Disease Severity and Mortality in Skin of Color

Numerous studies have reported that African American patients with SSc have greater disease severity and higher mortality than their Caucasian counterparts. One study reported that in the United States the death rate peaked 10 years earlier for African Americans (age 65–74) with SSc than Caucasians (age 75–84). The authors also reported a higher age-adjusted mortality rate for African Americans (7.1 deaths per million population per year) than Caucasians (4.4 deaths per million population per year) with SSc. Furthermore, age-adjusted mortality rate was highest for African American women (9.5 deaths per million population per year) with SSc [75]. Another study determined that African American patients were more likely to experience in-hospital deaths than Caucasians when hospitalized for complications of SSc [76]. Steen et al. found that African American patients with anti-topoisomerase antibody had more severe pulmonary fibrosis and decreased survival compared to Caucasian patients who were positive for the same antibody [57]. Overall, African Americans with scleroderma appear to be at greater risk for more severe disease including diffuse disease, younger age of onset, associated pulmonary disease, and overall worse prognosis [70, 77].

Treatment

Patients with cutaneous manifestations of SSc warrant evaluation for internal organ involvement [78]. Studies to evaluate for pulmonary disease include pulmonary function tests, high-resolution CT scan of the chest, and echocardiography [79]. A urinalysis is important to obtain for evaluation of renal involvement. For evaluation of gastrointestinal symptoms, an endoscopy and upper gastrointestinal series (i.e., barium swallow) can be ordered in consultation with a specialist particularly for patients who do not respond as expected to antireflux therapies [74].

The treatment of SSc is challenging and therapeutic interventions focus mainly on specific organ involvement. D-penicillamine, minocycline, and methotrexate have been trialed for cutaneous sclerosis with minimal success [80, 81]. UVA1 has also been reported to have a role in treating skin disease, similar to morphea [82]. Mycophenolate mofetil has been used as first-line therapy in expert reviews, with intravenous immunoglobulin and low-dose cyclophosphamide as second-line agents [74]. First-line treatment of Raynaud's phenomenon is behavioral and includes counseling on avoiding cold temperatures, keeping core body and extremities warm, stress management, and smoking cessation [83]. The most commonly used pharmacologic agents for Raynaud's include topical nitroglycerin, calcium channel blockers, angiotensin II receptor blockers, antidepressants, and phosphodiesterase-5 inhibitors [83]. Treatment of esophageal dysmotility usually includes symptomatic control with proton-pump inhibitors for gastroesophageal reflux [84].

Dermatomyositis in Skin of Color

Dermatomyositis (DM) is an idiopathic inflammatory myositis that presents with characteristic cutaneous signs in combination with symmetric, proximal inflammatory myopathy. It can occur in association with interstitial lung disease and internal malignancies.

Epidemiology

Estimates on the incidence of dermatomyositis range from 1.2 to 17 new cases per million [85]. Females are twice as likely to be affected compared to males and data suggests prevalence is 2–4 times greater in African Americans than Caucasians [86, 87]. The estimated incidence of juvenile DM is 2 per million for Caucasians and 7 per million for African Americans [88].

Pathogenesis

The exact etiology of DM is not known but is thought to be triggered by an autoimmune response to foreign antigens such as drugs, infectious agents, or malignancy in genetically predisposed individuals [89]. Numerous HLA types have been associated with DM including HLA-DR3, HLA-DR52, HLA-DR7, HLA-DRw53, HLA-B14, and HLA-B40. Several autoantibodies have been found in patients with DM, the more commonly described include anti-JO-1, anti-Mi-2, anti-MDA-5, anti-SAE, anti-TIF1γ, and anti-NXP2—all of which are associated with various clinical phenotypes [89, 90]. Mi-2 autoantibodies are associated with classic DM with both the characteristic cutaneous findings as well as muscle disease with an overall favorable prognosis [90]. Patients with MDA5 autoantibodies typically have mild or absent muscle disease and an increased risk of interstitial lung disease [90, 91]. Furthermore, patients with MDA5 autoantibodies also appear to have a specific cutaneous phenotype consisting of ulcerating skin lesions and/or tender palmar papules [92]. TIF1γ autoantibodies (formally classified as a p155/140 doublet) have been shown to have 89% specificity and 78% sensitivity for detecting cancer-associated DM [89, 93]. NXP-2 (formally p140) is found more frequently in juvenile DM with calcinosis along with polyarthritis, joint contractures, and intestinal vasculitis [90]. More recent studies of NXP-2 antibodies in adults have shown association with significant muscle disease and malignancy [90, 94]. Anti-JO-1 antibodies have classically been associated with the antisynthetase syndrome, which is characterized by Gottron's papules, mechanic's hands, myositis, arthritis, fever, Raynaud's phenomenon, and interstitial lung disease [89]. The more recently described anti-SAE antibodies have been associated with the presence of myositis and severe dysphagia [91].

Certain autoantibodies and HLA types specific to those with darker skin types have also been identified. The combination of anti-topoisomerase I antibody and anti-U1RNP was found to be more prevalent in African Americans and clinically more likely to be associated with an overlap between systemic sclerosis (with mild skin involvement) and systemic lupus erythematosus or polymyositis/dermatomyositis [95]. Certain HLA alleles have been identified as possible risk factors for idiopathic inflammatory myopathies in African Americans compared to ethnically matched controls and include HLA-A*6802, HLA- DQA1*0501, and

HLA-DRB1*03. For dermatomyositis, HLA-DQA1*0601 was identified as a novel risk factor for African Americans compared to other inflammatory myopathies [96]. Higher frequencies of anti-PL-12 autoantibodies were found in African American patients with idiopathic inflammatory myopathies compared to European American patients with idiopathic inflammatory myopathies [96].

Diagnosis of Dermatomyositis

The first criteria to diagnosing DM were developed by Bohan and Peter and include five components: (1) symmetric proximal muscle weakness determined by physical examination, (2) elevation of serum skeletal muscle enzymes, (3) abnormal characteristic electromyography, (4) characteristic abnormal muscle biopsy, and (5) the presence of the characteristic skin findings of DM [97, 98]. A possible, probable or definite diagnosis is made when a patient has the characteristic skin findings in addition to 1, 2, or 3 muscular criteria, respectively [97, 98]. These criteria have been widely used and are highly sensitive (94%), but do not include the more recently described entity "clinically amyopathic DM", wherein the cutaneous features of DM are present without involvement of muscle. Other more recent criteria have been proposed and include the use of autoantibodies and imaging modalities but have not been widely validated [99, 100].

Clinical Presentation

DM presents in a bimodal distribution in children ages 5–15 and then adults ages 40–65 [101]. Cutaneous findings may precede muscle disease by many months in one-third to one-half of patients; however, after 2 years without muscle involvement, the patient can be classified as having clinically amyopathic DM [102, 103]. The pathognomonic skin findings of DM include the heliotrope rash and Gottron's papules. The heliotrope rash is characterized by periorbital violaceous erythema with or without edema most often involving the upper eyelid. In African Americans, this may only present as periorbital edema [50]. Gottron's papules are erythematous to violaceous flat-topped scaly papules distributed over bony prominences, typically the interphalangeal joints of the dorsal fingers. Other cutaneous findings characteristic of DM include violaceous erythema on extensor extremities or lateral thighs ("holster sign"), photodistributed poikiloderma, centrofacial erythema, periungual telangiectasias and dystrophic cuticles, and diffuse alopecia. Skin lesions are frequently pruritic. Proximal muscle weakness is the predominant musculoskeletal presentation of DM. Myalgias, while infrequent, may precede weakness and muscle atrophy can occur late in the course of disease [85]. Typically, the muscle disease activity does not correlate with skin disease.

Other internal organs may also be involved in DM, such as pulmonary and cardiac systems, which lead to increased morbidity and mortality [102]. DM in adults has also been associated with an increased risk of internal malignancy, with an incidence ranging from 9 to 32%, and the risk remains elevated for three to five years after diagnosis [104]. Associated malignancies are typically detected within 1 year of symptom onset while the majority of associated malignancies are detected in the first 3 years. In African American women, the risk of DM associated malignancy is decreased compared to Caucasian women [50]. In those of Chinese decent, nasopharyngeal carcinoma composes 40–80% of associated malignancy with DM [105]. The most common associated malignancies include lymphomas, lung, ovary, colon, and genitourinary carcinomas [89].

Histology

Skin biopsies in DM reveal a vacuolar interface dermatitis with dermal mucin deposition similar to that of lupus erythematosus [102]. Muscle biopsies characteristically show a perivascular and perifascicular inflammatory infiltrate in addition to type II muscle fiber atrophy, necrosis, regeneration, and hypertrophy [106].

Prognosis and Mortality

The prognosis for DM has improved over time but there are still large ranges in mortality in the literature likely due to small sample sizes of studies and variation amongst patients. One-year survival varies from 83 to 95% while five year survival varies from 63 to 95%. Nine year or greater survival ranges from 53 to 100% [107]. Recent studies for juvenile DM found the mortality to range from 0 to 1.5% [108, 109]. Poor prognostic factors in DM include older age, malignancy, progressive disease, cardiac or pulmonary complications, longer duration of symptoms before treatment, and extensive cutaneous lesions on the trunk [107]. No studies have specifically looked at survival or prognosis in ethnic skin types.

Treatment

Treatment for dermatomyositis is largely based on retrospective studies and case series as few randomized controlled trials have been performed. For those with confirmed DM and active muscle disease, high dose systemic corticosteroids are the mainstay of therapy [110]. Initial doses usually range from 0.5 to 1.5 mg/kg and then are slowly tapered over the course of several months based upon disease response [111]. Steroid-sparing agents and adjunctive therapy for refractory disease include methotrexate, azathioprine, mycophenolate mofetil, and intravenous immunoglobulins (IVIg) among others [107].

The treatment of the skin manifestations of DM starts with strict sun protection and topical agents, including steroids and calcineurin inhibitors [110]. Control of pruritus is important and use of emollients and systemic antihistamines may be beneficial. Antimalarials, such as hydroxychloroquine, have been found to be effective in 41–75% of patients [107]. Additional systemic therapies include methotrexate (to be used with caution in patients with associated lung disease), mycophenolate mofetil, IVIg, dapsone, and rituximab, and have been reported for refractory skin manifestations of DM [107]. Most recently, tofacitinib has been described as effective in a small case series of three patients with multidrug-resistant cutaneous dermatomyositis [112].

Morphea in Skin of Color

Morphea, also known as localized scleroderma, is a rare inflammatory disease characterized by sclerosis of the skin. While the underlying etiology of morphea remains unclear, it is considered an autoimmune disease that is likely multifactorial in nature. Individuals with morphea are thought to have an underlying genetic predisposition coupled with an environmental trigger. Triggering events have been hypothesized to include infection, medications, trauma, or radiation. In the right setting, this combination of factors ultimately results in small vessel damage, the release of profibrotic cytokines and disruption of the balance of collagen production and destruction [113].

Prevalence in Skin of Color

Morphea has an estimated incidence of 2.7 per 100,000 individuals, with a female predominance ranging from 2.4 to 4.2:1 [114–116]. The few published population-based studies report morphea to more commonly affect Caucasians, who make up 73–83% of cases. Conversely, Hispanics make up 13–14% of morphea patients, African Americans comprise 3–7% and Asians comprise 2–3% [114, 115, 117].

Clinical Presentation

Morphea runs a variable and unpredictable course. Clinically, morphea is typically composed of an initial inflammatory stage with the appearance of erythematous to dusky-violaceous patches and plaques. Eventually, these lesions transition to a fibrotic stage in which they become white to hyperpigmented sclerotic plaques which can be both hairless and anhidrotic [113]. Specific manifestations have not been well characterized in skin of color, which may be a reflection of the rarity of the disease or nature of the presentation as with other inflammatory diseases in skin of color, the initial erythematous stage can be a more subtle hyperpigmentation.

Morphea has been described as having five variants, including: circumscribed, linear, generalized, pansclerotic, and mixed [118]. Circumscribed morphea, which can be superficial or deep, is most often localized to the trunk and is characterized by three or fewer discrete, indurated plaques. While the superficial variant is limited to the epidermis or dermis, the deep variant can affect the subcutaneous tissue including the underlying fascia and muscle.

Generalized morphea is defined as either having four or more indurated plaques or involving two or more body sites, typically sparing the face and hands in contrast with scleroderma. Generalized morphea can be differentiated from systemic sclerosis by the lack of Raynaud's phenomenon, digital sclerosis, or internal organ involvement.

Linear morphea more frequently affects children and can cause significant morbidity as it often leads to fibrosis and atrophy of the underlying tissue; when occurring over a limb, this can lead to contractures, limb length discrepancy, and significant functional disability. Lesions may also affect the scalp and face, potentially leading to significant disfigurement in addition to neurologic and ophthalmologic complications [119, 120]. The initial lesion may appear as a discrete plaque, which then extends longitudinally as multiple plaques that eventually coalesce. Linear variants include the trunk/limb variant, en coup de sabre and progressive hemifacial atrophy.

Pansclerotic morphea consists of circumferential involvement of the limbs and the underlying subcutaneous tissue, often involving tissue down to the bone. This deep involvement can cause atrophy and contractures, which ultimately results in significant morbidity, making it the most debilitating form of morphea. Mixed morphea is any combination of two or more of the above subtypes.

Histology

Histologically, early morphea is characterized by lymphocytic perivascular infiltration in the reticular dermis and swollen endothelial cells. Late morphea demonstrates thickened collagen bundles involving the entire dermis and extending into the subcutaneous fat. Additional features commonly seen include loss of eccrine glands and blood vessels as well as "fat trapping," where foci of fat are trapped between bands of thickened collagen [113].

Treatment

The treatment of morphea is mostly based on expert opinion as there have been very few randomized controlled studies, and the approach is based on extent and subtype of disease [117]. Treatment algorithms have been proposed by Zwischenberger et al. and Fett et al., which are similar in that they propose superficial morphea is best treated with localized therapy while deep or linear morphea should be treated more aggressively. Topical therapies for superficial morphea include tacrolimus, calcipotriene, imiquimod, or a high-potency corticosteroid. Other treatment options for superficial morphea include intralesional triamcinolone and phototherapy including UVA1, nbUVB, and UVA. Both Fett and Zwischenberger propose that initial therapy for generalized superficial morphea is whole-body phototherapy if available [121, 122].

The treatment of deep morphea, as well as superficial morphea that continues to progress despite the use of localized therapy, is best approached with more aggressive systemic therapy. This includes methotrexate with or without a systemic glucocorticoid, or mycophenolate mofetil [121, 122].

The use of methotrexate and pulsed-dose systemic glucocorticoids is commonly employed in the pediatric setting, and a randomized trial found relapse rates to be lower when employing this regimen as compared to prednisone alone [123]. Although similar randomized controlled trials are lacking in the adult population, this regimen may be employed to achieve disease control when there is rapidly progressive superficial disease or deeper involvement causing functional or cosmetic impairment. For inactive disease, the focus should be on correcting any functional or cosmetic defects with the use of measures such as surgery, fillers, physio- or occupational therapy, or orthotics [122].

Sarcoidosis in Skin of Color

Sarcoidosis is a multisystem inflammatory disorder that is characterized by the presence of noncaseating granulomas in involved tissues. Sarcoidosis predominantly involves the pulmonary system and skin, but can also affect the ocular, cardiovascular, musculoskeletal, endocrine, and neurologic systems. Sarcoidosis is more common, presents with more advanced disease, and has a poorer prognosis in skin of color.

Pathogenesis

The etiology of sarcoidosis is unknown but is thought to result from an exaggerated immune response in genetically susceptible individuals. Specifically, CD4+ T cells accumulate at the site of active disease and are thought to interact with antigen presenting cells through the human leukocyte antigen (HLA) class II pathway, with subsequent initiation of granulomatous inflammation [124]. In the HLA class II region of chromosome 6p, the various alleles of HLA-DRB1 have been found to have a strong association with developing sarcoidosis [125]. Several HLA alleles are associated with increased susceptibility to disease, though these vary between racial groups. The exception is HLA-DRB1*11:01, which is associated with a higher risk of developing sarcoidosis across different ethnic populations [126]. The presence of HLA-DRB1*03.01 in Europeans has been found to confer a high likelihood of self-limited disease. Similarly, the HLA-DRB1*03:02 allele is more likely found in American blacks with self-resolved sarcoidosis rather than persistent disease. In contrast, the HLA-DRB1 alleles *12:01 and *11:01 result in increased susceptibility to disease in blacks. The HLA-DRB1*08 and *09 alleles are strongly associated with disease in Japanese patients but have less of an association in the UK, Scandinavian, and Czech populations [124].

Incidence

In the United States, the estimated annual incidence of sarcoidosis is 10.0 per 100,000. It has been reported to be 3–4 times more common in blacks compared to whites, and blacks have a threefold higher prevalence of family history of sarcoidosis compared with whites [127]. A retrospective review of 311 sarcoidosis patients in New York City reported a racial distribution of 36% white, 47% black, and 17% Puerto Rican; in Los Angeles, the distribution in 150 patients was 11% white, 82% black, and 7% Mexican [128]. Another retrospective study of 156 patients in South London found that the incidence of sarcoidosis in Indo-Pakistan Asians was only slightly less than the incidence in the black West Indian/African population [129]. Japan, in contrast, has a very low incidence and prevalence of sarcoidosis, averaging 1.01 per 100,000 inhabitants [130]. Sarcoidosis may also have locational, temporal, and occupational clustering [131]. For instance, outbreaks of sarcoidosis have been reported in the UK, Japan, and Sweden where the affected individuals lived within close distances of one another. Seasonal clustering has also been noted, with increased diagnoses of sarcoidosis during the spring in Greece and the summer in Spain and Japan. In addition, there appears to be occupational clustering with higher percentage of cases observed in health care workers, firefighters, and naval aircraft servicemen in the United States.

Clinical Features

There is large variability in the clinical presentation, evolution, and prognosis of disease across individuals, thus explaining why sarcoidosis is known as the "great mimicker"—its many manifestations can be mistaken for different disease processes including various primary neoplasms, metastatic disease, vasculitis, and other granulomatous infections [132]. Most typically, sarcoidosis presents with lung and intrathoracic lymph node involvement. The lungs are affected in approximately 90% of patients, and the most frequent presenting symptoms are cough, dyspnea, or chest pain. Lymph node involvement results in the classic finding on chest X-ray of bilateral hilar adenopathy. However, nearly any organ system can be involved, and patients can present with extrathoracic manifestations.

The skin is the second most common organ affected, occurring in 25–30% of cases reported [133]. Cutaneous sarcoidosis may occur with or without systemic involvement, and there is a wide range of associated cutaneous findings (Table 12.1) [134, 135]. Cutaneous lesions of sarcoidosis can be classified as specific, showing noncaseating granulomas histologically, or nonspecific, in which noncaseating granulomas are not seen. Proper identification of specific skin lesions is necessary as certain variants can determine prognosis [133, 136]. Skin plaques (large erythematous lesions that appear predominantly on the head, limbs, and back), lupus pernio (violaceous firm plaques that occur on the cheeks, nose, and ears), and ichthyosiform sarcoidosis are associated with more severe systemic involvement and chronic disease, whereas maculopapules, subcutaneous nodules, and scar sarcoidosis tend to have a more benign or acute course. Erythema nodosum, a nonspecific manifestation of sarcoidosis presenting as erythematous tender nodules on the anterior lower extremities, usually represents benign disease and generally self-resolves [124]. An acute form of sarcoidosis, called Lofgren's Syndrome, is characterized by hilar lymphadenopathy, fever, erythema nodosum, and polyarthralgia.

Cutaneous findings can be affected by ethnicity and gender. Ulcerative lesions are more likely to occur in blacks and women than in whites and men [138]. Lupus pernio also occurs most commonly in black women [139]. Patients with darker skin also have a higher rate of hypopigmented sarcoid lesions. Erythema nodosum, in contrast, is seen significantly less frequently in black or Asian patients as compared to white patients and those of European, Puerto Rican, and Mexican descent [128, 129, 139]. Subcutaneous nodules also tend to occur more often in whites than those with skin of color [16].

Sarcoidosis can involve any organ system, particularly the ocular, cardiovascular, musculoskeletal, endocrine, and neurologic systems. Ocular sarcoidosis can involve any part of the eye and its adnexal tissues, but most commonly presents as uveitis, dry eye, and conjunctival nodules. Ocular disease occurs more frequently in women, blacks, and Japanese [137, 140]. In cardiac sarcoidosis, granulomatous inflammation and infiltration can affect any part of the heart. Clinically, it can present with arrhythmias, conduction defects, or sudden death, but a greater percentage of patients do not exhibit any symptoms [141]. The incidence of cardiac sarcoid granulomas and cardiac sarcoidosis-induced death was several times higher in the Japanese compared with Blacks and Whites [142]. Musculoskeletal symptoms generally include polyarthralgias or polyarthritis and neurologic involvement may affect the cranial nerves, hypothalamus, and pituitary gland [143].

Table 12.1 Cutaneous manifestations of sarcoidosis

Variant	Nonspecific versus specific	Description	Unique characteristics
Calcifications	Nonspecific	Subcutaneous calcium deposits	Reflects calcium homeostasis dysregulation that occurs in sarcoidosis
Erythema nodosum	Nonspecific	Tender, palpable, and erythematous nodules that appear predominantly on the anterior lower extremities	
Nail clubbing	Nonspecific	Thickening of the distal fingers resulting in a Lovibond angle (the angle between the nail plate and the proximal nail fold) that is greater than 180°	
Prurigo nodularis	Nonspecific	Pruritic nodules that usually affect the extensor surfaces of the limbs	
Hypopigmented lesions	Specific	Hypopigmented macules, papules, or nodules	Typically occur in darker skinned patients
Ichthyosiform	Specific	Large hyperpigmented polygonal scaling plaques that typically affects the anterior surface of the lower extremities	Majority of patients will have or develop systemic symptoms. Very rare
Lupus pernio	Specific	Indurated red-brown edematous changes on nose, cheeks, and ears	Most common in black women. Often associated with involvement of sinuses and oropharynx. Usually portends chronic and treatment-resistant course
Papules and plaques	Specific	Small, firm, red-brown to violaceous lesions that can be localized or generalized	Most common cutaneous finding. Apple jelly color on diascopy. Plaques infiltrate more deeply and can cause more scarring
Psoriasiform	Specific	Erythematous or hyperpigmented scaling plaques that predominantly affect the lower extremities	More commonly affects darker skinned individuals. Heals with scarring
Scar sarcoidosis	Specific	Scars or areas of previous skin trauma (injection, tattoos) become thickened and develop a more erythematous or violaceous hue	Isolated scar sarcoidosis usually self-resolves

(continued)

Table 12.1 (continued)

Variant	Nonspecific versus specific	Description	Unique characteristics
Subcutaneous nodules (Darier-Roussy sarcoidosis)	Specific	Firm mobile nodules that predominantly affect the trunk and upper extremities. Typically painless	Rare overall. Affects whites more than skin of color
Ulcerative	Specific	Ulcers with hyperpigmented or violaceous borders that can develop de novo or in existing cutaneous sarcoid lesions	Rare. More common in women and blacks

Data from [133, 137]

Diagnostic Workup and Histology

The elaboration of standard diagnostic criteria for sarcoidosis is challenging due to the high variability in clinical manifestations. At the present time, diagnosis is based on the following: (1) a compatible clinical and radiologic presentation, (2) histologic evidence of noncaseating granulomas, and (3) exclusion of other diseases with similar findings, such as infections or malignancy [144]. Chest radiography can be used to stage sarcoidosis, with stage 0 correlating with normal findings and stage IV representing pulmonary fibrosis.

Because cutaneous sarcoidosis has such a wide variety of morphologies that can mimic many other diseases, a skin biopsy is the diagnostic tool of choice. The most common histopathologic finding is a discrete noncaseating granuloma consisting of highly differentiated mononuclear phagocytes (such as epithelioid cells and giant cells) and lymphocytes [145]. These granulomas tend to have CD4+ lymphocytes in the central zone and CD8+ lymphocytes in the periphery, and they may develop fibrotic changes that begin in the periphery and move towards the center. Focal coagulative necrosis may also be seen within the granulomas. However, similar histologic features may be seen in other mycobacterial infections and some vasculitic disorders. In addition, not all sarcoid lesions have these histological findings —nonspecific cutaneous sarcoidosis lesions do not contain granulomas and are thought to represent a reactive process [146]. Thus, it is important to corroborate the histopathology with clinical findings consistent with sarcoidosis, as well as to exclude other disorders.

Laboratory tests are generally neither sensitive nor specific but can offer additional information that may aid in diagnosis. The complete blood count in sarcoidosis may show leukopenia, anemia, thrombocytopenia, or pancytopenia. In addition, both hypercalcemia and hypercalciuria can be seen secondary to secretion of 1,25 vitamin D by noncaseating granulomas. Men are more likely to have difficulties with calcium homeostasis than women and present with an elevated urinary calcium/Cr ratio rather than hypercalcemia [147]. Noncaseating granulomas also secrete angiotensin converting enzyme (ACE) and serum ACE levels are elevated in approximately 70% of patients. However, there is a high false-positive rate associated with serum ACE and thus elevated levels are not diagnostic of disease [147].

Additional testing varies based on the suspected organs involved. Cardiac sarcoidosis can exhibit conduction abnormalities on electrocardiogram ranging from benign arrhythmias to high-degree heart block [148]. Liver enzymes and alkaline phosphatase may be elevated, and pulmonary function testing can show a restrictive pattern with a decreased forced vital capacity (FVC) and diffusion impairment [147].

Morbidity and Mortality

The major causes of death are from cardiac and pulmonary complications. There is a striking racial difference in prognosis and mortality. Blacks tend to present with sarcoidosis at a younger age, have a more severe disease course, such as pulmonary fibrosis and cardiac involvement, and have more extrathoracic involvement than whites [149]. Similarly, Indo-Pakistan Asians were found to have more extrathoracic manifestations and more severe disease than Caucasians at presentation [129]. Mortality ranges from 1 to 8%, though this varies greatly depending on age, ethnicity, and gender. Mortality is highest in African Americans, women, and in older populations, with African Americans being eight times more likely to die from sarcoidosis-related causes as well as dying at a younger age [150, 151].

Treatment

Treatment is not always necessary as sarcoidosis can self-resolve or remain stable. Cutaneous sarcoidosis can be treated if manifestations are cosmetically distressing or symptomatic [152]. For rapidly progressive, generalized, or highly disfiguring disease, systemic corticosteroids can be started at 20–60 mg per day until the patient achieves good clinical response then tapered down to the lowest effective dose. Adjunctive therapy such as corticosteroid-sparing agents or intralesional and topical steroids may accelerate tapering or lower the needed maintenance dose of systemic corticosteroids. There is a lack of strong evidence supporting the efficacy of topical corticosteroids in treating cutaneous sarcoidosis, and intralesional injections of triamcinolone acetonide at concentrations of 3–20 mg/mL repeated every 3–4 weeks may be more effective than topicals. Other therapies include antimalarials (such as hydroxychloroquine and chloroquine), methotrexate, and tetracyclines, though there is limited evidence demonstrating their effectiveness. TNF-alpha antagonists are another potential therapy as TNF-alpha is critical for the formation and maintenance of granulomas. Symptom improvement has been reported after treatment in recalcitrant systemic and cutaneous sarcoidosis, and it may be useful as a second-line agent [153].

Indications for treatment of extracutaneous sarcoidosis include ocular disease, cardiac sarcoidosis, neurosarcoidosis, unremitting hypercalcemia, and progressive organ involvement [152]. For pulmonary disease, oral corticosteroids are the mainstay of treatment though they may not improve patient-oriented outcomes or affect disease progression [144]. Cardiac or neurosarcoidosis may require higher doses [145]. For steroid-refractory disease or medication toxicity, the use of immunosuppressive and biologic agents may be required [131].

Conclusion

Autoimmune and connective tissue diseases have unique profiles in skin of color populations with differing disease severity and prognosis compared to their Caucasian counterparts. Disease burden at presentation, skin manifestations, severity of disease, prognosis, and disease-specific mortality have been shown to differ in ethnic groups when compared to Caucasians.

References

1. Durosaro O, et al. Incidence of cutaneous lupus erythematosus, 1965–2005: a population-based study. Arch Dermatol. 2009;145(3):249–53.
2. Osio-Salido E, Manapat-Reyes H. Epidemiology of systemic lupus erythematosus in Asia. Lupus. 2010;19(12):1365–73.
3. Rees F, et al. The incidence and prevalence of systemic lupus erythematosus in the UK, 1999–2012. Ann Rheum Dis. 2016;75(1):136–41.
4. Flower C, et al. Systemic lupus erythematosus in an African Caribbean population: incidence, clinical manifestations, and survival in the Barbados National Lupus Registry. Arthritis Care Res (Hoboken). 2012;64(8):1151–8.
5. Borba EF, et al. Clinical and immunological features of 888 Brazilian systemic lupus patients from a monocentric cohort: comparison with other populations. Lupus. 2013;22(7): 744–9.
6. Castano-Rodriguez N, et al. Meta-analysis of HLA-DRB1 and HLA-DQB1 polymorphisms in Latin American patients with systemic lupus erythematosus. Autoimmun Rev. 2008;7(4): 322–30.
7. Alarcon GS, et al. Systemic lupus erythematosus in three ethnic groups: II. Features predictive of disease activity early in its course. LUMINA Study Group. Lupus in minority populations, nature versus nurture. Arthritis Rheum. 1998;41(7):1173–80.
8. Molineros JE, et al. Admixture in Hispanic Americans: its impact on ITGAM association and implications for admixture mapping in SLE. Genes Immun. 2009;10(5):539–45.
9. Lee YH, Ji JD, Song GG. Fcgamma receptor IIB and IIIB polymorphisms and susceptibility to systemic lupus erythematosus and lupus nephritis: a meta-analysis. Lupus. 2009;18(8): 727–34.

10. Yuan H, et al. Meta analysis on the association between FcgammaRIIa-R/H131 polymorphisms and systemic lupus erythematosus. Mol Biol Rep. 2009;36(5):1053–8.

11. Li LH, et al. Role of the Fcgamma receptor IIIA-V/F158 polymorphism in susceptibility to systemic lupus erythematosus and lupus nephritis: a meta-analysis. Scand J Rheumatol. 2010;39(2):148–54.

12. Chai HC, et al. Insight into gene polymorphisms involved in toll-like receptor/interferon signalling pathways for systemic lupus erythematosus in South East Asia. J Immunol Res. 2014;2014:529167.

13. Katkam SK, et al. Association of CTLA4 exon-1 polymorphism with the tumor necrosis factor-alpha in the risk of systemic lupus erythematosus among South Indians. Hum Immunol. 2016;77(2):158–64.

14. Chua KH, et al. Association between PDCD1 gene polymorphisms and risk of systemic lupus erythematosus in three main ethnic groups of the Malaysian population. Int J Mol Sci. 2015;16(5):9794–803.

15. Hochberg MC. Updating the American College of Rheumatology revised criteria for the classification of systemic lupus erythematosus. Arthritis Rheum. 1997;40(9):1725.

16. Petit A, Dadzie OE. Multisystemic diseases and ethnicity: a focus on lupus erythematosus, systemic sclerosis, sarcoidosis and Behcet disease. Br J Dermatol. 2013;169(Suppl 3):1–10.

17. Fabbri P, et al. Cutaneous lupus erythematosus: diagnosis and management. Am J Clin Dermatol. 2003;4(7):449–65.

18. Tebbe B, et al. Markers in cutaneous lupus erythematosus indicating systemic involvement. A multicenter study on 296 patients. Acta Derm Venereol. 1997;77(4):305–8.

19. Deng JS, Sontheimer RD, Gilliam JN. Relationships between antinuclear and anti-Ro/SS-A antibodies in subacute cutaneous lupus erythematosus. J Am Acad Dermatol. 1984;11(3):494–9.

20. Kuhn A, Landmann A. The classification and diagnosis of cutaneous lupus erythematosus. J Autoimmun. 2014;48–49:14–9.

21. Arrico L, et al. Ocular complications in cutaneous lupus erythematosus: a systematic review with a meta-analysis of reported cases. J Ophthalmol. 2015;2015:254260.

22. Wollina U, et al. Lupus erythematosus-associated red lunula. J Am Acad Dermatol. 1999;41(3 Pt 1):419–21.

23. Al-Refu K, Goodfield M. Hair follicle stem cells in the pathogenesis of the scarring process in cutaneous lupus erythematosus. Autoimmun Rev. 2009;8(6):474–7.

24. Fernandes MS, et al. Discoid lupus erythematosus with squamous cell carcinoma: a case report and review of the literature in Indian patients. Lupus. 2015;24(14):1562–6.

25. Keith WD, et al. Squamous cell carcinoma arising in lesions of discoid lupus erythematosus in black persons. Arch Dermatol. 1980;116(3):315–7.

26. Baltaci M, Fritsch P. Histologic features of cutaneous lupus erythematosus. Autoimmun Rev. 2009;8(6):467–73.

27. Harrist TJ, Mihm MC Jr. The specificity and clinical usefulness of the lupus band test. Arthritis Rheum. 1980;23(4):479–90.

28. Cozzani E, et al. Serology of lupus erythematosus: correlation between immunopathological features and clinical aspects. Autoimmune Dis. 2014;2014:321359.

29. Jakes RW, et al. Systematic review of the epidemiology of systemic lupus erythematosus in the Asia-Pacific region: prevalence, incidence, clinical features, and mortality. Arthritis Care Res (Hoboken). 2012;64(2):159–68.

30. Serdula MK, Rhoads GG. Frequency of systemic lupus erythematosus in different ethnic groups in Hawaii. Arthritis Rheum. 1979;22(4):328–33.

31. Hopkinson ND, Doherty M, Powell RJ. Clinical features and race-specific incidence/prevalence rates of systemic lupus erythematosus in a geographically complete cohort of patients. Ann Rheum Dis. 1994;53(10):675–80.

32. Samanta A, et al. High prevalence of systemic disease and mortality in Asian subjects with systemic lupus erythematosus. Ann Rheum Dis. 1991;50(7):490–2.

33. Deligny C, et al. Pure cutaneous lupus erythematosus in a population of African descent in French Guiana: a retrospective population-based description. Lupus. 2012;21(13):1467–71.

34. Molokhia M, et al. Systemic lupus erythematosus in migrants from west Africa compared with Afro-Caribbean people in the UK. Lancet. 2001;357(9266):1414–5.

35. Bajaj DR, Devrajani BR, Matlani BL. Discoid lupus erythematosus: a profile. J Coll Physicians Surg Pak. 2010;20(6):361–4.

36. Johnson SR, et al. Ethnic variation in disease patterns and health outcomes in systemic lupus erythematosus. J Rheumatol. 2006;33(10):1990–5.

37. Stoll T, Seifert B, Isenberg DA. SLICC/ACR damage index is valid, and renal and pulmonary organ scores are predictors of severe outcome in patients with systemic lupus erythematosus. Br J Rheumatol. 1996;35(3):248–54.

38. Patel M, et al. The prevalence and incidence of biopsy-proven lupus nephritis in the UK: evidence of an ethnic gradient. Arthritis Rheum. 2006;54(9):2963–9.

39. Alarcon GS, et al. Systemic lupus erythematosus in three ethnic groups: III. A comparison of characteristics early in the natural history of the LUMINA cohort. Lupus in minority populations: nature vs. nurture. Lupus. 1999;8(3):197–209.

40. Pons-Estel BA, et al. The GLADEL multinational Latin American prospective inception cohort of 1214 patients with systemic lupus erythematosus: ethnic and disease heterogeneity among "Hispanics". Medicine (Baltimore). 2004;83(1):1–17.

41. Tan TC, et al. Differences between male and female systemic lupus erythematosus in a multiethnic population. J Rheumatol. 2012;39(4):759–69.

42. Scalzi LV, Hollenbeak CS, Wang L. Racial disparities in age at time of cardiovascular events and cardiovascular-related death in patients with systemic lupus erythematosus. Arthritis Rheum. 2010;62(9):2767–75.

43. Wadee S, Tikly M, Hopley M. Causes and predictors of death in South Africans with systemic lupus erythematosus. Rheumatology (Oxford). 2007;46(9):1487–91.

44. Gómez-Puerta JA, Barbhaiya M, Guan H, Feldman CH, Alarcón GS, Costenbader KH. Racial/Ethnic variation in all-cause mortality among United States medicaid recipients with systemic lupus erythematosus: a Hispanic and asian paradox. Arthrit Rheumatol. 2015;67(3): 752–60.

45. Wang Z, et al. Long-term survival and death causes of systemic lupus erythematosus in China: a systemic review of observational studies. Medicine (Baltimore). 2015;94(17):e794.

46. Reveille JD, Bartolucci A, Alarcon GS. Prognosis in systemic lupus erythematosus. Negative impact of increasing age at onset, black race, and thrombocytopenia, as well as causes of death. Arthritis Rheum. 1990;33(1):37–48.

47. Korbet SM, et al. Severe lupus nephritis: racial differences in presentation and outcome. J Am Soc Nephrol. 2007;18(1):244–54.

48. Kaslow RA. High rate of death caused by systemic lupus erythematosus among U. S. residents of Asian descent. Arthritis Rheum. 1982;25(4):414–8.

49. Agbai ON, et al. Skin cancer and photoprotection in people of color: a review and recommendations for physicians and the public. J Am Acad Dermatol. 2014;70(4):748–62.

50. Kovacs SO, Kovacs SC. Dermatomyositis. J Am Acad Dermatol. 1998;39(6):899–920; quiz 921–2.

51. Marmor MF, et al. Recommendations on screening for chloroquine and hydroxychloroquine retinopathy (2016 revision). Ophthalmology. 2016;123(6):1386–94.

52. Pons-Estel GJ, et al. Lupus in Latin-American patients: lessons from the GLADEL cohort. Lupus. 2015;24(6):536–45.

53. Isenberg D, et al. Influence of race/ethnicity on response to lupus nephritis treatment: the ALMS study. Rheumatology (Oxford). 2010;49(1):128–40.

54. Arnett FC, et al. Familial occurrence frequencies and relative risks for systemic sclerosis (scleroderma) in three United States cohorts. Arthritis Rheum. 2001;44(6):1359–62.

55. Mayes MD, et al. Prevalence, incidence, survival, and disease characteristics of systemic sclerosis in a large US population. Arthritis Rheum. 2003;48(8):2246–55.

56. Laing TJ, et al. Racial differences in scleroderma among women in Michigan. Arthritis Rheum. 1997;40(4):734–42.

57. Steen V, et al. A clinical and serologic comparison of African American and Caucasian patients with systemic sclerosis. Arthritis Rheum. 2012;64(9):2986–94.

58. Steen VD, et al. Incidence of systemic sclerosis in Allegheny County, Pennsylvania. A twenty-year study of hospital-diagnosed cases, 1963–1982. Arthritis Rheum. 1997;40(3): 441–5.

59. Arnett FC, et al. Increased prevalence of systemic sclerosis in a Native American tribe in Oklahoma. Association with an Amerindian HLA haplotype. Arthritis Rheum. 1996;39(8): 1362–70.

60. Gabrielli A, Avvedimento EV, Krieg T. Scleroderma. N Engl J Med. 2009;360(19): 1989–2003.

61. Falanga V, Zhou L, Yufit T. Low oxygen tension stimulates collagen synthesis and COL1A1 transcription through the action of TGF-beta1. J Cell Physiol. 2002;191(1):42–50.

62. Silver RM, et al. Racial differences between blacks and whites with systemic sclerosis. Curr Opin Rheumatol. 2012;24(6):642–8.

63. He D, et al. Association of the HLA-DRB1 with scleroderma in Chinese population. PLoS ONE. 2014;9(9):e106939.

64. Tikly M, et al. Human leukocyte antigen class II associations with systemic sclerosis in South Africans. Tissue Antigens. 2004;63(5):487–90.

65. Beretta L, et al. Analysis of class II human leucocyte antigens in Italian and Spanish systemic sclerosis. Rheumatology (Oxford). 2012;51(1):52–9.

66. Arnett FC, et al. Major histocompatibility complex (MHC) class II alleles, haplotypes and epitopes which confer susceptibility or protection in systemic sclerosis: analyses in 1300 Caucasian, African-American and Hispanic cases and 1000 controls. Ann Rheum Dis. 2010;69(5):822–7.

67. Pope JE, Johnson SR. New classification criteria for systemic sclerosis (scleroderma). Rheum Dis Clin North Am. 2015;41(3):383–98.

68. Bolognia JL. Dermatology, vol. 3, 3rd ed. Elsevier/Saunders; 2012.

69. Schinke S, Riemekasten G. Systemic sclerosis. Dtsch Med Wochenschr. 2016;141(8):550–6.

70. Reveille JD, et al. Systemic sclerosis in 3 US ethnic groups: a comparison of clinical, sociodemographic, serologic, and immunogenetic determinants. Semin Arthritis Rheum. 2001;30(5):332–46.

71. Dadzie OE. Ushering in a new era for studying human cutaneous diversity. Br J Dermatol. 2013;169 Suppl 3:iii–iv.

72. Grassi W, et al. Microvascular involvement in systemic sclerosis: capillaroscopic findings. Semin Arthritis Rheum. 2001;30(6):397–402.

73. Allanore Y, Simms R, Distler O, Trojanowska M, Pope J, Denton CP, Varga J. Systemic sclerosis. Nat Rev Dis Primers. 2015;1:15053.

74. Shah AA, Wigley FM. My approach to the treatment of scleroderma. Mayo Clin Proc. 2013;88(4):377–93.

75. Mendoza F, Derk CT. Systemic sclerosis mortality in the United States: 1999–2002 implications for patient care. J Clin Rheumatol. 2007;13(4):187–92.

76. Nietert PJ, et al. Demographic and clinical factors associated with in-hospital death among patients with systemic sclerosis. J Rheumatol. 2005;32(10):1888–92.

77. Nietert PJ, et al. Racial variation in clinical and immunological manifestations of systemic sclerosis. J Rheumatol. 2006;33(2):263–8.

78. Persa OD, Moinzadeh P, Hunzelmann N. Systemic sclerosis. Current classification and diagnosis of organ involvement. Hautarzt. 2015;66(8):599–603.

79. Gladue H, et al. Screening and diagnostic modalities for connective tissue disease-associated pulmonary arterial hypertension: a systematic review. Semin Arthritis Rheum. 2014;43(4): 536–41.

80. Mayes MD, et al. Minocycline is not effective in systemic sclerosis: results of an open-label multicenter trial. Arthritis Rheum. 2004;50(2):553–7.

81. Pope JE, et al. A randomized, controlled trial of methotrexate versus placebo in early diffuse scleroderma. Arthritis Rheum. 2001;44(6):1351–8.
82. Kreuter A, Gambichler T. UV-A1 phototherapy for sclerotic skin diseases: implications for optimizing patient selection and management. Arch Dermatol. 2008;144(7):912–6.
83. Chatterjee S. Management of Raynaud's phenomenon in the patient with connective tissue disease. Curr Treat Options Cardiovasc Med. 2010;12(2):185–204.
84. Emmanuel A. Current management of the gastrointestinal complications of systemic sclerosis. Nat Rev Gastroenterol Hepatol. 2016;13(8):461–72.
85. Iaccarino L, et al. The clinical features, diagnosis and classification of dermatomyositis. J Autoimmun. 2014;48–49:122–7.
86. Hochberg MC. Epidemiology of polymyositis/dermatomyositis. Mt Sinai J Med. 1988;55(6):447–52.
87. Oddis CV, et al. Incidence of polymyositis-dermatomyositis: a 20-year study of hospital diagnosed cases in Allegheny County, PA 1963–1982. J Rheumatol. 1990;17(10):1329–34.
88. Reed AM, Stirling JD. Association of the HLA-DQA1*0501 allele in multiple racial groups with juvenile dermatomyositis. Hum Immunol. 1995;44(3):131–5.
89. Bolognia JL, Jorizzo JL, Schaffer JV. Dermatology, vol. 1, 3rd ed. Philadelphia, PA: Elsevier Saunders; 2012.
90. Casciola-Rosen L, Mammen AL. Myositis autoantibodies. Curr Opin Rheumatol. 2012;24(6):602–8.
91. Fujimoto M, et al. Recent advances in dermatomyositis-specific autoantibodies. Curr Opin Rheumatol. 2016;28(6):636–44.
92. Fiorentino D, et al. The mucocutaneous and systemic phenotype of dermatomyositis patients with antibodies to MDA5 (CADM-140): a retrospective study. J Am Acad Dermatol. 2011;65(1):25–34.
93. Trallero-Araguas E, et al. Usefulness of anti-p155 autoantibody for diagnosing cancer-associated dermatomyositis: a systematic review and meta-analysis. Arthritis Rheum. 2012;64(2):523–32.
94. Fiorentino DF, et al. Most patients with cancer-associated dermatomyositis have antibodies to nuclear matrix protein NXP-2 or transcription intermediary factor 1gamma. Arthritis Rheum. 2013;65(11):2954–62.
95. Satoh M, et al. Frequent coexistence of anti-topoisomerase I and anti-U1RNP autoantibodies in African American patients associated with mild skin involvement: a retrospective clinical study. Arthritis Res Ther. 2011;13(3):R73.
96. O'Hanlon TP, et al. HLA polymorphisms in African Americans with idiopathic inflammatory myopathy: allelic profiles distinguish patients with different clinical phenotypes and myositis autoantibodies. Arthritis Rheum. 2006;54(11):3670–81.
97. Bohan A, Peter JB. Polymyositis and dermatomyositis (first of two parts). N Engl J Med. 1975;292(7):344–7.
98. Bohan A, Peter JB. Polymyositis and dermatomyositis (second of two parts). N Engl J Med. 1975;292(8):403–7.
99. Dalakas MC, Hohlfeld R. Polymyositis and dermatomyositis. Lancet. 2003;362(9388):971–82.
100. Hoogendijk JE, et al. 119th ENMC international workshop: trial design in adult idiopathic inflammatory myopathies, with the exception of inclusion body myositis, 10–12 October 2003, Naarden, The Netherlands. Neuromuscul Disord. 2004;14(5):337–45.
101. Medsger TA Jr, Dawson WN, Masi AT Jr. The epidemiology of polymyositis. Am J Med. 1970;48(6):715–23.
102. Callen JP. Cutaneous manifestations of dermatomyositis and their management. Curr Rheumatol Rep. 2010;12(3):192–7.
103. Sontheimer RD. Would a new name hasten the acceptance of amyopathic dermatomyositis (dermatomyositis sine myositis) as a distinctive subset within the idiopathic inflammatory dermatomyopathies spectrum of clinical illness? J Am Acad Dermatol. 2002;46(4):626–36.
104. Dalakas MC. Inflammatory muscle diseases. N Engl J Med. 2015;372(18):1734–47.

105. Ee HL, Ng PP, Tan SH. Exacerbation of amyopathic dermatomyositis in orientals: a high alert for nasopharyngeal carcinoma. Australas J Dermatol. 2004;45(1):77–8.
106. Schwarz HA, et al. Muscle biopsy in polymyositis and dermatomyositis: a clinicopathological study. Ann Rheum Dis. 1980;39(5):500–7.
107. Iorizzo LJ 3rd, Jorizzo JL. The treatment and prognosis of dermatomyositis: an updated review. J Am Acad Dermatol. 2008;59(1):99–112.
108. Constantin T, et al. National registry of patients with juvenile idiopathic inflammatory myopathies in Hungary–clinical characteristics and disease course of 44 patients with juvenile dermatomyositis. Autoimmunity. 2006;39(3):223–32.
109. Huber AM, et al. Medium- and long-term functional outcomes in a multicenter cohort of children with juvenile dermatomyositis. Arthritis Rheum. 2000;43(3):541–9.
110. Drake LA, et al. Guidelines of care for dermatomyositis. American Academy of Dermatology. J Am Acad Dermatol. 1996;34(5 Pt 1):824–9.
111. Phillips BA, et al. Frequency of relapses in patients with polymyositis and dermatomyositis. Muscle Nerve. 1998;21(12):1668–72.
112. Kurtzman DJ, et al. Tofacitinib citrate for refractory cutaneous dermatomyositis: an alternative treatment. JAMA Dermatol. 2016;152(8):944–5.
113. Fett N, Werth VP. Update on morphea: part I. Epidemiology, clinical presentation, and pathogenesis. J Am Acad Dermatol. 2011;64(2):217–28; quiz 229–30.
114. Christen-Zaech S, et al. Pediatric morphea (localized scleroderma): review of 136 patients. J Am Acad Dermatol. 2008;59(3):385–96.
115. Leitenberger JJ, et al. Distinct autoimmune syndromes in morphea: a review of 245 adult and pediatric cases. Arch Dermatol. 2009;145(5):545–50.
116. Peterson LS, et al. The epidemiology of morphea (localized scleroderma) in Olmsted County 1960–1993. J Rheumatol. 1997;24(1):73–80.
117. Pequet MS, et al. Risk factors for morphoea disease severity: a retrospective review of 114 paediatric patients. Br J Dermatol. 2014;170(4):895–900.
118. Laxer RM, Zulian F. Localized scleroderma. Curr Opin Rheumatol. 2006;18(6):606–13.
119. Tollefson MM, Witman PM. En coup de sabre morphea and Parry-Romberg syndrome: a retrospective review of 54 patients. J Am Acad Dermatol. 2007;56(2):257–63.
120. Chak G, Wang HZ, Feldon SE. Coup de sabre presenting with worsening diplopia and enophthalmos. Ophthalmic Plast Reconstr Surg. 2011;27(4):e97–8.
121. Fett N, Werth VP. Update on morphea: part II. Outcome measures and treatment. J Am Acad Dermatol. 2011;64(2)231–42; quiz 243–4.
122. Zwischenberger BA, Jacobe HT. A systematic review of morphea treatments and therapeutic algorithm. J Am Acad Dermatol. 2011;65(5):925–41.
123. Zulian F, et al. Methotrexate treatment in juvenile localized scleroderma: a randomized, double-blind, placebo-controlled trial. Arthritis Rheum. 2011;63(7):1998–2006.
124. Foley PJ, et al. Human leukocyte antigen-DRB1 position 11 residues are a common protective marker for sarcoidosis. Am J Respir Cell Mol Biol. 2001;25(3):272–7.
125. Levin AM, et al. Association of HLA-DRB1 with sarcoidosis susceptibility and progression in African Americans. Am J Respir Cell Mol Biol. 2015;53(2):206–16.
126. Rossman MD, et al. HLA-DRB1*1101: a significant risk factor for sarcoidosis in blacks and whites. Am J Hum Genet. 2003;73(4):720–35.
127. Rybicki BA, et al. Racial differences in sarcoidosis incidence: a 5-year study in a health maintenance organization. Am J Epidemiol. 1997;145(3):234–41.
128. James DG, Neville E, Siltzbach LE. A worldwide review of sarcoidosis. Ann N Y Acad Sci. 1976;278:321–34.
129. Edmondstone WM, Wilson AG. Sarcoidosis in Caucasians, Blacks and Asians in London. Br J Dis Chest. 1985;79(1):27–36.
130. Morimoto T, et al. Epidemiology of sarcoidosis in Japan. Eur Respir J. 2008;31(2):372–9.
131. Baughman RP, Lower EE, du Bois RM. Sarcoidosis. Lancet. 2003;361(9363):1111–8.
132. Guidry C, et al. Imaging of Sarcoidosis: A Contemporary Review. Radiol Clin North Am. 2016;54(3):519–34.

133. Wanat KA, Rosenbach M. Cutaneous Sarcoidosis. Clin Chest Med. 2015;36(4):685–702.
134. Chong WS, Tan HH, Tan SH. Cutaneous sarcoidosis in Asians: a report of 25 patients from Singapore. Clin Exp Dermatol. 2005;30(2):120–4.
135. Elgart ML. Cutaneous sarcoidosis: definitions and types of lesions. Clin Dermatol. 1986;4 (4):35–45.
136. Mana J, et al. Granulomatous cutaneous sarcoidosis: diagnosis, relationship to systemic disease, prognosis and treatment. Sarcoidosis Vasc Diffuse Lung Dis. 2013;30(4):268–81.
137. Pasadhika S, Rosenbaum JT. Ocular Sarcoidosis. Clin Chest Med. 2015;36(4):669–83.
138. Albertini JG, Tyler W, Miller OF 3rd. Ulcerative sarcoidosis. Case report and review of the literature. Arch Dermatol. 1997;133(2):215–9.
139. Heath CR, David J, Taylor SC. Sarcoidosis: are there differences in your skin of color patients? J Am Acad Dermatol. 2012;66(1):121.e1–14.
140. Pietinalho A, et al. The frequency of sarcoidosis in Finland and Hokkaido. Japan. A comparative epidemiological study. Sarcoidosis. 1995;12(1):61–7.
141. Lynch JP 3rd, et al. Cardiac involvement in sarcoidosis: evolving concepts in diagnosis and treatment. Semin Respir Crit Care Med. 2014;35(3):372–90.
142. Iwai K, et al. Racial difference in cardiac sarcoidosis incidence observed at autopsy. Sarcoidosis. 1994;11(1):26–31.
143. Haimovic A, et al. Sarcoidosis: a comprehensive review and update for the dermatologist: part II. Extracutaneous disease. J Am Acad Dermatol. 2012;66(5):719.e1–10; quiz 729–30.
144. Soto-Gomez N, Peters JI, Nambiar AM. Diagnosis and Management of Sarcoidosis. Am Fam Physician. 2016;93(10):840–8.
145. Statement on sarcoidosis. Joint Statement of the American Thoracic Society (ATS), the European Respiratory Society (ERS) and the World Association of Sarcoidosis and Other Granulomatous Disorders (WASOG) adopted by the ATS Board of Directors and by the ERS Executive Committee, February 1999. Am J Respir Crit Care Med. 1999;160(2):736–55.
146. Fernandez-Faith E, McDonnell J. Cutaneous sarcoidosis: differential diagnosis. Clin Dermatol. 2007;25(3):276–87.
147. Heinle R, Chang C. Diagnostic criteria for sarcoidosis. Autoimmun Rev. 2014;13(4–5):383–7.
148. Sekhri V, et al. Cardiac sarcoidosis: a comprehensive review. Arch Med Sci. 2011;7(4):546–54.
149. Gerke AK. Morbidity and mortality in sarcoidosis. Curr Opin Pulm Med. 2014;20(5):472–8.
150. Mirsaeidi M, et al. Racial difference in sarcoidosis mortality in the United States. Chest. 2015;147(2):438–49.
151. Swigris JJ, et al. Sarcoidosis-related mortality in the United States from 1988 to 2007. Am J Respir Crit Care Med. 2011;183(11):1524–30.
152. Haimovic A, et al. Sarcoidosis: a comprehensive review and update for the dermatologist: part I. Cutaneous disease. J Am Acad Dermatol. 2012;66(5):699 e1–18; quiz 717–8.
153. Doty JD, Mazur JE, Judson MA. Treatment of sarcoidosis with infliximab. Chest. 2005; 127(3):1064–71.

Chapter 13
Disorders of Hyperpigmentation

Neeta Malviya and Amit Pandya

Disorders of hyperpigmentation appear more pronounced in individuals with skin of color and tend to be more challenging to treat. The exaggerated response of melanocytes in these individuals to cutaneous trauma is seen as a hallmark of skin of color [1]. A study with 1076 dermatology patients in Saudi Arabia found pigment disorders to be the fourth most common skin disease [2]. A study of 2000 Black patients in Washington, DC, found pigment disorders to be the third most common skin disorder [3]. The majority of these patients were noted to have post-inflammatory hyperpigmentation, with melasma being the second most frequent disorder [3]. The most common causes of hyperpigmentation are post-inflammatory hyperpigmentation, melasma, lichen planus pigmentosus, erythema dyschromicum perstans, drug-induced hyperpigmentation, and metabolic causes of hyperpigmentation.

Post-inflammatory Hyperpigmentation

Post-inflammatory hyperpigmentation (PIH) is a common acquired condition that is the result of increased production of melanin following inflammation, trauma, or injury to the skin (Fig. 13.1). This hyperpigmentation can be seen in numerous cutaneous disorders ranging from acne vulgaris to drug reactions, is particularly

N. Malviya
Department of Dermatology, University of Texas Southwestern Medical Center,
5323 Harry Hines Blvd., Dallas, TX 75390-9069, USA
e-mail: Neeta.Malviya@UTSouthwestern.edu

A. Pandya (✉)
Department of Dermatology, UT Southwestern Medical Center,
5939 Harry Hines Blvd., 4th Floor, Suite 100, Dallas, TX 75390-9191, USA
e-mail: amit.pandya@sbcglobal.net; Amit.Pandya@UTSouthwestern.edu

© Springer International Publishing AG 2017
N.A. Vashi and H.I. Maibach (eds.), *Dermatoanthropology of Ethnic Skin and Hair*, DOI 10.1007/978-3-319-53961-4_13

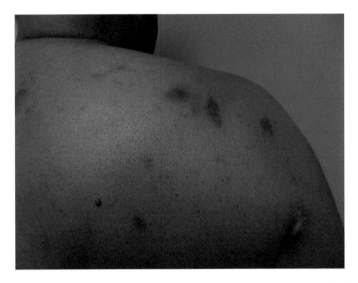

Fig. 13.1 Post-inflammatory hyperpigmentation after resolution of pemphigus vulgaris

pronounced in individuals of Fitzpatrick skin type IV–VI, and difficult to treat. It is the third most common chief complaint seen in African American patients presenting to dermatology [4].

Diagnosis and Clinical Presentation

Post-inflammatory hyperpigmentation presents as light brown to dark brown to black macules or patches that are present in the same area of a previous trauma or current trauma or inflammatory skin disorder. Lesions are typically asymptomatic. The lesions may also appear gray to blue in color if pigmentation is present in the dermis. The primary lesions leading to the hyperpigmentation may or may not be clearly evident, and are the determinants of the size, shape, and distribution of the hyperpigmentation.

Etiology

Common causes of post-inflammatory hyperpigmentation include acne vulgaris, atopic dermatitis, psoriasis, allergic and irritant contact dermatitis, and insect bites. Inflammatory mediators that lead to pigmentation include histamine, prostaglandins E2 and D2, and leukotrienes C4 and D4, thromboxane-2, IL-1, IL-6, and nitric oxide which all serve to increase the synthesis of melanin [5, 6]. Keratinocyte growth factor and interleukin-1α have been shown to induce hyperpigmented lesions and are thought to be involved in PIH [7]. There are two mechanisms behind the increased pigmentation seen in PIH. Epidermal hyperpigmentation is due to the increased activity of melanocytes whereas dermal hyperpigmentation entails melanin migration from the epidermis to the dermis due to defects in the basement membrane from an inflammatory process.

Histology

Microscopically, epidermal PIH reveals increased melanin in keratinocytes. Dermal PIH is characterized by the presence of melanophages within the dermis.

Management

The first step in the management of post-inflammatory hyperpigmentation is treatment of the underlying inflammatory skin disease. The use of a broad-spectrum sunscreen in combination with avoidance of the sun is also used in treatment of PIH as these measures prevent further darkening of the pigmented lesions. Topical skin lightening agents, chemical peels, and laser treatments can be used in treatment as well. Topical retinoids have shown benefit in patients with skin of color, both tretinoin and tazarotene demonstrated significant reduction of PIH in randomized, double-blind, controlled trials [8, 9]. Tretinoin is also thought to enhance the action of hydroquinone. A triple combination cream containing a topical retinoid, corticosteroid, and hydroquinone can be used in the treatment of PIH similar to treatment of melasma is discussed later. Chemical peels have shown mixed results in clinical studies. Some studies have failed to show statistically significant improvement in patients of darker skin types even though clinical improvement can be seen [10]. For darker skin types, superficial chemical peels provide notable clinical results and are well tolerated [1]. Caution should be used with chemical peels as side effects include worsened PIH as well as irritation.

Laser treatments are another option for patients with PIH, but should be used with great caution in patients with darker skin types. Lasers targeting pigment while employing longer wavelengths and cooling devices are viable options for those patients with skin of color. Considering the high risk of adverse events with inappropriate laser use, the safest laser to treat patients with skin of color are the long-pulsed and low-fluence Q-switched Nd:YAG (neodymium-doped yttrium aluminium garnet) lasers. Recent studies have shown the 755 nm picosecond alexandrine laser to be a safe and effective alternative to Q-switched lasers for treating pigmented lesions in patients with skin of color [11]. A study of this laser in Chinese patients showed it to be efficacious in treating benign pigmented lesions and it was found to be associated with a much lower risk of PIH [12].

Melasma

Melasma (chloasma), also referred to as the "mask of pregnancy," is a chronic acquired disorder of hyperpigmentation consisting of brown macules typically found on sun-exposed areas of the face of women of Fitzpatrick skin types III–VI (Fig. 13.2).

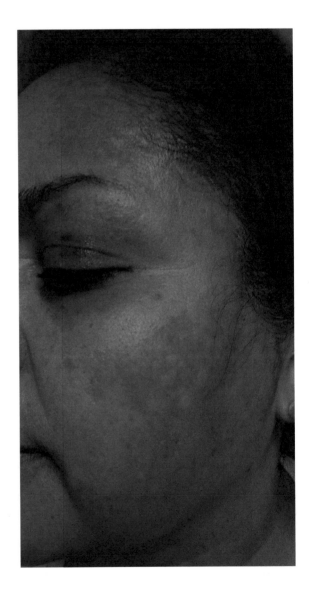

Fig. 13.2 Hispanic female with melasma of cheek and forehead

Diagnosis and Clinical Presentation

Melasma consists of tan, light to dark brown, or grayish-brown hyperpigmented macules to patches with well-defined but irregular borders found on the face in a symmetrical distribution. The lesions most commonly present in a centrofacial pattern but can also present less frequently in a malar and mandibular pattern [13]. Lesions can also rarely be found on the extensor aspect of the forearms as well as on the upper middle chest. The differential diagnosis includes post-inflammatory hyperpigmentation, acanthosis nigricans, solar lentigines, Hori nevi, and nevus of Ota and Ito.

Etiology

The pathogenesis of melasma is not entirely understood. Sun exposure, pregnancy, sex hormones, use of oral contraceptives, steroids, inflammation, and photosensitizing drugs are known triggers. Ultraviolet radiation (UV) leads to the stimulation of melanocytes within the involved areas of skin to produce increased melanin [14]. UV radiation is thought to be involved in the pathogenesis due to the distribution along sun-exposed areas of the face such as the cheeks, nose, and forehead with sparing of sun-protected areas such as the philtrum. Furthermore, the hyperpigmentation is noted to fade during the winter months and worsen in the summer months. The melanocytes in melasma lesions are more biologically active compared to non-lesional skin, evidenced by increased mitochondria, rough endoplasmic reticulum, Golgi complex, and dendrites [15]. This hyperactivity is thought to be triggered by UV radiation.

There is also a clear genetic component to melasma as greater than 40% of patients report having family members with the disease [16]. Melasma is found in all ethnic groups. Regardless of this, studies have shown a higher prevalence of melasma in more pigmented populations including Japanese, Korean, Chinese, Indian, Pakistani, Middle Eastern, Mediterranean-African, and Hispanic individuals [4, 17]. It is most common in patients with Fitzpatrick skin types III and IV, in addition, 54.7% of patients with melasma in Iran, and 70.4% of Latino patients were noted to have a family history of this disorder [18, 19].

Histology

Melasma can be divided into three main histologic patterns: epidermal, comprising 70% of cases, dermal, comprising 10–15% of cases, and mixed, which comprises 20% of cases [20]. A fourth pattern is indeterminate, which is reserved for patients with very dark pigmentation. These patterns can be detected with a combination of

Wood's light exam and skin biopsy [20]. Epidermal melasma is light brown in color and tends to have a better response to treatment with depigmenting agents compared to dermal melasma which is gray-brown in appearance and less responsive to treatment. Biopsies of melasma lesions reveal increased melanin deposition in all layers of the epidermis along with a possible increased number of melanophages. The number of melanocytes is not significantly changed from non-lesional skin, however, they are larger and have an increased number of dendritic processes as well as an increased number of melanosomes [14]. The dermal subset of melasma contains less pigment in the epidermis compared to the epidermal subset. As all subtypes of melasma show increased pigment deposition in both the epidermis and dermis, the value of a Wood's lamp examination in dictating the level of involvement in the skin and response to treatment may be minimal [14].

Management

The treatment of melasma includes topical agents, laser treatment, light therapy, and chemical peels. Bleaching agents containing hydroquinone are the gold standard treatment for melasma. A combination topical agent containing hydroquinone, tretinoin, and a topical corticosteroid is the most efficacious topical therapy for melasma.

Azelaic acid, arbutin, kojic acid, vitamin C, and methimazole are additional skin lightening therapies that can be used. Intralesional triamcinolone has been shown in one study to be a more efficacious treatment for melasma compared to a combination topical agent containing hydroquinone, tretinoin, and a topical corticosteroid, although this should be performed with caution given risks of atrophy [21]. A sunscreen with broad-spectrum UVA protection as well as protection from visible light should be used on a daily basis. The use of sunscreen moderately improves melasma when used on its own, but when combined with bleaching creams it serves to enhance their efficacy. Tranexamic acid, an antifibrinolytic agent, has been shown to decrease melanogenesis and was found to be effective in a recent retrospective study of 561 patients with melasma at a dose of 250 mg twice daily [22]. This medication is associated with an increased risk of thrombosis, therefore, a detailed past medical history and family history must be obtained prior to treatment [22].

Laser and light therapy should be utilized carefully in the treatment of melasma as it can cause side effects of irritation, hyperpigmentation, hypopigmentation, and scarring. Intense pulse light (IPL) is another treatment modality for melasma; however, it is associated with a high rate of recurrence as is low-fluence Q-switched Nd:YAG laser for treating melasma [23]. Pulse dye laser can be useful in combination with topical treatment such that prolonged improvement can be seen even following therapy. The use of laser therapy may result in both hypo- and hyperpigmentation.

Lichen Planus Pigmentosus

Lichen planus pigmentosus (LPP) is a rare variant of lichen planus found in patients with darker skin pigment and presents as hyperpigmented macules and patches on sun-exposed and flexural areas (Fig. 13.3). It is often found in patients from South Asia, East Asia, the Middle East, and Latin America. A rare subset of this disorder includes lichen planus pigmentosus inversus (LPP inversus), which consists of LPP lesions in intertriginous areas.

Fig. 13.3 Lichen planus pigmentosus

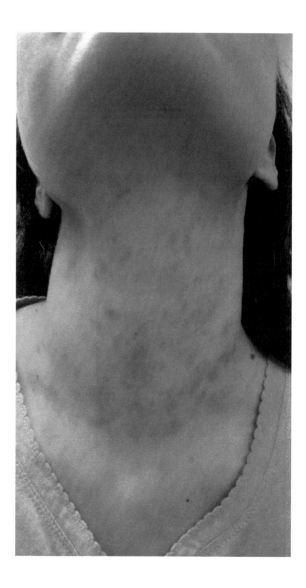

Diagnosis and Clinical Presentation

The lesions of LPP present as asymptomatic, small, brown, ashy-brown or brownish-black hyperpigmented macules to patches with a predilection for the sun-exposed areas of the body such as the face and neck as well as flexural areas, most commonly in skin types III–V. The distribution of lesions is most often symmetrical; however, a linear, unilateral variant has been described. The lesions tend to develop in middle-aged women. LPP follows a prolonged clinical course in the form of chronic relapsing and remitting lesions that may be associated with mild pruritus. LPP inversus presents as well-circumscribed violaceous-brownish black macules within intertriginous areas, affecting primarily the axillae, inframammary folds, and inguinal folds [24]. The main entity on the differential diagnosis of LPP is erythema dyschromicum perstans (EDP), also referred to as ashy dermatosis. While these conditions have overlapping features, EDP is distinguished by an inflammatory phase. LPP can be distinguished from EDP by lack of an erythematous border and presence of mucosal lesions. The differential diagnosis for LPP inversus also includes erythema dyschromicum perstans in addition to acanthosis nigricans, figurate erythema, and post-inflammatory hyperpigmentation [25].

Etiology

The etiology of LPP is yet to be elucidated. UV radiation is thought to play a role in the pathogenesis given the distribution of lesions in sun-exposed areas as well as the triggering of disease activity following the use of photosensitizers such as mustard oil, hair dyes, and cosmetic fragrances [26].

Histology

Histologically, LPP exhibits a lichenoid lymphohistiocytic infiltrate in a perivascular distribution located in the upper dermis and dermoepidermal junction, epidermal atrophy, basal cell degeneration, as well as dermal melanophages [27]. The histologic findings are identical for LPP inversus [28].

Management

Treating LPP can be quite difficult due to the unpredictable clinical course and uncertain etiology. A primary mode of treatment includes the use of sunscreen coupled with sun avoidance in order to prevent further darkening of the lesions.

Tacrolimus has been shown to have a beneficial effect in improving the pigmentation, with half of patients in one study showing lightening of lesions [29]. A combination of topical tacrolimus and oral dapsone was shown to be efficacious in a case series of 5 patients [30]. A nonrandomized, prospective study of 27 patients showed stabilization of lesions as well as a decrease in pigmentation with the use of low-dose isotretinoin, with stabilization of disease seen in 4–6 weeks which was gauged by improvement in histopathologic findings [31]. Topical corticosteroids and tacrolimus have been shown to be of variable benefit in patients with LPP inversus [32–34].

Erythema Dyschronicum Perstans

Erythema dyschromicum perstans (EDP), also referred to as ashy dermatosis, is an acquired disorder of hypermelanosis that is found worldwide, but with a greater prevalence in Central Americans and Asians.

Diagnosis and Clinical Presentation

EDP presents as asymptomatic, ashy brown to gray-blue, oval to irregularly shaped macules to patches. The lesions develop slowly and are most frequently found on the trunk with spread to the proximal upper extremities and neck. The lesions tend to be asymptomatic, however mild pruritus can occur. Early lesions can have a raised, erythematous border and this serves as a distinguishing feature between lichen planus pigmentosus. The clinical course of EDP is chronic with slow progression, and regression does not usually occur in adults though it has been seen in some studies of children [35]. EDP can present across the spectrum of ages, but tends to be rarer in children and has a predilection for the second decade of life. It is unclear whether a gender predilection exists as some studies have noted both genders to be equally affected while others note an increased prevalence in women [36–38]. An HLA-DR4 association was found in Mexican patients with EDP, and this may suggest a genetic susceptibility [36].

Etiology

The cause of EDP remains unknown, though associations have been noted. Previous reports have shown a relation with the consumption of ammonium nitrate, oral contrast media, certain pesticides, and medications. Malfunctioning cell-mediated immunity involving cell adhesion and activation molecules is also thought to be involved in the pathogenesis of EDP, and that an antigen response leads to its development [39]. The predominance of CD8+ T cells in the dermis along with HLA-DR and ICAM-1 positivity in the epidermal keratinocytes points to this mechanism, along with the exocytosis of cutaneous lymphocyte antigen positive cells in the basement membrane zone [39].

Histology

EDP is characterized by a dermal lymphocytic infiltrate, the presence of melano-phages, the vacuolization of the basement membrane zone, colloid bodies, and the exocytosis of lymphocytes [39]. The lymphocytic infiltrate is noted to be perivas-cular in contrast with lichen planus and its subsets [40]. EDP lesions also have increased expression of ICAM-1 (CD54), which suggests an underlying inflam-matory etiology of the disease. Inactive lesions present later in the course of the disease show an increased number of dermal melanophages with an absence in basal cell layer changes. Furthermore, later lesions have a reduced dermal lym-phocytic infiltrate as compared to early lesions.

Management

The treatment of EDP is challenging as the efficacy of various modalities is quite variable. Presently, there are no randomized controlled trials for EDP therapies. Clofazimine, corticosteroids, dapsone, and vitamin A have all been used with varying degrees of success. The management of EDP can also include the use of topical tacrolimus, which was shown in a two-patient case series to resolve all lesions within 3 months and prevented recurrence [38]. The mechanism for the efficacy of tacrolimus in EDP is thought to be related to its immunomodulatory effects in relation to the malfunctioning cell-mediated immunity postulated to be causing EDP.

Drug-Induced Hyperpigmentation

A wide variety of medication and chemical exposure can lead to the development of hypermelanosis with resolution seen upon discontinuation of the drug or exposure. It accounts for 10–20% of cases of acquired hyperpigmentation [41]. A prolonged course can be seen particularly in skin of color leading to cosmetic disfigurement.

Diagnosis and Clinical Presentation

Systemic and topical medications can both lead to hyperpigmentation in the skin, and therefore it is crucial to obtain a detailed medication history from patients. The drugs most often associated with hyperpigmentation reactions include chemotherapy agents, antimalarials, nonsteroidal anti-inflammatory drugs, amiodarone, antipsychotic drugs, antiepileptics, tetracycline antibiotics, and heavy metals (Table 13.1). The resulting pigmentation can be discrete and well circumscribed or diffuse. If sun exposure is also involved in the development, it is referred to as a phototoxic reaction. Exposure to certain foods and plants in conjunction with exposure to sunlight produces a similar response, which is called phytophotodermatitis. Typically, patients who exhibit drug-induced hyperpigmentation demonstrate a diffuse hypermelanosis. The hyperpigmentation may be preceded by erythema, representing an allergic reaction. Drug-induced hyperpigmentation can also initially present as a bullous reaction in sun-exposed areas due to inflammation. The clinical features of drug-induced hyperpigmentation are quite varied and depend upon the triggering substance along with the location of the pigment within

Table 13.1 Medications or chemicals that cause direct hyperpigmentation

ACTH/MSH	Hydroxychloroquine
Arsenic	Hydroxyurea
Amiodarone	Imatinib
Amitriptyline	Imipramine
Azidothymidine	Iron
Bismuth	Lead
Bleomycin	Mechlorethamine
Busulfan	Mercury
Carmustine	Methotrexate
Chloroquine	Minocycline
Chlorpromazine	Nitrogen mustard (topical)
Clofazimine	Non-steroidal anti inflammatory drugs
Cyclophosphamide	Oral contraceptives
Dactinomycin	Phenothiazines
Daunorubicin	Phenacetin
Desipramine	Procarbaine
Diltiazem	Psoralens
Dioxins	Quinacrine
Doxorubicin	Silver
5-Fluorouracil	Thioridazine
Gold	Zidovudine
Hydantoins	

the skin. A wide range of patterns and colorations exist and these may sometimes be associated with that of the inciting drug.

Diltiazem, for example, produces a gray to brownish-gray discoloration in photodistributed areas. This drug reaction has a predilection for patients with skin types IV–VI, individuals of African American and Asian descent are much more likely to experience this discoloration [42]. Distinguishing hyperpigmentation in a patient with a darker skin type can be difficult due to the need to differentiate the normal pigment from the abnormal coloration. The differential diagnosis for drug-induced hyperpigmentation also includes melasma, Addison's disease, hemochromatosis, diabetes mellitus, and cirrhosis as these are all conditions linked to pigmentary changes.

Etiology

The pathogenesis of drug-induced hyperpigmentation is varied depending upon the implicated substance. One mechanism is the accumulation of melanin either in the dermis or in the dermal macrophages, which is a result of increased production from melanocytes due to stimulation from the drug or from a lack of melanin clearance due to complex formation. A second mechanism entails the accumulation of the offending medication itself within the skin in the form of granules or within macrophages in the dermis. A third mechanism for drug-induced hyperpigmentation entails the synthesis of unique pigments as a direct result of the drug, an example of which is lipofuscin. A fourth mechanism for drug-induced hyperpigmentation is the damage of dermal vessels by the medication, which results in the extravasation of red blood cells into the dermis, leading to the deposition of hemosiderin.

Histology

Drug-induced hyperpigmentation is variable in its histologic appearance. Pigment is usually found to be concentrated in dermal macrophages, but can also be found in a free form. The pigment can be distributed in a distinct, recognizable pattern depending on the culprit drug or chemical. Associated inflammation or an unusual pigment induced by the drug, either free or included in dermal macrophages may also be seen.

Management

The first step in management of drug or chemical induced hyperpigmentation is discontinuation of the drug or cessation of the exposure. This will usually lead to resolution of the discoloration. In cases where a drug cannot be stopped, adjustment of the dose may be beneficial in reducing the risk for pigmentation. Sun exposure should be minimized to prevent worsening of pigmentation and to prevent the stimulation of phototoxic reactions. The use of sun protective clothing and sunscreens should be encouraged. Phototoxic reactions can be treated with topical lightening agents similar to the treatment of melasma such as hydroquinone along with the use of sunscreen. The Alexandrite 755 nm laser was shown to be an effective treatment for minocycline hyperpigmentation and resulted in resolution of the pigmentation after 2 treatments in one study [43]. The Q-Switched 755-nm laser was found to be an effective treatment for hemosiderin hyperpigmentation as has the Q-switched 650-nm wavelength laser, both in case studies [44, 45].

Metabolic Causes of Hyperpigmentation

Metabolic causes are a common etiology of diffuse hyperpigmentation and include vitamin B12 and folic acid deficiencies, cortisol deficiency, ACTH excess, disruption of thyroid function, and diabetes (Table 13.2).

Table 13.2 Metabolic causes of hyperpigmentation

Diagnosis	Clinical presentation	Histology	Etiology
Hyperpigmentation due to B12 and folic acid deficiency	Typically presents on the dorsal hands and feet and is particularly prominent on the interphalangeal joints and terminal phalanges. Pigmentation can also be present on the oral mucosa	Increased melanin present in basal keratinocytes and dermal macrophages	The pathogenesis of hyperpigmentation due to vitamin B12 deficiency is uncertain, however it is postulated that vitamin B12 deficiency causes decreased intracellular levels of reduced-type glutathione, which serves to inhibit tyrosinase and leads to the stimulation of melanin production by epidermal melanocytes [46]

(continued)

Table 13.2 (continued)

Diagnosis	Clinical presentation	Histology	Etiology
Hyperpigmentation due to hypocortisolism, or Addison's disease	Presents in a generalized fashion with an increased prominence of normal pigment distribution. It has a predilection for mucosal surfaces, nipples, areola, axillae, genitalia, elbows, knees, and palmar creases	Increased melanin present in basal keratinocytes and dermal macrophages	The pathogenesis of hyperpigmentation in Addison's disease is related to the deficiency of cortisol which leads to increased levels of melanocyte-stimulating hormone (MSH) and adrenocorticotropic hormone (ACTH). Paraneoplastic production of ACTH also leads to hyperpigmentation, due to the homology of alpha MSH and the first 13 amino acids of ACTH
Hyperpigmentation due to hyperthyroidism	A wide spectrum of hyperpigmentation can be seen in hyperthyroidism. These patients can present with localized or generalized distribution of hyperpigmentation that can be clinically similar to that seen in Addison's disease	Hemosiderin pigment was noted to be present around dermal vasculature and sweat glands in two cases of Japanese patients [47]. The presence of basal cell hypermelanosis was also noted	Hyperpigmentation in hyperthyroidism is thought to be the result of perivascular hemosiderin deposition in the dermis. A hypothesis as to why this occurs is the increased capillary fragility in thyrotoxicosis leading to extravasation of red blood cells [48]
Diabetic dermopathy	Presents as atrophic, light brown to reddish, hyperpigmented macules to patches with a predilection for the extensor surfaces of the lower extremities. Red macules, papules or plaques may also be present along with the hyperpigmentation	Atrophy of rete ridges in the epidermis along with hyperkeratosis with a variable amount of pigment in basal cells. The papillary dermis reveals telangiectasias, fibroblast proliferation, hyaline mircroangiopathy, extravasated erythrocytes, and hemosiderin deposits	The pathogenesis of diabetic dermopathy currently remains unknown. The hyperpigmented appearance of the lesions is the result of the extravasation of red blood cells which leads to hemosiderin deposition, a similar mechanism to the hyperpigmentation seen in hyperthyroidism

(continued)

Table 13.2 (continued)

Diagnosis	Clinical presentation	Histology	Etiology
Acanthosis nigricans	Presents as hyperpigmented plaques with a velvet-like appearance which is the result of thickened superficial epithelium. It commonly presents in the skin folds such as the neck, axilla, and groin and can be associated with acrochordons	Characterized by hyperkeratosis and papillomatosis along with mild acanthosis [49]. The hyperpigmented appearance of the lesions is the result of the hyperkeratosis even though some hyperpigmentation may be present in the basal layer	Insulin resistance results in hyperinsulinemia, which leads to increased amounts of insulin interacting with insulin-like growth factor-1 receptors (IGFR). Increased binding of insulin to these receptors results in the proliferation of keratinocytes and fibroblasts [50]. This leads to the hyperkeratosis that gives the hyperpigmented appearance of these lesions

Conclusion

Disorders of hyperpigmentation range widely in their etiologies, but much overlap can be observed in their treatment. Treatment of these disorders in patients with skin of color continues to pose a challenge, but advancements in laser therapy and oral agents have added to the dermatologist's armamentarium. An understanding of pathophysiology and treatment of hyperpigmentation is important, particularly in this population in which it is a very common chief complaint and a source of psychological and emotional distress that negatively impacts the quality of life of patients. As more research is performed on the underlying causes of these disorders, more targeted and efficacious therapies may be discovered.

References

1. Grimes PE. Management of hyperpigmentation in darker racial ethnic groups. In: Seminars in cutaneous medicine and surgery, vol. 2. WB Saunders; 2009. p. 77–85.
2. Alakloby OM. Pattern of skin diseases in Eastern Saudi Arabia. Saudi Med J. 2005;26 (10):1607–10.
3. Halder RM, Grimes PE, McLaurin CI, Kress MA, Kenney JA Jr. Incidence of common dermatoses in a predominantly black dermatologic practice. Cutis. 1983;32(4):388, 390.
4. Taylor SC. Epidemiology of skin diseases in ethnic populations. Dermatol Clin. 2003;21 (4):601–7.

5. Tomita Y, Maeda K, Tagami H. Melanocyte-stimulating properties of arachidonic acid metabolites: possible role in postinflammatory pigmentation. Pigment Cell Res. 1992;5 (5):357–61.
6. Davis EC, Callender VD. Postinflammatory hyperpigmentation a review of the epidemiology, clinical features, and treatment options in skin of color. J Clin Aesthetic Dermatol. 2010;3(7).
7. Cardinali G, Kovacs D, Picardo M. Mechanisms underlying post-inflammatory hyperpigmentation: lessons from solar lentigo. Ann Dermatol Venereol. 2012;139(Suppl 4):S148–52. doi:10.1016/s0151-9638(12)70127-8.
8. Grimes P, Callender V. Tazarotene cream for postinflammatory hyperpigmentation and acne vulgaris in darker skin: a double-blind, randomized, vehicle-controlled study. Cutis. 2006;77 (1):45–50.
9. Bulengo-Ransby SM, Griffiths CE, Kimbrough-Green CK, Finkel LJ, Hamilton TA, Ellis CN, Voorhees JJ. Topical tretinoin (retinoic acid) therapy for hyperpigmented lesions caused by inflammation of the skin in black patients. N Eng J Med. 1993;328(20):1438–43.
10. Burns RL, Prevost-Blank PL, Lawry MA, Lawry TB, Faria DT, Ftvenson DP. Glycolic acid peels for postinflammatory hyperpigmentation in black patients. Dermatol Surg. 1997;23 (3):171–5.
11. Levin MK, Ng E, Bae YS, Brauer JA, Geronemus RG. Treatment of pigmentary disorders in patients with skin of color with a novel 755 nm picosecond, Q-switched ruby, and Q-switched Nd:YAG nanosecond lasers: a retrospective photographic review. Lasers Surg Med. 2016;48 (2):181–7.
12. Chan JC, Shek SY, Kono T, Yeung CK, Chan HH. A retrospective analysis on the management of pigmented lesions using a picosecond 755-nm alexandrite laser in Asians. Lasers Surg Med. 2016;48(1):23–9.
13. Pandya AG, Guevara IL. Disorders of hyperpigmentation. Dermatol Clin. 2000;18(1):91–8.
14. Grimes PE, Yamada N, Bhawan J. Light microscopic, immunohistochemical, and ultrastructural alterations in patients with melasma. Am J Dermatopathol. 2005;27(2):96–101.
15. Kang WH, Yoon KH, Lee ES, Kim J, Lee KB, Yim H, Sohn S, Im S. Melasma: histopathological characteristics in 56 Korean patients. Br J Dermatol. 2002;146(2):228–37.
16. Handel AC, Miot LDB. Melasma: a clinical and epidemiological review. 2014;89(5):771–82.
17. Sheth VM, Pandya AG. Melasma: a comprehensive update: part I. J Am Acad Dermatol. 2011;65(4):689–97; quiz 698.
18. Goh C, Dlova C. A retrospective study on the clinical presentation and treatment outcome of melasma in a tertiary dermatological referral centre in Singapore. Singapore Med J. 1999;40 (7):455–8.
19. Vázquez M, Maldonado H, Benmamán C, Sanchez JL. Melasma in men. Int J Dermatol. 1988;27(1):25–7.
20. Rigopoulos D, Gregoriou S, Katsambas A. Hyperpigmentation and melasma. J Cosmet Dermatol. 2007;6(3):195–202.
21. Eshghi G, Khezrian L, Esna Ashari F. Comparison between Intralesional triamcinolone and Kligman's formula in treatment of melasma. Acta Med Iranica. 2016;54(1):67–71.
22. Lee HC, Thng TG, Goh CL. Oral tranexamic acid (TA) in the treatment of melasma: a retrospective analysis. J Am Acad Dermatol. 2016;75(2):385–92.
23. Hofbauer Parra CA, Careta MF, Valente NY, de Sanches Osorio NE, Torezan LA. Clinical and histopathologic assessment of facial melasma after low-fluence Q-switched neodymium-doped yttrium aluminium garnet laser. Dermatol Surg: Official Publication for American Society for Dermatologic Surgery [et al]. 2016;42(4):507–12.
24. Pock L, Jelínková L, Drlík L, Abrhámová S, Vojtechovská Š, Sezemská D, Borodácová I, Hercogová J. Lichen planus pigmentosus–inversus. J Eur Acad Dermatol Venereol. 2001;15 (5):452–4. doi:10.1046/j.1468-3083.2001.00347.x.
25. Barros HR. Lichen planus pigmentosus inversus. 2013;88(6 Suppl 1):146–9.
26. Kanwar A, Dogra S, Handa S, Parsad D, Radotra B. A study of 124 Indian patients with lichen planus pigmentosus. Clin Exp Dermatol. 2003;28(5):481–5.

27. Rieder E, Kaplan J, Kamino H, Sanchez M, Pomeranz MK. Lichen planus pigmentosus. Dermatol Online J. 2013;19(12).
28. Murzaku EC, Bronsnick T, Rao BK. Axillary lichen planus pigmentosus-inversus: dermoscopic clues of a rare entity. Diagnosis: lichen planus pigmentosus (LPP). J Am Acad Dermatol. 2014;71(4):e119–20.
29. Al-Mutairi N, El-Khalawany M. Clinicopathological characteristics of lichen planus pigmentosus and its response to tacrolimus ointment: an open label, non-randomized, prospective study. J Eur Acad Dermatol Venereol. 2010;24(5):535–40.
30. Verma P, Pandhi D. Topical tacrolimus and oral dapsone combination regimen in lichen planus pigmentosus. Skinmed. 2015;13(5):351–4.
31. Muthu SK, Narang T, Saikia UN, Kanwar AJ, Parsad D, Dogra S. Low-dose oral isotretinoin therapy in lichen planus pigmentosus: an open-label non-randomized prospective pilot study. Int J Dermatol. 2016;55(9):1048–54.
32. Mohamed M, Korbi M, Hammedi F, Youssef M, Soua Y, Akkari H, Lahouel I, Belhadjali H, Zili J. Lichen planus pigmentosus inversus: a series of 10 Tunisian patients. Int J Dermatol. 2016;55(10):1088–91.
33. Bennassar A, Mas A, Julia M, Iranzo P, Ferrando J. Annular plaques in the skin folds: 4 cases of lichen planus pigmentosus-inversus. Actas Dermo-Sifiliograficas. 2009;100(7):602–5.
34. Gaertner E, Elstein W. Lichen planus pigmentosus-inversus: case report and review of an unusual entity. Dermatol Online J. 2012;18(2):11.
35. Silverberg NB, Herz J, Wagner A, Paller AS. Erythema dyschromicum perstans in prepubertal children. Pediatr Dermatol. 2003;20(5):398–403.
36. Correa MC, Memije EV, Vargas-Alarcon G, Guzman RA, Rosetti F, Acuna-Alonzo V, Martinez-Rodriguez N, Granados J. HLA-DR association with the genetic susceptibility to develop ashy dermatosis in Mexican Mestizo patients. J Am Acad Dermatol. 2007;56(4):617–20.
37. Schwartz RA. Erythema dyschromicum perstans: the continuing enigma of Cinderella or ashy dermatosis. Int J Dermatol. 2004;43(3):230–2.
38. Mahajan VK, Chauhan PS, Mehta KS, Sharma AL. Erythema dyschromicum perstans: response to topical tacrolimus. Indian J Dermatol. 2015;60(5):525.
39. Vasquez-Ochoa LA, Isaza-Guzman DM, Orozco-Mora B, Restrepo-Molina R, Trujillo-Perez J, Tapia FJ. Immunopathologic study of erythema dyschromicum perstans (ashy dermatosis). Int J Dermatol. 2006;45(8):937–41.
40. Gadenne BM, Camisa C. Lichenoid dermatitides (lichen planus, keratosis lichenoides and erythema dischromicum perstans). Cutan Med Surg. 1ᵃ ed. Philadelphia: WB Saunders; 1996. p. 241.
41. Dereure O. Drug-induced skin pigmentation. Epidemiology, diagnosis and treatment. Am J Clin Dermatol. 2001;2(4):253–62.
42. Campbell M, Ahluwalia J, Watson AC. Diltiazem-associated hyperpigmentation. J Gen Intern Med. 2013;28(12):1676.
43. Nisar MS, Iyer K, Brodell RT, Lloyd JR, Shin TM, Ahmad A. Minocycline-induced hyperpigmentation: comparison of 3 Q-switched lasers to reverse its effects. Clin Cosmet Investig Dermatol. 2013;6:159–62.
44. Hamilton HK, Dover JS, Arndt KA. Successful treatment of disfiguring hemosiderin-containing hyperpigmentation with the Q-switched 650-nm wavelength laser. JAMA Dermatol. 2014;150(11):1221–2.
45. Gan SD, Orringer JS. Hemosiderin hyperpigmentation: successful treatment with Q-switched 755-nm laser therapy. Dermatol Surg: Official Publication for American Society for Dermatologic Surgery [et al]. 2015;41(12):1443–4.
46. Gilliam JN, Cox AJ. Epidermal changes in vitamin B 12 deficiency. Arch Dermatol. 1973;107 (2):231–6.

47. Banba K, Tanaka N, Fujioka A, Tajima S. Hyperpigmentation caused by hyperthyroidism: differences from the pigmentation of Addison's disease. Clin Exp Dermatol. 1999;24(3): 196–8.
48. Thomson JA. Alterations in capillary fragility in thyroid disease. Clin Sci. 1964;26:55–60.
49. Brown J, Winkelmann RK. Acanthosis nigricans: a study of 90 cases. Medicine. 1968;47 (1):33–51.
50. Cruz PD Jr, Hud JA Jr. Excess insulin binding to insulin-like growth factor receptors: proposed mechanism for acanthosis nigricans. J Invest Dermatol. 1992;98(6).

Chapter 14
Disorders of Hypopigmentation and Depigmentation

Trisha J. Patel, Ife J. Rodney and Rebat M. Halder

There are a vast number of disorders characterized by hypopigmentation or depigmentation that can be simply subdivided into one of two main categories based on pathogenesis: those that are melanopenic, referring to disorders of decrease pigment production; and those that are melanocytopenic, characterized by a reduction or an absence of melanocytes. Clinically, melanopenic processes present as lightening of the skin, whereas melanocytopenic processes present as milky white discoloration, with accentuation of affected areas on illumination with Wood's lamp, which is a handheld ultraviolet A (UVA) emitting device. In this chapter, those disorders of hypopigmentation and depigmentation that are clinically relevant, including tinea versicolor (TV), idiopathic guttate hypomelanosis (IGH), pityriasis alba (PA), postinflammatory hypopigmentation, hypopigmented variant of mycosis fungoides (MF), progressive macular hypomelanosis (PMH), piebaldism, oculocutaneous albinism (OCA) type 2B, and vitiligo will be discussed.

Tinea Versicolor

Tinea versicolor (TV), formally known as pityriasis versicolor, is a superficial infection caused by the fungus *Pityrosporum ovale* (also known as *Microsporum furfur*, *Malassezia furfur*, or *Pityrosporum orbiculare*) that manifests as hypopigmented or hyperpigmented, ivory to tan, slightly scaly macules and patches predominantly on the trunk, arms, neck, and face. Although there is no known racial predilection [1], the dyschromia that results from the infection is more apparent in skin of color due to the greater contrast between the individual's normal skin and

T.J. Patel · I.J. Rodney · R.M. Halder (✉)
Department of Dermatology, Howard College of Medicine, 2041 Georgia Avenue, Washington, DC 20060, USA
e-mail: rhalder@howard.edu

© Springer International Publishing AG 2017
N.A. Vashi and H.I. Maibach (eds.), *Dermatoanthropology of Ethnic Skin and Hair*, DOI 10.1007/978-3-319-53961-4_14

the affected areas. The pathogenesis of TV can be classified as both melanopenic and melanocytopenic, attributed to the organism's lipoxygenase property. The process by which *P. ovale* oxidizes oleic acid to azelaic acid has been shown to inhibit tyrosinase and damage melanocytes in tissue cultures [2]. It is also known that *P. ovale* acts on unsaturated fatty acids to produce lipoperoxidases that are theorized to be toxic to melanocytes, leading to depigmentation [3]. Some authors have hypothesized that that the abnormally small melanosomes seen within TV lesions in conjunction with lipids in the stratum corneum allow for the dispersion of ultraviolet light, which is partly responsible for the hypopigmentation that is observed [3–5]. On histology, TV changes are mild and consist of hyperkeratosis and slight acanthosis with round, budding yeast with short, septate hyphae in the stratum corneum. In hypopigmented lesions, the basal layer will display reduced numbers of melanosomes [6]. In the superficial dermis, a slight perivascular lymphohistiocytic infiltrate may be observed. Diagnosis is typically made clinically. Examination of affected skin with Wood's lamp displays a greenish hue, and potassium hydroxide (KOH) preparation of the scale of a lesion shows the characteristic "spaghetti and meatballs" appearance, representing hyphae and spores. First line treatments include topical antifungal shampoos, creams, or lotions, such as selenium sulfide, terbinafine, or ketoconazole. Oral antifungal agents such as ketoconazole, fluconazole, and itraconazole have also been shown to be effective. Interestingly, oral terbinafine has not displayed efficacy in treatment of TV. Prophylactic therapy may be helpful in cases of relapse such as once monthly application of 2% ketoconazole shampoo to the affected area for 10–15 min, followed by rinsing. It is important to note, that even after the fungal infection has cleared, it may take many months for the hypopigmentation to resolve which can be of great concern in patients of color. The resulting hypopigmentation can be treated with phototherapy including narrow band ultraviolet B (UVB) or topical psoralen with UVA therapy.

Idiopathic Guttate Hypomelanosis

Idiopathic guttate hypomelanosis (IGH) is a common acquired leukoderma of unclear etiology. It occurs in individuals of all races but is more apparent in skin of color and has a female predominance. IGH has been reported to occur in up to 80% of people over the age of 70 years old with lesions increasing over time [7]. Typically, lesions present as less than 5 mm, symmetric, discrete, asymptomatic, porcelain-white macules distributed most commonly on the extensor surfaces of the extremities, but can also involve the trunk and rarely the face (Fig. 14.1). Once formed, they do not spontaneously regress [8]. The exact pathogenesis is unknown; however, genetic and racial factors, trauma, and autoimmunity have all been postulated [7]. Additionally, IGH has been hypothesized to be induced by UV exposure and can be considered a form of skin photoaging, especially in darker racial and ethnic groups [7]. IGH is classified as both a melanopenic and melanocytopenic process, owing to decreased tyrosinase activity, lower levels of melanin and fewer melanocytes as detected by electron microscopy [9–11]. There are two variants of IGH, the first being actinic IGH in which sunlight plays a role in the distribution of lesions on the body, and the second, hereditary IGH that usually affects darker skinned individuals on sun-protected areas of the body. On histology, there is a flattening of the rete ridges with marked reduction in melanosomes which are irregularly distributed. A significant reduction in the number of DOPA-positive melanocytes can also be observed [12]. Treatment is not necessary, but IGH can be of cosmetic concern, especially in skin of color. Reassurance that lesions will remain small and will not coalesce should be emphasized in patients seeking treatment. As sun exposure may be a precipitating factor, sun protection including sunscreens and physical barriers should be used. There is no definitive treatment; however, anecdotal accounts of cryotherapy, intralesional corticosteroids, topical calcineurin inhibitors, topical and oral PUVA, skin grafts, and superficial dermabrasion have all been reported [13–15]. Cryotherapy, the most frequently used treatment modality, is thought to be effective through irritation of the skin, with stimulation of subsequent migration of melanocytes from the surrounding normal skin [14]. Caution must be exercised given the risk of leukoderma of surrounding normal skin induced by freezing with liquid nitrogen. Histologic examination of repigmented skin demonstrates increased DOPA-positive melanocytes compared with untreated skin [14]. Through a similar mechanism, localized superficial dermabrasion has also been shown to be an effective treatment when targeting larger surface areas [15]. There has been less success with intralesional steroid therapy and skin grafts [7]. Cosmetic camouflage products and concealers may also be used.

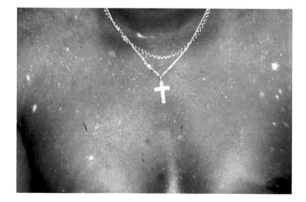

Fig. 14.1 Idiopathic guttate hypomelanosis. Multiple, discrete, 1–5 mm, porcelain-white macules on the trunk

Pityriasis Alba

Pityriasis alba (PA) is a common self-limiting eczematous disorder that presents as hypopigmented, round to oval, scaly patches on the face, neck, and trunk, being more apparent in the summer months. While PA has been reported in all races, there is a predilection for individuals of African, Hispanic, and Asian origin [16]. This disorder affects both sexes equally and is most commonly observed in children and adolescents. Lesions consist of erythematous macules to patches with slightly raised borders which fade over weeks and result in ill-discrete hypopigmented patches with an overlying whitish scale. Most lesions are asymptomatic, but some patients may complain of pruritus and burning. Although most individuals only have one or two lesions, some patients have presented with many more lesions. There are several variations of PA. In extensive PA, which usually affects adults, involvement is widespread (located mostly on the trunk), symmetric, and asymptomatic. Because there is no preceding erythema or history of atopy, some authors believe this form of PA to be a distinct entity. In the pigmented variant of PA, involvement is much more localized, especially on the face, and appears as bluish hyperpigmentation surrounded by scaly hypopigmentation. The blue hue observed in pigmented PA is attributed to melanin deposition in the dermis. A superficial dermatophyte infection has been reported in up to 65% of patients with pigmented PA [17]. The patho-genesis of PA remains unclear, but several mechanisms have been proposed. Given that the prevalence of PA in the general population is estimated to be 1%, while the prevalence in atopic patients is estimated to be up to 30%, there is believed to be a relationship between PA and atopic dermatitis [18, 19]. PA is characterized as an eczematous dermatitis which results in hypomelanosis after the initial inflammation has subsided [20, 21]. The hypomelanosis that is observed in these patients is attributed to the impairment of pigment transfer from melanocytes to keratinocytes, in addition to a decreased number and size of melanosomes, [22]. The xerosis that is often seen in PA is associated with a reduction in the water-holding capacity of the stratum corneum of affected skin. Other proposed mechanisms include nutri-tional and vitamin deficiencies such as copper deficiency, which plays a vital role in tyrosinase activity needed for melanin synthesis [19, 23–25]. On histologic examination, the appearance of chronic spongiotic dermatitis with decreased mel-anin pigment in the basal layer is observed. While PA is usually asymptomatic with the exception of mild pruritus, treatment may be warranted given the striking appearance sometimes seen in skin of color. Management includes emollients, such as petroleum jelly or 12% ammonium lactate lotion, as well as avoidance of sun-exposure and hot water bathing. Other reported therapies include tar emulsions, topical corticosteroids, topical calcineurin inhibitors, and photochemotherapy [26]. Tar emulsions twice daily have been shown to be beneficial as a melanogenic agent and are commercially available as a 6% cream or compounded with 5 or 10% liquor carbonis detergents (LCD) in a variety of vehicles. Topical corticosteroids have been used with limited success. Once weekly PUVA at a starting dose of 0.5 J/cm^2 and increasing by 0.3 J/cm^2 on a weekly basis as tolerated until repigmentation occurs can also be attempted in these patients. Narrow band UVB (NB-UVB) phototherapy at 311 nm up to three times weekly may also be used starting at 75–200 mJ/cm^2, increasing by 20% with each treatment as tolerated.

Post-inflammatory Hypopigmentation

Post-inflammatory hypopigmentation (PIHypo) is an acquired pigmentary disorder characterized by localized partial or total loss of pigmentation following a cutaneous inflammatory or traumatic process. While it can occur in patients of all ages and skin types, it is more striking in those with darker skin attributable to the greater color contrast between the affected lesions and the individual's normal skin. A variety of conditions may result in PIHypo including papulosquamous diseases, such as atopic dermatitis and seborrheic dermatitis, vesiculobullous disorders, such as herpes simplex, inflammatory conditions, including acne and pityriasis lichenoids chronica, connective tissue dermopathies, such as lupus erythematosus, and after exogenous trauma to the skin. The size and shape of the hypopigmented lesion mimics the original inflammatory or traumatic dermatosis, and in severe cases, complete depigmentation may be observed (Fig. 14.2). PIHypo can also be seen after therapeutic interventions such as those with topical retinoids, benzoyl peroxide, liquid nitrogen, and procedures, such as chemical peels, dermabrasion, and laser therapy. In PIHypo, hypopigmentation is thought to result from decreased melanin production [27], loss or blockage of melanosome transfer, or destruction of bystander melanocytes. One proposed mechanism is decreased melanin production through various inflammatory mediators, such as interferon-γ (IFN-γ), tumor necrosis factor-α (TNF-α), TNF-β, and interleukins (IL-6 and IL-7) [28, 29]. Another proposed theory is the blockage of melanosome transfer through epidermal edema and rapid cell turnover. Additionally, the adhesion of leukocytes to melanocytes via cell-surface expression of intracellular adhesion molecule (ICAM-1), ultimately resulting in destruction of innocent bystander melanocytes has been proposed [27]. Histopathological evaluation reveals decreased melanin in the epidermis with a mild lymphohistiocytic infiltrate in the upper dermis. There may also be histologic evidence of the underlying disorder. While findings are nonspecific, histology is typically useful in excluding many dermatoses that present with hypopigmentation, such as sarcoidosis, leprosy, and MF. PIHypo can be differentiated from melanocytopenic conditions such as vitiligo with the use of Wood's lamp as this tool will accentuate lesions devoid of melanin but will not accentuate lesions with melanin. However, Wood's lamp is less helpful in severe cases of PIHypo when melanocyte destruction occurs. Mild PIHypo may resolve within

Fig. 14.2 Postinflammatory
hypopigmentation secondary
to seborrheic dermatitis.
Multiple ill-defined,
hypopigmented macules and
patches to the face

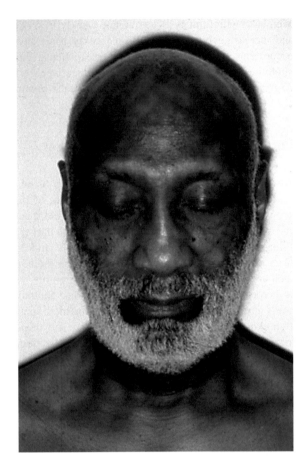

weeks; however, severe hypopigmentation or depigmentation may require years to repigment, if at all. Identification of the underlying dermatosis is imperative in the treatment and prevention of PIHypo. As long as inflammation persists, repigmentation remains an obstacle. Once the inciting condition is controlled, stimulation of melanogenesis can be attempted through the use of topical corticosteroids, topical immunomodulators, such as tacrolimus, topical or oral PUVA, and/or NB-UVB phototherapy. For weekly topical PUVA, 8-methoxypsoralen (8-MOP) is applied to the hypopigmented skin at concentrations of 0.1% or lower, and after 30 min, the patient is exposed to UVA light starting at a dose of 0.2–0.5 J/cm^2 and increasing by 0.2–0.5 J/cm^2 with each treatment as tolerated [30]. In more generalized lesions, oral PUVA at a dose of 0.3 mg/kg of 8-MOP twice weekly is used. NB-UVB phototherapy at 311 nm up to three times weekly may also be used starting at 75–100 mJ/cm^2 and increasing by 20% with each treatment as tolerated [30].

Mycosis Fungoides

Mycosis fungoides (MF) is the most common type of primary cutaneous T-cell lymphoma (CTCL). This uncommon disorder usually presents as hyperpigmented patches, plaques, nodules, and tumors presenting in the fifth and sixth decades of life. However, the hypopigmented variant of MF (HMF) is a rare presentation that usually occurs in younger individuals (including children and adolescents) of darker skin types and is typically associated with an indolent clinical course [31, 32]. The presentation may vary from an eruption of multiple hypopigmented macules to a single large patch with multihued regions. The pathogenesis leading to the hypopigmentation is attributed to blockage of melanosome transfer within melanocytes [33]. Histologically, hypopigmented MF is identical to classic MF. Atypical lymphocytes surrounded by a clear halo in the lower epidermis and papillary dermis can be observed. In more advanced disease, Pautrier microabcesses may also be detected as clusters of atypical lymphocytes in the epidermis [33]. However, unlike classic MF, immunophenotype examination usually reveals a predominance of CD 8^+ T-cells in the epidermal infiltrate as opposed to a predominance of CD 4^+ T-cells. Skin biopsy with histologic confirmation is needed for diagnosis; however, histologic findings typically are subtle and subsequently may require serial biopsies until diagnosis can be confirmed. The initial treatment depends on the stage of the disease as well as the general health condition and age of the patient. Nonetheless, hypopigmented MF is treated similarly to classic MF. For patients with an early-stage disease of the HMF, topical therapy may be sufficient for treatment. Topical therapies include corticosteroids, retinoids such as tazarotene, as well as immune response modifiers such as imiquimod. In cases unresponsive to topical therapy or in more advanced stages of hypopigmented MF, PUVA is a superior alternative with high success rates. NB-UVB phototherapy at 311 nm has also been shown to be effective in treating hypopigmented MF. Additionally, NB-UVB can be used both in disease remission to prevent recurrence as well as to aid in repigmenting affected skin patches. Other therapies that have been tried, especially in refractory cases, include combination bexarotene and PUVA, carmustine, and topical nitrogen mustard [34, 35]. Prognosis is generally favorable in hypopigmented MF, especially with early disease recognition; however, while progression beyond patch stage is rare, serial monitoring for skin lesions is recommended.

Progressive Macular Hypomelanosis

Progressive macular hypomelanosis (PMH) is a relatively common, yet under-recognized, skin disorder characterized by ill-defined hypopigmented macules symmetrically located on the trunk and rarely the face, neck, and extremities (Fig. 14.3). It is most commonly seen in young women of darker skin types who

Fig. 14.3 Progressive
macular hypomelanosis.
Multiple coalescing circular,
poorly defined,
hypopigmented, non-scaly
macules on the back

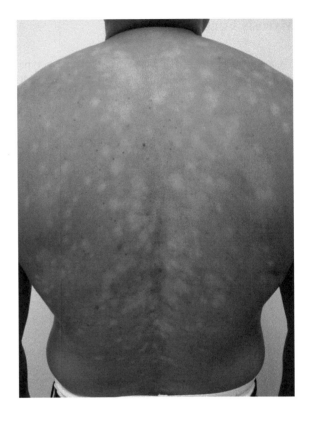

originate from tropical climates but may be seen in all ethnicities [36]. The natural evolution of PMH, although not certain, appears to be an active phase with slow progression over decades followed by spontaneous disappearance after mid-life [37]. This finding is supported by the rarity of PMH to occur in the elderly. The hypopigmented macules are asymptomatic and are not preceded by prior inflammation. The exact pathogenesis of PMH is unknown, but the hypopigmentation is believed to be due to a melanopenic process. *Westerhof* and *Relyveld* have hypothesized that various strains of the bacteria, *Propionibacterium acnes*, may produce a factor that interferes with melanogenesis and subsequently causes hypopigmentation [37]. It is hypothesized that this *Propionibacterium strain* may also produce porphyrins that causes a red follicular fluorescence seen with Wood's lamp examination. Histologic examination shows decreased melanin pigment in the epidermis with a normal number of melanocytes at the basal layer. Electron microscopic examination of patients with Fitzpatrick skin types V and VI show a shift from large, stage IV single melanosomes in keratinocytes seen in normal skin, to small, stage I–III aggregates of membrane-bound melanosomes seen in affected skin [37–39]. On Wood's lamp examination of affected skin, macular accentuation and red follicular fluorescence is seen. The treatment of PMH is challenging and typically delayed, which can be upsetting in those in which dyspigmentation is more evident. There is no first line or single effective treatment for this disorder. Given the probable bacterial etiology, therapy is typically begun with antimicrobials, with many reported cases of successful treatment with oral and topical antibiotics. Furthermore, success has been observed with once daily 5% benzoyl peroxide hydrogel with once daily clindamycin 1% lotion application in combination with NB-UVB irradiation [40]. It is hypothesized that this therapy combination allows for the inhibition of *P. acnes* while also stimulating melanogenesis [37]. There are reports of improvement with PUVA phototherapy; however, upon discontinuation, the hypopigmented lesions reoccur [41]. Patients undergoing therapy may need maintenance treatments to prevent relapse.

Piebaldism

Piebaldism is a rare autosomal dominant disorder that affects all races and genders. The most characteristic manifestation, seen in about 80–90% of individuals with piebaldism, is a white forelock that is present at birth [42]. The forelock is located on the anterior midline scalp in a triangular or diamond shaped distribution, with depigmentation of both the affected hairs and the underlying skin. In severe cases, depigmentation may also be observed in the medial third of the eyebrows and eyelashes [43]. Nonprogressive leukoderma, distributed on the central forehead, central anterior trunk, and the anterior mid-extremities may also be observed (Fig. 14.4). Most individuals with this condition are otherwise healthy with no systemic involvement. About 75% of individuals with piebaldism possess a mutation in the *c-kit* protooncogene, which encodes tyrosine kinase transmembrane receptors found on the surface of melanoblasts in the neural crest [44–46]. Ultimately, a mutated *c-kit* gene leads to a failure of melanoblast proliferation, differentiation, and migration to their location in the skin [47]. While there have been numerous mutation sites found in the gene coding for *c-kit* that result in piebaldism, a Val620Ala mutation has been reported to result in progression of depigmented patches, uncharacteristic of typical piebaldism [48]. In individuals that do not possess a *c-kit* mutation, a mutation in the *slug* gene, which encodes a zinc-finger neural crest transcription factor, has been reported [49]. The differential diagnosis includes Waardenburg syndrome, vitiligo, Vogt-Koyanagi-Harada syndrome, Alezzandrini syndrome, alopecia areata, and tuberous sclerosis. While most cases of piebaldism are isolated to cutaneous depigmentation, piebaldism is rarely associated with other disorders such as Hirschsprung's disease, neurofibromatosis type 1, Grover's disease, and deafness. On histology, piebaldism is characterized by the absence of melanocytes in amelanotic skin. The adjacent normal skin or the hyperpigmented macules within the depigmented skin reveals numerous melanosomes in the melanocytes and keratinocytes. Treatment options are limited as piebaldism rarely responds to topical medications or phototherapy. Surgical procedures such as split thickness grafts, autografts of normal skin to affected skin, and transplantation of autologous cultured melanocytes can be used with variable

Fig. 14.4 Piebaldism. Large, irregular, depigmented patches with islands of pigmentation to the face, trunk, and upper extremities. Note the midline predominance

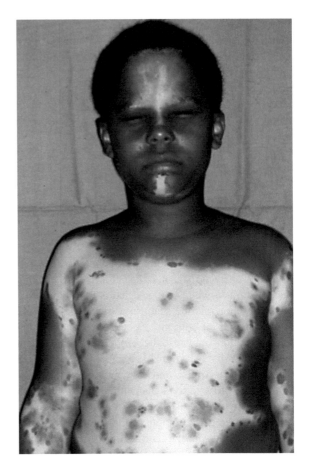

success. Furthermore, there have been reports of successful repigmentation in patients with piebaldism via the destruction of amelanotic skin with an erbium: YAG laser followed by transplantation of cultured epidermal grafts [50]. Nonetheless, in all patients with this condition, aggressive sun protection should be practiced.

Oculocutaneous Albinism

Oculocutaneous albinism (OCA) is a group of autosomal recessive genetic disorders characterized by diffuse depigmentation of skin, hair, and iris due to the partial or total absence of melanin within melanocytes [51]. Four types of OCA have been identified. Type 1 OCA is attributed to mutations in the *TYR* gene resulting in reduced or absent tyrosinase activity needed for melanin production [52]. Type 2

OCA arises from mutations in the OCA2 or *P* gene located on the long arm of chromosome 15 and encodes for the *P* protein [53]. While the exact function of *P* protein is not fully understood, it is believed to play an integral role in melanin synthesis and transport. Several proposed mechanisms for the role of the *P* protein include a membrane transporter of substrates such as tyrosine [54], a sorter of tyrosinase to the melanosome [55], a stabilizer of melanosomal protein complexes [56], and a regulator in melanosomal pH [57]. Additionally, OCA2 has been observed in approximately 1% of individuals with Prader–Willi syndrome and Angelman syndrome, attributed to their chromosome 15 linkage [58]. Type 3 OCA is attributed to a mutation in the *TYRP1* gene which encodes the tyrosinase-related protein 1 [59]. The exact function of this protein is unknown, but it is believed to play a role in tyrosinase stabilization. Type 4 OCA is associated with a mutation in the *MATP* or *SLC45A2* gene which encodes for a membrane-associated transporter proteins needed for normal melanin synthesis [60].

The phenotypic presentation of OCA2 is variable with a spectrum of pigmentary changes of the hair, skin, and iris. In these individuals, eumelanin is almost completely absent, but pheomelanin is normal or increased [61]. Consequently, those affected with this disorder have pale skin (but to a lesser degree than those affected by OCA1), an inability to tan, blonde to brown hair, and blue eyes (most commonly). With time, pigmented nevi and lentigines may develop in sun-exposed areas of the skin. It is also not unusual for patients with OCA2 to have strabismus, nystagmus, or lack of binocular vision attributed to a misrouting of optic nerve fibers during development [62]. OCA2 is the most common type of OCA to develop in individuals of African descent. A variant of OCA2 known as the African brown variant has a phenotypic appearance of light brown hair and skin with gray to tan irides at birth [63]. The differential diagnosis of OCA2 is varied and includes OCA1, 3, and 4, Hermansky-Pudlak syndrome, Chédiak–Higashi syndrome, Menkes syndrome, Griscelli syndrome, Cross syndrome, Tietz syndrome, phenylketonuria, homocystinuria, and histidinemia. On histopathologic examination, there is a reduction in melanin content, but the number of epidermal and follicular melanocytes remains normal. There is no specific treatment for OCA, but aggressive sun protection is mandatory. Individuals with this condition are at increased risk of skin carcinomas [64, 65], specifically squamous cell carcinoma, thus sun avoidance, the use of sun-protective clothing, and frequent application of broad spectrum sunscreens and physical blockers are essential.

Vitiligo

Vitiligo is a relatively common, acquired, multifactorial disorder that results in the destruction of mucomembranous, ocular, follicular, and cutaneous melanocytes [66]. This disorder has been reported to affect approximately 0.5–2% of the global population, with the highest reported prevalence in Gujarat, India, affecting 8.8% of the population [67]. There is no gender, racial, or ethnic predilection; however, this condition can be more physically devastating in individuals with darker skin types due to the greater color contrast between unaffected normal skin and affected depigmented skin. Vitiligo can present at any age, but in nearly 50% of people affected, onset occurs before the age of 20 [68]. Clinical features include fairly discrete, round to oval, amelanotic macules or patches distributed anywhere on the body (Fig. 14.5). There are three general types of vitiligo: (1) localized-further divided into focal, segmental/unilateral, or mucosal, (2) generalized-further divided into vulgaris, acrofacial, or mixed, and (3) Universal, involving more than 80% body surface area. Generalized vitiligo is the most common presentation [66]. Clinical variants occur including trichrome vitiligo, quadrichrome vitiligo, blue vitiligo, and inflammatory vitiligo. Quadrichrome vitiligo is more common in darker skin types, defined by a tan zone between normal and depigmented skin along with marginal or perifollicular hyperpigmentation. The exact pathogenesis of vitiligo is not fully understood; however, it is believed that etiology is multifactorial with genetics and autoimmunity playing large roles. The inheritance pattern can be characterized by incomplete penetrance, multiple susceptibility loci, and genetic heterogeneity [63]. The role of immunity is supported by the association of vitiligo with other autoimmune endocrinopathies, such as hypo- and hyper-thyroidism, pernicious anemia, and Addison's disease. In new onset vitiligo patients, thyroid screening is recommended. Other proposed mechanisms include an intrinsic defect of melanocytes, defective free radical defenses, reduced melanocyte survival, transepidermal melanocytorrhagy (altered melanocyte responses to stress prompting their detachment and subsequent loss), deficiency of melanocyte growth factors, destruction of melanocytes by neurochemical substrates, and aberrant response to viral infections [63]. Diagnosis is almost exclusively made based on clinical examination. On Wood's lamp examination, there is accentuation of vitiliginous lesions with a white fluorescence observed. Treatment modalities for vitiligo are broad. For small, localized lesions, first line therapy includes topical corticosteroids. If no improvement is seen within 2 months, topical steroids should be discontinued to minimize potential adverse effects. Topical immunomodulators such as tacrolimus ointment can also be implemented as steroid-sparing agents. For more generalized lesions, NB-UVB or PUVA therapy are ideal treatments. NB-UVB phototherapy is typically used two to three times weekly at a starting dose of 75–200 mJ/cm^2 and increased by 10–20% with each treatment as tolerated [69, 70]. Oral or topical psoralen with UVA light is generally conducted weekly at a starting dose of 0.5–1 J/cm^2 and gradually increasing by 0.3 J/cm^2 as tolerated [69]. The excimer laser at 308 nm twice weekly for 24–48 treatments has also been reported to be efficacious and can work particularly well in patients with skin of color compared to conventional phototherapy [71, 72]. For rapidly progressive disease, a short course of systemic corticosteroids may be considered; however, guidelines on optimal dosing parameters have not been established. In patients with stable vitiligo lesions for approximately 4–6 months, autologous minigrafts can be implemented. This modality involves harvesting 1–2 mm punch grafts from a donor site and transplanting them to the recipient site at a distance of 3–4 mm apart. Other grafting

Fig. 14.5 Generalized
vitiligo. Fairly discrete,
symmetrical, large,
amelanotic patches with
surrounding smaller, round to
oval amelanotic macules to
the face, trunk, and upper
extremities. Note the
depigmentation of facial hair

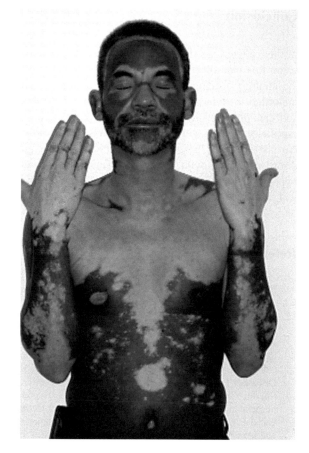

methods include autologous thin Thiersch grafting which allows for grafting large areas of the body via a process similar to dermabrasion and Suction-blister grafting which involves covering depigmented skin with denuded blisters that are formed via liquid nitrogen assault or dermabrasion [72, 73]. Lastly, autologous, non-cultured, melanocyte-keratinocyte cell transplantation is an effective repigmentation technique that involves injecting normally pigmented melanocytes and keratinocytes into the epidermis of affected skin. In patients with diffuse disease and who fail traditional repigmentation therapies, depigmentation with topical monobenzyl ether of hydroquinone may be beneficial. As with many individuals affected by depigmented disorders, aggressive photoprotection is necessary. Given, the psychologically devastating nature of the disease, physicians should have a lower threshold to advance therapy. In addition, psychological support and counseling may be necessary.

Conclusion

In this chapter, we discuss various disorders of hypopigmentation and depigmentation that can affect individuals of all racial and ethnic backgrounds. We discuss the etiology, pathogenesis, diagnosis, and management of these conditions. It is important to remain mindful that many of these dyschromias can be long-lasting and can pose serious physical and psychological disturbances to those affected especially to those with darker skin tones. Fortunately, dermatological research over the last 50 years has allowed for a better understanding and treatment of these disorders today, with the correct identification of the primary cause of the hypopigmentation or depigmentation, we can adequately manage these conditions with a variety of therapies and improve the quality of life of these patients.

References

1. Halder RM, Nandedkar MA, Neal KW. Pigmentary disorders in ethnic skin. Dermatol Clin. 2003;21:617–28.
2. Nazzaro-Porro M, Passi S. Identification of tyrosinase inhibitor in culture of *Pityrosporum*. J Invest Dermatol. 1978;71:389–402.
3. Karaoui R, Bou-Resli M, Alzaid NS, Mousa A. Tinea versicolor: ultrastructural studies on hypopigmented and hyperpigmented skin. Dermatologica. 1981;162:69–73.
4. Odom RB, James WD, Berger TG, editors. Disorders resulting from fungi and yeast. In: Diseases of the Skin, 12th ed. Philadelphia, PA: Elsevier; 2011. p. 285–318.
5. Charles CR, Sire DJ, Johnson BL, Beidler JG. Hypopigmentation in tinea versicolor: a histochemical and electron microscopic study. Int J Dermatol. 1973;12:48–58.
6. Galadari I, el Komy M, Mousa A, Hashimoto K, Mehregan AH. Tinea versicolor: histologic and ultrastructural investigation of pigmentary changes. Int J Dermatol. 1992;31(4):253–6.
7. Falabella R, Escobar C, Giraldo N, Rovetto P, Gil J, Barona MI, Acosta F, Alzate A. On the pathogenesis of idiopathic guttate hypomelanosis. J Am Acad Dermatol. 1987;16(pt 1):35–44.
8. Cummings KI, Cottel WI. Idiopathic guttate hypomelanosis. Arch Dermatol. 1966;93:184.
9. Savall R, Ferrandiz C, Ferrer I, Peyri J. Idiopathic guttate hypomelanosis. Br J Dermatol. 1980;103:635.
10. Ortonne J-P. Idiopathic guttate hypomelanosis: ultrastructural study. Arch Dermatol. 1980;116:664.
11. Wilson PD, Lavker RM, Kligman AM. On the nature of idiopathic guttate hypomelanosis. Acta Dermatol Venereol. 1982;62:301.
12. Wallace ML, Grichnik JM, Prieto VG, et al. Numbers and differentiation status of melanocytes in idiopathic guttate hypomelanosis. J Cutan Pathol. 1998;25:375–9.
13. Golhar A, Pillar T, Eidelman S, Etzioni A. Vitiligo and idiopathic guttate hypomelanosis. Repigmentation of skin following engraftment onto nude mice. Arch Dermatol. 1989;125 (10):1363–6.
14. Ploysangam T, Dee-Ananlap S, Suvanprakorn P. Treatment of idiopathic guttate hypomelanosis with liquid nitrogen: light and electron microscopic studies. J Am Acad Dermatol. 1990;23(4 Pt 1):681–4.
15. Hexsel DM. Treatment of idiopathic guttate hypomelanosis by localized superficial dermabrasion. Dermatol Surg. 1999;25(11):917–8.

16. Halder RM. Pigmentary disorders in pigmented skins. In: Halder RM, editor. Dermatology and dermatological therapy of pigmented skins. Boca Raton, FL: CRC Press; 2005.
17. Dhar S, Kanwar AJ, Dawn G. Pigmenting pityriasis alba. Pediatr Dermatol. 1995;12:197–8.
18. Watkins DB. Pityriasis alba: a form of atopic dermatitis. A preliminary report. Arch Dermatol. 1961;83:915–9.
19. Diepgen TL, Fartasch M, Hornstein OP. Evaluation and relevance of atopic basic and minor features in patients with atopic dermatitis and in the general population. Acta Derm Venereol Suppl (Stockh). 1989;144:50–4.
20. Bassaly M, Miale A Jr, Prasad AS. Studies on pityriasis alba: a common facial skin lesion in Egyptian children. Arch Dermstol. 1963;88:272–5.
21. Martin RF, Lugo-Somolinos A, Sanchez JL. Clinicopathologic study on pityriasis alba. Bol Asoc Med PR. 1990;82:463–5.
22. Zaynoun ST, Aftimos BG, Tenekjian KK, et al. Extensive pityriasis alba: a histological, histochemical and ultrastructural study. Br J Dermatol. 1983;108:83–90.
23. Wells BT, Whyte HJ, Kierland RR. Pityriasis alba: a ten year survey and review of the literature. Arch Dermatol. 1960;82:183–9.
24. Galan EB, Janniger CK. Pityriasis alba. Cutis. 1998;61:11–3.
25. Galadari E, Helmy M, Ahmed M. Trace elements in serum of pityriasis alba patients. Int J Dermatol. 1992;31:525–6.
26. Lin A. Topical immunotherapy. In: Wolverton SE, editor. Comprehensive dermatological therapy. Philadelphia, PA: Saunders; 2001. p. 617–9.
27. Morelli JG, Norris DA. Influence of inflammatory mediators and cytokines on human melanocyte function. J Invest Dermatol. 1993;100(2 Suppl):191S–5S.
28. Ellis DA, Tan AK. How we do it: management of facial hyperpigmentation. J Otolaryngol. 1997;26(4):286–9.
29. Ortonne JP, Bahadoran P, Fitzpatrick TB, et al. Hypomelanoses and hypermelanoses. In: Freedberg IM, Eisen AZ, Wolff K, et al., editors. Fitzpatrick's dermatology in general medicine, 6th ed. New York City, NY: McGraw-Hill; 2003. p. 857.
30. Vachiramon V, Thadanipon K. Postinflammatory hypopigmentation. Clin Exp Dermatol. 2011;36(7):708–14.
31. Tang M, Tan SH, Lim LC. Leukoderma associated with Sézary syndrome: a rare presentation. J Am Acad Dermatol. 2003;49:S247–9.
32. Whitmore SE, Simmons-O'Brien E, Rotler FS. Hypopigmented mycosis fungoides. Arch Dermatol. 1994;130:476–80.
33. Whittaker SJ, MacKie RM. Cutaneous lymphomas and lymphocytic infiltrates. In: Burns T, Breathnach S, Cox N, et al., editors. Rook's textbook of dermatology, vol. 3, 7th ed. Oxford, England: Blackwell; 2004. p. 51–3.
34. Singh F, Lebwohl MG. Cutaneous T-cell lymphoma treatment using bexarotene and PUVA: a case series. J Am Acad Dermatol. 2004;51:570–3.
35. Knobler E. Current management strategies for cutaneous T-cell lymphoma. Clin Dermatol. 2004;22:197–208.
36. Relyveld GN, Kingswijk MM, Reitsma JB, Menke HE, Bos JD, Westerhof W. Benzoyl peroxide/clindamycin/UVA is more effective than fluticasone/UVA in progressive macular hypomelanosis: a randomized study. J Am Acad Dermatol. 2006;55:836–43.
37. Relyveld GN, Menke HE, Westerhof W. Progressive macular hypomelanosis: an overview. Am J Clin Dermatol. 2007;8(1):13–9.
38. Guillet G, Helenon R, Gauthier Y, et al. Progressive macular hypomelanosis of the trunk: primary acquired hypopigmentation. J Cutan Pathol. 1988;15:286–9.
39. Guillet G, Helenon R, Guillet MH, et al. Hypomelanose maculeuse confluente et progressive du metis melanoderme. Ann Dermatol Venereol. 1992;119(1):19–24.
40. Relyveld GN, Kingswijk M, Reitsma JB, et al. Benzoyl peroxide/clindamycin/ultraviolet A is more effective than fluticasone/ultraviolet A in progressive macular hypomelanosis: a randomized study. J Am Acad Dermatol. 2006;55(5):836–43.

41. Menke HE, Ossekoppele R, Dekker SK, et al. Nummulaire en confluerende hypomelanosis van de romp. Ned Tijdsch Dermatol Venereol. 1997;7:117–22.
42. Ward KA, Moss C, Sanders DS. Human piebaldism: relationship between phenotype and site of kit gene mutation. Br J Dermatol. 1995;132:929–35.
43. Thomas I, Kihiczac GG, Fox MD, et al. Piebaldism: an update. Int J Dermatol. 2004;43:716–9.
44. Spritz RA. The molecular basis of human piebaldism. Pigment Cell Res. 1992;5:340–3.
45. Giebel LB, Strunk KM, Holmes SA, Spritz RA. Organization and nucleotide sequence of the human KIT (mast/stem cell growth factor receptor) proto-oncogene. Oncogene. 1992;7:2207–17.
46. Boissy RE, Nordlund JJ. Molecular basis of congenital hypopigmentary disorders in humans: a review. Pigment Cell Res. 1997;10:2–24.
47. Syrris P, Heathcote K, Carrozzo R, et al. Human piebaldism: six novel mutations of the proto-oncogene KIT. Hum Mutat. 2002;20:234.
48. Richards KA, Fukai K, Oiso N, et al. A novel KIT mutation results in piebaldism with progressive depigmentation. J Am Acad Dermatol. 2001;44:288–92.
49. Sanchez-Martin M, Perez-Losada J, Rodriguez-Garcia A, et al. Deletion of the SLUG(SNAI2) gene results in human piebaldism. Am J Med Genet A. 2003;122:125–32.
50. Mahakrishnan A, Srinivasan MS. Piebaldism with Hirschprung's disease. Arch Dermatol. 1980;116:1102.
51. Passeron T, Mantoux F, Ortonne JP. Genetic disorders of pigmentation. Clin Dermatol. 2005;23:56–67.
52. Toyofuku K, Wada I, Spritz RA, Hearing VJ. The molecular basis of oculocutaneous albinism type 1 (OCA1): sorting failure and degradation of mutant tyrosinases results in a lack of pigmentation. Biochem J. 2001;355:259–69.
53. Brilliant MH. The mouse p (pink-eyed dilution) and human P genes, oculocutaneous albinism type 2 (OCA2), and melanosomal pH. Pigment Cell Res. 2001;14:86–93.
54. Rosemblat S, Sviderskaya EV, Easty DJ, Wilson A, Kwon BS, Bennett DC, Orlow SJ. Melanosomal defects in melanocytes from mice lacking expression of the pink-eyed dilution gene: correction by culture in the presence of excess tyrosine. Exp Cell Res. 1998;239:344–52.
55. Puri N, Gardner JM, Brilliant MH. Aberrant pH of melanosomes in pink-eyed dilution (p) mutant melanocytes. J Invest Dermatol. 2000;115:607–13.
56. Manga P, Orlow SJ. Inverse correlation between pink-eyed dilution protein expression and induction of melanogenesis by bafilomycin A1. Pigment Cell Res. 2001;14:362–7.
57. Brilliant MH. The mouse p (pink-eyed dilution) and human P genes, oculocutaneous albinism type 2 (OCA2), and melanosomal pH. Pigment Cell Res. 2001;14:86–93.
58. Spritz RA. The molecular basis of human piebaldism. Pigment Cell Res. 1992;5:340–3.
59. Sarangarajan R, Boissy RE. Tyrp1 and oculocutaneous albinism type 3. Pigment Cell Res. 2001;14:437–44.
60. Newton JM, Cohen-Barak O, Hagiwara N, et al. Mutations in the human orthologue of the mouse underwhite gene (uw) underlie a new form of oculocutaneous albinism, OCA4. Am J Hum Genet. 2001;69:981–8.
61. Bothwell JE. Pigmented skin lesions in tyrosinase-positive oculocutaneous albinos: a study in black South Africans. Int J Dermatol. 1997;36(11):831–6.
62. Witkop CJ Jr, Hill CW, Desnick S, Theis JK, Thorn HL, Jenkins M. Ophthalmologic, biochemical, platelet and ultrastructural defects in the various types of oculocutaneous albinism. J Invest Dermatol. 1973;60:443–56.
63. Ortonne JP. Vitiligo and other disorders of hypopigmentation. In: Bolognia JL, Jorizzo JL, Rapini RP, editors. Dermatology. 2nd ed. Spain: Mosby Elsevier; 2003. p. 913–38.
64. Kromberg JGR, Castle D, Zwane EM, Jenkins T. Albinism and skin cancer in Southern Africa. Clin Genet. 1989;36:43–52.
65. Perry PK, Silverberg NB. Cutaneous malignancy in albinism. Cutis. 2001;67(5):427–30.
66. Kovac S. Vitiligo. J Am Acad Dermatol. 1998;38:647–66.

67. Alikhan A, Felsten LM, Daly M, et al. Vitiligo: a comprehensive overview Part I. Introduction, epidemiology, quality of life, diagnosis, differential diagnosis, associations, histopathology, etiology, and work-up. J Am Acad Dermatol. 2011;65(3):473–91.
68. Halder RM, Chappell JL. Vitiligo update. Semin Cutan Med Surg. 2009;28(2):86–92.
69. Westerhof W, Nieuweboer-Krobotova L. Treatment of vitiligo with UVB radiation vs topical psoralen plus UVA. Arch Dermatol. 1997;133(12):1525–8.
70. Scherschun L, Kim JJ, Lim HW. Narrow-band ultraviolet B is a useful and well-tolerated treatment for vitiligo. J Am Acad Dermatol. 2001;44:999–1003.
71. Passeron T, Ortonne JP. Use of the 308-nm excimer laser for psoriasis and vitiligo. Clin Dermatol. 2006;24:33–42.
72. Ortonne JP, Passeron T. Melanin pigmentary disorders: treatment update. Dermatol Clin. 2005;23:209–26.
73. Bose SK. Modified Thiersch grafting in stable vitiligo. J Dermatol. 1996;23(5):362–4.

Chapter 15
Keloids and Hypertrophic Scarring

Shalini Thareja and Roopal V. Kundu

Keloid and hypertrophic scarring are diseases of excessive dermal fibrosis that occur during and beyond the wound healing process. These lesions are difficult to treat as they have a high tendency to recur. Affected individuals often deal with physical disfigurement, discomfort, and negative psychological impact. Keloid scarring was initially documented in Western literature in 1806. However, the Yoruban culture of Nigeria had described the typical characteristics of keloids in 3000 B.C. in both oral literature and art. Their descriptions demonstrated an understanding of the genetic nature of keloids, their tendency for unchecked growth, and their lack of response to attempted treatment [1].

Human conceptions of scarring are often deeply tied to social and cultural beliefs. While individuals in Western societies often strive to minimize scarring, cultures in regions throughout sub-Saharan Africa view cicatrization as a valued symbolic process or respected ornamentation. Both men and women intentionally prolong the healing process of inflicted wounds through regular reinjuring, packing of wounds with foreign agents, and superficial exposure to environmental substances, such as tree sap and wood [2].

Though research is slowly elucidating the pathophysiology of this condition, much still remains to be understood about keloid scarring and effective treatment options.

S. Thareja
Emory School of Medicine, 1648 Pierce Dr NE, Atlanta, GA 30307, USA
e-mail: shalini.thareja@emory.edu

R.V. Kundu (✉)
Department of Dermatology, Northwestern University Feinberg School of Medicine, 676 N. St. Clair St., Suite 1600, Chicago, IL 60611, USA
e-mail: rkundu@nm.org; Roopal.Kundu@nm.org

© Springer International Publishing AG 2017
N.A. Vashi and H.I. Maibach (eds.), *Dermatoanthropology of Ethnic Skin and Hair*, DOI 10.1007/978-3-319-53961-4_15

Epidemiology

The highest rate of occurrence of keloid scarring is between the ages of 10 and 30 years old, with men and women affected equally [3, 4]. Although keloid scarring can occur in any skin type, it most commonly occurs in darker pigmented skin. The highest incidence has been reported in the African and Hispanic population at 16% [5, 6]. Rates have been found to increase during pregnancy and puberty [4].

Clinical Presentation

Keloids typically develop after trauma, including cuts, surgical wounds, burns, and inflammatory lesions such as acne (Fig. 15.1). Spontaneous keloids also can occur. Early on, keloid lesions are soft and erythematous. However, over time, they become firm [7]. While darker skin type keloids tend toward hyperpigmentation, lighter skin type keloids can be more telangiectatic [8] (Fig. 15.2).

Keloids most commonly develop on the central chest, upper back, ears, and shoulders. Those in areas of high tension, such as the central chest, tend to be flat and more broadly based. However, shoulder and back keloids generally grow larger than other areas. Keloids on the face, neck, wrist, and lower extremities are less common. The jawline, however, is still at high risk for keloid and keloid-variant development. Scalp keloids tend to be papulonodular [9].

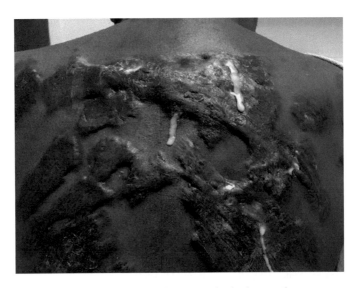

Fig. 15.1 Extensive firm hyperpigmented plaques on the back secondary to severe acne in a FST V woman

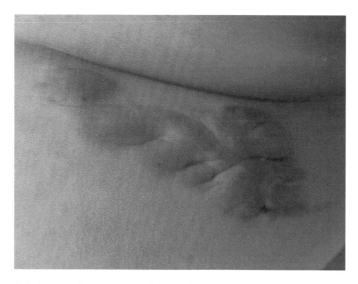

Fig. 15.2 Pink brown telangiectactic and hyperpigmented multilobulated plaque in a FST III Asian woman

There are four morphologies of keloids that develop on the earlobe. The button-shaped keloid is a single nodule that occurs on the anterior or posterior aspect of the earlobe. In the dumbbell morphology, both anterior and posterior keloid nodules are present, and a central stalk connects them. In contrast, in the wraparound presentation, the keloid is "U-shaped" so there is no central stalk (Fig. 15.3). Finally, the lobular form is complete replacement of the lobe by a single large lesion due to recurrent keloids [7].

The consideration of keloids and hypertrophic scars as more than a matter of appearance has grown in recent years, since both conditions can be quite symptomatic. They can become pruritic and painful, particularly during periods of growth. The pruritus can be attributed to the increased quantity of mast cells and histamine within HTS and keloid tissue [10]. Twenty-five percent of affected individuals state their symptoms are severe. Further, these symptoms can have a negative impact on quality of life, most severely in emotional well-being. Pruritus and pain have been found to have the strongest effect on quality of life, beyond that of cosmetic issues such as color, thickness, and irregularity [11].

Hypertrophic Scars Versus Keloids

Hypertrophic scarring is an important clinical entity to differentiate from keloids. Both types of conditions are triggered by injury, including cuts, surgical wounds, burns, and inflammatory lesions such as acne [7].

Fig. 15.3 Wraparound firm
hyperpigmented auricular
keloid in a FST V man

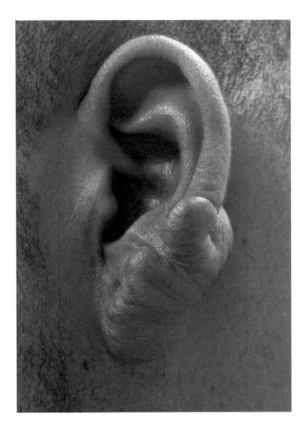

Like keloids, hypertrophic scars are elevated and often erythematous scars. However, they typically appear pink or white and remain confined to the borders of the original wound. Further, after a period of growth they tend to stabilize in size or shrink over time.

On the other hand, keloids are a more aggressive form of scarring. They typically are a deep red or purple color and extend beyond the borders of the original wound in an irregular fashion [5], giving rise to the originally described "claw-like" borders [12]. Keloids tend to have more erratic growth patterns. Periods of stability in size and inflammation can quickly be followed by reactivation and growth [3].

Predisposing Factors

Trauma is the most well-documented trigger for keloid development, and as such vaccinations, tattoos, and piercings can all lead to keloid scarring. Individuals with a predisposition to acne and keloids are at particularly high risk for keloid development on the chest, back, and jawline. Thus, it is important to aggressively manage acne early in at-risk individuals [13].

Hormonal influences can also contribute to keloid and HTS development, which explains their increased incidence during puberty and pregnancy [3]. Prolonged wound healing, through infection, injury, or presence of foreign material in the wound, can also predispose to pathologic scarring. The most important identified extrinsic risk factor, aside from any initial inciting trauma, is mechanical tension and strain. Scars that are perpendicularly oriented to the direction of skin tension from underlying muscle contraction are at high risk for becoming hypertrophied. As a result, the chest, particularly the presternal area, shoulder, and back are particularly prone to the development of these scars [3]. The earlobes are also at high risk to develop keloid scarring, likely related to the common practice of ear piercing. Early piercing can minimize the risk in this highly reactive area.

Histology

Both keloids and hypertrophic scars are processes of increased dermal extracellular matrix deposition. In young lesions, type III collagen predominates; however, over time replacement with type I collagen occurs [5].

In normal skin, collagen is arranged in bundles that lie parallel to the skin surface in an organized pattern. In hypertrophic scars, collagen bundles maintain this directionality but are more loosely organized, shorter, and arranged in a wavy pattern [14]. In keloids, the collagen is even less organized, with apparent loss of bundle structure, larger fibril size, increased fibril density [15], random orientation of collagen fibrils, and unpatterned connections between fibers [14].

Hypertrophic scars and keloids both have increased vascularity compared to normal skin and normal scars. The vessels have greater volume density, are dilated, and take longer and more tortuous paths in the papillary and reticular dermis [14, 16].

Hypertrophic scars have a thickened epidermis and increased cellularity [16]. Myofibroblasts are characteristically increased. Collagen, fibroblasts, and small vessels are randomly organized within nodular structures in the deep dermis [14, 16, 17]. Both keloids and HTS have absent dermal papillae and cutaneous appendages. In keloids, rarely, nodular collagen structures can be seen [16].

Genetics

As there are high rates of occurrence in pigmented populations, increased rates of concordance in identical twins, and reports of familial clustering, a genetic link is suspected for keloid scarring [18–20]. Autosomal dominant inheritance with incomplete penetrance and variable expression is the most commonly reported pattern, although autosomal recessive and autosomal dominant with complete penetrance has also been described [20–24].

Many major histocompatibility (MHC) alleles have recently been implicated in keloid scarring, particularly DRB1*15, HLA-DQA1*0104, DQB1*0501, and DQB1*0503 [25]. SMAD-3, 6, and 7, genes reported to be involved in other fibrotic disorders, did not correlate with risk for keloid scarring in Jamaican patients [18]. However, a Chinese pedigree linkage study showed keloid association with 19q21.1, potentially involving SMAD in keloid pathogenesis [26]. Other studies have found varying levels of SMAD subtypes associated with keloids [27]. A systematic review showed several commonly significantly dysregulated genes in keloids. The top processes controlled by the most commonly implicated genes were related to skeletal development, biological adhesion, and cell adhesion. Meanwhile, the top processes controlled by the gene mutations in HTS were ossification, extracellular matrix structural constituents, and the extracellular region [28].

Pathophysiology

The pathogenesis of keloids is poorly understood. Multiple studies have shown abnormal levels of transforming growth factor-β (TGF-β) in keloids and HTS. The pro-scarring forms, TGF-β1, TGF-β2, and their receptors, are increased, and the anti-scarring form, TGF-β3 and its receptor, is decreased in this tissue [29]. Fibroproliferative cytokines, such as IL-6, have increased expression and levels [30]. Aberrant Wnt signaling and platelet-derived growth factor levels have been found in keloids and HTS, while IL-8, homeobox13, and early growth response-1 all increase fibroplasia [31].

Other drivers may include increased levels of S100A8/9 proteins [32], elevated p53 levels [33], high-mobility group box protein-1 (a pro-fibroblastic proliferation cytokine), imbalanced levels of matrix metalloproteinases (collagenases), and altered Vitamin D levels or cellular signaling relating to it [34]. Systemic hypertension and elevated body mass index have also recently been postulated to contribute to keloid scarring [35, 36].

In vitro, fibroblasts in the superficial and basal regions of keloids have been found to have similar population doubling times and saturation densities as normal fibroblasts. However, central keloid fibroblasts have half the apoptotic rate of normal fibroblasts and reach higher cell densities [37]

Variants

Keloid variants including acne keloidalis nuchae (AKN) and pseudofolliculitis barbae will be discussed in brief below. Please refer to the chapter on adnexal disorders a full review.

Acne Keloidalis Nuchae

AKN is a keloid variant that was initially coined in 1869 as dermatitis papillaris capillitii [38]. Most commonly, black men under the age of 50 are affected, and after the age of 50 affected individuals usually do not develop new lesions [39]. Similar to true keloids, they present with pain and pruritus [39]. The condition begins after puberty as an acute folliculitis and perifolliculitis; however, with time, it progresses into a chronic condition. Initially, the condition presents with 2–4 mm firm papules, which resemble keloids, and pustules on the base of scalp and back of the neck. The pustules often break open from pruritus-induced scratching or hair brushing. Over time, the papules can merge to form large horizontally oriented plaques. Complications include subcutaneous abscesses with draining sinuses and a scarring alopecia of the affected skin. The keloid-like papules and plaques are nonresponsive to antibiotic therapy, which can treat the underlying folliculitis [38].

The pathogenesis of AKN is unknown. Short tightly curled hair, which is common in the African American population, is believed to be the incriminating factor in AKN. As the hair shaft grows beyond the surface of the epidermis, it curls back and pierces the skin surface. This triggers an inflammatory reaction in the epidermis leading to the development of the characteristic papules and pustules. Other triggers include constant rubbing in the area from shirt collars, a chronic folliculitis, and an autoimmune condition [38].

Histologic evidence in one study found AKN to be a scarring alopecia. Foreign antigens, such as the demodex mite and normal skin flora, and autologous antigens, such as sebum, on the follicular epithelium and intrafollicular canal can trigger an inflammatory cascade. This leads to damaged and fragmented hair unit structures that can encourage HTS and keloid scarring [40]. AKN has also been described as a transepithelial elimination disorder [41], a form of lichen simplex chronicus [42], and associated with the male seborrheic constitution, increased fasting blood testosterone, and early reproductive years [43].

Pseudofolliculitis Barbae (PFB)

The term pseudofolliculitis of the beard was first coined in 1956 [44]. The condition primarily occurs in African American men as well, likely because of its association with tightly curled coarse hair types. The prevalence in this population is 45–83%. However, women and other ethnicities can also be affected. In fact, women of African or Hispanic lineage with hypertrichosis or hirsutism have similar incidence of PFB [39].

PFB presents with inflammatory papules and pustules in the beard area. The papules can be flesh-colored, erythematous, or hyperpigmented. Typically, the upper lip and lateral margin of the face are spared. Other shaved areas can also develop PFB, such as the scalp and leg [38]. In fact, in predisposed women, these lesions may occur in the axilla and groin [39].

As PFB is a result of epidermal and dermal inflammation from curled hair shaft growth, shaving is the precipitating factor in its development. Two mechanisms explain its pathogenesis: extrafollicular penetration and transfollicular penetration. Transfollicular penetration occurs when the hair is shaved against the grain with the skin held taught. Once the stretch on the skin is released, the hair tip withdraws below the skin surface. Curved hair regrowth results in penetration of the follicle wall, leading to the development of papules and pustules. Hair removal techniques that can cause midshaft hair breakage, such as tweezing and electrolysis, can also lead to transfollicular penetration. In extrafollicular penetration, the shaved tip grows in a curved fashion beyond the hair follicle, repierces the epidermis, and then grows into the dermis. The inflammatory response that occurs on epidermal penetration is significantly heightened with the hair shaft's presence in the dermis. This gives rise to the characteristic papules and pustules. The hair springs back out of the skin once it has grown roughly 10 mm long [38]. Injury of PFB lesions from shaving can lead to secondary bacterial infection, abscesses, hypertrophic scarring, and keloids [38].

Prevention

Primary Prevention

Minimizing trauma is the most important method of prevention. High-risk patients, including those with a greater degree of skin pigmentation, family history, or personal history of keloids, should avoid tattoos, piercings, and other surgical procedures [45]. To avoid auricular keloid development, ear piercing before 11 years of age is advantageous [46]. The senior author, however, prefers piercing before seven years of age given the changing hormonal milieu of earlier onset puberty may increase the risk for keloid formation.

Prevention plays a major role in the treatment of AKN and pseudofolliculitis barbae. For AKN, patients should avoid high-collared shirts and hats, which can irritate the scalp. Also, short hairstyles and razor/hair clipper use along the occipital scalp should be avoided [39]. For PFB, patients should not pull the skin taught when shaving and should shave in the direction of hair growth. Regular brushing of the beard can help free embedded tips [38].

Secondary Prevention

Ear Keloids

Ear lobe keloids typically respond well to postsurgical pressure therapy. The recommended regimen is continuous pressure of 24–30 mm Hg for eight to 24 hours over 6- to 12-months [6]. In 1436 keloids, magnets as a form of pressure therapy worn 12 hours daily for 6 months showed a recurrence rate of 11.6% after 18 months. Interestingly, recurrence was associated with high body mass index, prior treatment, and slow keloid growth rate [36]. Postsurgical "sandwich" radiotherapy and triple therapy with surgical excision, intralesional steroid, and silicone sheeting have also been utilized [47, 48].

Pressure Dressings

Pressure has been postulated to lead to collagen and fibroblast degeneration in HTS via creation of a hypoxic environment [19]. Changes in cytokine expression may underlie structural changes induced by pressure garments in HTS [49]. In an animal model study, 2 weeks of pressure treatment led to 51.9% decreased collagen levels in HTS, most significantly through reductions in collagen I and III [50]. Rearrangement of collagen fibers from nodular to wave-like patterns also occurs. Increased dermal layer apoptotic indices, reductions in dermal cell layer density, and significant reductions in myofibroblast and α-smooth muscle actin levels have also been found [51].

For years, compression garments have been standard practice in many institutions for the prevention of burn-induced HTS [52]. However, a 2009 meta-analysis found little convincing evidence for the effectiveness of pressure garment treatment [53]. Optimum pressure requirements are also unknown. Some papers have shown 15 mmHg is required at minimum for improvement [54, 55] and 40 mmHg can lead to complications [55]. A 12-year randomized control trial published in 2011 did find efficacy of pressure therapy as a preventative modality for burn induced moderate to severe HTS [56]. Further, studies in keloids specifically are limited.

Silicone Gel Sheets

Silicone gel sheets (SGS) are often used as preventative treatment of high-risk wounds. Primarily, SGS provide occlusion and hydration to the healing wound, key components of wound healing. Transepidermal water loss in the stratum corneum, which is increased in unoccluded scar, stimulates keratinocyte production of cytokines. These active fibroblasts produce exaggerated amounts of collagen, which assist in water retention. Occlusion of the developing scar with SGS therefore stunts excessive collagen and cytokine production [57–59]. Specifically, TGF-β1, TGF-β2, bFGF, and PDGF are decreased with preventative SGS use in early scars [58, 60]. It is important to note that excessive occlusion and hydration can impair wound healing [57]. SGS provide a similar level of occlusion as normal skin, explaining their ability to improve collagen structures and cytokine profiles.

Secondly, wound tension is lowered with SGS application. Tension is transferred from the wound to the sheet through the sheet's adhesion to the surrounding skin [57]. Thirdly, friction between the scar and SGS produces a negatively charged electric field that improves collagen orientation and encourages scar involution

[61]. Finally, decreased injury may be incurred on healing skin with the gentle adhesive of SGS [57, 62, 63].

Application of SGS is recommended for 12–24 hours daily with twice daily washing for at least 1 month. Application should be initiated 2–3 weeks after wound formation to allow for wound epithelialization. SGS use as preventative treatment has been shown to improve scar size, induration, pruritus, and pain [64–66]. However, a recent systematic review, concluded that the benefit of preventative SGS in high-risk patients does not currently exist as most studies are of poor quality [67].

Silicone gel preparations form a clear, gas-permeable, water-impermeable, silicone covering on the skin. Several advantages exist for gel preparations over SGS, including ease of application over large areas of skin, near joints, and on cosmetically sensitive areas such as the face. Compliance tends to be higher as patients prefer the decreased visibility of gel preparations to SGS. Further, there is less risk of infection and rash with gel since the need for regular washing and cleaning of a reusable sheet has been removed [59]. Prospective RCTs have found decreased scar elevation, erythema, pliability, and symptoms with the preventative use of gel preparations in high-risk lesions [68–71]. Further, no significant difference in the efficacy between SGS and silicone gel has been found [70]. Silicone gel formulation efficacy is still debated given the unclear overall benefit of SGS use [67].

Radiation

Improvements in keloids with postoperative radiation therapy are believed to be via regulation of the fibroblast cell cycle. Radiotherapy extends the G0/G1 phase of the cell cycle and normalizes the rate of fibroblast apoptosis [37, 72]. Further, expression of genes associated with cellular senescence, mainly p16, p21, and p27, is upregulated with treatment [72].

Concerns about the carcinogenic potential of radiation have limited the use of radiotherapy for keloids [73]. External beam radiotherapy is the most commonly utilized technique for postoperative treatment. However, it is difficult to treat long wounds and wounds on uneven skin surface through this technique. Interstitial and superficial brachytherapy are alternative methods in which the radiation source, an applicator, is placed within or just above the lesion, respectively. These are well suited for irregularly contoured lesions, such as those on the scapula or jaw. Interstitial treatment allows for a smaller irradiated area, thus less involvement of healthy issue. However, radiation schedules must be much shorter given the implanted applicator must be removed to prevent wound dehiscence and keloid recurrence. On the other hand, superficial brachytherapy allows for more cost-effective and shorter treatment regimens, as well as more consistent radiation dosage to changing wound shapes secondary to postoperative edema and hematoma [74, 75].

Overall, high-level randomized studies are lacking [76]. Prospective clinical studies have shown recurrence rates with radiotherapy after surgical excision from 2.2 to 38.0% [74, 75, 77–81]. Improved long-term control has been demonstrated with radiotherapy initiation within 24 hours of surgery [80]. Rates of improvement in pruritus and pain are notable. Side effects include hypopigmentation, hyperpigmentation, erythema, pruritus, skin atrophy, telangiectasia, and subcutaneous fibrosis [75, 78]. There may be heightened risk of the development of pigment abnormalities in higher Fitzpatrick skin types [81]. It has been reported that a dosage range of 10–30 Gy for keloids has a low risk of carcinogenesis while maintaining efficacy in keloid treatment [82]. However, a dosage of 15 Gy is reported effective for 90% of keloids [79], and total doses above 21 Gy increase the risk of side effects such as abnormal pigmentation [83]. None of the reviewed studies reported any incidences of cancer; however, follow-up time periods ranged from 18 to 46.5 months [74, 75, 77–81]. Additional well-structured randomized control trials with longer follow-up periods are still needed to assess the efficacy and carcinogenesis risk of radiation therapy. The elevated risks in adolescents and children must be considered prior to decision for radiation treatment.

Treatment

Corticosteroids

Although there are only a small number of well-designed studies on corticosteroid efficacy, intralesional corticosteroid injections have continued as the gold standard in keloid treatment since the 1960s [6, 84]. By inhibiting expression of TGF-β, VEGF, and IGF-1, corticosteroid treatment is able to prevent overgrowth of fibroblast populations and excessive collagen formation [6]. Corticosteroids induce G1 cell cycle arrest but do not promote apoptosis [85].

Typically, the regimen is a 10–40-mg/mL injection every 1–2 months (Table 15.1). Response rates range from 50 to 100% with recurrence rates of 9–50% [86]. Topical steroids have not shown the same efficacy and are therefore not preferred [84]. Recently, delivery of topical steroid through fractional ablative laser has shown potential for post-acne keloids [87]. Side effects of corticosteroid therapy include dermal and epidermal atrophy, telangiectasia, hyper- and hypopigmentation. As children are most at risk for developing Cushing's syndrome from intralesional corticosteroids, total dosage should not exceed 30 mg per month in children [88]. For post-excision prophylaxis in helix keloids, no significant advantage was found in recurrence rate with the addition of two postoperative injections of triamcinolone to a single intraoperative injection [89].

Surgical Excision

Because recurrence rates range from 45 to 100%, surgical excision as a monotherapy is discouraged [90–92]. AKN is the only type of keloid that typically

Table 15.1 Clinical practice—intralesional corticosteroids

---

1. Pain control
   a. Options: topical or combination anesthetics, intralesional or perilesional anesthetic, cryotherapy
   b. Senior author prefers to avoid IL lidocaine as injections are painful and IL anesthetic can limit the volume of injected corticosteroid
   c. Cryotherapy should be used with care. Epidermal melanocytes are more sensitive to cryotherapy destruction than keratinocytes or fibroblasts. Excessive cryotherapy can lead to hypopigmentation

---

2. Preparation
   a. 27–30 gauge needle on a 1 cc syringe. Larger needle sizes may exacerbate injection pain and lead to leakage of injected medication
   b. Use of luer lock needle syringe that is fully locked to the needle. High backpressure is exerted from the dense keloid tissue during injection. This can cause needle separation from the syringe
   c. Begin with triamcinolone 10 mg/mL. Increase by 10 mg/mL if there is not adequate response
   d. Always wear a mask
3. Injection procedure
   a. The needle should be inserted bevel down
   b. Senior author prefers a fan technique: several tracks within the body of the keloid should be made with each needle insertion. Deliberate medication injection should be done at the edges of the keloid
   c. Throughout the entire injection, medication should be released against the resistance of the keloid tissue only. Any superficial or deep release of corticosteroid may lead to epidermal or subcutaneous atrophy, respectively, and hypopigmentation
   d. To avoid injection pain from dulled needle, the needle should be changed every four to five injections
4. Patient counseling
   a. Patients should be educated that treatment will involve a series of at least five to six injections every four to eight weeks
   b. Side effects should be discussed: depressions secondary to atrophy, color changes, telangiectasia
   c. If side effects occur, there is an option to skip an injection in the series or continue onwards depending on patient preference

---

has low recurrence rates after excision, even with secondary intention healing [6]. Intraoperative pathologic examination is not routinely performed for keloids. However, incomplete excision of keloid tissue, either at peripheral or deep margins, and ill-defined keloid tissue borders pose an increased risk of recurrence [93]. In certain situations such as auricular keloids, intralesional excision with rind flap use has shown benefit in areas where total scar excision and closure will distort structural anatomy. This method also reduces wound tension and leaves behind rich vasculature for the healing wound [47, 94]. Combined treatment with surgical excision and intralesional corticosteroids, pressure devices, magnets, or postoperative radiation improves recurrence risk. Auricular keloids respond particularly well to surgical excision with adjuvant therapy (See Section on Ear Keloids).

Cryotherapy

By inducing blood stasis and coagulation, cryotherapy destroys the microvasculature supplying keloid tissue [95]. It also can cause directly cellular damage, although the fibrous tissue itself has been found to be relatively resistant to freezing [95, 96]. Histologic analyses have found cryotherapy normalizes collagen synthesis, orientation, and fibroblast differentiation [96, 97]. Small keloids tend to respond best and multiple sessions may be required for adequate keloid response. Side effects include pain, atrophy, and ulceration. Given melanocyte sensitivity to cooler temperatures, there is also a high risk of hypopigmentation, particularly in higher Fitzpatrick groups [98, 99].

In contrast to surface cryotherapy, intralesional cryotherapy, a relatively recent method, enables more direct damage to dermal fibrous tissue with sparing of superficial tissues. Thus, there is a decreased risk of melanocyte damage and hypopigmentation. Keloid and hypertrophic scars have shown improvements of 47–89% with monotherapy [97, 99–102]. Combination treatment with topical silicone gel sheeting has not improved success rates [101], although a recent study with addition of intralesional corticosteroids demonstrated a volume reduction of 93.5% [95].

Lasers

Both ablative and non-ablative lasers have been utilized for keloid treatment, including pulsed dye laser (PDL) (585–595 nm), neodymium-doped yttrium aluminum garnet (Nd:YAG) (1064 nm), erbium-doped yttrium aluminum garnet (Er: YAG), and CO_2. The use of ablative lasers, including Er:YAG and CO_2, have been limited due to high recurrence rates. There is no agreement on the mechanism of action for each of the lasers, although multiple theories exist. A level 1 systematic review recently found the evidence for laser treatment for keloids was not strong enough to endorse its efficacy during the treatment and follow-up periods [103].

Pulsed Dye Laser (PDL)

By the late 1980s, PDL had become a leading treatment for vascular lesions, including port-wine stains and telangiectasias. Soon after, a landmark study by Alster et al. paved the way for its use in HTS and keloids [104, 105]. Multiple mechanisms have been suggested for scar improvement with PDL use. The leading theory is based on the selective targeting of hemoglobin, which causes local thermal injury to the blood vessel with minimal energy dispersion to surrounding tissues [106, 107]. Coagulation and occlusion of the microvasculature in the papillary and reticular dermis follows. The ischemia and nutrient deprivation of the scar tissue inhibits its growth and collagen production. PDL is also believed to stimulate matrix breakdown via inhibition of TGF-β and PDGF and stimulation of MMP and IL-6 [106]. Collagen fiber structural realignment through heat-induced modifications of disulfide bonds has also been suggested [108].

Both 585 and 595 nm are utilized for keloid treatment, although more studies have been done utilizing 585 nm [107]. PDL should be used cautiously in darker pigmented patients, as it can target the epidermal pigmentation and lead to greater risk of complications. For these patients and those with scars in high-risk areas, the energy density should be decreased by 10%. Posttreatment purpura is the most common side effect, which typically resolves within 10 days [109]. No correlation has been found between energy density and treatment outcome. Thus, higher fluence may pose unnecessary risk for irritation without additional treatment benefits [103]. A recent systematic review of PDL treatment in HTS and keloids included studies with PDL of 585 nm wavelength, duration of 250–1500 ms, spot size of 5–10 mm, and fluences of 3.5–9 J/cm^2. PDL was superior to conventional modalities in improving overall scar appearance and scar pigmentation. Issues with incomplete outcomes, selective reporting, blinding, and/or randomization in these studies limited the ability to formulate a strong conclusion about PDL for HTS and keloids [108].

Nd:YAG

Nd:YAG treatment is believed to function through heat generation. This initiates an inflammatory cascade, elevating vascular permeability, MMP production, and collagen degradation [106]. The resulting tissue infarction causes skin sloughing with underlying wound healing. 532-nm lasers are the most efficient frequency for use, possibly because this energy level is close to the absorption peak of oxyhemoglobin (542 nm). This leads to the greatest energy absorption by hemoglobin and consequent vascular destruction. A recently published retrospective case series on use of 1064 nm Nd:YAG laser in 102 patients with HTS or keloids found both scar types significantly improved in subjective and objective parameters. However, keloid recurrence rates 6 months after a 1-year regimen were still high—4% on the abdomen, 25% on the scapula, 35.7% on the upper arms, and 52.9% on the anterior chest [110].

Other Lasers

CO_2 treatment induces reorganization of collagen bundle structures [111, 112], decreases in type I collagen, and may increase type III collagen [113]. CO_2 laser treatment may also improve keloids through modulation of MMP9 levels [111]. Further high level studies are needed for CO_2 and copper bromide lasers.

Onion Extract

The exact mechanism of onion extract, *Allium cepa*, activity is still unknown. In vitro fibroblast studies have shown onion extract inhibits fibroblast proliferation, decreases β1 integrin, and can induce fibroblast apoptosis. β1 integrin is an adhesion protein important in fibrogenesis. It may also inhibit IL-6 and VEGF [114], upregulate MMP-1 production [115], and modulate histamine levels by increasing mast cell stability [116]. Results of onion extract studies have been mixed. While unchanged rates of keloid development with topical 10% onion extract in silicone gel have been found [117], improved scar volume and induration has also been found in combination with 0.5% hydrocortisone [118]. Topical mixtures of onion extract with other compounds have improved pain, sensitivity, pruritus, elevation, and neoangiogenesis [119, 120]. These improvements may be confounded by a large representation of HTS in study participants and impact of heparin on collagen fibril structure [119].

Chemotherapeutics

Multiple chemotherapeutics have been utilized for keloid treatment, including 5-fluorouracil (5-FU), mitomycin, and bleomycin. 5-FU is a pyrimidine analogue with antimetabolite activity. It induces G2-cycle arrest and apoptosis, perhaps through p53 activation [85]. Theoretically, its antimetabolite activity should be greatest on fibroblasts stimulated to proliferate and secrete collagen. Thus, 5-FU as a preventative modality may be more efficacious than as a treatment modality. Excessive 5-FU can lead to erythema, scar widening, ulceration, and wound dehiscence [121, 122]. In a recent study, the prophylactic use of post-excisional 5-FU (50 mg/mL) and botulinim A toxin injections in treatment-resistant keloids had a recurrence rate of 3.75% after 2 years [122]. As a treatment modality, treatment with 5-FU tattoo (50 mg/mL) elicited greater reduction in keloid height, induration, and pruritus than intralesional triamcinolone alone (40 mg/mL) [123]. 5-FU treatment is effective in 45–79% of patients and up to 96% of patients with combination 5-FU and triamcinolone [121]. Of note, low doses of triamcinolone have been used, from 1:45 to 4:45 triamcinolone:5-FU. The current evidence cannot define a maximum allowed dose per scar area or total. However, most studies have investigated weekly injections, 80–100 mg of 5-FU per session, and a 4:45 mg/mL ratio of TAC:5-FU. This is therefore the current recommended frequency, concentration, and dose [124].

Bleomycin and mitomycin are both cytotoxic proteins produced by *Streptomyces* species [125, 126]. However, studies on both are limited. There is some evidence of the efficacy of intralesional bleomycin in flattening keloids and providing symptomatic control [127–129]. When used intralesionally with electroporation, which increases medication absorption by over 10,000-fold, bleomycin has also improved keloid scar [127]. Atrophy and hyperpigmentation have been reported as long-term side effects [127]. Systemic side effects of bleomycin, mainly pulmonary, renal, and cutaneous fibrosis have not been found with keloid treatment [128, 130, 131].

Calcium Antagonists

Intralesional verapamil was initially harnessed for burn scar therapy in 1994 [132]. In vitro studies with fibroblasts have shown calcium antagonists slow extracellular matrix growth by hindering proline incorporation [133], inhibiting IL-6 and VEGF production [134], and inducing collagen degradation [133–136]. A recent systematic review and meta-analysis agreed on lack of high quality studies examining calcium antagonist efficacy [137, 138]. In the three existing high-level studies, verapamil had efficacy equal to or greater than that of intralesional triamcinolone [139–141]. While verapamil had a slower rate of improvement, it also had a significantly decreased rate of complications and a lower drug cost [139, 141].

Botulinum Toxin Type A

There has been some recent interest in intralesional botulinum toxin type A as a treatment modality. Although it can eliminate the constant wound margin tension that induces fibroblast growth [86], in vitro studies have shown conflicting evidence of any adjusted expression of chemical messengers [142, 143]. Independently, it has shown efficacy in improving scar size [144], and it may be equally as efficacious as corticosteroids with a lower risk of side effects [145].

Key Points

1. High-risk groups for keloid development include adolescents, young adults, pregnant women, and darkly pigmented populations, including blacks and Hispanics.
2. Acne lesions and areas of high tension, such as the chest, shoulder, and back, are also at higher risk for keloid development. Aggressive management of acne in predisposed populations is important in prevention.
3. AKN and pseudofolliculitis barbae are keloid variants in which curled hair shaft growth leads to cutaneous injury and inflammation.
4. Ear piercing below 11 years of age is preferable to prevent auricular keloids.
5. Intralesional triamcinolone (10–40 mg/mL) is the gold standard in treatment. Auricular keloids often respond well to combination therapy with surgical excision.

References

1. Omo-Dare P. Yoruban contributions to the literature on keloids; (1943-4693 (Print)).
2. Ayeni OA, Ayeni OO, Jackson R. Observations on the procedural aspects and health effects of scarification in sub-Saharan Africa. J Cutan Med Surg. 2007;11(6):217–21.
3. Roseborough IE, Grevious MA, Lee RC. Prevention and treatment of excessive dermal scarring. J Natl Med Assoc. 2004;96(1):108–16.
4. Alhady SM, Sivanantharajah K. Keloids in various races. A review of 175 cases. Plast Reconstr Surg. 1969;44(6):564–6.
5. Dadzie OE, Alexis A, Petit A. Ethnic dermatology: principles and practice. Somerset, NJ, USA: John Wiley & Sons; 2013.
6. Shockman S, Paghdal KV, Cohen G. Medical and surgical management of keloids: a review. J Drugs Dermatol. 2010;9(10):1249–57.
7. Schwarzenberger K, Werchniak AE, Ko CJ, editors. General dermatology. Edinburgh; New York: Saunders Elsevier; 2009.
8. Sobec R, et al. Ear keloids: a review and update of treatment options. Clujul Med. 2013;86 (4):313–7.
9. Bayat A, et al. Description of site-specific morphology of keloid phenotypes in an Afrocaribbean population. Br J Plast Surg. 2004;57(2):122–33.
10. Wulff BC, Wilgus TA. Mast cell activity in the healing wound: more than meets the eye? Exp Dermatol. 2013;22(8):507–10.
11. Kouwenberg CA, et al. Emotional quality of life is severely affected by keloid disease: pain and itch are the main determinants of burden. Plast Reconstr Surg. 2015;136(4 Suppl):150–1.
12. Addison T. On the keloid of Alibert, and on true keloid. Med Chir Trans. 1854;37:27–47.
13. Yin NC, McMichael AJ. Acne in patients with skin of color: practical management. Am J Clin Dermatol. 2014;15(1):7–16.
14. Rockwell WB, Cohen IK, Ehrlich HP. Keloids and hypertrophic scars: a comprehensive review. Plast Reconstr Surg. 1989;84(5):827–37.
15. Kischer CW. Comparative ultrastructure of hypertrophic scars and keloids. Scan Electron Microsc. 1984(Pt 1):423–31.
16. Amadeu T, et al. Vascularization pattern in hypertrophic scars and keloids: a stereological analysis. Pathol Res Pract. 2003;199(7):469–73.
17. Ehrlich HP, et al. Morphological and immunochemical differences between keloid and hypertrophic scar. Am J Pathol. 1994;145(1):105–13.
18. Brown JJ, et al. Genetic susceptibility to keloid scarring: SMAD gene SNP frequencies in Afro-Caribbeans. Exp Dermatol. 2008;17(7):610–3.
19. Love PB, Kundu RV. Keloids: an update on medical and surgical treatments. J Drugs Dermatol. 2013;12(4):403–9.
20. Marneros AG, et al. Clinical genetics of familial keloids. Arch Dermatol. 2001;137 (11):1429–34.
21. Shih B, Bayat A. Genetics of keloid scarring. Arch Dermatol Res. 2010;302(5):319–39.
22. Marneros AG, et al. Genome scans provide evidence for keloid susceptibility loci on chromosomes 2q23 and 7p11. J Invest Dermatol. 2004;122(5):1126–32.
23. Omo-Dare P. Genetic studies on keloid. J Natl Med Assoc. 1975;67(6):428–32.
24. Bloom D. Heredity of keloids; review of the literature and report of a family with multiple keloids in five generations. N Y State J Med. 1956;56(4):511–9.
25. Brown JJ, Bayat A. Genetic susceptibility to raised dermal scarring. Br J Dermatol. 2009;161(1):8–18.
26. Yan X, et al. Preliminary linkage analysis and mapping of keloid susceptibility locus in a Chinese pedigree. Zhonghua Zheng Xing Wai Ke Za Zhi. 2007;23(1):32–5.
27. Seifert O, Mrowietz U. Keloid scarring: bench and bedside. Arch Dermatol Res. 2009;301 (4):259–72.

28. Huang C, et al. A snapshot of gene expression signatures generated using microarray datasets associated with excessive scarring. Am J Dermatopathol. 2013;35(1):64–73.

29. Liu W, Wang DR, Cao YL. TGF-beta: a fibrotic factor in wound scarring and a potential target for anti-scarring gene therapy. Curr Gene Ther. 2004;4(1):123–36.

30. Ghazizadeh M, et al. Functional implications of the IL-6 signaling pathway in keloid pathogenesis. J Invest Dermatol. 2007;127(1):98–105.

31. Profyris C, Tziotzios C, Do Vale I. Cutaneous scarring: pathophysiology, molecular mechanisms, and scar reduction therapeutics Part I. The molecular basis of scar formation. J Am Acad Dermatol. 2012;66(1):1–10; quiz 11–2.

32. Zhong A, et al. S100A8 and S100A9 are induced by decreased hydration in the epidermis and promote fibroblast activation and fibrosis in the dermis. Am J Pathol. 2016;186(1):109–22.

33. Tanaka A, et al. Expression of p 53 family in scars. J Dermatol Sci. 34(1):17–24.

34. Lee DE, et al. High-mobility group box protein-1, matrix metalloproteinases, and vitamin D in keloids and hypertrophic scars. Plast Reconstr Surg Glob Open. 2015;3(6):e425.

35. Huang C, Ogawa R. The link between hypertension and pathological scarring: does hypertension cause or promote keloid and hypertrophic scar pathogenesis? Wound Repair Regen. 2014;22(4):462–6.

36. Park TH, et al. Outcomes of surgical excision with pressure therapy using magnets and identification of risk factors for recurrent keloids. Plast Reconstr Surg. 2011;128(2):431–9.

37. Luo S, et al. Abnormal balance between proliferation and apoptotic cell death in fibroblasts derived from keloid lesions. Plast Reconstr Surg. 2001;107(1):87–96.

38. Kelly AP. Pseudofolliculitis barbae and acne keloidalis nuchae. Dermatol Clin. 2003;21 (4):645–53.

39. Madu P, Kundu RV. Follicular and scarring disorders in skin of color: presentation and management. Am J Clin Dermatol. 2014;15(4):307–21.

40. Sperling LC, et al. Acne keloidalis is a form of primary scarring alopecia. Arch Dermatol. 2000;136(4):479–84.

41. Goette DK, Berger TG. Acne keloidalis nuchae. A transepithelial elimination disorder. Int J Dermatol. 1987;26(7):442–4.

42. Burkhart CG, Burkhart CN. Acne keloidalis is lichen simplex chronicus with fibrotic keloidal scarring. J Am Acad Dermatol. 1998;39(4 Pt 1):661.

43. George AO, et al. Clinical, biochemical and morphologic features of acne keloidalis in a black population. Int J Dermatol. 1993;32(10):714–6.

44. Kligman AM, Strauss JS. Pseudofolliculitis of the beard. AMA Arch Derm. 1956;74 (5):533–42.

45. Nuovo J, Sweha A. Keloid formation from levonorgestrel implant (Norplant System) insertion. J Am Board Fam Pract. 1994;7(2):152–4.

46. Lane JE, Waller JL, Davis LS. Relationship between age of ear piercing and keloid formation. Pediatrics. 2005;115(5):1312–4.

47. De Sousa RF, et al. Efficacy of triple therapy in auricular keloids. J Cutan Aesthet Surg. 2014;7(2):98–102.

48. Stahl S, et al. Treatment of earlobe keloids by extralesional excision combined with preoperative and postoperative "sandwich" radiotherapy. Plast Reconstr Surg. 2010;125 (1):135–41.

49. Reno F, et al. In vitro mechanical compression induces apoptosis and regulates cytokines release in hypertrophic scars. Wound Repair Regen. 2003;11(5):331–6.

50. Tejiram S, et al. Compression therapy affects collagen type balance in hypertrophic scar. J Surg Res. 2016;201(2):299–305.

51. Li-Tsang CW, et al. A histological study on the effect of pressure therapy on the activities of myofibroblasts and keratinocytes in hypertrophic scar tissues after burn. Burns. 2015;41 (5):1008–16.

52. Yagmur C, et al. Mechanical receptor-related mechanisms in scar management: a review and hypothesis. Plast Reconstr Surg. 2010;126(2):426–34.

53. Anzarut A, et al. The effectiveness of pressure garment therapy for the prevention of abnormal scarring after burn injury: a meta-analysis. J Plast Reconstr Aesthet Surg. 2009;62 (1):77–84.
54. Giele H, et al. Anatomical variations in pressures generated by pressure garments. Plast Reconstr Surg 1998;101(2):399–406; discussion 407.
55. Naismith RS. Hypertrophic scar therapy: pressure-induced remodelling and its determinants. Glasgow: University of Strathclyde; 1980.
56. Engrav LH, et al. 12-Year within-wound study of the effectiveness of custom pressure garment therapy. Burns. 2010;36(7):975–83.
57. Bleasdale B, et al. The use of silicone adhesives for scar reduction. Adv Wound Care (New Rochelle). 2015;4(7):422–30.
58. Kuhn MA, et al. Silicone sheeting decreases fibroblast activity and downregulates TGFbeta2 in hypertrophic scar model. Int J Surg Investig. 2001;2(6):467–74.
59. Mustoe TA. Evolution of silicone therapy and mechanism of action in scar management. Aesthetic Plast Surg. 2008;32(1):82–92.
60. Choi J, et al. Regulation of transforming growth factor beta1, platelet-derived growth factor, and basic fibroblast growth factor by silicone gel sheeting in early-stage scarring. Arch Plast Surg. 2015;42(1):20–7.
61. Borgognoni L. Biological effects of silicone gel sheeting. Wound Repair Regen. 2002;10 (2):118–21.
62. Nickoloff BJ, Naidu Y. Perturbation of epidermal barrier function correlates with initiation of cytokine cascade in human skin. J Am Acad Dermatol. 1994;30(4):535–46.
63. O'Shaughnessy KD, et al. Homeostasis of the epidermal barrier layer: a theory of how occlusion reduces hypertrophic scarring. Wound Repair Regen. 2009;17(5):700–8.
64. Berman B, Flores F. Comparison of a silicone gel-filled cushion and silicon gel sheeting for the treatment of hypertrophic or keloid scars. Dermatol Surg. 1999;25(6):484–6.
65. de Oliveira GV, et al. Silicone versus nonsilicone gel dressings: a controlled trial. Dermatol Surg. 2001;27(8):721–6.
66. Fulton JE Jr. Silicone gel sheeting for the prevention and management of evolving hypertrophic and keloid scars. Dermatol Surg. 1995;21(11):947–51.
67. O'Brien L, Jones J. Daniel Silicone gel sheeting for preventing and treating hypertrophic and keloid scars. Cochrane Database Syst Rev. 2013;. doi:10.1002/14651858.CD003826.pub3.
68. Chan KY, et al. A randomized, placebo-controlled, double-blind, prospective clinical trial of silicone gel in prevention of hypertrophic scar development in median sternotomy wound. Plast Reconstr Surg. 2005;116(4):1013–20; discussion 1021–2.
69. van der Wal MB, et al. Topical silicone gel versus placebo in promoting the maturation of burn scars: a randomized controlled trial. Plast Reconstr Surg. 2010;126(2):524–31.
70. Chernoff WG, Cramer H, Su-Huang S. The efficacy of topical silicone gel elastomers in the treatment of hypertrophic scars, keloid scars, and post-laser exfoliation erythema. Aesthetic Plast Surg. 2007;31(5):495–500.
71. Signorini M, Clementoni MT. Clinical evaluation of a new self-drying silicone gel in the treatment of scars: a preliminary report. Aesthetic Plast Surg. 2007;31(2):183–7.
72. Ji J, et al. Ionizing irradiation inhibits keloid fibroblast cell proliferation and induces premature cellular senescence. J Dermatol. 2015;42(1):56–63.
73. Botwood N, Lewanski C, Lowdell C. The risks of treating keloids with radiotherapy. Br J Radiol. 1999;72(864):1222–4.
74. Kuribayashi S, et al. Post-keloidectomy irradiation using high-dose-rate superficial brachytherapy. J Radiat Res. 2011;52(3):365–8.
75. Jiang P, et al. Perioperative interstitial high-dose-rate brachytherapy for the treatment of recurrent keloids: feasibility and early results. Int J Radiat Oncol Biol Phys. 2016;94(3):532–6.
76. van Leeuwen MC, et al. Surgical excision with adjuvant irradiation for treatment of keloid scars: a systematic review. Plast Reconstr Surg Glob Open. 2015;3(7):e440.

77. Duan Q, et al. Postoperative brachytherapy and electron beam irradiation for keloids: a single institution retrospective analysis. Mol Clin Oncol. 2015;3(3):550–4.
78. Emad M, et al. Surgical excision and immediate postoperative radiotherapy versus cryotherapy and intralesional steroids in the management of keloids: a prospective clinical trial. Med Princ Pract. 2010;19(5):402–5.
79. Ogawa R, et al. Is radiation therapy for keloids acceptable? The risk of radiation-induced carcinogenesis. Plast Reconstr Surg. 2009;124(4):1196–201.
80. Shen J, et al. Hypofractionated electron-beam radiation therapy for keloids: retrospective study of 568 cases with 834 lesions. J Radiat Res. 2015;56(5):811–7.
81. van Leeuwen MC, et al. High-dose-rate brachytherapy for the treatment of recalcitrant keloids: a unique, effective treatment protocol. Plast Reconstr Surg. 2014;134(3):527–34.
82. McKeown SR, et al. Radiotherapy for benign disease; assessing the risk of radiation-induced cancer following exposure to intermediate dose radiation. Br J Radiol. 1056;2015 (88):20150405.
83. Sakamoto T, et al. Dose-response relationship and dose optimization in radiotherapy of postoperative keloids. Radiother Oncol. 2009;91(2):271–6.
84. Tziotzios C, Profyris C, Sterling J. Cutaneous scarring: pathophysiology, molecular mechanisms, and scar reduction therapeutics Part II. Strategies to reduce scar formation after dermatologic procedures. J Am Acad Dermatol. 2012;66(1):13–24; quiz 25–6.
85. Huang L, et al. A study of the combination of triamcinolone and 5-fluorouracil in modulating keloid fibroblasts in vitro. J Plast Reconstr Aesthet Surg. 2013;66(9):e251–9.
86. Heppt MV, et al. Current strategies in the treatment of scars and keloids. Facial Plast Surg. 2015;31(4):386–95.
87. Cavalie M, et al. Treatment of keloids with laser-assisted topical steroid delivery: a retrospective study of 23 cases. Dermatol Ther. 2015;28(2):74–8.
88. Fredman R, Tenenhaus M. Cushing's syndrome after intralesional triamcinolone acetonide: a systematic review of the literature and multinational survey. Burns. 2013;39(4):549–57.
89. Bashir MM, et al. Comparison of single intra operative versus an intra operative and two post operative injections of the triamcinolone after wedge excision of keloids of helix. J Pak Med Assoc. 2015;65(7):737–41.
90. Berman B, Flores F. Recurrence rates of excised keloids treated with postoperative triamcinolone acetonide injections or interferon alfa-2b injections. J Am Acad Dermatol. 1997;37(5 Pt 1):755–7.
91. Lawrence WT. In search of the optimal treatment of keloids: report of a series and a review of the literature. Ann Plast Surg. 1991;27(2):164–78.
92. Sclafani AP, et al. Prevention of earlobe keloid recurrence with postoperative corticosteroid injections versus radiation therapy: a randomized, prospective study and review of the literature. Dermatol Surg. 1996;22(6):569–74.
93. Tan KT, et al. The influence of surgical excision margins on keloid prognosis. Ann Plast Surg. 2010;64(1):55–8.
94. Lee Y, et al. A new surgical treatment of keloid: keloid core excision. Ann Plast Surg. 2001;46(2):135–40.
95. Weshahy AH, Abdel Hay R. Intralesional cryosurgery and intralesional steroid injection: a good combination therapy for treatment of keloids and hypertrophic scars. Dermatol Ther. 2012;25(3):273–6.
96. Dalkowski A, et al. Cryotherapy modifies synthetic activity and differentiation of keloidal fibroblasts in vitro. Exp Dermatol. 2003;12(5):673–81.
97. Har-Shai Y, Amar M, Sabo E. Intralesional cryotherapy for enhancing the involution of hypertrophic scars and keloids. Plast Reconstr Surg. 2003;111(6):1841–52.
98. van Leeuwen MC, et al. A new argon gas-based device for the treatment of keloid scars with the use of intralesional cryotherapy. J Plast Reconstr Aesthet Surg. 2014;67(12):1703–10.
99. van Leeuwen MC, et al. Intralesional cryotherapy for treatment of keloid scars: a prospective study. Plast Reconstr Surg. 2015;135(2):580–9.

144. Zhibo X, Miaobo Z. Intralesional botulinum toxin type A injection as a new treatment measure for keloids. Plast Reconstr Surg. 2009;124(5):275e–7e.
145. Shaarawy E, Hegazy RA, Abdel Hay RM. Intralesional botulinum toxin type A equally effective and better tolerated than intralesional steroid in the treatment of keloids: a randomized controlled trial. J Cosmet Dermatol. 2015;14(2):161–6.

Chapter 16
Skin Cancer

Ali Al-Haseni and Debjani Sahni

Skin cancer is the most common malignancy in the United States, though the actual incidence is difficult to estimate as the most common form, non-melanoma skin cancer (NMSC), is not tracked by central cancer registries. In addition, interpretation of data comparing skin cancer between races is challenging, as there is limited data in people of color (POC) due to a lack of large population-based studies. Skin cancers are more prevalent in Caucasians than POC, accounting for approximately 40% of all neoplasms in whites, 5% in Hispanics, 4% in Asians, and 2% in blacks. The low incidence of skin cancer in POC has been attributed for the most part to their increased epidermal melanin. The differences in color observed in darker individuals is not the result of higher number of melanocytes, but rather the increased melanocyte activity. Melanocytes in darker skin are larger and produce more melanin and melanosomes, and they are dispersed evenly between keratinocytes rather than as aggregates, when compared to white skin [1]. The epidermis of dark skin can thus absorb and scatter more light energy than white skin, providing inherent photoprotection, and filtering at least twice as much ultraviolet radiation (UVR) compared to the epidermis of Caucasians [2]. It is noteworthy that POC encompass a diverse group of individuals displaying a spectrum of skin pigmentation and possessing a wide range of phototypes. It is therefore conceivable that POC may show variation in etiopathogenesis, clinical presentation, and prognosis of skin cancers among them. Despite the lower incidence of skin cancer in POC compared to whites, the morbidity and mortality from skin cancer in the former is disproportionately high [3, 4]. This will have increasing significance to public health concerns given the evolving demographics in the US, where it is

A. Al-Haseni · D. Sahni (✉)
Department of Dermatology, Boston University Medical Center,
609 Albany St, Boston MA 02120, USA
e-mail: debjani.sahni@bmc.org

A. Al-Haseni
e-mail: Ali.Al-Haseni@bmc.org

© Springer International Publishing AG 2017
N.A. Vashi and H.I. Maibach (eds.), *Dermatoanthropology of Ethnic Skin and Hair*, DOI 10.1007/978-3-319-53961-4_16

estimated that an international immigrant arrives in the US every 28 s [5]. By the year 2050, it is predicted that POC will represent approximately 50% of the US population, compared to 38% in 2014 [3, 6, 7]. It is therefore critically important that physicians become familiar with the varied presentation and characteristics of skin cancer within this heterogeneous group, so enabling them to manage these patients appropriately and be able to provide the necessary photoprotection and skin surveillance recommendations.

Non-melanoma Skin Cancer (NMSC)

NMSC encompasses both squamous cell carcinoma (SCC) and basal cell carcinoma (BCC). Epidemiologic studies suggest that individuals of all races with NMSCs are at an increased risk of developing a second primary malignancy. This appears to be more significant in POC as demonstrated in the Women's Health Initiative Observational Study, where women with a history of NMSC were 2.3 times more likely to develop a second primary malignancy with breast cancer being the most common. When subgroup analysis was done in the same study within racial groups, it demonstrated a higher likelihood of developing a second malignancy in POC with NMSC versus those without, with odds ratios of: 7.46 in blacks, 5.64 in Asian/Pacific Islanders, 4.51 in American Indians, 3.67 in Hispanics, and 2.27 in white [8]. The increased risk of a second malignancy has been attributed to UVR-induced suppression of cell-mediated immunity and UVR-induced P53 mutations [3]. The greater risk in POC may be explained by subtle differences in immunology, for example, in comparison to whites, blacks have a higher concentration of total skin urocanic acid, a photoimmune-suppressive receptor. This might explain why blacks have more photoimmune suppression, which may contribute to the greater risk of developing a second malignancy [9, 10].

Squamous Cell Carcinoma

SCC is the second most common skin cancer in Caucasians representing 15–25% of cutaneous neoplasms. In blacks and Asian Indians, however, SCC is the most common cutaneous malignancy, comprising 30–65% of skin cancers respectively in both races [3]. Despite this, the actual incidence of SCC in blacks is still lower than in whites and is reported to be ~3.4 per 100,000 versus ~125 per 100,000 in whites [11]. Unlike blacks and Asian Indians, but comparable to Caucasians, SCC ranks as the second most common skin cancer in Japanese, Chinese, and Hispanics [3, 12–14]. Although the incidence of SCC in POC is low, it tends to present with more advanced stage and in different anatomical sites from that seen in whites, posing a diagnostic and therapeutic challenge.

Pathogenesis

It is known that cumulative long-term ultraviolet light exposure and sunburns during childhood increase the risk of SCC and actinic keratoses (AKs) in Caucasians. This is demonstrated in studies showing the higher incidence of NMSCs in individuals who were born in countries with high UVR, versus the lower incidence in individuals with similar genetic background who migrated from countries with low to high UVR later in life [15, 16]. As mentioned earlier, dark skinned individuals have better inherent photoprotection than whites. It must however be emphasized that this does not completely prevent UV related damage in blacks, as epidermal changes (atypia and atrophy) and dermal collagen and elastin damage are evident in dark skinned individuals with history of sun exposure [17, 18].

To date, the information about SCC in ethnic groups is limited due to inconsistent reporting of NMSCs in tumor registries and most of the data focusing on blacks [3, 4, 6]. Therefore, the remainder of this section on SCC will concentrate on the black population.

Although a prior US study showed increasing incidence of NMSCs in blacks with decreasing latitudes [19], the role of UVR in the development of SCC in blacks is likely to be less important than in whites, as blacks typically develop SCC in non-sun-exposed areas [13, 20–23]. In addition, AKs which represent the most common precursor to SCC in sun-exposed skin, are very rare in blacks [24]. When AKs do occur, they tend to present in individuals with fairer complexion [11]. Risk factors for the development of SCC in blacks are outlined below with the first two being the most important:

(1) *Chronic scarring*: this is present in 20–40% of cases of SCC in blacks and includes previous burns, past physical or thermal trauma, and areas of prior radiation treatment [3, 20, 21, 23, 25, 26].
(2) *Chronic inflammation*: most notably in chronic ulcers, but also in discoid lupus erythematosus, granuloma annulare, hidradenitis suppurativa, osteomyelitis, and areas of chronic skin infections such as lupus vulgaris, leprosy, and lymphogranuloma venereum [20, 21, 25–27].
(3) *UVR:* this is felt to be the major risk factor for lesions that less commonly develop on the head and neck region.
(4) *Other risk factors* include: albinism, vitiligo, immunosuppression, epidermodysplasia verruciformis (EDV), human papilloma virus (HPV) infection, smegma of the uncircumcised penis, and exposure to carcinogenic chemicals like arsenic and tar [3, 6, 20, 25, 26, 28].

It should be noted however that given the limited data about these risk factors taken from isolated reports and small case series, it is difficult to draw firm conclusions about them.

Clinical Presentation

In whites, SCC typically presents as an erythematous scaly plaque. In blacks, however, it commonly manifests as a non-healing ulcer or indurated nodule developing in or adjacent to the area of preexisting disease such as a chronic leg ulcer or hidradenitis suppurativa (Fig. 16.1). The areas of predilection for SCC is also quite different in blacks, as SCCs tend to develop more commonly on non-sun-exposed sites of the lower limbs and the anogenital region, although lesions on the head and neck area do also occur. SCC of the nail bed is another location that is uncommon in whites but appears to be relatively common in blacks [11, 20, 26, 29, 30]. Squamous cell carcinoma in situ (SCCis) is less common in blacks, and like SCC, typically develop in non-sun-exposed areas, especially the

Fig. 16.1 Squamous cell carcinoma (SCC) arising within a chronic burn scar on the lower leg. Ulcerated vegitating tumor with thick yellow crust

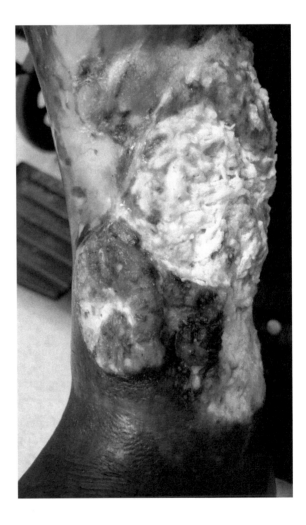

lower limbs. They are frequently pigmented, which can pose a diagnostic challenge due to its resemblance to melanoma. Most studies show that SCCis affects individuals later in life, after the 6th decade, with males being affected more commonly than females. One study suggested arsenic as an important risk factor as 3 of 7 patients with SCCis had a history of exposure to this [28]. The risk of progressing to invasive SCC is estimated to be between 3 and 11% [3, 20, 25, 28, 31].

In black individuals, it is important to note the more aggressive behavior of SCCs and their increased tendency to metastasize in areas of chronic scarring—20–40% risk of metastasis compared to 1–4% of SCCs in sun-exposed sites [3]. In addition, several studies report an increased mortality from SCC in blacks compared to whites [20, 21, 23, 32], with the highest mortality being observed in perianal SCC [21]. The high mortality and morbidity seen in blacks has been attributed to biologically more aggressive tumors, an advanced stage at diagnosis, delays in seeking medical attention due to a combination of lower socioeconomic status and education level, and association with other comorbidities. Given the atypical clinical presentation together with increased morbidity and mortality in this population, a high index of suspicion and low threshold for biopsy are required, with emphasis on checking non-sun-exposed areas when performing a skin exam.

Treatment

An aggressive approach is recommended for SCC in blacks, as tumors tend to carry a worse prognosis than in Caucasians [23]. Factors such as histological type, tumor size, location, primary versus recurrent or metastatic, patient's general health, patient's preference, and cost all play a role in determining treatment. Therapeutic options include surgical excision, Mohs micrographic surgery, electrodessication, and curettage (ED&C), cryosurgery, topical chemotherapy/immunotherapy, photodynamic therapy (PDT), radiation, conventional chemotherapy, and biologic agents such as epidermal growth factor receptor inhibitors (EGFRi) e.g. cetuximab [23, 31, 33, 34].

Basal Cell Carcinoma

BCC is the most common skin cancer among Caucasians, Hispanics, and Asians (excluding Asian Indians) [3, 6, 25, 35]. It can be locally destructive if left untreated, yet it has a very low metastatic potential. Hispanics are six times more likely to have BCC than SCC, and they are more likely to have multiple rather than solitary BCC [6]. On the other hand, BCC is the second most common skin cancer in blacks and Asian Indians [3, 25]. The incidence of BCC per 100,000 population in different races is estimated to be 1–2 in blacks, 5.8–6.4 in Chinese, 15–16.5 in

Japanese, 50–91 in Southeastern Arizona Hispanics, 113–171 in New Mexican Hispanics, and 212–250 in whites.

Pathogenesis

The most important risk factor for BCC is chronic UV exposure regardless of race or skin color, with the vast majority (>70%) of BCCs occurring in older individuals on sun-exposed skin in all races [3, 6, 20]. This highlights the importance of emphasizing sun protection in POC. The adverse effect of UVR is more significant in people with lighter skin with lower inherent photoprotection, as evidenced by the incidence of BCC directly correlating with the degree of skin pigmentation, being most common in Caucasians, and least common in African blacks [3, 6, 25] (BCC represents 65–75% of skin cancer in Caucasians, 20–30% in Asian Indians, 12–35% in African Americans blacks, and 2–8% in African blacks) [3]. In addition, BCC occurs more commonly in lighter complexioned blacks compared to darker blacks [20]. In all races, BCC can also occur on non-sun-exposed sites. There is conflicting data as to whether the incidence of BCC in sun-exposed rather than non-sun-exposed sites is the same in Caucasians and blacks [20], versus a higher incidence of BCC in non-sun-exposed sites in blacks compared to Caucasians [36]. Interestingly, BCCs rarely occur on the dorsal hands and forearms, two areas that are heavily sun damaged [37].

UVR causes activating mutations in the Sonic Hedgehog (SHH) pathway, which is critical in embryonic development, cellular proliferation and differentiation, and cell fate. During adult life, this pathway is largely silenced in all cells except for hair follicles and sebaceous glands, where it functions in maintaining stem cells [38]. The SHH pathway is activated in BCCs, mostly by inactivating mutations in Patched (PTCH) or rarely due to activating mutations in Smoothened (SMO) genes. Basal cell nevus syndrome (BCNS), also called Gorlin syndrome, is an autosomal dominant condition caused by a mutation in the human PTCH gene, resulting in the development of multiple BCCs at a young age. Other features of BCNS include odontogenic keratocysts of the jaw, palmoplantar pits, calcification of the falx cerebri, and various skeletal anomalies with affected individuals being prone to various neoplasms including medulloblastomas, cardiac fibromas, bilateral ovarian fibromas, and meningiomas [39, 40]. BCNS is rare in POC contributing to only 5% cases [41], and when it occurs in POC, individuals develop fewer BCCs and at a later age compared to Caucasians. An example is the case of a black man with Gorlin syndrome, who presented with his first BCC at the age of 77 [39, 42]. This emphasizes the importance of UVR in the pathogenesis of BCC and the UV protective nature of dark skin [43].

Other risk factors for the development of BCCs in POC include radiation and scars. The risk of developing BCC in previously irradiated skin is higher in Caucasians than in blacks [44], and in the case of BCC arising in scars, this typically occurs in sun-exposed older individuals [45]. Both observations suggest a synergistic effect of UVR with either trauma or radiation.

Clinical Presentation

In whites, BCCs clinically present as asymptomatic, translucent, erythematous to skin colored papules with a rolled pearly border and central ulceration or telangiectasia. In POC, the darker skin can make it difficult to appreciate the rolled pearly border and telangiectasia explaining why these lesions may be mistaken for seborrheic keratoses, melanocytic nevi, or malignant melanoma. Whereas pigmentation occurs in only 5% of BCCs in Caucasians, it occurs in over 50% of BCCs in POC, and they are characteristically described as a "black pearly" papule (Fig. 16.2) [20, 36, 45–51]. Other clinical presentations include nodules, plaques, non-healing ulcers, or if left untreated, indurated or pedunculated masses [46, 47, 52]. BCCs rarely metastasize in whites, and the same is true in POC with only a handful of cases reported in the literature [3, 36, 53]. Unlike SCCs, BCCs in blacks are not associated with increased morbidity in comparison to whites [20, 25].

Pathology

The histological features of BCCs in POC are similar to those in whites. Nodular BCC is the most common histologic type in whites, blacks, and Asians [3]. Adenoid BCC is relatively more common in blacks and Asians, while morpheaform BCC appears less frequently in blacks in comparison to whites [3]. Furthermore, compared with whites, BCCs in blacks tend to stain positive with carcinoembryonic

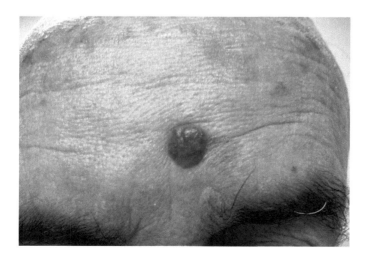

Fig. 16.2 Pigmented basal cell carcinoma (BCC) on central forehead. Single pearly nodule with pigmentation and mild erosion

antigen in a higher percentage of patients, indicating a tendency towards follicular, eccrine, or sebaceous differentiation [54].

Treatment

The management of BCCs in POC is no different to that in whites. Treatment options include surgical excision, Mohs surgery, cryotherapy, ED&C, topical chemotherapy, PDT, topical imiquimod, laser surgery, and radiotherapy. Although the incidence of metastatic BCC is very low, being approximately 0.0028%, these cases carry a poor prognosis, with mean survival ranging between 8 months and 3.6 years [33, 35, 54, 55]. Advancement in understanding the pathogenesis of BCC has led to the development of targeted therapies that inhibit SMO (e.g., vismodegib and sonidegib) which are approved for the treatment of metastatic BCC, locally advanced BCC that have recurred after surgery, or in patients who are not candidates for surgery or radiation therapy [56, 57].

Melanoma

Melanoma is the most lethel type of skin cancer in all races, with an estimated 76,380 new cases and 10,130 deaths in 2016 [4, 58]. The incidence of melanoma has been increasing at a rate of 3–7% per year in the past 30 years in Caucasians and Hispanics, but it is relatively stable in Asians and blacks. Currently, melanoma is the 3rd most common type of skin cancer in all ethnicities, and the 6th most common type of cancer in the US [3, 58]. Recent data predicts the lifetime probability of developing melanoma in the general population is 3% for males and 1.9% for females [58]. Melanoma incidence varies among different races, with an inverse relationship between melanoma incidence and degree of skin pigmentation, so that the white to black ratio in melanoma incidence is 16:1. The number of melanoma cases among Hispanics is midway between that of whites and blacks, a finding that reflects their intermediate skin pigmentation [3, 59–61]. Melanoma incidence is similar between Asians and blacks [60], and it is approximately twice as common in Japanese compared to the other Asian races occurring more frequently in women than in males [14]. According to the United States National Cancer Institute Surveillance, Epidemiology, and End Results (SEER) data, the age-adjusted melanoma incidences per 100,000 persons by different ethnic groups and sex from 2008 to 2012 were 38.2 in white non-Hispanic males, 24.2 in white non-Hispanic females, 4.8 in Hispanic males, 4.5 in Hispanic females, 1.6 in Asian males, 1.1 in Asian females, 1.2 in black males, and 1.0 in black females [62].

Pathogenesis and Risk Factors

Melanoma is a multifactorial tumor that develops in genetically predisposed individuals when exposed to certain environmental factors. Genetic factors predisposing to melanoma are evident phenotypically in the form of inability to tan, having red/ blond hair, blue eyes, fair skin, large number of melanocytic nevi, presence of atypical/ dysplastic nevi, personal or family history of melanoma, and various genetic disorders resulting in the inability to repair DNA defects. Various genetic mutations have been described in the pathogenesis of melanoma including gain-of-function oncogenic mutations (BRAF, NRAS, KIT, or GNAQ/GNA11) and loss-of-function tumor suppressor gene mutations (CDKN2A, PTEN, NF1, or BAP1). Melanomas in non-severely sun-damaged skin often harbor BRAF or NRAS mutations, while melanomas arising on severely sun-damaged skin, as well as acral and mucosal melanomas, commonly carry a mutation in KIT gene as well as BRAF and NRAS. Environmental factors associated with increased risk of melanoma appear to differ in whites compared to POC. DNA damage caused by UVR specifically from intermittent heavy sun exposure, blistering childhood sunburns, history of indoor tanning, or large cumulative UVR doses from chronic sun exposure (outdoor workers) play a major role in whites [4, 59, 63–67]. Other environmental risk factors include immunosuppression, PUVA treatment, and residence in equatorial latitudes [59, 63–66, 68]. The main etiologic factor for the development of melanoma in POC is yet to be defined, and given that it tends to occur most commonly on acral skin in POC, suggests that UVR is not as important in the pathogenesis of melanoma in this group as it is in Caucasians. A study using SEER data looking at the relationship between age-adjusted melanoma incidence rates and the UV index or latitude within racial and ethnic groups concluded there was no evidence to support the association of UV exposure and melanoma incidence in black or Hispanic populations [69]. Nevertheless, there are reports of increased risk of melanoma in black patients with albinism or those with prior radiation treatment. In addition, another study looking at 6 US state cancer registries found that for both Hispanics and blacks, the incidence of melanoma was positively associated with the UV index and negatively associated with the latitude of residency. A statistically significant correlation between melanoma and the UV index ($R = 0.93$; $P = 0.01$) and latitude ($R = -0.80$; $P = 0.05$) was observed in black males. The authors concluded that exposure to solar radiation appears to play a role in the development of melanoma in both Hispanics and blacks [59]. These observations suggest a potential though perhaps less significant role for UVR in the pathogenesis of melanoma in POC [14, 60, 61, 70–78]. Other risk factors implicated in POC include burn scars, immunosuppression, and preexisting pigmented lesions (especially on acral and mucosal regions) [79–81].

Clinical Presentation

Clinically, melanoma in POC presents similarly to Caucasians, most commonly appearing as an asymmetric, rapidly spreading, dark brown-black macule or patch with irregular borders and various shades of pigmentation. Melanoma in Hispanics commonly has the appearance of flecked, gray-white areas; while papillomatous, verrucous, or hyperkeratotic lesions in blacks have been reported [11]. A significant proportion of acral lentiginous melanoma (ALM) present with unusually large diameters >3 cm, often with signs of advanced local disease, such as pain, bleeding, and ulceration.

Melanoma varies in its clinical and pathological features among the different ethnicities. In Caucasians, melanomas most commonly present on intermittently sun-exposed areas such as the trunk in males and legs in females, with superficial spreading melanoma (SSM) being the most common histological variant and ALM being the least common [82]. SSM is also the most commonly encountered melanoma in Hispanics, though the incidence of ALM is greater than in Caucasians [3, 4]. In contrast, Asians and blacks are more likely to develop melanomas on non-sun-exposed areas of acral skin, with ALM being the most common histological variant in both groups. Seventy five percent of melanomas in POC are acral tumors, in comparison to only 5% of melanomas in whites. The plantar foot is the most common site (Fig. 16.3) (with plantar:palmar ratio of 17:1), and the ratio of palmoplantar:subungual lesions is 4:1. In addition, in 25–50% of cases, the tumor arises within a preexisting pigmented lesion [11, 61, 72, 74, 75, 81, 83]. Given the higher incidence of melanoma particularly on the pressure bearing areas of the heel and the ball of the foot, trauma has been postulated to be a predisposing factor in acral melanomas [79, 84, 85]. Another possible explanation for the increased risk of acral melanomas in POC is based on the distribution of melanocytic nevi. POC tend to have a lower density of melanocytic nevi and lower incidence of melanoma compared to Caucasians, in whom the melanoma risk is higher and the number of melanocytic nevi is directly proportional to the risk of developing melanoma [4]. However, the risk of developing melanoma in a specific body region is more closely related to the number of melanocytic nevi at that site, rather than the total number of nevi in the whole body [86, 87]. This may explain the high prevalence of acral melanomas in blacks, who tend to have melanocytic nevi predominantly on acral locations [80, 88]. Interestingly, one study showed that both blacks and whites have similar incidences of plantar melanomas (1.7 and 2 per million per year for blacks and whites, respectively), and attributed the reported predominance of plantar lesions in blacks to the low overall incidence of melanomas at other sites, rather than a true increased incidence of plantar melanomas [84]. Benign-appearing acral lesions in POC should be examined carefully, as 39% of acral melanomas have been shown to imitate the appearance of benign hyperkeratotic dermatoses (verrucae, calluses, or dermatophyte infections) in one case series [11]. Subungual melanomas are most commonly seen on the thumb or the first toe and represent 15–20% of melanomas in blacks, 10–31% in Asians, 2.5% in Hispanics, and 0.31% in

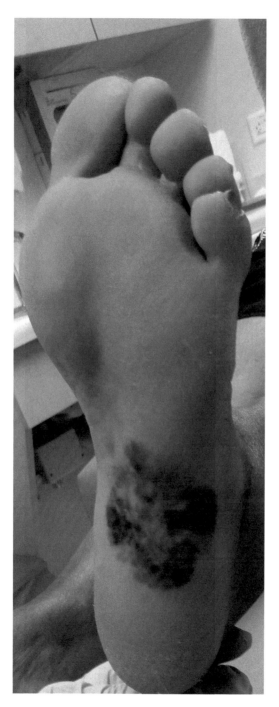

Fig. 16.3 Acral lentiginous melanoma (ALM) on the plantar surface of the foot. Irregularly shaped large hyperpigmented patch with variation in color

Fig. 16.4 Subungual melanoma of the middle finger. Single pigmented band showing evidence of Hutchinson's sign and nail dystrophy

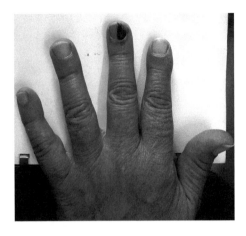

whites. Although the vast majority of blacks aged over 50 years have longitudinal melanonychia, subungual melanoma should be suspected when a pigmented band on the nail is wider than 3 mm, pigment extends to the proximal nail fold (Hutchinson sign), there is pigment variation, there is a rapid change in size, the onset is after mid-adulthood, and/or there is presence of a solitary lesion (Fig. 16.4). Further progression may cause nail damage, revealing a friable hemorrhagic mass [4, 11, 89]. The most common mimickers of subungual melanoma are hematoma and onychomycosis [11]. Another common location for the development of melanoma in POC, though uncommon in whites, is mucous membrane sites, with approximately two thirds of these tumors developing from preexisting oral melanosis [3, 4, 75, 90]. The typical body regions affected by melanoma in Hispanics seem to vary, with some studies suggesting it is similar to Caucasians, while others suggest similarities to blacks and Asians. The discordance between the studies may be explained by the varying degree of pigmentation in Hispanic people, with lighter skinned Hispanics following a more Caucasian distribution and darker skinned Hispanics following a black/Asian distribution [60, 61, 91].

Treatment and Prognosis

The standard treatment for melanoma involves wide local excision with 0.5–2 cms margins, dependent on Breslow thickness, and a sentinel lymph node biopsy (SLNB). The latter is offered based on histopathological criteria that include Breslow thickness and presence/ absence of ulceration. Early stage melanoma has a favorable prognosis with 5-year survival over 95%, whereas metastatic melanoma has a dismal prognosis. For decades, advanced melanoma had been refractory to conventional chemotherapy agents that had low response rates with no demonstrable overall survival benefit. The roadmap for melanoma therapy changed drastically from 2011 onwards following the discovery of novel targets after years of researching the molecular biology and immunology of melanoma. Approved therapeutic options for metastatic melanoma now include a number of biological modalities that include: *immunotherapeutic agents*: including interleukin-2 (IL-2), inhibitors of key immune checkpoint molecules, such as cytotoxic T-lymphocyte (CTLA-4) and programmed cell death protein 1 (PD-1) and oncolytic viral therapy; *targeted therapy agents*: these target and inhibit a number of mutated oncogenes with constitutive kinase activity in the mitogen activated protein kinase (MAPK) pathway. These oncogenes play a key role in melanomagenesis and include BRAF and MEK [92].

Between 1973 and 1992, mortality from melanoma increased by 34.1%, the third highest increase of all cancers [72]. However, death rates have been largely stable from 2004 to 2013 [62]. Advanced stage melanoma is seen more commonly in POC (52% in blacks and 26% in Hispanics), in comparison to whites (16%) [4, 21, 72, 76, 81, 83, 93–96]. Multiple studies have demonstrated that melanomas in POC are more likely to be thicker [75, 89, 97, 98], present with ulceration [72, 99], advanced stage 3 or 4 disease [70, 72, 75, 77, 83, 89, 94, 96, 97, 100–102] or metastatic disease [60, 89, 94, 103], all contributing to a worse prognosis in this group and survival rate. ALM is also more common in POC and typically carries a worse prognosis given its propensity for deeper invasion at presentation.

This lower survival in POC has been associated with the frequent presence of thick primary lesions at the time of diagnosis attributed to delay in seeking medical attention. There are many possible reasons that could contribute to the delay in diagnosis of melanoma in POC. These include difficulty in accessing medical care and preventative screening; a misconception that certain races do not develop skin cancer, leading to a low level of awareness and a lack of public and physician education; and finally the predominance of lesions in unexpected sites, such as the palms, soles, subungual areas, and mucosal regions. These areas of the body are rarely emphasized in skin screening programs, and there may be a tendency to overlook dark lesions in dark skinned individuals, especially with the ubiquity of hyperpigmented macules of the palms and soles and normal longitudinal melanonychia in blacks. Thus, patients and physicians do not typically suspect melanomas in these areas. The identification of high-risk body areas in POC and suspicious signs in longitudinal melanonychia are of extreme importance to prevent delays in diagnosis. Although public awareness campaigns focusing on risk factors, such as red hair, susceptibility to burn, and inability to tan, are of extreme importance for the health of the majority of the population, they may unintentionally suggest that melanoma is not a health concern in POC. All these combined factors lead to delay in diagnosis and could contribute to subsequent increased mortality [3, 76] Of note, some studies have found that blacks with early stage melanoma (stage 1 and 2) have a shorter survival time than whites with the equivalent stages [70, 72, 83]. In addition, other studies have found higher rates of death in blacks in comparison to whites even after adjusting for sex, age, stage, histology, anatomic site, socioeconomic status, and treatment [4, 104]. This suggests the lower survival from melanoma may be due to biologically more aggressive tumors, which are therefore likely to present at an advanced stage.

Improving the survival of melanoma patients is a goal that will only be achieved by collaborative efforts between both patients and care providers. Patients should be encouraged to perform self-skin examinations, with special attention to high-risk areas as suggested by their skin types. Physicians should keep a high index of suspicion for melanoma regardless of a patient's ethnic background. This will facilitate earlier diagnosis of melanoma in all races and potentially improve survival. In addition, public education programs for skin cancer and melanoma should be directed to all ethnic groups in addition to high-risk individuals.

Cutaneous Lymphoma

Cutaneous lymphoma is an umbrella term used to describe a heterogeneous group of non-Hodgkin lymphomas (NHL) either T or B cell type, that originate primarily within the skin [105]. After the gastrointestinal tract, the skin is the second most common site of extranodal NHL. Primary cutaneous lymphomas have a distinct clinical behavior and outcome from their histologically similar systemic counterparts, which can present secondarily on the skin. The World Health Organization (WHO) and European Organization for Research and Treatment of Cancer (EORTC) classification system therefore define primary cutaneous lymphomas as separate entities in their classification of NHL. Primary cutaneous T-cell lymphoma (CTCL) represents the majority ($\sim 75\%$) of primary cutaneous lymphomas, while primary cutaneous B-cell lymphoma (CBCL) make up the other $\sim 25\%$ of cases [105]. There is considerable variation in incidence and survival patterns of both CTCL and CBCL by race. The annual incidence rate (IR) of CTCL is highest among blacks (IR = 10.0/1,000,000 personyears) followed by whites (8.1) and Asians and Hispanics (both 5.1). In contrast to this, CBCL has the highest IR in whites (3.5/1,000,000 person-years), followed by Hispanics (2.8) and Asians (1.9), with the lowest IR being in blacks (1.5) [106].

The most common CTCL is mycosis fungoides (MF) which makes up $\sim 50\%$ of CTCL. This is followed by CD30+ lymphoproliferative disorder (CD30+ LPD) and Sezary syndrome, and together these three entities make up more than 90% of CTCL. MF is characterized by the evolution of patches, plaques, and tumors (Fig. 16.5a–c). In early stage disease, the lesions are often confined to the skin, but the tumor cells have the propensity to spread to lymph nodes, blood, and viscera with disease advancement [105]. The incidence and prognosis of MF varies with race. Blacks are 1.6 times more likely to be affected and have a higher mortality of 2.4 times that of whites [3, 4, 105, 107–109]. Furthermore, blacks tend to be diagnosed at a later stage in their disease which is typically harder to treat and may explain why their mortality is higher. Contrary to this, Asians and Hispanics have a lower incidence and reduced mortality compared to whites, with incidence in Asians being 0.6 and mortality ratio being 0.5 that of whites [4, 11]. The reason for this variation remains unknown. Blacks and Hispanics tend to develop the disease earlier in life, with early-onset MF (defined as onset before the age of 40) being

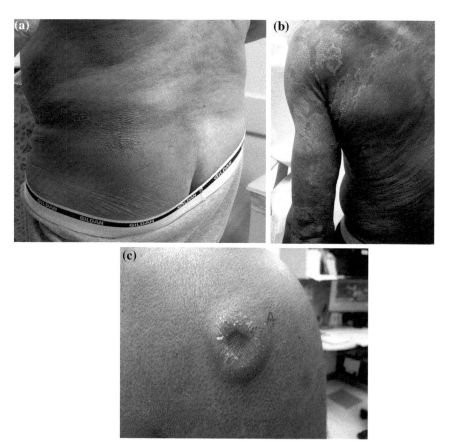

Fig. 16.5 Classic mycosis fungoides. **a** Patch stage on the flank. Erythematous patch with cigarette-paper like wrinkling. **b** Plaque stage. Widespread hyperpigmented polymorphic plaques with irregular, arcuate borders. **c** Tumor stage on the shoulder. Single annular pink scaly tumor with central depression

especially more common in black and Hispanic women. Furthermore, black women with early-onset MF had the highest rate of disease progression (38%), in comparison to white (10%) and Hispanic (5%) women [109]. Classic MF presents most commonly with erythematous atrophic patches or scaly plaques, often with atypical arcuate/horse-shoe shaped borders. There are also less common variants of MF that include hypopigmented MF, granulomatous MF, poikilodermatous MF, folliculotropic MF, pagetoid reticulosis, and granulomatous slack skin [110, 111]. The hypopigmented variant of MF typically presents with ill-defined hypopigmented macules and patches in younger patients (Fig 16.6). Almost three quarters of these patients have a prolonged history of an eczematous or psoriasiform dermatitis, and the diagnosis can be difficult to make, as this condition can be mistaken for pityriasis alba, vitiligo, pityriasis versicolor, hypopigmented sarcoidosis, and postinflammatory hypopigmentation [25, 111] Hypopigmented MF appears almost

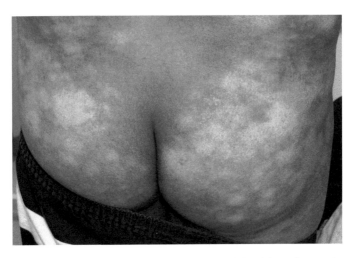

Fig. 16.6 Hypopigmented mycosis fungoides. Multiple ill-defined hypopigmented patches on bathing trunk distribution

exclusively in POC and tends to carry an excellent prognosis in comparsion to classic MF [110–112]. In contrast to MF, the IR for primary cutaneous CD30+ LPD is similar among whites and blacks, and significantly lower among Hispanics and Asians compared to whites and blacks [106].

CBCL is much rarer than CTCL and consists of 3 main subtypes: follicle center lymphoma (11% of all cutaneous lymphomas), marginal zone B-cell lymphoma (7%), and diffuse large B-cell lymphoma-leg type (DLBCL) (4%) [105]. Compared with other races, whites have the highest IR for CBCL overall, and also the highest IR for cutaneous marginal zone B-cell lymphoma and follicle center lymphoma subtypes. In contrast, Asians have a significantly lower IR than whites for all CBCL subtypes except for primary cutaneous (pc) DLBCL where, it is higher [106]. In fact, pcDLBCL has been previously reported as the most frequent (89%) CBCL subtype in Japanese patients [113].

Kaposi Sarcoma

In 1872, Moritz Kohn, who changed his name to Moritz Kaposi to resemble his hometown of Kaposvar/Hungary, first described 'idiopathisches multiples Pigmentsarkom der Haut,' which later became known as Kaposi sarcoma (KS). KS is among the most common cutaneous soft tissue sarcomas. The clinical presentation of KS ranges from an indolent disease limited to the skin to rapidly progressive multifocal disease involving skin and visceral organs. It is still unclear whether to consider KS as a hyperplasia, neoplasia, or both. Furthermore, ultrastructural and immunohistochemical testing have firmly established the endothelial nature of KS, but it remains a matter of debate whether this endothelial proliferation is derived from vascular or lymphatic origin as it tends to express antigens from both. Early KS shows a reactive pattern with polyclonal nature, which can progress to sarcoma later on. Human herpes virus-8 (HHV-8) and virally induced cytokines have been implicated in the pathogenesis of KS. HHV-8 infection is present in all patients with KS. The virus contains a homolog of cellular genes that can stimulate proliferation and tumorigenesis. It spreads via sexual intercourse, blood, saliva, and vertical transmission. Although HHV-8 infection is necessary, it is not sufficient on its own for the development of KS. The second factor contributing to the pathogenesis of KS is cytokines produced by virally infected cells as a host immune response, which may further support tumor growth in an autocrine/paracrine fashion.

KS is divided into four major types based on the population affected and all four types are associated with HHV-8. **Classic KS**—typically affects elderly men (male to female ratio of $\sim 10{:}1$) from Ashkenazi Jewish or Mediterranean/ Eastern European descent. It typically presents in the 6th decade of life with asymptomatic, slowly growing, dusky, red-violaceous macules/patches that evolve over time into larger plaques or dome-shaped nodules with the lower extremities being involved in the majority of cases. **Endemic KS**—is seen in Africans representing 10% of cancers in central Africa. It is further subdivided into four subtypes (nodular, florid, infiltrative, and lymphadenopathic), which tend to be more aggressive than classic KS. The lymphadenopathic type is the predominant form in African children and involves primarily lymph nodes. **Transplantation-related KS**—includes individuals receiving immunosuppressive medications. It resembles classic KS and usually resolves upon removal of immune suppressive therapy. The incidence of KS in transplant patients is ~ 500 times that of the general population, with certain immunosuppressive medications, particularly prednisone and cyclosporine, being the most common culprits for reactivation of HHV-8. **Acquired immune deficiency syndrome (AIDS)-related KS**—constitutes the fourth type (Fig. 16.7). HIV infection is thought to increase HHV-8 pathogenicity in many ways, including through immunosuppression, priming of target cells for HHV-8 infection, and by exerting direct effects on HHV-8 gene expression and viral replication [6, 114]. AIDS-related KS tends to affect HIV-infected individuals when CD4+ T-cell counts drop below 500 cell/mm^3 and is characterized by an aggressive course. Lesions are frequently oval in shape and follow the lines of cleavage of skin with a predilection for the trunk and face. In KS, any visceral organ can be involved, with gastrointestinal tract, lymph nodes (LN), and lungs being most commonly affected. Generalized lymphedema may rarely be the presenting sign of KS.

Historically, KS occurred most commonly in Mediterranean and Eastern European elderly men, or as an endemic form in equatorial Africa, and was rare in the US before the onset of AIDS in 1981. The incidence of KS increased dramatically with the AIDS epidemic in the early 1980s, peaked around the mid 1990s, and subsequently declined following the introduction of highly active antiretroviral therapy (HAART): IR of KS was 24.7/1000 personyears follow-up (PYFU) in 1997 and dropped to less than 10% of its original value (1.7/1000 PYFU) in 2002 and

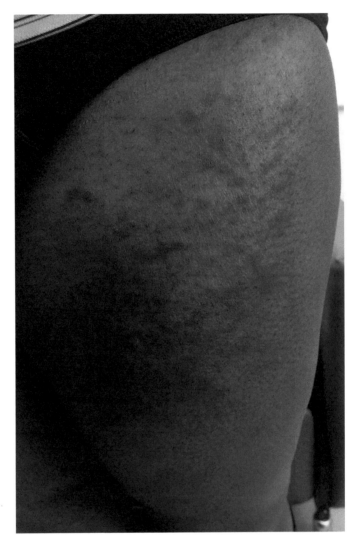

Fig. 16.7 Kaposi sarcoma in a patient with HIV. Multiple hyperpigmented papules coalescing into a large constricting plaque on the thigh causing surrounding lymphedema

beyond. During the 1980s, KS rates among white men were the highest, but the rates among black men exceeded those of white men after the mid-1990s. The KS rates in Asians showed the most dramatic decrease after the mid-1990s [115].

Overall, KS shows a higher incidence in blacks (23.5/1,000,000 personyears) in comparison to whites (17.5/1,000,000 person-years) with Asians having the lowest incidence (4.0/1,000,000 persons-years) [3, 6, 114]. Age-specific KS rate has a bimodal pattern with rates being elevated in early adulthood and at older ages, and this pattern is evident in both whites and blacks. However, the rates are higher among blacks compared to whites in the <70 age-group and higher among whites than blacks in the >70 age-group. Asians show a similar but lower incidence peak in early adulthood also, but the data is insufficient to provide an incidence in the older age group [115].

Treatment of KS is based on the disease stage, distribution, clinical type, and immune status. As the natural history of KS is variable and tends to carry a high recurrence rate even after successful treatment, realistic expectations should be discussed with patients. Management modalities for localized KS include nonintervention, surgical excision, laser surgery, cryotherapy, PDT, radiotherapy, intralesional chemotherapy, topical immunotherapy (imiquimod 5% cream), antiviral drugs (e.g., cidofovir), and cessation/alteration of immunosuppressive medication in iatrogenically immunosuppressed patients. The latter can prove challenging in many organ transplant recipient patients, and one option is substituting sirolimus for other immunosuppressive agents, which has been shown to improve KS lesions without sacrificing the much needed immune suppression required in these patients. For patients with symptomatic visceral involvement, or rapidly progressive cutaneous disease, systemic chemotherapies (e.g., doxorubicin, vincristine, etoposide, bleomycin, or docetaxel), systemic retinoid, or immunotherapy (e.g., interferon-alpha) are used. For AIDS-related KS, although initial disease progression may occur at initiation of HAART, the KS tends to improve with proper control of AIDS [20, 25, 114, 116].

Dermatofibrosarcoma Protuberans

Dermatofibrosarcoma protuberans (DFSP) is a rare cutaneous soft tissue sarcoma that accounts for less than 0.1% of all malignancies [3, 117]. It is characterized by an indolent growth and tendency to recur after excision. It has an overall good prognosis with a 10-year relative survival of 99% [118]. Although locally aggressive, DFSPs rarely metastasize (<5% of cases). Metastases typically arise from lesions with multiple local recurrences, and spread is predominantly to the lungs via the hematogenous route [117, 119]. DFSP typically occurs on the trunk as an asymptomatic, solitary, slowly growing, skin colored/red-brown or violaceous indurated plaque that can develop a bulging (protuberant) surface over the course of months to years (Fig. 16.8). The size usually ranges from 1 to 5 cm; however, neglected lesions may grow to more than 20 cm in diameter and develop satellite nodules. Initially, it is fixed only to the overlying skin, but it can invade fascia, muscle, and bone if left untreated [117]. The majority (∼95%) of DFSP harbor a translocation between 17q22 and 22q13 chromosomal regions leading to the fusion of collagen 1A1 (COL1A1) and platelet-derived growth factor β-chain (PDGFB) genes. This results in upregulation of a COL1A1–PDGFB fusion protein, leading to activation of the PDGF receptor and subsequent cellular proliferation [119].

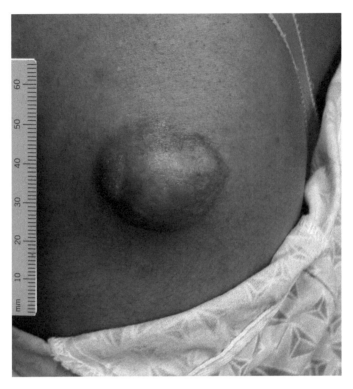

Fig. 16.8 Dermatofibrosarcoma protuberans. A large firm pink-brown nodule on the shoulder

The overall incidence of DFSP is 4.1 per 1,000,000 person-years, [118] with a peak incidence in the 40 s. Recent large-scale studies consistently show that DFSP incidence rates in blacks are higher than whites or Asians: incidence rate in blacks is 6.4/1,000,000 person-years versus whites 4.4/1,000,000 person-years versus Asians 2.7/1,000,000 person-years. In addition, higher mortality rates are associated with the black race [6]. Pigmented DFSPs, also known as Bednar tumors, are a rare variant making up <5% of DFSPs. They contain melanin-bearing dendritic cells with Schwann cell differentiation and occur most commonly in black individuals [3, 4, 117].

Given the locally aggressive nature of DFSP, adequate histopathological clearance of margins is the most important prognostic factor for local disease control. The treatment of choice is excision with wide local margins (2–4 cm) or Mohs surgery. Other treatment options in advanced disease include adjuvant radiation or systemic medication (e.g., imatinib mesylate, a tyrosine kinase inhibitor that targets many receptors including the PDGF receptor) [119, 120].

Merkel Cell Carcinoma

Merkel cell carcinoma (MCC) is an uncommon neoplasm caused by a malignant proliferation of highly anaplastic cells with features suggestive of neuroendocrine origin. The tumor has an aggressive biological behavior, with only 0.08% of cases diagnosed as in situ disease in the literature [121]. There is some controversy regarding the cellular origin of MCC. Tumor cells share various morphological, immunohistochemical, and ultrastructural features with Merkel cells, a mechanoreceptor in the basal layer of the epidermis. However, differences in the expression of phenotypic markers exist as MCC express c-kit (CD117) and neural cell adhesion molecule L1 (CD171), and it lacks the expression of vasoactive intestinal peptide and metenkephalin which are specific to Merkel cells [122]. Furthermore, polyomavirus, a critical etiologic factor in the development of MCC, does not seem to infect Merkel cells. Lastly, extracutaneous neuroendocrine tumors display characteristics similar to MCC. Thus, some pathologists use the term 'primary neuroendocrine carcinoma of the skin' over MCC. Although there is no definitive evidence supporting the cell of origin of MCC, in the last two decades, MCC has been shown to demonstrate various lines of differentiation (e.g., epithelial, eccrine, sarcomatous, lymphocytic, and other non-endocrine epithelial elements) [122, 123]. This suggests the possibility of MCC being derived from a progenitor cell (stem cell) capable of differentiating along these lines [122, 124].

Merkel cell polyomavirus (MCPyV) is an important etiologic agent in the pathogenesis of MCC and is identified in ~80% of cases, although perhaps significantly less commonly in Australian patients [122]. The viral genome is clonally integrated into the host genome, and all tumor progenitor cells, both early stage and metastases, display the same viral genome, suggesting that viral infection happens early during tumorigenesis [123]. The virus is ubiquitous in the general population and is thought to be acquired in childhood as an asymptomatic infection. MCPyV+ and MCPyV− tumors demonstrate biological differences. MCPyV− tumors have been associated with a number of mutations including p53, often associated with UV-damage, as well as NOTCH, NF1, FGFR2 and PI3/AKT pathway. MCPyV+ tumors tend to have a relatively lower mutational burden and lack UV-signature mutations [125]. Phylogenetic analyses has demonstrated the existence of 5 major MCPyV genotypes which relate to different ethnic/geographical backgrounds and include (i) Europe/North America/Caucasian, (ii) Africa [sub-Saharan], (iii) Oceania, (iv) South America/Amerindian, and (v) Asia/Japan. Further analyses over time may shed more light as to the significance of these genotypes in the pathogenesis of MCC in different ethnic groups and whether this may have any biological significance [126]. Immune suppression, particularly in cellular immunity, is also felt to play a role in the pathogenesis of MCC. The tumor is more frequently seen in the elderly, in AIDS and chronic lymphocytic leukemia patients, and in organ transplant recipients. In addition, withdrawal of immunosuppression has been shown to lead to complete tumor regression [121]. There is also evidence suggesting that sun exposure, as well as PUVA treatment, is associated with the development of MCC. UV light may cause local immunomodulation by reducing epidermal T cells and Langerhans cells and inducing hapten tolerance [122].

MCC usually presents in the elderly (over 70 years) and is more common in men. The most common site of presentation is the sun-exposed area of the head and neck in whites and Asians, while in blacks it tends to occur on the lower extremities [3, 121, 127]. Clinically it presents as a solitary, rapidly growing, non-tender, red-violaceous, firm, dome-shaped, nodule or plaque, with a shiny surface and overlying telangiectasia that may ulcerate [124]. Diagnosis is confirmed with a skin biopsy and immunohistochemical staining with neuroendocrine markers and cytokeratins. Thyroid transcription factor 1 (TTF-1) and CK7 are negative in MCC, which helps to differentiate it from cutaneous metastasis of small cell carcinoma of the lung which can also show similar morphology and expression of neuroen-docrine markers and cytokeratins [122].

Most reported patients from 1973-2006 SEER database are white ($\sim$95% of cases), with the tumor being very rare in Asians, American Indians and Pacific Islanders ($\sim$4% of cases), and blacks ($\sim$1% of cases) [121]. A large series found the annual age-adjusted incidence rate of MCC from 1986-1994 to be 0.01 in blacks compared with 0.23 in whites per 100,000 [3]. According to SEER data, there was an increase in the incidence of MCC between 1986 and 2011 by 8% per year, though it is unclear whether this increase is due to an increasingly aging population versus better detection of the cancer [122].

MCC is a locally aggressive tumor with significant risk of recurrence. It is treated surgically with wide local excision of 1–2 cm margins down to fascia with the goal of achieving clear surgical margins. Mohs micrographic surgery can be considered when tissue sparing is critical due to the anatomic location of the tumor. In the past, SLNB was controversial in MCC patients, but recent data shows pathologically node negative disease has a better prognosis than clinically node negative MCC irre-spective of tumor size, and hence SLNB is recommended in nearly all clinically node negative cases in the most recent NCCN guidelines. Pathologically involved nodes are managed with complete lymph node dissection with or without radiation. MCC is very radiosensitive and radiation can be useful as adjunctive treatment and can improve locoregional control, though it may not improve overall survival. It does not offer much benefit in SLNB negative cases but is useful for locoregional control in inoperative cases. Chemotherapy using platinum-based agents +/− etoposide may be utilized palliatively in advanced cases, though it is hard to achieve a durable response, and treatment can be associated with significant toxicity. More recently, immunotherapy has been an emerging therapeutic option in MCC with immune checkpoint inhibitors demonstrating durable responses in some patients by reacti-vating antitumor cellular immune responses [125].

Conclusion

Skin cancer is less common in persons of color compared to Caucasians. When it does occur, however, it often carries a poorer prognosis with higher morbidity and mortality. This has been attributed to many factors including: atypical location or appearance of skin cancer, lack of public awareness campaigns targeting non-white persons, false cultural convictions that darker skinned individuals do not develop skin cancer, and low socioeconomic status with difficulty accessing healthcare, all of which can lead to a delay in diagnosis and advanced disease at the time of presentation. In addition, it is possible that at least some of the skin cancers in POC have inherently biologically more aggressive behavior. As the US demographics evolve over time with greater representation of the ethnic minorities, skin cancer in POC will prove to be an increasingly more significant public health concern. It is therefore important for clinicians to familiarize themselves with the characteristic presentation and behavior of skin cancer in POC, particularly as they can vary in their clinical appearance and as the body areas involved by skin cancer in this group often tend to be overlooked during routine skin exams. Public education programs should be expanded to take into account the diversity in culture, beliefs, and languages among this growing heterogeneous group and to stress the importance of photoprotection, avoidance of tanning beds, and routine self-conducted examination to allow early detection and treatment of skin cancer. A collaborative endeavor from physicians, patients, and healthcare officials is needed to help decrease the morbidity and mortality caused by skin cancer in POC.

References

1. Jimbow K, et al. Some aspects of melanin biology: 1950–1975. J Invest Dermatol. 1976;67(1):72–89.
2. Montagna W, Carlisle K. The architecture of black and white facial skin. J Am Acad Dermatol. 1991;24(6 Pt 1):929–37.
3. Gloster HM Jr, Neal K, Skin cancer in skin of color. J Am Acad Dermatol. 2006;55(5):741–60; quiz 761-4.
4. Agbai ON, et al. Skin cancer and photoprotection in people of color: a review and recommendations for physicians and the public. J Am Acad Dermatol. 2014;70(4):748–62.
5. US Census Bureau. 2010 Census. Accessed March 20, 2016. Available from: http://www.census.gov.
6. Bradford PT. Skin cancer in skin of color. Dermatol Nurs. 2009;21(4):170–7, 206; quiz 178.
7. Weishaupt C, et al. Skeletal muscle involvement in early-onset mycosis fungoides. J Am Acad Dermatol. 2011;64(6):e118–20.
8. Rosenberg CA, et al. Association of nonmelanoma skin cancer with second malignancy. Cancer. 2004;100(1):130–8.
9. Norval M. Effects of solar radiation on the human immune system. J Photochem Photobiol, B. 2001;63(1–3):28–40.
10. Stab F, et al. Urocanic acid and its function in endogenous antioxidant defense and UV-protection in human skin. J Invest Dermatol. 1994;102(4):666.

11. Taylor S, et al. Taylor and Kelly's dermatology for skin of color. 2nd ed (Edmonson KG, Brown RY, editors). New York: McGraw-Hill Education; 2016.
12. Gray DT, et al. Trends in the population-based incidence of squamous cell carcinoma of the skin first diagnosed between 1984 and 1992. Arch Dermatol. 1997;133(6):735–40.
13. Scotto J, Fears TR, Fraumeni JF. Incidence of nonmelanoma skin cancer in the United States. U.S. Dept. Health and Human Services, Public Health Service, National Institute of Health, National Cancer Institute. NIH Publication No. 83–2433 (1983), 1983.
14. Ishihara K, et al. Updated statistical data for malignant melanoma in Japan. Int J Clin Oncol. 2001;6(3):109–16.
15. Almahroos M, Kurban AK. Ultraviolet carcinogenesis in nonmelanoma skin cancer. Part I: incidence rates in relation to geographic locations and in migrant populations. Skinmed 2004;3(1):29–35; quiz 35-6.
16. Almahroos M, Kurban AK. Ultraviolet carcinogenesis in nonmelanoma skin cancer part II: review and update on epidemiologic correlations. Skinmed. 2004;3(3):132–9.
17. Kotrajaras R, Kligman AM. The effect of topical tretinoin on photodamaged facial skin: the Thai experience. Br J Dermatol. 1993;129(3):302–9.
18. Battie C, et al. Skin cancer in skin of color: an update on current facts, trends, and misconceptions. J Drugs Dermatol. 2013;12(2):194–8.
19. Scotto J, et al. Nonmelanoma skin cancer. In: Schottenfeld D, Fraumeni JF Jr, editors. Cancer epidemiology and prevention. 2nd ed. New York: Oxford University Press; 1996. pp. 1313–30.
20. Halder RM, Bang KM. Skin cancer in blacks in the United States. Dermatol Clin. 1988;6(3):397–405.
21. Mora RG, Perniciaro C. Cancer of the skin in blacks. I. A review of 163 black patients with cutaneous squamous cell carcinoma. J Am Acad Dermatol. 1981;5(5):535–43.
22. Mora RG, Perniciaro C, Lee B. Cancer of the skin in blacks. III. A review of nineteen black patients with Bowen's disease. J Am Acad Dermatol. 1984;11(4 Pt 1):557–62.
23. Fleming ID, et al. Skin cancer in black patients. Cancer. 1975;35(3):600–5.
24. Hale EK, et al. Current concepts in the management of actinic keratosis. J Drugs Dermatol. 2004;3(2 Suppl):S3–16.
25. Halder RM, Bridgeman-Shah S. Skin cancer in African Americans. Cancer. 1995;75(2 Suppl):667–73.
26. McCall CO, Chen SC. Squamous cell carcinoma of the legs in African Americans. J Am Acad Dermatol. 2002;47(4):524–9.
27. Schoeman BJ. Squamous cell carcinoma in neuropathic plantar ulcers in leprosy: another example of Marjolin's ulcer. S Afr Med J. 1996;86(8):966–9.
28. Rosen T, Tucker SB, Tschen J. Bowen's disease in blacks. J Am Acad Dermatol. 1982;7(3):364–8.
29. Amir H, Mbonde MP, Kitinya JN. Cutaneous squamous cell carcinoma in Tanzania. Cent Afr J Med. 1992;38(11):439–43.
30. Yakubu A, Mabogunje OA. Squamous cell carcinoma of the skin in Africans. Trop Geogr Med. 1995;47(2):91–3.
31. Rudolph R, Zelac DE. Squamous cell carcinoma of the skin. Plast Reconstr Surg. 2004;114(6):82e–94e.
32. Mora RG. Surgical and aesthetic considerations of cancer of the skin in the black American. J Dermatol Surg Oncol. 1986;12(1):24–31.
33. Preston DS, Stern RS. Nonmelanoma cancers of the skin. N Engl J Med. 1992;327(23):1649–62.
34. Della Vittoria Scarpati G, et al. Concomitant cetuximab and radiation therapy: a possible promising strategy for locally advanced inoperable non-melanoma skin carcinomas. Mol Clin Oncol. 2016;4(4):467–471.
35. Rubin AI, Chen EH, Ratner D. Basal-cell carcinoma. N Engl J Med. 2005;353(21):2262–9.
36. Abreo F, Sanusi ID. Basal cell carcinoma in North American blacks. Clinical and histopathologic study of 26 patients. J Am Acad Dermatol. 1991;25(6 Pt 1):1005–11.

37. Nguyen AV, Whitaker DC, Frodel J. Differentiation of basal cell carcinoma. Otolaryngol Clin North Am. 1993;26(1):37–56.
38. Blanpain C, Fuchs E. Epidermal homeostasis: a balancing act of stem cells in the skin. Nat Rev Mol Cell Biol. 2009;10(3):207–17.
39. Kimonis VE, et al. Clinical manifestations in 105 persons with nevoid basal cell carcinoma syndrome. Am J Med Genet. 1997;69(3):299–308.
40. Kimonis VE, et al. Clinical and radiological features in young individuals with nevoid basal cell carcinoma syndrome. Genet Med. 2013;15(1):79–83.
41. Hall J, et al. Nevoid basal cell carcinoma syndrome in a black child. J Am Acad Dermatol. 1998;38(2 Pt 2):363–5.
42. Martin S, Waisman M. Basal cell nevus syndrome in a black patient: report of a case and review of the literature. Arch Dermatol. 1978;114(9):1356–7.
43. Gorlin RJ. Nevoid basal cell carcinoma (Gorlin) syndrome: unanswered issues. J Lab Clin Med. 1999;134(6):551–2.
44. Shore RE, et al. Skin cancer after X-ray treatment for scalp ringworm. Radiat Res. 2002; 157(4):410–8.
45. Dhir A, et al. Basal cell carcinoma on the scalp of an Indian patient. Dermatol Surg. 1995; 21(3):247–50.
46. Altman A, et al. Basal cell epithelioma in black patients. J Am Acad Dermatol. 1987;17(5 Pt 1): 741–5.
47. Kikuchi A, Shimizu H, Nishikawa T. Clinical histopathological characteristics of basal cell carcinoma in Japanese patients. Arch Dermatol. 1996;132(3):320–4.
48. Kalter DC, Goldberg LH, Rosen T. Darkly pigmented lesions in dark-skinned patients. J Dermatol Surg Oncol. 1984;10(11):876–81.
49. Bigler C, et al. Pigmented basal cell carcinoma in Hispanics. J Am Acad Dermatol. 1996; 34(5 Pt 1):751–2.
50. Cheng SY, Luk NM, Chong LY. Special features of non-melanoma skin cancer in Hong Kong Chinese patients: 10-year retrospective study. Hong Kong Med J. 2001;7(1):22–8.
51. Tan ES, et al. Basal cell carcinoma in Singapore: a prospective study on epidemiology and clinicopathological characteristics with a secondary comparative analysis between Singaporean Chinese and Caucasian patients. Australas J Dermatol. 2015;56(3):175–9.
52. Zhang B, Wang N, He W. Clinicopathologic analysis of 60 cases of basal cell carcinoma. Chin Med Sci J. 1993;8(2):121–2.
53. Lanehart WH, et al. Metastasizing basal cell carcinoma originating in a stasis ulcer in a black woman. Arch Dermatol. 1983;119(7):587–91.
54. Kidd MK, et al. Carcinoembryonic antigen in basal cell neoplasms in black patients: an immunohistochemical study. J Am Acad Dermatol. 1989;21(5 Pt 1):1007–10.
55. Kauvar AN, et al. Consensus for nonmelanoma skin cancer treatment: basal cell carcinoma, including a cost analysis of treatment methods. Dermatol Surg. 2015;41(5):550–71.
56. Basset-Seguin N, et al. Vismodegib in patients with advanced basal cell carcinoma (STEVIE): a pre-planned interim analysis of an international, open-label trial. Lancet Oncol. 2015;16(6):729–36.
57. Migden MR, et al. Treatment with two different doses of sonidegib in patients with locally advanced or metastatic basal cell carcinoma (BOLT): a multicentre, randomised, double-blind phase 2 trial. Lancet Oncol. 2015;16(6):716–28.
58. Siegel RL, Miller KD, Jemal A. Cancer statistics, 2016. CA Cancer J Clin. 2016;66(1):7–30.
59. Hu S, et al. UV radiation, latitude, and melanoma in US Hispanics and blacks. Arch Dermatol. 2004;140(7):819–24.
60. Cress RD, Holly EA. Incidence of cutaneous melanoma among non-Hispanic whites, Hispanics, Asians, and blacks: an analysis of california cancer registry data, 1988–93. Cancer Causes Control. 1997;8(2):246–52.
61. Bergfelt L, et al. Incidence and anatomic distribution of cutaneous melanoma among United States Hispanics. J Surg Oncol. 1989;40(4):222–6.

62. Surveillance, Epidemiology, and End Results (SEER) Program. SEER Stat Database: National Cancer Institute, Division of Cancer Control and Population Sciences, Surveillance Research Program, Cancer Statistics Branch. Available at http://seer.cancer. gov. Accessed March 28, 2016; SEER 18 2008–2012, Age-Adjusted.

63. Jemal A, et al. Cancer statistics, 2005. CA Cancer J Clin. 2005;55(1):10–30.

64. Rhodes AR, et al. Risk factors for cutaneous melanoma. A practical method of recognizing predisposed individuals. JAMA. 1987;258(21):3146–54.

65. Holly EA, et al. Cutaneous melanoma in women. I. Exposure to sunlight, ability to tan, and other risk factors related to ultraviolet light. Am J Epidemiol. 1995;141(10):923–33.

66. Whiteman DC, Whiteman CA, Green AC. Childhood sun exposure as a risk factor for melanoma: a systematic review of epidemiologic studies. Cancer Causes Control. 2001;12(1): 69–82.

67. Griewank KG, et al. Genetic alterations and personalized medicine in melanoma: progress and future prospects. J Natl Cancer Inst. 2014;106(2):djt435.

68. Elwood JM. Melanoma and sun exposure. Semin Oncol. 1996;23(6):650–66.

69. Eide MJ, Weinstock MA. Association of UV index, latitude, and melanoma incidence in nonwhite populations—US Surveillance, Epidemiology, and End Results (SEER) Program, 1992 to 2001. Arch Dermatol. 2005;141(4):477–81.

70. Hudson DA, Krige JE. Plantar melanoma in black South Africans. Br J Surg. 1993;80(8): 992–4.

71. Giraud RM, Rippey E, Rippey JJ. Malignant melanoma of the skin in Black Africans. S Afr Med J. 1975;49(16):665–8.

72. Bellows CF, et al. Melanoma in African-Americans: trends in biological behavior and clinical characteristics over two decades. J Surg Oncol. 2001;78(1):10–6.

73. Reintgen D, et al. Malignant melanoma: staging and treatment of localized and advanced disease. Cancer Control. 1999;6(4):398–404.

74. Muchmore JH, Mizuguchi RS, Lee C. Malignant melanoma in American black females: an unusual distribution of primary sites. J Am Coll Surg. 1996;183(5):457–65.

75. Collins RJ. Melanoma in the Chinese of Hong Kong. Emphasis on volar and subungual sites. Cancer. 1984;54(7):1482–8.

76. Rahman Z, Taylor SC. Malignant melanoma in African Americans. Cutis. 2001;67(5): 403–6.

77. Rippey JJ, Rippey E. Epidemiology of malignant melanoma of the skin in South Africa. S Afr Med J. 1984;65(15):595–8.

78. Coleman WP 3rd, et al. Acral lentiginous melanoma. Arch Dermatol. 1980;116(7):773–6.

79. Bang KM, et al. Skin cancer in black Americans: a review of 126 cases. J Natl Med Assoc. 1987;79(1):51–8.

80. Schreiber MM, et al. The incidence of skin cancer in southern Arizona (Tucson). Arch Dermatol. 1971;104(2):124–7.

81. Reintgen DS, et al. Malignant melanoma in black American and white American populations. A comparative review. JAMA. 1982;248(15):1856–9.

82. Slingluff CL Jr, Vollmer R, Seigler HF. Acral melanoma: a review of 185 patients with identification of prognostic variables. J Surg Oncol. 1990;45(2):91–8.

83. Byrd KM, et al. Advanced presentation of melanoma in African Americans. J Am Acad Dermatol. 2004;50(1):21–4; discussion 142-3.

84. Stevens NG, Liff JM, Weiss NS. Plantar melanoma: is the incidence of melanoma of the sole of the foot really higher in blacks than whites? Int J Cancer. 1990;45(4):691–3.

85. Durbec F, et al. Melanoma of the hand and foot: epidemiological, prognostic and genetic features. A systematic review. Br J Dermatol. 2012;166(4):727–39.

86. Swerdlow AJ, et al. Benign melanocytic naevi as a risk factor for malignant melanoma. Br Med J (Clin Res Ed). 1986;292(6535):1555–9.

87. Rodenas JM, et al. Melanocytic nevi and risk of cutaneous malignant melanoma in southern Spain. Am J Epidemiol. 1997;145(11):1020–9.

88. Coleman WP 3rd, et al. Nevi, lentigines, and melanomas in blacks. Arch Dermatol. 1980;116(5):548–51.
89. Black WC, Goldhahn RT Jr, Wiggins C. Melanoma within a southwestern Hispanic population. Arch Dermatol. 1987;123(10):1331–4.
90. Pennello G, Devesa S, Gail M. Association of surface ultraviolet B radiation levels with melanoma and nonmelanoma skin cancer in United States blacks. Cancer Epidemiol Biomarkers Prev. 2000;9(3):291–7.
91. Pathak DR, et al. Malignant melanoma of the skin in New Mexico 1969–1977. Cancer. 1982;50(7):1440–6.
92. (NCCN), N.C.C.N. NCCN Guidlines Melanoma. Melanoma Version 2.2016 2016 [cited 2016 5.30.2016]; Available from: https://www.nccn.org/.
93. Vayer A, Lefor AT. Cutaneous melanoma in African-Americans. South Med J. 1993;86(2): 181–2.
94. Hudson DA, Krige JE, Stubbings H. Plantar melanoma: results of treatment in three population groups. Surgery. 1998;124(5):877–82.
95. Hudson DA, Krige JE. Melanoma in black South Africans. J Am Coll Surg. 1995;180(1): 65–71.
96. Hu S, et al. Comparison of stage at diagnosis of melanoma among Hispanic, black, and white patients in Miami-Dade County, Florida. Arch Dermatol. 2006;142(6):704–8.
97. Johnson DS, et al. Malignant melanoma in non-Caucasians: experience from Hawaii. Surg Clin North Am. 2003;83(2):275–82.
98. Cockburn MG, Zadnick J, Deapen D. Developing epidemic of melanoma in the Hispanic population of California. Cancer. 2006;106(5):1162–8.
99. Crowley NJ, et al. Malignant melanoma in black Americans. A trend toward improved survival. Arch Surg. 1991;126(11):1359–64; discussion 1365.
100. Swan MC, Hudson DA. Malignant melanoma in South Africans of mixed ancestry: a retrospective analysis. Melanoma Res. 2003;13(4):415–9.
101. Chen YJ, et al. Clinicopathologic analysis of malignant melanoma in Taiwan. J Am Acad Dermatol. 1999;41(6):945–9.
102. Hu S, et al. Disparity in melanoma: a trend analysis of melanoma incidence and stage at diagnosis among whites, Hispanics, and blacks in Florida. Arch Dermatol. 2009;145(12): 1369–74.
103. Kosary C, Ries L, Miller B. SEER cancer statistics review, 1973–1992: tables and graphs. Bethesda (MD): National Cancer Institute; 1995.
104. Zell JA, et al. Survival for patients with invasive cutaneous melanoma among ethnic groups: the effects of socioeconomic status and treatment. J Clin Oncol. 2008;26(1):66–75.
105. Willemze R, et al. WHO-EORTC classification for cutaneous lymphomas. Blood. 2005; 105(10):3768–85.
106. Bradford PT, et al. Cutaneous lymphoma incidence patterns in the United States: a population-based study of 3884 cases. Blood. 2009;113(21):5064–73.
107. Weinstock MA, Horm JW. Mycosis fungoides in the United States. Increasing incidence and descriptive epidemiology. JAMA. 1988;260(1):42–6.
108. Akaraphanth R, Douglass MC, Lim HW. Hypopigmented mycosis fungoides: treatment and a 6(1/2)-year follow-up of 9 patients. J Am Acad Dermatol. 2000;42(1 Pt 1):33–9.
109. Sun G, et al. Poor prognosis in non-caucasian patients with early-onset mycosis fungoides. J Am Acad Dermatol. 2009;60(2):231–5.
110. Lambroza E, et al. Hypopigmented variant of mycosis fungoides: demography, histopathology, and treatment of seven cases. J Am Acad Dermatol. 1995;32(6):987–93.
111. Stone ML, et al. Hypopigmented mycosis fungoides: a report of 7 cases and review of the literature. Cutis. 2001;67(2):133–8.
112. Agar NS, et al. Survival outcomes and prognostic factors in mycosis fungoides/Sezary syndrome: validation of the revised International Society for Cutaneous Lymphomas/European Organisation for Research and Treatment of Cancer staging proposal. J Clin Oncol. 2010;28(31):4730–9.

113. Morton LM, et al. Lymphoma incidence patterns by WHO subtype in the United States, 1992–2001. Blood. 2006;107(1):265–76.
114. Schwartz RA, et al. Kaposi sarcoma: a continuing conundrum. J Am Acad Dermatol. 2008;59(2):179–206; quiz 207-8.
115. Rouhani P, et al. Cutaneous soft tissue sarcoma incidence patterns in the U.S.: an analysis of 12,114 cases. Cancer. 2008;113(3):616–27.
116. Stallone G, et al. Sirolimus for Kaposi's sarcoma in renal-transplant recipients. N Engl J Med. 2005;352(13):1317–23.
117. Gloster HM Jr. Dermatofibrosarcoma protuberans. J Am Acad Dermatol. 1996;35(3 Pt 1): 355–74; quiz 375-6.
118. Kreicher KL, et al. Incidence and survival of primary dermatofibrosarcoma protuberans in the United States. Dermatol Surg. 2016;42(Suppl 1):S24–31.
119. Wang C, et al. Target therapy of unresectable or metastatic dermatofibrosarcoma protuberans with imatinib mesylate: an analysis on 22 Chinese patients. Medicine (Baltimore). 2015; 94(17):e773.
120. Ugurel S, et al. Neoadjuvant imatinib in advanced primary or locally recurrent dermatofibrosarcoma protuberans: a multicenter phase II DeCOG trial with long-term follow-up. Clin Cancer Res. 2014;20(2):499–510.
121. Albores-Saavedra J, et al. Merkel cell carcinoma demographics, morphology, and survival based on 3870 cases: a population based study. J Cutan Pathol. 2010;37(1):20–7.
122. Czapiewski P, Biernat W. Merkel cell carcinoma—recent advances in the biology, diagnostics and treatment. Int J Biochem Cell Biol. 2014;53:536–46.
123. Prieto Munoz I, et al. Merkel cell carcinoma from 2008 to 2012: reaching a new level of understanding. Cancer Treat Rev. 2013;39(5):421–9.
124. Ratner D, et al. Merkel cell carcinoma. J Am Acad Dermatol. 1993;29(2 Pt 1):143–56.
125. Cassler NM, et al. Merkel cell carcinoma therapeutic update. Curr Treat Options Oncol. 2016;17(7):36.
126. Martel-Jantin C, et al. Molecular epidemiology of merkel cell polyomavirus: evidence for geographically related variant genotypes. J Clin Microbiol. 2014;52(5):1687–90.
127. Song PI, et al. The clinical profile of Merkel cell carcinoma in mainland China. Int J Dermatol. 2012;51(9):1054–9.

Chapter 17
Pediatric Dermatology

Lubna H. Suaiti, Yasin A. Damji and Margaret S. Lee

A major theory regarding the evolution of skin pigmentation is defense against folate photoproteolysis, as folate is necessary for normal nucleic acid biosynthesis [1]. Thousands of years of migration from our origins in Africa, the distance from the equator, and different environmental parameters are believed to play roles in genetic selection and variations in skin color [2–5]. This chapter will discuss skin conditions that are commonly observed in patients with skin of color or that phenotypically differ compared to presentations in light skin; for example, erythema is not as easily distinguished or might have a violaceous or brown hue in dark-skinned patients. Also, pigmented skin may demonstrate variant responses to skin disease, including pigment lability, follicular vs hyperkeratotic presentations, mesenchymal (granulomatous or keloidal) reactions, and bullous lesions [6, 7]. Normal pigmented skin findings, birthmarks, and pediatric hair disorders will also be discussed. We end with a brief review of the psychosocial impact of congenital and acquired skin conditions, a fundamental aspect of the patient and family experience in pediatric dermatology.

L.H. Suaiti
Department of Dermatology, Boston University Medical Center,
609 Albany St., Boston, MA 02120, USA
e-mail: lsuaiti@gmail.com

Y.A. Damji
Boston University School of Medicine, 72 East Concord St.,
Boston, MA 02118, USA
e-mail: ydamji@bu.edu

M.S. Lee (✉)
Department of Dermatology, Boston University School of Medicine,
609 Albany St., Boston, MA 02118, USA
e-mail: margaret.lee@bmc.org

© Springer International Publishing AG 2017
N.A. Vashi and H.I. Maibach (eds.), *Dermatoanthropology of Ethnic Skin and Hair*, DOI 10.1007/978-3-319-53961-4_17

Birthmarks

Congenital pigmentary lesions vary according to race, sex, and type of birthmark. Birthmarks are either localized and limited to having potential psychosocial impact (discussed later in this chapter) or are extensive and might signify systemic involvement [8–11]. In this chapter, we will review birthmarks that are due to pigment changes, as they are more common among dark-skinned newborns. There is generally no treatment available for pigmented birthmarks, although laser therapy is sometimes helpful.

Dermal Melanocytosis

Between the 11th and 14th weeks of gestation, dermal melanocytes migrate from the neural crest to the epidermis or undergo apoptosis; however, some dermal melanocytes persist at the time of birth and produce melanin within the dermis [12]. Hepatocyte growth factor and other gene mutations, i.e., GNA11 (G protein subunit alpha 11) and GNAQ (G protein subunit alpha G), are believed to play a role in dermal melanocyte survival in head and neck, distal extremities, and sacral skin area resulting in Nevus of Ota, Nevus of Ito, blue nevus, and Mongolian spots. The Tyndall effect, an optical phenomenon, results from reflection of dermal pigment giving the bluish appearance of dermal melanin [12–14].

Mongolian Spots

The most common form of congenital dermal melanocytosis is usually referred to as Mongolian spots, occurring in approximately 90% of infants of color all over the world [15, 16]. They typically are observed at birth as blue-gray or slate gray patches on the lumbosacral region, and fade partially or completely over a period of years. "Aberrant" Mongolian spots can be found in extra-sacral locations. Superimposed Mongolian spots have been reported (a darker macule or patch overlying a lighter colored patch) [13]. Extensive Mongolian spots at birth or persistent Mongolian spots in older children may be associated with lysosomal storage diseases, i.e., Hurler disease, GM1(monosialotetrahexosylganglioside) gangliosidosis, Mucopolysaccharidosis type II, and Niemann–Pick disease [17]. Extensive Mongolian spots are also seen in phakomatosis pigmentovascularis; careful physical exam is crucial to identify coexisting vascular birthmarks, which might be difficult to appreciate in darkly pigmented patients [13, 16, 17]. It is important to note uniformity of color and chronicity, to avoid confusing these birthmarks with ecchymoses due to child abuse or neglect (Fig. 17.1).

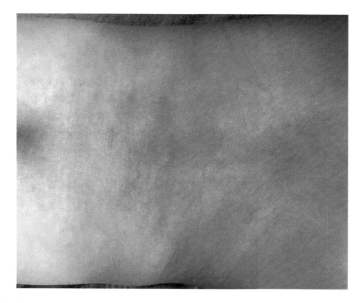

Fig. 17.1 Dermal melanocytosis on an infant's back mimicking ecchymoses

Nevus of Ota (Oculodermal Melanocytosis/Nevus Fuscoceruleus Ophthalmomaxillaris)

Nevus of Ota is common among Asians and other females with skin of color [18]. It is usually a unilateral blue-gray or brown mottled patch, located on skin and mucous membranes innervated by the ophthalmic and maxillary branches of the trigeminal nerve. Approximately 5% are bilateral [19]. Up to 70% of patients have ipsilateral scleral involvement. It presents shortly after birth and darkens around puberty or may not be obvious until puberty, when it is thought that hormones stimulate pigmentation [18, 20–23]. Although rare, cutaneous, choroidal or leptomeningeal melanoma has been reported within nevus of Ota [24, 25].

Nevus of Ito (Nevus Fuscoceruleus Acromiodeltoideus)

Clinically and histologically similar to nevus of Ito, this form of dermal melanocytosis is located on the posterior supraclavicular, scapular, and deltoid areas (lateral cutaneous nerve distribution) [19, 26]. Malignant melanoma transformation within nevus of Ito has been reported [27]. Coexistence of nevus of Ito with nevus spilus [26] or nevus of Ito with nevus of Ota [19] have been described.

Blue Nevus (Dermal Melanocytoma)

Blue nevi are congenital in 25% of cases, and 75% are acquired during childhood or later in life. They are usually solitary, blue or blue-black papules on the scalp, sacral, and extensor distal extremities [23, 28]. Giant congenital blue nevi are rare, commonly seen on the scalp, with risk of malignant transformation during childhood or later in life [28, 29]. Blue nevi are categorized as common (1 cm or less, often located on the dorsal hand), cellular (1–3 cm, most often on the buttock and sacral area), or epithelioid (sporadic or in association with Carney complex, usually on trunk and extremities) [23, 28–30]. It is challenging to differentiate atypical cellular blue nevi from malignant blue nevi histologically.

Café-Au-Lait Macules

Café-au-lait macules (CALMs) are a very common finding in the general population; prevalence of CALMs in large cohort studies range from 0.3 to 2.7% of newborns [11, 31, 32]. In one large cohort study, 18.3% of black infants versus 0.3% of white infants were found to have CALMs at birth [11]. These are solitary or multiple, well-defined, evenly pigmented brown macules or patches. Smooth borders are described as "coast of California" while serrated borders are described as "coast of Maine." Average size is 0.2–4 cm in newborns and 1.5–30 cm in older children [32]. Histopathologic examination reveals increased melanin content in the basal layer as well as in melanocytes, with no evidence of increased melanocytic infiltration. Multiple CALMs could be a normal finding with no other systemic disease association (1.9% of normal children with skin of color reportedly have more than 2 CALMs) or might signify systemic involvement in the context of several genetic disorders. Neurofibromatosis 1, neurofibromatosis 2, ring chromosome syndrome, and Watson syndrome are most closely associated with multiple CALMs, and McCune Albright syndrome with large/segmental CALMs [32]. Other systemic disorders with questionable association with CALMs include tuberous sclerosis, ataxia-telangiectasia, Bloom, and Silver–Russell Syndromes [31, 32]. Full discussion of associated genodermatoses is beyond the scope of this chapter.

Patterned Pigmentation (Pigmentary Mosaicism)

Patterned pigmentation refers to hyper- or hypopigmentation that results from two different cell clones (chromosomal mosaicism) [33–35]. A wide range of clinically distinct presentations include linear Blaschkoid, broad checkerboard (flag-like), and phylloid (leaf-like) hyper- and hypopigmentation. Patterned pigmentation is rarely associated with cutaneous, skeletal, and neurological abnormalities. Cases are sporadic; however, a few familial cases due to functional (epigenetic) modification of autosomal genes have been described [34, 35].

Linear Nevoid Hypomelanosis Versus Linear and Whorled Nevoid Hypermelanosis

Linear nevoid hypomelanosis, also known as hypomelanosis of Ito (HI), describes hypopigmented Blaschkoid linear swirls and streaks [36, 37]. It presents at birth or during childhood as a result of somatic mosaicism with two clones of cells, where one clone produces less melanin. It affects males and females with no racial predilection; however, it is easier to appreciate in darker skinned patients [36, 38]. Reported association with neurologic, ocular, and musculoskeletal abnormalities varies widely, between 30 and 94% of patients; it is now believed that the lower estimates are more likely [37].

Conversely, linear and whorled nevoid hypermelanosis (LWNH) involves hyperpigmented linear swirls that follow Blaschko's lines due to pigmentary mosaicism causing increased melanin in one clone. Similar to HI, it has been associated with ocular, musculoskeletal, and neurological abnormalities, but in both conditions the risk of extracutaneous abnormalities should not be overemphasized to patients and parents. In one case review of 16 cases with LWNH, only one out of six patients with extensive LWNH had extracutaneous abnormalities [39]. Dermoscopic exam shows linear and circular streak-like pigmentation organized in a parallel linear manner [40]. Differential diagnoses include incontinentia pigmenti and macular/early epidermal nevus. Histopathology reveals increased basal layer hyperpigmentation with no melanophages [33].

Pigmentary Demarcation Lines

Pigmentary demarcation lines, also known as Futcher's lines or Voight's lines, are normal in skin of color and persist through adulthood [41]. They represent an abrupt transition of pigmentation established during fetal development [42–44]. The most commonly observed lines are found on the anterolateral upper arms and postero-medial legs (Fig. 17.2a, b).

Transient Infantile Patterned Hyperpigmentation

An often-overlooked diagnosis, transient infantile patterned hyperpigmentation is a benign condition that fades over a few months [45]. Skin examination reveals multiple transverse, parallel pigmented thin lines on the extremities and/or torso. In contrast to hormonal hyperpigmentation of the genitals and areolar skin, transient infantile patterned hyperpigmentation is believed to be due to intrauterine fetal position and friction [45, 46].

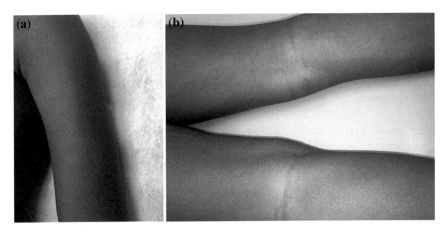

Fig. 17.2 **a** Futcher's line on the upper arm. **b** Futcher's line on the posterior leg

Pigmented Nevi

Many pigmented lesions are benign and more frequently observed in children of color. Mucosal hyperpigmentation has been reported in 72–100% of darker skinned populations, with 25% onset before the age of 10. Positive family history is usually elicited. Scleral hyperpigmentation is reported in 78%, 8% before the age of 10 [6]. Hyperpigmented palms, melanonychia (pigmented nail plate), and congenital melanocytic nevi are also common.

Melanonychia and Nevi of the Nail Matrix

Longitudinal melanonychia, also known as melanonychia striata, represents melanin deposition within the nail plate. While 5–10% of longitudinal melanonychia in adults are due to malignant melanoma, no cases of invasive melanoma have been reported in association with pediatric longitudinal melanonychia [47]. Melanonychia presents as a longitudinal hyperpigmented band with variable widths (up to complete involvement of the nail plate) affecting fingernails, especially thumbs, more often than toenails [47, 48]. Color can vary from bluish-gray, brown, to black. Melanonychia of childhood is predominantly caused by benign lentigines and melanocytic nevi, much less commonly due to atypical melanocytic nevi or malignant melanoma in situ. Biopsy or surgical excision is recommended only for lesions with concerning signs: irregularity of pigmentation or borders, width of the pigmentation exceeding 3 mm, hazy border, Hutchinson's sign (pigmented proximal or lateral nail bed), irregular pigmented lines on dermoscopy, and rapid evolution [48].

Congenital Melanocytic Nevi (CMN)

Congenital melanocytic nevi are melanocytic neural crest-derived hamartomas, common in skin of color. They occur as a result of unregulated melanoblast growth between the 5th and 24th weeks of gestation. Approximately 1% of newborns are affected, with slightly higher female prevalence [49]. Giant CMN have different histological elements because they originate from pluripotent stem cells and are difficult to evaluate using dermoscopy, as the cells extend deeper into the dermis and subcutaneous tissue [49, 50]. Hypertrichosis, perifollicular hypo/hyperpigmentation, pseudomilia, and vascular structures are common dermoscopic findings of CMN [50]. Neurocutaneous melanosis (NCM) is a melanocytic proliferation of the leptomeninges (brain and/or spinal cord) that occurs in association with larger and axial CMN [50]. Diagnosis and management is the same for all skin phototypes.

Disorders of Late-Onset and Secondary Hyperpigmentation

Hyperpigmented lesions occurring beyond infancy include entities of congenital origin. Dermal melanocytosis can manifest later in life, i.e., Nevus of Ito, Ota-like (Hori nevus), and acquired dermal melanocytosis of the hands [51, 52]. Also, late-onset linear and whorled nevoid hypermelanosis in a zosteriform distribution has been reported [53].

Becker's Nevus (Pigmented Hairy Epidermal Nevus)

Becker's nevus is thought to be a hamartomatous congenital lesion of ectodermal and mesodermal origin where the pigmentation usually presents years later, although congenital cases have been described [54]. A pigmented patch may appear during childhood then darken during puberty along with coarse hair development. Males are more often affected. Androgen is believed to play a major role in its development. It is usually unilateral, on chest, shoulder, lateral arm, and scapular regions. Hypertrichosis and acneiform lesions may be seen within Becker's nevus. Rare cases have been reported involving hands, feet, and segmental face with mucosa [55]. Becker's nevus syndrome is characterized by association with musculoskeletal abnormalities such as ipsilateral mammary hypoplasia or odontomaxillary dysplasia [56, 57]. Treatment is mainly reassurance and camouflage. Laser treatment of the hypertrichosis may be attempted with low-fluence high-repetition-rate diode lasers (808–810 nm) [58], and the pigmentation has been treated with long-pulsed ruby laser [59] and fractional resurfacing [60], although greater risk of dyspigmentation exists for patients of color.

Postinflammatory Hyperpigmentation

Many dermatologic diseases heal with hyperpigmentation or hypopigmentation, especially in darker skinned patients [61, 62]. The exact mechanism is not fully understood; however, many inflammatory mediators have been found to increase melanogenesis, such as interleukin 1 and 6 [62]. Other studies have suggested that epithelial–mesenchymal interactions via growth factors such as keratinocyte growth factor and fibroblast-derived growth factor modulate melanogenesis [63].

Friction Hypermelanosis

Friction hypermelanosis is an acquired hyperpigmentation resulting from continuous rubbing of the skin [64, 65]. Friction hypermelanosis is common in darker skin but it is not commonly observed in infants or young children. Unique curvilinear hyperpigmented patches were described in infants wearing tight socks and mittens for a prolonged length of time, also known as sock-line and mitten-line hyperpigmentation. The differential diagnosis includes child abuse and amniotic band syndrome [66]. Vertically oriented, round, discrete, hyperpigmented patches overlying the lumbosacral area have been described in an institutionalized orphan as a result of repetitive backward and forward movement, inspiring the name "orphan rocker tracks" [67]. A similar hyperpigmentation, Davener's dermatosis, has been described among young orthodox Jewish males who perform repetitive rocking motions during religious rituals [65].

Idiopathic Eruptive Macular Pigmentation

This condition presents in children and adolescents with sudden onset of multiple brown nonconfluent macules on the trunk, neck, face, and proximal extremities with no preceding inflammatory skin disease or medication administration [68, 69]. The pathogenesis in unknown, although hormonal etiology, has been suggested [68]. Histopathologic exam reveals basal cell layer hyperpigmentation and occasional dermal melanophages without structural changes in the basal layer or lichenoid inflammatory infiltrate. It is important to differentiate it from ashy dermatosis in which the macules are gray, sometimes with erythema, and basal layer vacuolization. Other differential diagnoses include pityriasis versicolor, urticaria pigmentosa, café-au-lait macules, and postinflammatory hyperpigmentation [68, 70]. It resolves over the course of a few months to years [68].

Reticulate Hyperpigmentation

Skin disorders with reticulate hyperpigmentation (net-like pattern) are not very common, and they can be idiopathic, genetic, or drug-induced. Family history, age of onset, race, sex, and distribution as well as full hair and skin exam are important when approaching the patient [71]. Confluent and reticulated papillomatosis (CARP) usually affects peripubertal females, presenting with reticulated hyperpigmented patches, papules, and plaques on the chest and upper back, sometimes axillae [72]. Prurigo pigmentosa, which has a similar distribution to CARP but affects young Japanese females, presents with pruritic inflammatory papules that heal with reticulate hyperpigmentation [73]. Both disorders have shown response to oral minocycline [74] and other tetracyclines.

Genetic disorders with reticulate hyperpigmentation are rare [75]. They can be generalized, flexural, and acral. Genital reticulate hyperpigmentation in association with vitiligo on the same skin area has been described [71, 75].

Disorders with Later Onset Hypopigmentation and Depigmentation

Postinflammatory Hypopigmentation and Depigmentation

Although acquired partial or total pigment loss affects all skin types, it is more noticeable and troublesome for darker skinned patients. Certain skin diseases have a tendency to resolve with postinflammatory hypopigmentation, including lichen striatus and pityriasis lichenoides chronica; infections such as impetigo, pityriasis versicolor, and chicken pox; and skin injuries such as burns and cryotherapy [76]. Leukotriene C4 released during inflammation was found to reduce melanogenesis [62].

Vitiligo

Vitiligo is a common disorder of acquired depigmentation, affecting 1–2% of the world population [77]. About half of the cases occur before the age of 20 and about one-fourth of total cases occur before the age of 8. No gender or skin phototype predilection is known [77, 78]. The underlying pathogenesis includes autoimmunity, genetic, neurologic, and biochemical events resulting in destruction of melanocytes [77–79]. Hypopigmented and depigmented macules or patches with focal, generalized, or segmental distribution is observed [77]. Trichrome vitiligo represents the combination of hypopigmentation, depigmentation, and normal skin pigment in the same patient [80]. Treatment of childhood vitiligo remains challenging; about one-third of patients do not respond to treatment [77–79]. Topical treatment is preferred in childhood vitiligo if less than 20% of body surface area (BSA) is involved, and includes topical steroids, topical calcineurin inhibitors, and calcipotriol. A combination of these may yield a better response in patients who have failed monotherapy [78]. Camouflage is a good option for small lesions or when side effects are a concern. Other treatment options include narrow-band UVB, excimer laser, surgical approaches including epidermal autotransplantation, intralesional steroid injection, and total depigmentation for the most extensive involvement [78, 79]. Many of these are difficult to perform on children without sedation.

Pityriasis Alba

Pityriasis alba is a common skin disorder affecting children 3–16 years of age, with higher incidence reported in patients of color and the atopic population [81–83]. It may be a mild form of atopic dermatitis, with spontaneous relapse and remission. Clinically, it can present with subtly erythematous and scaly, poorly defined small patches, typically on the cheeks, then hypopigmented patches with minimal to no scale [83]. Most patients present with poorly defined hypopigmentation and deny preceding inflammation. Differential diagnosis includes postinflammatory hypopigmentation and pityriasis versicolor. Photoprotection, emollients, topical tacrolimus [84], and low potency topical steroids may improve pityriasis alba [81].

Progressive Macular Hypomelanosis

Progressive macular hypomelanosis manifests as hypopigmented, non-scaly macules coalescing over the trunk. It usually affects adolescents, with no gender predilection [85]. Pathology shows only reduced melanin content compared to normal skin. The etiology remains unknown, although a *Propionibacterium* species is thought to play a role, causing red fluorescence under Wood's lamp and in some cases improving after treatment with benzoyl peroxide 5% gel with or without clindamycin 1% lotion [86–88]. Other treatment options include psoralen and Ultraviolet A (PUVA), narrow-band Ultraviolet B, and oral tetracycline derivatives [85, 87]. It is important to counsel the patient regarding the course and the outcome of the disease, as recurrence after successful treatment is often reported, and it may take up to 5 years before spontaneous regression, if any, is observed [85].

Clear Cell Papulosis

Clear cell papulosis is a rare entity predominantly affecting Asian children, between 4 months and 5 years of age. It presents with multiple asymptomatic non-scaly hypopigmented macules or thin papules on the lower abdomen and tends to follow mammary lines [89–92]. Pathology shows normal basal keratinocytes admixing with larger keratinocytes characterized by pale cytoplasm that stain positive for cytokeratin 7, EMA, CEA, and AE; therefore, some authors consider it a benign form of extramammary Paget disease [93]. Not all cases display reduced basal pigmentation, so the exact etiology of hypopigmentation remains unknown. Spontaneous regression has been reported [93].

Dermatitis

Atopic Dermatitis

Atopic dermatitis (AD) is the most common pediatric skin disorder; more than two-thirds of patients present before the age of 5 years [94, 95]. Genetic predisposition, barrier dysfunction, and cytokine signaling along with immunoglobulin switching are thought to contribute to etiology, and interestingly, recent studies have concluded that pediatric AD differs from adult AD in their pathophysiology [96, 97]. For example, pediatric AD patients display increased expression of CD69 on T cells soon after CD4 and CD8 are activated, but lower levels of IL-22, which increases susceptibility to infection [97]. IL-22 is believed to induce epidermal hyperplasia, suggesting that it plays an important role in chronic lesions, seen more in adults than in children with AD. About two-thirds of pediatric patients outgrow their AD within 10 years, likely due to upregulation of T_H1 and T_H17, resulting in decreased T_H2 and T_H22 levels [97].

African American (AA) patients reportedly have a higher incidence rate of AD, and of greater severity, compared to Asians and Caucasians [96]. Although studies on the structure and function of ethnic skin are limited and somewhat controversial, with conflicting results, some have shown that AA patients have the lowest ceramide-to-cholesterol ratio in the stratum corneum, higher transepidermal water loss, lower response to capsaicin, and decreased itch signaling due to lower pH levels in their skin [95, 98]. Genetic susceptibility also seems to differ in AA patients. Fewer AA patients have filaggrin mutations than their Caucasian counterparts, where filaggrin mutation is linked to AD susceptibility and severity [95]. Caucasian AD patients tend to develop eczematous plaques on extremity flexor surfaces while AA patients tend to alternatively or additionally develop discrete follicular papules, prurigo nodularis and lichen simplex chronicus or lichen planus-like lesions on the extensor extremities (Fig. 17.3). The infraorbital crease (commonly referred to as Dennie–Morgan lines) is a minor feature of AD often seen in AA and Asian patients, but is common among darker skinned children regardless of atopy, so its presence should not be overemphasized in diagnosing AD in these patients [99].

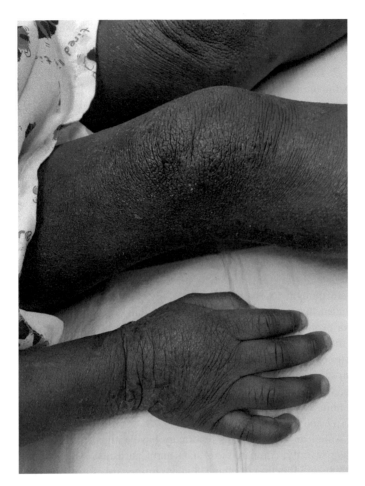

Fig. 17.3 Atopic dermatitis in a child with thick, lichenified plaques

Clinicians should tailor management toward individual symptoms and severity of skin findings (including degree of lichenification or presence of prurigo nodules), as well as comorbidities such as food and environmental allergies or superinfections. First-line therapy always involves optimization of baseline skin care using bland, hypoallergenic emollients, and cleansing regimens, and the safe but effective use of topical corticosteroids. Alternative or adjunctive strategies include wet wraps, antihistamines, calcineurin inhibitors, other nonsteroidal anti-inflammatory topicals, nb-UVB phototherapy, and systemic immunosuppressants [94, 95]. Phototherapy and systemic medications are reserved for severe, recalcitrant cases. Cyclosporine is often used as a first-line systemic agent due to its relatively rapid effect, and stopped upon resolution of clinical flaring or after transitioning to safer long-term systemic agents such as methotrexate, azathioprine, or mycophenolate mofetil [100, 101]. Several biologics are in clinical trials at the time of this printing.

Treatment of pediatric AD patients is the same regardless of skin pigmentation; however, while managing AA patients with AD, a few points should be considered. Hypopigmentation is usually postinflammatory but patient/parent concerns over corticosteroid-related hypopigmentation may affect compliance. Thicker plaques usually require more potent corticosteroids or topical treatment under occlusion [95]. Risk of azathioprine toxicity is higher in the AA population due to altered dosing requirements; there is reportedly a 20–30% decreased oral bioavailability and 17% reduction in thiopurine methyltransferase activity in these patients [102]. And finally, higher doses of nb-UVB may be needed to treat AA patients with AD [95].

Allergic Contact Dermatitis

Allergic contact dermatitis (ACD) in children is not uncommon and may even occur in early infancy [103]. Females are affected more than males [104]. Nickel remains the number one antigenic culprit; other common allergens include fragrance mix, lanolin, thimerosal, and neomycin [103, 104]. ACD in skin of color may be missed by clinicians unfamiliar with cultural practices, such as henna body art and early skin piercing, and undertreated by those unfamiliar with lichenification or lichenoid dermatitis as features of ACD in skin of color, or those who do not look for subtle erythema in pigmented skin [6]. Intricate skin art using traditional red henna (leaves of the plant *Lawsonia inermis* crushed into essential oils) is common in the Indian subcontinent and the Middle East, but ACD to red henna is rare; allergic contact dermatitis is more often caused by adulterated products termed 'black henna' in which p-phenylenediamine (PPD) is admixed with red henna [105]. Keloidal lesions, an erythema multiforme-like targetoid reaction, bullous, and generalized dermatitis due to black henna have been reported [105]. Patch testing may be needed to confirm a contact allergen [104], but patients should be cautioned about dyspigmentation in patch test sites. Education, allergen avoidance, and topical corticosteroids or steroid sparing agents for active dermatitis are all important in the management of ACD [106].

Seborrheic Dermatitis

Seborrheic dermatitis (SD) is a very common skin disorder that affects patients of all ages [107]. Incidence in infants reaches 42% [108]. *Malassezia furfur* overgrowth and/or hypersensitivity are thought to contribute to the etiology of SD, especially in adults, but the etiology of infantile SD remains uncertain; metabolic disturbance of essential fatty acids is assumed to play a role in the pathogenesis [109] while other studies have concluded that *Pityrosporum ovale* is likely to be the cause of infantile SD [110]. SD presents with nonpruritic, scaly, erythematous lesions on the scalp, face (eyebrows and paranasal skin), retro-auricular folds, flexures, and diaper region [107]. In dark-skinned patients, the erythema is not easily distinguished, and patients may present with scalp dandruff and hyperkeratosis that can be mistaken for tinea capitis, atopic dermatitis, or scalp psoriasis [111]. Also, they may present with hyper- or hypopigmented scaly lesions. Topical preparations are usually used to treat infantile SD, e.g., mineral oil or bland emollients to loosen scale, 2% ketoconazole shampoo, and topical steroids used with caution to prevent systemic absorption or atrophy [110].

Papulosquamous Disorders

Psoriasis

Psoriasis is a common chronic inflammatory skin disorder that affects children with an annual incidence of 40.8/100,000 found in one study of the US Midwest [112]. Similar to adults, the most common type of psoriasis in children is plaque-type psoriasis [113, 114]. Guttate, inverse, palmoplantar, and pustular psoriasis are also seen in pediatric patients [114, 115]. Guttate psoriasis is more often seen in children, tends to follow streptococcal infection more often than in plaque-type pediatric psoriasis, and tends to predict more severe psoriatic disease [116]. Scalp psoriasis was found to be more prevalent in girls while nail psoriasis was more common among boys. Nail psoriasis does not correlate with disease severity in pediatric patients, in contrast to what is observed in adults [113, 115]. Darker skin pigmentation may complicate the assessment of psoriasis severity beyond the greater difficulty observing erythema; one study found thicker plaques and more dyspigmentation in psoriasis in patients of color as compared to Caucasians [117]. Also, scalp psoriasis lesions in dark-skinned children may be more hyperkeratotic than in patients with lighter skin [111].

Pediatric psoriasis is generally treated with emollients, keratolytics, corticosteroids, and steroid sparing agents [118]. No standard guidelines exist for phototherapy, systemic, and biologic drugs for pediatric psoriasis [118]; many protocols are derived from adult psoriasis treatment regimens and other specialists' experience with biologics and systemic drugs used to treat children with rheumatoid arthritis, hematological malignancies, and Crohn's disease [118–120]. Psychological support is crucial for children with psoriasis, given that it is associated with obesity, hypertension, diabetes mellitus, and psychosocial stress [118, 121].

Pityriasis Rosea

Pityriasis rosea (PR) is a papulosquamous skin disorder of uncertain etiology that affects young individuals worldwide [122, 123]. It may be associated with human herpes virus 6 and 7. PR typically manifests as mildly pruritic erythematous thin papules and plaques with few scales on the trunk, erupting within a few weeks of the appearance of a *herald patch*—a single, relatively larger patch or plaque with raised scaly margins [122]. Atypical variants have been described, including inverse, unilateral, erythema multiforme-like, and generalized papular and papulovesicular PR [124–127]. Case reports and studies of dark-skinned individuals with this eruption have reported reduced or absent erythema, thicker scale, and significant itching in comparison to PR in light-skinned patients [123]. In addition, generalized papular, follicular, and erythema multiforme-like variants were noticed to be more prevalent among dark-skinned and Indian patients [124, 126, 127]. Facial distribution is also observed among African Americans with pityriasis rosea [123, 125]. About two-thirds of dark-skinned patients with PR heal with hyperpigmentation while postinflammatory hypopigmentation tends to be noticed after the papular variant resolves [123]. Pityriasis rosea tends to heal spontaneously; treatment is mainly to control the itching using antihistamines, emollients, and topical steroids. Phototherapy, systemic antibiotics, and antivirals have been used in severe and recalcitrant cases with different results [123, 128, 129]. The dyspigmentation left by this benign condition can be very obvious and quite upsetting to patients and parents.

Lichen Planus

Lichen planus (LP) is a chronic pruritic skin disorder that mainly affects adults [130]; however, studies from different countries have shown increasing rates among children, reaching ~ 11% of cases [130–134]. In one study of 36 children from the United States, childhood LP affected females twice as often as males, and 72% were African American [135]. Childhood lichen planus is not uncommon in India, Middle East, and Mexico [131, 133, 135]; a retrospective study in the United Kingdom showed that more than two-thirds of the children with lichen planus came from Indian descent [134]. The exact etiology remains unknown and many theories including autoimmune, infectious, genetic, Hepatitis B infection, and/or vaccination triggers have been suggested [130, 136]. Classic LP is the most common presentation of childhood lichen planus [135], but linear, annular, mucosal, bullous, and lichen planopilaris subtypes are also reported [133, 135, 137, 138]. In darker skinned patients, lichen planus lesions tend to be gray in color rather than violaceous, with persistent and severe postinflammatory hyperpigmentation [139]. Actinic lichen planus predominates in tropical areas [130, 132]. Treatment of childhood lichen planus is mainly achieved by the use of topical corticosteroids under occlusion and topical tacrolimus. Systemic drugs and phototherapy are reserved for eruptive, bullous, and recalcitrant cases [130, 138].

Acneiform Eruptions

Acne Vulgaris

Acne vulgaris is one of the most common skin disorders, affecting patients from all ethnic backgrounds and skin pigmentation [7, 140–142]. Due to the practice of applying heavy oils and thick pomades to their hair, African American patients tend to have more comedonal acne on the forehead, also known as *pomade acne* [143]. Newer trends in African American hair care practices such as chemical relaxation led to a reduction in the use of thick hair oils, eventually decreasing the incidence of pomade acne [139]. Postinflammatory hyperpigmentation is very common among patients with darker skin, and the application of cosmetic products used to cover the hyperpigmentation can lead to acne cosmetica among those groups [140–142]. Treatment of acne vulgaris in skin of color does not differ from that for other ethnic groups; however, patient education and counseling are crucial, as well as sensitivity toward the psychological impact of the hyperpigmentation and/or acne-related keloidal scarring [141, 144].

Periorificial Dermatitis

Periorificial dermatitis is an eruption of erythematous, flesh-colored papules in association with skin desquamation and rare pustules around the mouth, eyes, nose, and occasionally the vulva or perineum [145–147]. Topical corticosteroid application may play a role in the pathogenesis [145]. Histology may reflect a granulomatous dermatitis, as seen in reports of childhood granulomatous periorificial dermatitis, sarcoid-like granulomatous dermatitis, and facial Afro-Caribbean childhood eruption [145, 147]. Treatment includes discontinuing steroid application, topical 0.75% metronidazole [148], topical calcineurin inhibitors, and mupirocin [145]. Oral antibiotics such as tetracycline, doxycycline, and erythromycin have been used [145, 147].

Hair Disorders

Human hair can be categorized based on sulfur protein content, keratin type, and amino acid composition, but it is generally classified based on ethnic background, differentiating Caucasian, Asian and African American (AA) hair. AA hair shafts are elliptical in cross section, with a variable diameter along the hair shaft, and also characterized by random reversals and twisting. AA hair follicles are curved, with less elastic fiber content attaching it to the dermis, resulting in spiral, curly hair and higher risk for hair shedding and breakage [149]. AA hair dryness is due to decreased sebaceous gland activity and lower moisture content compared with other ethnic groups [149].

Trichorrhexis Nodosa

Trichorrhexis Nodosa is a congenital or acquired hair shaft disorder. Congenital cases are seen among various genetic diseases including trichothiodystrophy and Menkes kinky hair syndrome, while acquired cases are caused by excessive heat, forceful combing and prolonged chemical use. Patients usually present with complaints of brittle, dull hair appearance, and white spots along the hair shaft. Microscopic hair shaft exam reveals what looks like two paintbrushes facing each other, which represent the whitish dots along the hair shaft. Treatment of acquired trichorrhexis nodosa is mainly through reducing chemical and physical hair shaft trauma [149].

Traction Alopecia

Traction is a common cause of hair loss that occurs as a result of prolonged tension applied on the hair, leading to clinical or subclinical inflammation of the hair follicles. It usually starts during childhood and might progress to permanent loss of the hair follicles. Traction alopecia predominantly affects AA females, with onset reportedly as young as 8 months of age. In one clinic population the prevalence of traction alopecia in AA females between the ages of 5 and 14.5 years was 18% [150]. Another study showed that African schoolchildren with traction alopecia increased from 8.6% in the first year of school to 21.7% in the last year of high school [151]. Traction alopecia is usually marginal frontal and/or temporal, with the presence of fringe hair. Hair casts in a biopsy indicate ongoing traction alopecia. Treatment is mainly through prevention and education.

Tinea Capitis

Tinea capitis is the most common fungal infection affecting the pediatric population. AA children have the highest incidence rate, in males more than females. *Trichophyton tonsurans* is an anthropophilic organism; it remains the most common causative agent of tinea capitis in North America. *Microsporum canis* is the most frequent cause of zoophilic tinea capitis [152]. In AA patients, tinea capitis may manifest as non-inflammatory disease with patches of hair loss, hyperkeratosis, or breakage of the hair shaft at the scalp surface (black dot tinea). Another clinical presentation is kerion, a tender, boggy, sometimes purulent plaque in a patient who may also have fever, malaise, and occipital lymphadenopathy. Bright green fluorescence with Wood's lamp is seen only in ectothrix fungi such as *M. canis*. It is negative in the presence of *T. tonsurans*, an endothrix infection. Dermoscopic examination reveals comma-shaped and corkscrew hair shafts. Hair culture is negative in up to 50% of cases [111, 153] so clinical features and history are important. Differential diagnoses of non-inflammatory tinea capitis with scalp hyperkeratosis include seborrheic dermatitis and atopic dermatitis, or rarer cause such as collagen vascular diseases and Langerhans cell histiocytosis, where erythema is difficult to appreciate in dark skin [111].

Tinea capitis is frequently undertreated and physicians tend to prescribe low doses of antifungal medication, resulting in frequent relapses once treatment is discontinued. While terbinafine, fluconazole, and pulsed itraconazole can be used for shorter or more convenient regimens, griseofulvin is still widely used by pediatric dermatologists due to its cost and safety profile. In cases of *M. canis* fungal infection, a longer duration of therapy is usually required [153].

Piedra

Piedra is a superficial fungal infection characterized by easily detachable gritty white or yellowish nodules (white piedra) or black nodules (black piedra) on hair shafts, usually of the axilla or scalp [154–156]. Black piedra is caused by *Piedraia hortae* while white piedra is caused by *Trichosporon* species. Most reported cases in the United States have been in immigrants from tropical regions [155]. Piedra affects females more than males, although in genital hair white piedra is more prevalent in black males [156]. Humid climate, poor hygiene, and the practice of veil hair covering have been implicated in the pathogenesis [157, 158]. They present easily detachable gritty nodules on the scalp, facial, or genital hair [154–156]. Diagnosis is based on the clinical presentation, KOH, and fungal cultures [152, 153]. Treatment is mainly achieved through hair shaving, although this is usually not desirable for scalp involvement. Oral azoles and topical antifungal shampoos have been successfully used with variable reported recurrence rates [154–157].

Vesicular and Pustular Diseases in Newborns

Transient neonatal pustular melanosis and infantile acropustulosis are seen more often in skin of color. Conversely, miliaria is less common, due to more efficient body temperature regulation with less sweating compared to white skin [6].

Transient Neonatal Pustular Melanosis

Transient neonatal pustular melanosis (TNPM) predominantly affects black new-borns with a 4.4–15% incidence rate [6, 159, 160]. It usually presents at birth as innumerable, superficial pustules without surrounding erythema. Pustular lesions last up to 2 days, and then heal leaving delicate collarettes of scale around hyperpigmented macules, which take from 2 weeks to months to fade [159]. Pustules may not be seen due to disruption perinatally. An infant born with multiple hyperpigmented macules that fade away over weeks to months (unlike true lentigines that do not fade) can be presumed to have had TNPM pustules in utero [160]. A smear of pustular contents yields abundant neutrophils with rare eosino-phils and Gram's stain is negative (ruling out staphylococcus bullous impetigo) [6]. Biopsy is rarely necessary for diagnosis but shows corneal and subcorneal pustules with abundant neutrophils and rare eosinophils, while hyperpigmented macular lesions show basal layer hyperpigmentation and hyperkeratosis [6, 159]. The main differential diagnosis is erythema toxicum neonatorum (ETN), which can be differentiated by the presence of erythema surrounding the pustules, although this may be difficult to recognize in darkly pigmented infants [6]. In ETN, eosinophils predominate on smear and histopathologic exams [6, 160].

Infantile Acropustulosis

Infantile acropustulosis (IA) is a rare disorder that primarily affects black males 2–10 months of age [6, 159]. It presents with recurrent 1–3 mm acral vesicles and pustules that appear in crops, occasionally at non-acral sites [160]. Lesions are intensely pruritic, last for 1–2 weeks, and then spontaneously remit until the next crop of lesions appears. IA eventually resolves within 2–3 years [159]. It is frequently misdiagnosed as scabies; other differential diagnoses include dyshidrotic eczema, hand–foot–mouth disease, transient neonatal pustular melanosis, and erythema toxi-cum neonatorum [159, 161]. If biopsied, histopathologic exam reveals subcorneal and intraepidermal neutrophilic pustules, mild perivascular lymphohistiocytic infiltrate and rare eosinophils [160]. Treatment includes topical steroids and antihistamines for intense pruritus [160, 162]. IA has been successfully treated with dapsone 2 mg/kg/day with tapering over the following few months to prevent relapse [6, 162].

Pediatric Malignancies

Skin cancers are rare in children. Most of the malignancies in darker skinned patients are described in the literature as case reports. Hypopigmented mycosis fungoides (MF) is more prevalent in patients of color. It has a chronic course that rarely progresses and responds well to topical steroids and phototherapy; however, recurrence after successful treatment is often seen [163]. Malignant melanoma has been reported within nevus of Ito [27] and nevus of Ota [25]. Malignant blue nevus arising within giant blue nevus in an infant has been described [28]. Childhood subungual malignant melanoma in situ is rare; no case of invasive subungual melanoma has been reported in children [47]. It has been argued that these reported cases of childhood subungual malignant melanoma in situ may in fact have been atypical melanocytic nevi because pediatric pigmented lesions in general display more atypia compared to lesions in adults [48].

Conclusion and Psychosocial Considerations

For the pediatric patient of color, skin conditions that alter pigmentation primarily, such as vitiligo or albinism [164, 165] and birthmarks (Figs. 17.4 and 17.5), or secondary to inflammation, as in atopic dermatitis, psoriasis, or ichthyosis, can significantly impair quality of life [165]. Devastating effects have been recorded cross-culturally and interracially. Children with visible differences are vulnerable to discrimination and bullying [166]. They often face other social challenges involving peer relationships during games and sports, as well as reduced academic performance [165, 167, 168]. These incidents influence future social engagement; fear of reliving a traumatizing event sometimes results in "safety-seeking behaviors" such as concealing the affected area with clothing or camouflage make-up, and avoiding activities that require skin exposure, such as swimming [169]. In addition, these conditions have an impact upon confidence, self-consciousness, shyness, and general happiness [165, 167, 168, 170, 171]. If prolonged, negative social and psychological experiences may precipitate mental illness; Picardi et al. found that 25% of patients with diverse skin conditions experience significant psychological distress and psychiatric morbidity [172]. While some children and young adults with skin conditions are remarkably confident and resilient, others may experience depressive symptoms, true clinical depression, anxiety, and suicidal ideation [165, 168, 173–178]. It is important to keep in mind that a clinician's objective assessment of a patient's skin condition does not correlate with the patient's self-perception and distress [179].

In children with atopic dermatitis there is a direct relationship between dermatologic disease severity and psychological disturbances [176]. Maladaptive effects may be due to a combination of the physical lesions, the signature pruritus, and secondary dyspigmentation. In some cultures, postinflammatory hyperpigmentation on the neck is sometimes called "atopic dirty neck," which adds the misperception of poor hygiene to the already challenging social experience of this condition [180]. Chronic pruritus can also cause fussiness, irritability, and significant problems with sleep and concentration [176, 181].

58. Lapidoth M, et al. Hypertrichosis in Becker's nevus: effective low-fluence laser hair removal. Lasers Med Sci. 2014;29(1):191–3.

59. Nanni CA, Alster TS. Treatment of a Becker's nevus using a 694-nm long-pulsed ruby laser. Dermatol Surg. 1998;24(9):1032–4.

60. Glaich AS, et al. Fractional resurfacing: a new therapeutic modality for Becker's nevus. Arch Dermatol. 2007;143(12):1488–90.

61. Taylor SC. Skin of color: biology, structure, function, and implications for dermatologic disease. J Am Acad Dermatol. 2002;46(2 Suppl Understanding):S41–62.

62. Halder RM, Nootheti PK. Ethnic skin disorders overview. J Am Acad Dermatol. 2003; 48(6, Supplement):S143–8.

63. Cardinali G, Kovacs D, Picardo M. Mechanisms underlying post-inflammatory hyperpigmentation: lessons from solar lentigo. Ann Dermatol Venereol. 2012;139(Suppl 4):S148–52.

64. Magaña M, Herrera-Goepfert R. Friction hypermelanosis: other variants. J Am Acad Dermatol. 2002;47(3):454.

65. Naimer SA, et al. Davener's dermatosis: a variant of friction hypermelanosis. J Am Acad Dermatol. 2000;42(3):442–5.

66. Ciliberto H, et al. Heel-line hyperpigmentation: a variant of sock-line hyperpigmentation after the use of heel-length socks. Pediatr Dermatol. 2013;30(4):473–5.

67. Diamond G, Ben D. Amitai, Orphan rocker tracks: a variant of friction melanosis in an institutionalized child. Pediatr Dermatol. 2013;30(6):e198–9.

68. Jang K-A, et al. Idiopathic eruptive macular pigmentation: report of 10 cases. J Am Acad Dermatol. 2001;44(2, Part 2):351–3.

69. Rodríguez VG, et al. Idiopathic eruptive macular pigmentation: a diagnostic challenge. J Am Acad Dermatol. 2011;64(2, Supplement 1):AB132.

70. Abbas O. Asymptomatic hyperpigmented macules. Pediatr Dermatol. 2015;32(5):733–4.

71. Chang MW. Disorders of hyperpigmentation. In: Bolognia J, Jorizzo JL, Schaffer JV, editors. Dermatology. Philadelphia: Elsevier Saunders. 2012. p. 1 online resource (2 v. in 1).

72. Wiesenborn A, Hengge U, Megahed M. Confluent and reticulated papillomatosis. Gougerot-Carteaud disease. Hautarzt. 2004;55(10):976–8.

73. Beutler BD, Cohen PR, Lee RA. Prurigo pigmentosa: literature review. Am J Clin Dermatol. 2015;16(6):533–43.

74. Ilkovitch D, Patton TJ. Is prurigo pigmentosa an inflammatory version of confluent and reticulated papillomatosis? J Am Acad Dermatol. 2013;69(4):e193–5.

75. Alfadley A, et al. Reticulate acropigmentation of Dohi: a case report of autosomal recessive inheritance. J Am Acad Dermatol. 2000;43(1, Part 1):113–7.

76. Vachiramon V, Thadanipon K. Postinflammatory hypopigmentation. Clin Exp Dermatol. 2011;36(7):708–14.

77. Phiske MM. Childhood vitiligo. Curr Rheumatol Rev. 2015.

78. Tamesis MEB, Morelli JG. Vitiligo treatment in childhood: a state of the art review. Pediatr Dermatol. 2010;27(5):437–45.

79. Ezzedine K, Silverberg N. A practical approach to the diagnosis and treatment of vitiligo in children. Pediatrics. 2016;138(1).

80. Hann SK, et al. Clinical and histopathologic characteristics of trichrome vitiligo. J Am Acad Dermatol. 2000;42(4):589–96.

81. Miazek N, et al. Pityriasis alba—common disease, enigmatic entity: up-to-date review of the literature. Pediatr Dermatol. 2015;32(6):786–91.

82. Jadotte YT, Janniger CK. Pityriasis alba revisited: perspectives on an enigmatic disorder of childhood. Cutis. 2011;87(2):66–72.

83. Blessmann Weber M, et al. Pityriasis alba: a study of pathogenic factors. J Eur Acad Dermatol Venereol. 2002;16(5):463–8.

84. Rigopoulos D, et al. Tacrolimus ointment 0.1% in pityriasis alba: an open-label, randomized, placebo-controlled study. Br J Dermatol. 2006;155(1):152–5.

85. Martínez-Martínez ML, et al. Progressive macular hypomelanosis. Pediatr Dermatol. 2012;29(4):460–2.

86. Cavalcanti SM, et al. The use of lymecycline and benzoyl peroxide for the treatment of progressive macular hypomelanosis: a prospective study. An Bras Dermatol. 2011;86(4):813–4.
87. Kim MB, et al. Narrowband UVB treatment of progressive macular hypomelanosis. J Am Acad Dermatol. 2012;66(4):598–605.
88. Cavalcanti SM, et al. Investigation of *Propionibacterium acnes* in progressive macular hypomelanosis using real-time PCR and culture. Int J Dermatol. 2011;50(11):1347–52.
89. Taylor S, Kircik L. Community-based trial results of combination acne therapy in subjects with skin of color: postinflammatory hyperpigmentation. J Am Acad Dermatol. 2008;58(2, Supplement 2):AB13.
90. Wysong A, Sundram U, Benjamin L. Clear-cell papulosis: a rare entity that may be misconstrued pathologically as normal skin. Pediatr Dermatol. 2012;29(2):195–8.
91. Tseng FW, et al. Long-term follow-up study of clear cell papulosis. J Am Acad Dermatol. 2010;63(2):266–73.
92. Kim SW, Roh J, Park CS. Clear cell papulosis: a case report. J Pathol Transl Med. 2016.
93. Sim JH, Do JE, Kim YC. Clear cell papulosis of the skin: acquired hypomelanosis. Arch Dermatol. 2011;147(1):128–9.
94. Eichenfield LF, et al. Guidelines of care for the management of atopic dermatitis: Section 1. Diagnosis and assessment of atopic dermatitis. J Am Acad Dermatol. 2014;70(2):338–51.
95. Vachiramon V, et al. Atopic dermatitis in African American children: addressing unmet needs of a common disease. Pediatr Dermatol. 2012;29(4):395–402.
96. Shaw TE, et al. Eczema prevalence in the United States: data from the 2003 National Survey of Children's Health. J Invest Dermatol. 2011;131(1):67–73.
97. Czarnowicki T, et al. Early pediatric atopic dermatitis shows only a cutaneous lymphocyte antigen (CLA)(+) TH2/TH1 cell imbalance, whereas adults acquire CLA(+) TH22/TC22 cell subsets. J Allergy Clin Immunol. 2015;136(4):941–951.e3.
98. Wang H, et al. Ethnic differences in pain, itch and thermal detection in response to topical capsaicin: African Americans display a notably limited hyperalgesia and neurogenic inflammation. Br J Dermatol. 2010;162(5):1023–9.
99. Williams HC, Pembroke AC. Infraorbital crease, ethnic group, and atopic dermatitis. Arch Dermatol. 1996;132(1):51–4.
100. Slater NA, Morrell DS. Systemic therapy of childhood atopic dermatitis. Clin Dermatol. 2015;33(3):289–99.
101. Galli E, et al. Consensus conference on clinical management of pediatric atopic dermatitis. Ital J Pediatr. 2016;42:26.
102. McLeod HL, et al. Thiopurine methyltransferase activity in American white subjects and black subjects. Clin Pharmacol Ther. 1994;55(1):15–20.
103. Sharma VK, Asati DP. Pediatric contact dermatitis. Indian J Dermatol Venereol Leprol. 2010;76(5):514–20.
104. Mortz CG, et al. Prevalence of atopic dermatitis, asthma, allergic rhinitis, and hand and contact dermatitis in adolescents. The Odense Adolescence Cohort Study on Atopic Diseases and Dermatitis. Br J Dermatol. 2001;144(3):523–32.
105. Almeida PJ, et al. Quantification of p-phenylenediamine and 2-hydroxy-1,4-naphthoquinone in henna tattoos. Contact Dermatitis. 2012;66(1):33–7.
106. Lee PW, Elsaie ML, Jacob SE. Allergic contact dermatitis in children: common allergens and treatment: a review. Curr Opin Pediatr. 2009;21(4):491–8.
107. Sampaio AL, et al. Seborrheic dermatitis. An Bras Dermatol. 2011;86(6):1061–71; quiz 1072–4.
108. Borda LJ, Wikramanayake TC. Seborrheic dermatitis and dandruff: a comprehensive review. J Clin Investig Dermatol. 2015;3(2).
109. Tollesson A, Frithz A, Stenlund K. Malassezia furfur in infantile seborrheic dermatitis. Pediatr Dermatol. 1997;14(6):423–5.
110. Gupta AK, Bluhm R. Seborrheic dermatitis. J Eur Acad Dermatol Venereol. 2004;18(1):13–26.

111. Silverberg NB. Scalp hyperkeratosis in children with skin of color: diagnostic and therapeutic considerations. Cutis. 2015;95(4):199–204, 207.
112. Tollefson MM, et al. Incidence of psoriasis in children: a population-based study. J Am Acad Dermatol. 2010;62(6):979–87.
113. Mercy K, et al. Clinical manifestations of pediatric psoriasis: results of a multicenter study in the United States. Pediatr Dermatol. 2013;30(4):424–8.
114. Arese V, et al. Juvenile psoriasis: an epidemiological study of 69 cases in the universitary dermatology clinic in Turin. G Ital Dermatol Venereol. 2016 Jun 30 (Epub ahead of print).
115. Morris A, et al. Childhood psoriasis: a clinical review of 1262 cases. Pediatr Dermatol. 2001;18(3):188–98.
116. Conrado LA, et al. Body dysmorphic disorder among dermatologic patients: prevalence and clinical features. J Am Acad Dermatol. 2010;63(2):235–43.
117. McMichael AJ, et al. Psoriasis in African-Americans: a caregivers' survey. J Drugs Dermatol. 2012;11(4):478–82.
118. Bronckers IM, et al. Psoriasis in children and adolescents: diagnosis, management and comorbidities. Paediatr Drugs. 2015;17(5):373–84.
119. Napolitano M, et al. Systemic treatment of pediatric psoriasis: a review. Dermatol Ther (Heidelb). 2016;6(2):125–42.
120. Saikaly SK, Mattes M. Biologics and pediatric generalized pustular psoriasis: an emerging therapeutic trend. Cureus. 2016;8(6):e652.
121. Gutmark-Little I, Shah KN. Obesity and the metabolic syndrome in pediatric psoriasis. Clin Dermatol. 2015;33(3):305–15.
122. Gündüz Ö, Ersoy-Evans S, Karaduman A. Childhood pityriasis rosea. Pediatric Dermatol. 2009;26(6):750–1.
123. Amer A, Fischer H, Li X. The natural history of pityriasis rosea in black American children: how correct is the "classic" description? Arch Pediatr Adolesc Med. 2007;161(5):503–6.
124. Zawar V, Chuh A. Follicular pityriasis rosea. A case report and a new classification of clinical variants of the disease. J Dermatol Case Rep. 2012;6(2):36–9.
125. Vano-Galvan S, et al. Atypical Pityriasis rosea in a black child: a case report. Cases J. 2009;2:6796.
126. Sinha S, Sardana K, Garg VK. Coexistence of two atypical variants of pityriasis rosea: a case report and review of literature. Pediatr Dermatol. 2012;29(4):538–40.
127. Das A, et al. A case series of erythema multiforme-like pityriasis rosea. Indian Dermatol Online J. 2016;7(3):212–5.
128. Jairath V, et al. Narrowband UVB phototherapy in pityriasis rosea. Indian Dermatol Online J. 2015;6(5):326–9.
129. Drago F, Rebora A. Treatments for pityriasis rosea. Skin Therapy Lett. 2009;14(3):6–7.
130. Kumar V, et al. Childhood lichen planus (LP). J Dermatol. 1993;20(3):175–7.
131. Nanda A, et al. Childhood lichen planus: a report of 23 cases. Pediatr Dermatol. 2001;18(1): 1–4.
132. Luis-Montoya P, Dominguez-Soto L, Vega-Memije E. Lichen planus in 24 children with review of the literature. Pediatr Dermatol. 2005;22(4):295–8.
133. Kanwar AJ, De D. Lichen planus in children. Indian J Dermatol Venereol Leprol. 2010;76(4): 366–72.
134. Balasubramaniam P, Ogboli M, Moss C. Lichen planus in children: review of 26 cases. Clin Exp Dermatol. 2008;33(4):457–9.
135. Walton KE, et al. Childhood lichen planus: demographics of a U.S. population. Pediatr Dermatol. 2010;27(1):34–8.
136. Limas C, Limas CJ. Lichen planus in children: a possible complication of hepatitis B vaccines. Pediatr Dermatol. 2002;19(3):204–9.
137. Kabbash C, et al. Lichen planus in the lines of Blaschko. Pediatr Dermatol. 2002;19(6):541–5.
138. Cohen DM, et al. Childhood lichen planus pemphigoides: a case report and review of the literature. Pediatr Dermatol. 2009;26(5):569–74.

139. Nnoruka EN. Lichen planus in African children: a study of 13 patients. Pediatr Dermatol. 2007;24(5):495–8.
140. Taylor SC, et al. Acne vulgaris in skin of color. J Am Acad Dermatol. 2002;46(2 Suppl Understanding):S98–106.
141. Davis EC, Callender VD. A review of acne in ethnic skin: pathogenesis, clinical manifestations, and management strategies. J Clin Aesthet Dermatol. 2010;3(4):24–38.
142. Alexis AF, Sergay AB, Taylor SC. Common dermatologic disorders in skin of color: a comparative practice survey. Cutis. 2007;80(5):387–94.
143. Arfan ul, Bari, Khan MB. Dermatological disorders related to cultural practices in black Africans of Sierra Leone. J Coll Physicians Surg Pak. 2007;17(5):249–52.
144. Shah SK, Alexis AF. Acne in skin of color: practical approaches to treatment. J Dermatolog Treat. 2010;21(3):206–11.
145. Nguyen V, Eichenfield LF. Periorificial dermatitis in children and adolescents. J Am Acad Dermatol. 2006;55(5):781–5.
146. Kuflik JH, Janniger CK, Piela Z. Perioral dermatitis: an acneiform eruption. Cutis. 2001;67 (1):21–2.
147. Knautz MA, Lesher JL. Childhood granulomatous periorificial dermatitis. Pediatr Dermatol. 1996;13(2):131–4.
148. Rodriguez-Caruncho C, et al. Childhood granulomatous periorificial dermatitis with a good response to oral metronidazole. Pediatr Dermatol. 2013;30(5):e98–9.
149. Rodney IJ, et al. Hair and scalp disorders in ethnic populations. J Drugs Dermatol. 2013; 12(4):420–7.
150. Mirmirani P, Khumalo NP. Traction alopecia: how to translate study data for public education—closing the KAP gap? Dermatol Clin. 2014;32(2):153–61.
151. Khumalo NP, et al. Hairdressing is associated with scalp disease in African schoolchildren. Br J Dermatol. 2007;157(1):106–10.
152. Mirmirani P, Tucker L-Y. Epidemiologic trends in pediatric tinea capitis: a population-based study from Kaiser Permanente Northern California. J Am Acad Dermatol. 2013;69(6): 916–21.
153. Gupta AK, et al. Tinea capitis: an overview with emphasis on management. Pediatr Dermatol. 1999;16(3):171–89.
154. Bonifaz A, et al. Tinea versicolor, tinea nigra, white piedra, and black piedra. Clin Dermatol. 2010;28(2):140–5.
155. Kiken DA, et al. White piedra in children. J Am Acad Dermatol. 2006;55(6):956–61.
156. Kalter DC, et al. Genital white piedra: epidemiology, microbiology, and therapy. J Am Acad Dermatol. 1986;14(6):982–93.
157. Viswanath V, et al. White piedra of scalp hair by *Trichosporon inkin*. Indian J Dermatol Venereol Leprol. 2011;77(5):591–3.
158. Desai DH, Nadkarni NJ. Piedra: an ethnicity-related trichosis? Int J Dermatol. 2014;53 (8):1008–11.
159. Van Praag MCG. et al. Diagnosis and Treatment of Pustular Disorders in the Neonate. Pediatric Dermatology. 1997;14(2):131–143.
160. Ghosh S. Neonatal pustular dermatosis: an overview. Indian J Dermatol. 2015;60(2):211.
161. Jennings JL, Burrows WM. Infantile acropustulosis. J Am Acad Dermatol. 1983;9(5):733–8.
162. Mancini AJ, Frieden IJ, Paller AS. Infantile Acropustulosis Revisited: History of Scabies and Response to Topical Corticosteroids. Pediatric Dermatology. 1998;15(5):337–341.
163. Castano E, et al. Hypopigmented mycosis fungoides in childhood and adolescence: a long-term retrospective study. J Cutan Pathol. 2013;40(11):924–34.
164. Westhoff W. A psychosocial study of albinism in a predominately mulatto Caribbean community. Psychol Rep. 1993;73(3):1007–10.
165. Dertlioğlu SB, Cicek D, Balci DD, Halisdemir N. Dermatology life quality index scores in children with vitiligo: comparison with atopic dermatitis and healthy control subjects. Int J Dermatol. 2012;52(1):96–101.

166. Magin P, Adams J, Heading G, Pond D, Smith W. Experiences of appearance-related teasing and bullying in skin diseases and their psychological sequelae: results of a qualitative study. Scand J Caring Sci. 2008;22(3):430–6.
167. Noor Aziah MS, Rosnah T, Mardziah A, Norzila MZ. Atopic dermatitis: a measurement of quality of life and family impact. Med J Malaysia. 2002;57(3):329–39.
168. Ganemo A, Lindholm C, Lindberg M, Sjoden P-O, Vahlquist A. Quality of life in adults with congenital ichthyosis. J Adv Nurs. 2003;44(4):412–9.
169. Thompson AR. Body issues in dermatology. In: Cash TF, Smolak L, editors. Body image, a handbook of science, practice, and prevention. New York: Guilford Press; 2012.
170. Thompson A, Kent G. Adjusting to disfigurement: processes involved in dealing with being visibly different. Clin Psychol Rev. 2001;21(5):663–82.
171. Nguyen CM, Koo J, Cordoro KM. Psychodermatologic effects of atopic dermatitis and acne: a review on self-esteem and identity. Pediatr Dermatol. 2016;33(2):129–35.
172. Picardi A, Abeni D, Melchi C, Puddu P, Pasquini P. Psychiatric morbidity in dermatological outpatients: an issue to be recognized. Br J Dermatol. 2000;143(5):983–91.
173. Bilgiç Ö, Bilgiç A, Akiş HK, Eskioğlu F, Kiliç EZ. Depression, anxiety and health-related quality of life in children and adolescents with vitiligo. Clin Exp Dermatol. 2010;36(4):360–5.
174. Alghamdi KM. Beliefs and perceptions of Arab vitiligo patients regarding their condition. Int J Dermatol. 2010;49(10):1141–5.
175. Mattoo S, Handa S, Kaur I, Gupta N, Malhotra R. Psychiatric morbidity in vitiligo: prevalence and correlates in India. J Eur Acad Dermatol Venereol. 2002;16(6):573–8.
176. Absolon CM, Cottrell D, Eldridge SM, Glover MT. Psychological disturbance in atopic eczema: the extent of the problem in school-aged children. Br J Dermatol. 1997;137(2):241–5.
177. Kimata H. Prevalence of suicidal ideation in patients with atopic dermatitis. Suicide Life Threat Behav. 2006;36:120–4.
178. Tareen RS, Tareen AN. Psychiatric disorders frequently encountered in dermatology practices. In: Tareen RS, Gredanus DE, Jafferany M, Patel DR, Merrick J, editors. Pediatric psychodermatology: a clinical manual of child and adolescent psychocutaneous disorders. Boston: De Gruyter; 2013.
179. Richards HL, Fortune DG, Weidmann A, Sweeney SK, Griffiths CE. Detection of psychological distress in patients with psoriasis; low consensus between dermatologist and patient. Br J Dermatol. 2004;151:1227–33.
180. Seghers AC, et al. Atopic dirty neck or acquired atopic hyperpigmentation? An epidemiological and clinical study from the National Skin Centre in Singapore. Dermatology. 2014;229(3):174–82.
181. Chamlin SL, Frieden IJ, Williams ML, Chren M. Effects of atopic dermatitis on young american children and their families. Pediatrics. 2004;114(3):607–11.
182. Naqvi H, Saul K. Culture and ethnicity. In: Rumsey N, Harcourt D, editors. The Oxford handbook of the psychology of appearance. Oxford: Oxford University Press; 2012.
183. Papadopoulos L, Bor R, Walker C, Flaxman P, Legg C. Different shades of meaning: illness beliefs among vitiligo sufferers. Psychol Health Med. 2002;7(4):425–33.
184. Ersser SJ, et al. Psychological and educational interventions for atopic eczema in children. Cochrane Database Syst Rev. 2015;4:CD009660.
185. Mitchell AE, et al. Childhood atopic dermatitis: a cross-sectional study of relationships between child and parent factors, atopic dermatitis management, and disease severity. Int J Nurs Stud. 2015;52(1):216–28.

Chapter 18
The Anthropology of Human Scalp Hair

Ophelia E. Dadzie, Tina Lasisi and Nina G. Jablonski

Hair is predominantly a proteinaceous fiber that originates from hair follicles located within the subcutis and/or dermis of the skin. It is one of the defining features of mammals, serving important functions, such as thermoregulation and endothermy. Among mammals, humans are exceptional in lacking a full covering of body hair [1]. Instead the growth of terminal hairs is limited to specific body regions, such as the scalp, axillae, and groin.

Our aim in this chapter is to provide an overview of the anthropology of human scalp hair. We will explore the diversity of human scalp hair and its evolutionary history. We will also discuss:

- Approaches to the study of variation in human scalp hair phenotypes
- The genetic basis of human scalp hair diversity

O.E. Dadzie (✉)
Departments of Dermatology and Histopathology, The Hillingdon Hospitals
NHS Foundation Trust, Pield Heath Road, Uxbridge, UK
e-mail: Opheliadadzie@nhs.net

O.E. Dadzie
Imperial College London, University of London, London, UK

T. Lasisi
Department of Anthropology, The Pennsylvania State University,
409 Carpenter Building, University Park, State College, PA 16802, USA
e-mail: tpl5158@psu.edu

N.G. Jablonski
Department of Anthropology, Center for Human Evolution and Diversity, The Huck
Institutes of the Life Sciences, The Pennsylvania State University, 409 Carpenter
Building, University Park, State College, PA 16802, USA
e-mail: ngj2@psu.edu

© Springer International Publishing AG 2017
N.A. Vashi and H.I. Maibach (eds.), *Dermatoanthropology of Ethnic Skin and Hair*, DOI 10.1007/978-3-319-53961-4_18

315

- The biology of human scalp hair, with emphasis on quantitative and qualitative differences among populations
- Hair grooming practices taking into account hair fiber characteristics and societal/cultural influences.

We have omitted discussions about the anthropology of human non-scalp hair. This is deliberate because the scientific literature about this topic is confusing and controversial.

Approaches to the Study of Variation in Human Scalp Hair Phenotypes

Scalp hair varies in appearance between human populations, and has long interested philosophers, systematists, naturalists, and anthropologists [2, 3]. Since the eighteenth century, characteristics of scalp hair color and texture were used along with other physical traits such as skin color, and some perceived behavioral attributes, to define races. Despite the complete discrediting of the concept of biological race, classifications of human scalp hair "types" associated with these obsolete race definitions have stuck, namely "African," "Asian," and "Caucasian." This race-based classification system is simplistic, archaic, and misleading because it does not account for the diversity within and between populations. These names given to these types, far from capturing the nature of existing variation in human hair, reflect a history of choices made by researchers with regard to the populations studied and the differences noted. In reality, the various aspects of hair morphology (i.e., thickness, shaft curvature, and color) each exist in a continuous spectrum that can be found in numerous combinations around the world. There are no discrete hair "types."

Variation in human hair has been measured by a range of methods and techniques. Hair color has been, and is still, predominantly visually assessed and described [4]. However, other methods of evaluating hair color have been used. For example, the Fischer-Saller scale (comparable to the Von Luschan scale for skin color) is a comparative method of assessing hair pigmentation on the basis of a set of hair swatches in a gradation of colors [5]. Reflectance spectrometry has been increasingly used to provide a quantitative measure of hair color, because it allows for a more accurate representation of the continuous nature of hair color [6, 7]. Studies of the chemical composition of hair, involving quantification of pheomelanin and eumelanin content, have also helped to shed light on how variation in melanin coloration is related to color phenotype [8]. Forensic anthropologists, among others, have also noted variation in the distribution of pigment granules within the hair shaft, which provides yet another method by which variation in hair color can be evaluated [9]. Anthropological research on normal variation in hair color has focused mostly on populations of European descent because variation in light-colored hair is readily perceptible [10, 11]. Populations of non-European descent are frequently considered as homogenously dark-haired even though measurable variation exists.

Hair form, like hair color, has mostly been assessed by visual means [12]. The two main aspects of hair form of interest have been cross-sectional geometry and (longitudinal) degree of curvature or curling. While many descriptive typologies have been proposed for classifying hair from straight to curly, a method for quantification of the curvature of the shaft was not developed until the 1970s [13]. Since the nineteenth century, cross-sectional geometry of the hair shaft has been assessed under the microscope with particular attention being paid to differences between populations in cross-sectional area (thickness), as well as cross-sectional shape [14]. The lack of discrete population groupings in hair shape, and the emergence of new hair shape phenotypes as the result of recent population admixture prompted Loussouarn and coworkers to develop a novel classification system based on objective criteria of human scalp hair fibers [3]. This includes:

- Curve diameter
- Curl index
- The highest number of waves
- The number of twists.

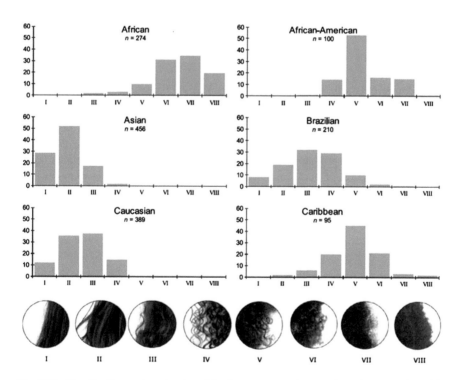

Fig. 18.1 Classification system developed by Loussouarn and co-workers demonstrating eight distinct phenotypes independent of ethnicity and race. From Salam et al. [56] with permission

This system divides human scalp hair phenotypes into eight distinct groups independent of ethnicity and race (Fig. 18.1). Future classification systems must explore human scalp hair phenotypes beyond hair fiber curvature and consider other attributes, such as pigmentation and texture.

Differences in the cross-sectional shape of hair between East Asians, (West) Africans and (Northern) Europeans were noted early on by anthropologists. Due to the co-occurrence of these differences in shape with degree of curl in the hair, the notion arose that cross-sectional shape determined hair curl, with circular hair shafts leading to straight hair and flattened or oblong hair shafts leading to curled hair [13]. However, it has been noted that whilst these cross-sectional differences exist between populations, they do not seem to correlate with curvature within populations [13].

Slight differences in hair form, growth characteristics, and susceptibility to breakage exist but have not been documented systematically. Sub-Saharan Africans generally exhibit tightly curled or Afro-textured hair and northern populations less tightly or loosely curled hair, but in all African populations, the hair shaft is elliptical in cross section. The curliness of the hair shaft is caused by retrocurvature of the hair bulb, which gives rise to an asymmetrical S-shape of the hair follicle [15]. The continent-wide distribution of Afro-textured hair indicates that this is the ancestral condition for modern humans. Hrdy, who was one of the first to systematically characterize the morphology of human hair, speculated that hair form was determined by multiple genes, and that tightly curly hair form had evolved convergently in African and Melanesian populations [13, 16].

The Genetic Basis of Human Scalp Hair Diversity

Research on the genetic basis of variation in human scalp hair phenotypes is still in its infancy. Most research to date has focused on the genetic basis of hair color, with the identification of polymorphisms in the *MC1R* locus being associated with decreased production of eumelanin and increased production of pheomelanin [2]. Non-red variation in European hair color (i.e., eumelanin content only) is likely influenced by a number of genes, some of which have been implicated through genome-wide association studies, e.g., *KITLG, SLC24A4, SLC45A2, IRF4, TYR, OCA2* [4, 7, 17, 18]. As for color variation in non-European hair, little is known except that in Melanesians, blond hair is due to a mutation in the *TYRP1* locus [19]. The lack of color variation in 'dark-haired populations' may be more apparent than real, and chemical methods may be able to detect unseen variation related to underlying genotypic variation [7]. Rigorous scientific assessment of subtle differences in the color phenotypes in 'dark-haired populations' is needed in conjunction with correlation of phenotypic variation with specific genotypes in order to understand how often and under what evolutionary conditions (e.g., natural selection or genetic drift) dark hair phenotypes evolved.

Despite the interest of early anthropologists in the cross-sectional shape of scalp hair, the genetic basis for the trait has been poorly explored. Cross-sectional area, specifically, increased thickness, has been associated with a mutation in *EDAR* that was under positive selection in East Asian populations. Studies on humans and mice have confirmed the thickening effect of the *EDAR* mutation on the hair shaft [20–22], but it is unclear whether selection was acting on hair thickness or whether this was a pleiotropic effect of selection for other traits.

While there is a great deal of variation in hair curl around the world [3], this trait has mainly been studied in Europeans because there exists the notion that they exhibit the widest range of variation [23]. Likely due, in part, to the frequent qualitative approach to the study of this continuous trait, few of the genes underlying this complex trait have been uncovered. In Europeans, variants in *TCHH* have been associated with straight hair through an effect on keratins of the inner root sheath of the hair follicle [23]. More recently, research on a population of admixed Latin Americans has identified a mutation in *PRSS53* in relation to hair curl variation, which is a protein expressed also in the inner root sheath of the hair follicle. However, paradoxically, African hair form is among the least studied by anthropologists, and, as such, there is currently no knowledge on the genetics underlying this phenotype.

Evolution of Human Scalp Hair

In light of the psychological importance of scalp hair, it is remarkable that so little rigorous research has been devoted to why and how humans evolved it. During ontogeny, in all primates, scalp hair appears first [24]. In nonhuman primates, development of a full-body covering of terminal hairs proceeds during infancy, but in humans this process is discontinued, as part of the process once described by Louis Bolk as "fetalization" [24]. Attempts to relate the evolutionary developmental biology of human hair zonation patterns to the activity of homeobox gene complexes or other genes that describe regional patterns of development in the body have been unsuccessful so far, although a theoretical argument has been put forward that this may be due to combined activity of several *WNT* loci [24].

The loss of most of the terminal body hairs in hominins was probably due to the increased importance of heat loss during prolonged and strenuous physical exercise under hot environmental conditions [25–27]. Scalp hair was retained probably also for thermoregulatory reasons, specifically, for protecting the scalp and head from overhead solar radiation while bipedal [26, 28, 29]. Causal and evolutionary explanations for the evolution of specific scalp hair forms are mostly conjectural. In the single experimental study examining the effect of hair form and length on body temperature, hair length and style were found to affect sweat rate when people were exposed to high environmental temperatures in a climate chamber [30]. Individuals with short straight hair and shorter permed hair had lower sweat rates and experience less loss of total body mass after heat exposure [30]. When this evidence is considered together with that from studies of heat gain and loss in birds and nonhuman mammals [31, 32], it suggests that short, curly, Afro-textured hair may have evolved because it can maintain a boundary layer of cooler, dryer air near the scalp, and thereby protect the thermogenic and thermosensitive brain.

Overview of Human Scalp Hair Biology

Hair follicles are autonomous self-renewing mini-organs [33]. They develop from the ectoderm at weeks 8–9 and maturation is complete by week 18 [34]. The morphogenesis of hair follicles occurs through the interaction of signals between the ectoderm and mesoderm [33]. Examples of these communicating signals include homeobox gene products, transcription factors, signaling and adhesion molecules, Wnt, β-catenin, sonic hedgehog, notch, tenascin, cadherins, epimorphin, nuclear receptors, extracellular matrix, and proteoglycans [33]. Thus, fully formed human scalp hair follicles have both epithelial and mesenchymal components (Fig. 18.2).

Human scalp hair follicles also exhibit an asynchronous cyclical pattern of growth: anagen (active hair fiber production), telogen (resting phase), catagen (tissue regression), and neogen (regeneration) phases [33, 34]. This is a well-controlled process involving a complex and dynamic network of interacting signals, including a variety of signaling pathways, cytokines, neuropeptides, hormones, prostaglandins, and growth factors [33, 34].

Scalp follicles produce hair fibers with three main regions: cuticle, cortex, and medulla.

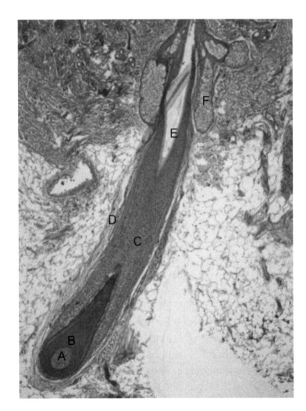

Fig. 18.2 The morphological features of a terminal anagen follicle (H&Ex4). A = Dermal papilla; B = Matrix; C = Outer root sheath; D = Perifollicular fibrous sheath; E = Inner root sheath; F = Sebaceous glands. NB: Hair follicles have three main regions: Lower segment (bulbar and suprabulbar regions): extends from the base of the follicle to insertion of arrector pili muscle; Middle segment (isthmic region): from insertion of arrector pili muscle to entrance of sebaceous gland duct; Upper segment (infundibular region): entrance of sebaceous gland duct to follicular orifice at the surface epidermis (not seen in this figure)

The cuticle is the outermost layer of the hair fiber. It comprises of multiple layers of imbricated corneocytes; the outer surface epicuticle is cysteine-rich, while the opposite is true for the inner layer endocuticle. 18-methyleicosanoic acid is also an important lipid constituent of the cuticular cell membrane complex. It forms a lipid film, which confers low friction and hydrophobic character to the hair fiber surface. Overall, the cuticle provides mechanical support to hair fibers [35].

The cortex is composed of spindle-shaped cortical cells packed with keratin filaments and their associated matrix. There are two types of keratin in human cortical cells: type I (acidic amino acid residues) and type II (basic amino acid residues). Within cortical cells, keratin filaments (composed of both type I and II keratins) form increasingly complex aggregates, resulting in macrofibrils. Variations in the packaging and arrangement of macrofibrils in cortical cells results in different regions of the cortex: orthocortex and paracortex.

Keratin filaments in cortical cells are associated with a matrix rich in keratin-associated proteins (KAPs), primarily through disulphide bonds and/or hydrophobic interactions. Human KAP genes may exhibit polymorphisms, although their functional significance has not yet been fully determined [36].

The medulla is composed of polygonal cells. It is often absent or fragmented in human hair fibers and its presence is highly correlated with thickness of the hair fiber [1, 37, 38].

Variations in Human Scalp Hair Biology Among Populations

As discussed previously, the bulk of human scalp hair fiber is proteinaceous in nature, with structural lipids and other components forming only a minor fraction. Among people of different geographic ancestral origin, the chemical composition of their hair fibers is similar. This is so, even when biological variability, dietary habits, sampling techniques and environmental factors are taken into consideration [35].

However, differences do exist in relation to material specific attributes of hair fibers (geometry, curvature, tensile strength and pigmentation), behavior of assemblies of hair fibers (combability, growth rate), as well as other quantitative and qualitative features of hair fibers and follicles [35].

Hair Growth Parameters

Published studies indicate that Africans have slower scalp hair growth rates compared to Europeans and Asians (mean $\pm$ SD: $280 \pm 50, 367 \pm 56$ and 411 ± 43 µm/day) [39–41]. Several lines of evidence also show that there are variations in scalp hair follicle and fiber density among people of different geographic origins. First, Sperling and coworkers demonstrated that African–Americans (AA) have a lower number of scalp follicles (mean of 21.4) compared to age-matched Caucasian subjects (mean of 35.5) [42]. Their study involved evaluating 4-mm scalp punch biopsies and was limited by the small number of study subjects (22 AA vs. 12 Caucasian). Second, Bernstein and Rassman also reported that AA have a lower scalp hair follicle density compared to Caucasians (1.6 vs. 2 hairs/mm^2) [43]. Their observation was made during scalp hair transplant procedures. Finally, Loussouarn and co-workers also demonstrated a lower hair fiber density in Africans compared to Caucasians [39, 40]. Their observation was based on a phototrichogram study of a 1 cm^2 area of scalp hair of age and sex-matched subjects. This group also demonstrated that subjects of African descent have a greater number of telogen follicles, especially in the occipital and temporal scalp regions [39].

These aforementioned studies are limited by the small number of subjects, and also by the use of biological races to define the groups studied. Nevertheless, the results of these studies imply that there are quantitative differences in human scalp hair follicle and fiber density among different populations. This has practical implications for the histological interpretation of scalp biopsies by Dermatopathologists/Pathologists.

Hair Fiber Geometry and Curvature

Broadly speaking, hair fibers of Asians are significantly thicker compared to other populations [1, 41]. In particular, East Asians exhibit a large cross-sectional area of their hair fibers [1]. This trait has been unequivocally linked with the *EDAR 370A* gene variant in this group [20–22]. In contrast, people of African descent exhibit an elliptical cross-sectional shape of their hair fibers [1, 44]. They also exhibit curled hair fibers, although significant within group variation to this curl pattern has also been observed, e.g., differences between East and West Africans [1].

Traditional concepts about the biological basis of hair fiber curvature have focused primarily on cross-sectional parameters of hair fibers [45]. However, this cannot be the only explanation for hair fiber curvature because not all published studies have showed the presence of a direct correlation between hair fiber curvature and cross-sectional parameters. Recently, Thibaut and co-workers have demonstrated that human scalp hair fiber shape is intrinsically programmed by the lower half of the hair follicle and is associated with a lack of axial symmetry in the lower part of the bulb, affecting the connective tissue sheath, outer and inner root sheaths, as well as hair fiber cuticle [45, 46]. Future work must also explore the gene(s) underlying hair fiber curvature among different populations.

Hair Fiber Pigmentation

Melanocytes are located in the hair follicle matrix. They synthesize melanin pigment, which is packaged into melanosomes and are subsequently transferred to the cortical region of hair fibers. The main melanin pigment variants in human hair fibers are eumelanin and pheomelanin.

A number of published studies have explored the variation of hair fiber pigmentation among different populations [1]. Most of these studies have focused on European populations and have used qualitative tools (spectrometry and colometric evaluation) to assess hair fiber pigmentation [1]. These former studies have reported a greater variability in hair fiber pigmentation of Europeans compared to non-Europeans and have identified several genes, including *OCA2/HERC2* and *IRF4* as contributors to this variation in Europeans [1, 6, 47–50].

Qualitative tools may not detect subtle variations in hair fiber pigmentation occurring in non-Europeans. In this setting, quantitative measurements of total melanin content and melanin pigment subtypes may be preferable [1]. This assertion is supported by the findings of Lasisi and co-workers who have demonstrated a comparable amount of variation in hair fiber pigmentation of non-Europeans when total melanin content is objectively measured [1]. More research is required to further define the variation in hair fiber pigmentation of non-Europeans. It is also important to consider quantitative differences in melanin pigment subtypes, as well as to explore potential genes that may be driving this variability.

Tensile Properties and Combability

Hair fibers with a lower curl diameter (and therefore a higher visual curl degree) have been shown to have a lower Young's modulus (a measure of elasticity), break strain and break stress, making them more susceptible to breakage [51, 52]. Syed et al. [53] have also showed that break stress and break elongation of untreated African–American hair is lower than that of Europeans and that this tensile strength is even lower in wet hair states. Thus, the hair fiber of people of African descent are fragile, especially in the wet state, although given the slight relaxation in curl pattern in the wet state, Afro-textured hair is much easier to comb in the wet state. This has implications in relation to grooming of Afro-textured hair in its natural state.

Another characteristic feature of the hair fibers of people of African descent, when compared to Europeans is the presence of both complex- and single-strand knots [54]. This leads to significant resistance when combing this hair type, with possible breakage of the hair fiber [35].

Moisture Content of Hair Fibers

The moisture content of hair fibers of African–Americans is much lower compared to those of European populations [53]. This former hair type is therefore more susceptible to breakage, especially during grooming.

The Scalp Microbiome

Exploration of the diversity of the human skin microbiome has only begun, and only one study to date has compared the scalp microbiome in different human populations [55]. Scalp microbiota from people of diverse ancestries appear to differ little, and the variation that does exist appears to be related to differences in shampooing practices [55].

Hair Grooming Practices Among Populations

Among different populations, hair grooming practices may vary, and this is dependent upon cultural/societal factors, as well as intrinsic biological differences of human scalp hair types. Given the established link between specific hair grooming practices, and hair and scalp disorders [56], understanding the differences in hair grooming practices among different populations is important in facilitating culturally appropriate discussions with patients about hair loss prevention/minimization. Table 18.1 provides an overview of pertinent hair grooming practices and their link with specific hair and scalp disorders.

Table 18.1 Overview of pertinent hair grooming practices among different populations and link with specific hair and scalp disorders

Hair grooming practice	Adverse effects
Braids Can be undertaken either using no extensions or with synthetic or human hair extensions. The hair can be braided onto the scalp (cornrows) or as individual plaits. The braids are left in place for variable periods of time (typically 3 months) Braiding of hair is a common practice in people of African ancestry	[a]Traction Alopecia CCCA (link with braiding has been suggested)
Brazilian keratin treatment (keratin smoothening or straightening) Protein keratin/formaldehyde solution is infused into the hair using heat, leading to cross-linking of amino acid side chains and straightening of the hair Can be applied to already relaxed or color-treated hair Effect lasts for 6 weeks to 5 months, depending on type of product used Brazilian keratin treatment can be undertaken on all hair phenotypes *Safe keratin treatments are non-formaldehyde containing keratin-straightening products.*	Eye, nose, throat, and respiratory irritation due to release of formaldehyde Contact dermatitis Formaldehyde is a known human carcinogen, therefore unregulated use may pose potential hazards to stylists

(continued)

Table 18.1   (continued)

Hair grooming practice	Adverse effects
They have hydrolyzed keratin with a combination of glyoxyloyl carbocysteine, glyoxyloyl keratin amino acids, silicone derivatives, and fatty acids	
Chemical Straightening (relaxers) Traditional salon relaxers ('lye relaxers') are emulsions of 3.5% sodium hydroxide. 'No-lye' relaxers Contain potassium hydroxide, lithium hydroxide or guanidine hydroxide and are available for home use Use of chemical relaxers results in breakage of disulfide bonds and softening and stretching of the hair shaft Regular 'touch ups' are advised (preferably not more frequently than 8 weekly) to new growth Chemical straightening is an engrained cultural practice in people of African descent	Hair fragility and breakage Contact dermatitis (irritant) Stevens Johnson syndrome [a]Traction alopecia
Dreadlocks Intentionally allowing own natural hair to tangle over time will result in progressive matting or 'locking' of the hair. Very long lengths are often achieved. The style can also be created in hair salons and is produced easier in those with tighter curls prone to tangling Dreadlocks can be undertaken in all hair phenotypes, but it is more commonly associated with Afro-textured hair	[a]Traction alopecia
Hot combs Lubricating "pressing oil" or "hair grease" is applied to the hair and then a hot metal comb (heated to 300–500 °F) is used to straighten the hair. This occurs through temporary rearrangement of the hydrogen bonds in the hair shaft, thus straightening reverts upon exposure of hair to moisture Hot combs use is more commonly associated with Afro-textured hair	Thermal burns Acquired trichorrhexis nodosa
Weaves Artificial hair is sewn into braided (cornrowed) natural hair. Sometimes glues/adhesives can be used to attach the artificial hair to the natural hair Weaves can be undertaken on all hair phenotypes	Allergic contact dermatitis Anaphylactic reactions from glues/adhesives used during weaves CCCA (link with use of sewn-in hair weaves has been suggested)

CCCA Central centrifugal cicatricial alopecia
[a]A link between traction alopecia (TA) and hairstyles that induce prolonged tension on the hair root, e.g., dreadlocks, weaves, and braiding. The risk is highest in the setting of combined hairstyles, i.e., braiding chemically relaxed hair

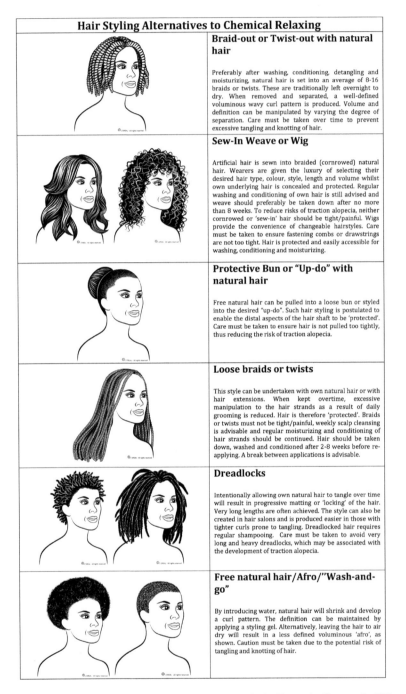

Fig. 18.3 Hairstyling alternatives to chemical straightening). From Aryiku et al. [51] with permission

Broadly speaking, women of African descent tend to wear a greater number of hairstyles throughout their lifetime (up to five different hairstyles reported in a recent study by Dadzie et al.) [57]. This may be because within certain societies, Afro-textured hair in its natural state is opposite to the dominant aesthetic norms [51]. Furthermore, in many European, American and international business contexts, Afro-textured hair is associated with negative stereotypes and lowered expectations [51]. Thus, women of African descent may wear different hairstyles as part of the covering and shifting behavior that allows them to manage their image to avoid discrediting themselves, especially in professional contexts [51]. Less widely acknowledged is the fact that "looking better" with straightened hair implies internalization of a hierarchy of appearance, which assumes superiority of naturally straight hair, a remnant of past social injustice [51]. In light of this, there is now a decline in certain hair grooming practices among women of African descent (e.g., use of chemical straighteners), concurrently with an increase in alternative hairstyles that celebrate Afro-textured hair in its natural form [57] (Fig. 18.3).

Conclusions

Human scalp hair varies in appearance between populations, and it is important that scientists continue to explore the biological and evolutionary basis of this diversity. Knowledge gained from such endeavors may lead to a greater understanding and acceptance of different hair phenotypes within societies, thereby helping to minimize/prevent adverse hair care practices which are undertaken to facilitate greater social acceptance.

References

1. Lasisi T, Ito S, Wakamatsu K, Shaw CN. Quantifying variation in human scalp hair fiber shape and pigmentation. Am J Phys Anthropol. 2016;160(2):341–52.
2. Rees JL. Genetics of hair and skin color. Annu Rev Genet. 2003;37:67–90.
3. Loussouarn G, Garcel A-L, Lozano I, Collaudin C, Porter C, Panhard S, et al. Worldwide diversity of hair curliness: a new method of assessment. Int J Dermatol. 2007;46(S1):2–6.
4. Sulem P, Gudbjartsson DF, Stacey SN, Helgason A, Rafnar T, Magnusson KP, et al. Genetic determinants of hair, eye and skin pigmentation in Europeans. Nat Genet. 2007;39(12): 1443–52.
5. Suter D. Hair colour in the Faroe and Orkney Islands. Ann Hum Biol. 1979;6(1):89–93.
6. Candille SI, Absher DM, Beleza S, Bauchet M, McEvoy B, Garrison NA, et al. Genome-wide association studies of quantitatively measured skin, hair, and eye pigmentation in four European populations. PLoS ONE. 2012;7(10):e48294.
7. Norton HL, Werren E, Friedlaender J. MC1R diversity in Northern Island Melanesia has not been constrained by strong purifying selection and cannot explain pigmentation phenotype variation in the region. BMC Genet. 2015;16(1):1–15.

8. Ito S, Wakamatsu K. Diversity of human hair pigmentation as studied by chemical analysis of eumelanin and pheomelanin. J Eur Acad Dermatol Venereol. 2011;25(12):1369–80.

9. Deedrick DW, Koch SL. Microscopy of hair part I: a practical guide and manual for human hairs. Forensic Sci Commun. 2004;6(1).

10. Trotter M. The form, size, and color of head hair in American whites. Am J Phys Anthropol. 1930;14(3):433–45.

11. Frost P. European hair and eye color: a case of frequency-dependent sexual selection? Evol Hum Behavior. 2006;27(2):85–103.

12. Medland SE, Zhu G, Martin NG. Estimating the heritability of hair curliness in twins of European ancestry. Twin Res Hum Genet. 2009;12(05):514–8.

13. Hrdy D. Quantitative hair form variation in seven populations. Am J Phys Anthropol. 1973;39 (1):7–17.

14. Vernall DG. A study of the size and shape of cross sections of hair from four races of men. Am J Phys Anthropol. 1961;19(4):345–50.

15. Westgate GE, Botchkareva NV, Tobin DJ. The biology of hair diversity. Int J Cosmet Sci. 2013;35(4):329–36.

16. Hrdy DB, Baden HP, Lee LD, Kubilus J, Ludwig KW. Frequency of an electrophoretic variant of hair alpha keratin in human populations. Am J Hum Genet. 1977;29(1):98–100.

17. Branicki W, Liu F, van Duijn K, Draus-Barini J, Pośpiech E, Walsh S, et al. Model-based prediction of human hair color using DNA variants. Hum Genet. 2011;129(4):443–54.

18. Guenther CA, Tasic B, Luo L, Bedell MA, Kingsley DM. A molecular basis for classic blond hair color in Europeans. Nat Genet. 2014;46(7):748–52.

19. Kenny EE, Timpson NJ, Sikora M, Yee MC, Moreno-Estrada A, Eng C, et al. Melanesian blond hair is caused by an amino acid change in TYRP1. Science. 2012;336(6081):554.

20. Fujimoto A, Kimura R, Ohashi J, Omi K, Yuliwulandari R, Batubara L, et al. A scan for genetic determinants of human hair morphology: EDAR is associated with Asian hair thickness. Hum Mol Genet. 2008;17(6):835–43.

21. Fujimoto A, Ohashi J, Nishida N, Miyagawa T, Morishita Y, Tsunoda T, et al. A replication study confirmed the EDAR gene to be a major contributor to population differentiation regarding head hair thickness in Asia. Hum Genet. 2008;124(2):179–85.

22. Mou C, Thomason HA, Willan PM, Clowes C, Harris WE, Drew CF, et al. Enhanced ectodysplasin-a receptor (EDAR) signaling alters multiple fiber characteristics to produce the East Asian hair form. Hum Mutat. 2008;29(12):1405–11.

23. Medland SE, Nyholt DR, Painter JN, McEvoy BP, McRae AF, Zhu G, et al. Common variants in the trichohyalin gene are associated with straight hair in Europeans. Am J Hum Genet. 2009;85(5):750–5.

24. Held LI. The evo-devo puzzle of human hair patterning. Evol Biol. 2010;37(2):113–22.

25. Jablonski NG. The evolution of human skin and skin color. Annu Rev Anthropol. 2004;33:585–623.

26. Jablonski NG. Skin: a natural history. Berkeley: University of California Press; 2006. p. 266.

27. Lieberman DE, Bramble DM, Raichlen DA, Shea JJ. Brains, brawn, and the evolution of human endurance running capabilities. In: Grine FE, Fleagle J, Leakey RE, editors. The first humans: origin and early evolution of the genus Homo. Vertebrate paleobiology and paleoanthropology series. New York: Springer; 2009. p. 77–92.

28. Coelho LGM, Ferreira-Junior JB, Martini ARP, Borba DA, Coelho DB, Passos RLF, et al. Head hair reduces sweat rate during exercise under the sun. Int J Sports Med. 2010;31 (11):779–83.

29. Jablonski NG, Chaplin G. The evolution of skin pigmentation and hair texture in people of African ancestry. Dermatol Clin. 2014;32(2):113–21.

30. Kim MJ, Choi JW, Lee HK, editors. Effect of hair style on human phsyiological responses in a hot environment. In: Environmental ergonomics: proceedings of the 13th international conference on environmental ergonomics. Boston, MA: University of Wollongong; Aug 2–7 Aug 2009.

31. Walsberg GE. Consequences of skin color and fur properties for solar heat gain and ultraviolet irradiance in two mammals. J Comp Physiol. 1988;158(2):213–21.

32. Wolf BO, Walsberg GE. The role of the plumage in heat transfer processes of birds. Am Zool. 2000;40(4):575–84.

33. Bernard BA. Advances in understanding hair growth. F1000Res. 2016; 5(F1000 Faculty Rev).

34. Bernard BA. Hair shape of curly hair. Am Acad Dermatol. 2003;48(6, Supplement 1): S120–6.

35. Wolfram LJ. Human hair: A unique physicochemical composite. Am Acad Dermatol. 2003;48(6, Supplement):S106–14.

36. Shimomura Y, Ito M. Human hair keratin-associated proteins. J Investigative Dermatol Symp Proc. 2005;10(3):230–3.

37. Banerjee AR. Variations in the medullary structure of human head hair. Proc Indian Natl Sci Acad Part B Biol Sci. 1963;29:309–16.

38. Das-Chaudhuri AB, Chopra VP. Variation in hair histological variables: medulla and diameter. Hum Hered. 1984;34(4):217–21.

39. Loussouarn G. African hair growth parameters. Br J Dermatol. 2001;145(2):294–7.

40. Loussouarn G, El Rawadi C, Genain G. Diversity of hair growth profiles. Int J Dermatol. 2005;44(s1):6–9.

41. Loussouarn G, Lozano I, Panhard S, Collaudin C, El Rawadi C, Genain G. Diversity in human hair growth, diameter, colour and shape. An in vivo study on young adults from 24 different ethnic groups observed in the five continents. Eur J Dermatol. 2016;26(2):144–54.

42. Sperling LC. Hair density in Afican Americans. Arch Dermatol. 1999;135(6):656–8.

43. Bernstein RM, Rassman WR. The aesthetics of follicular transplantation. Dermatol Surg. 1997;23(9):785–99.

44. Franbourg A, Hallegot P, Baltenneck F, Toutaina C, Leroy F. Current research on ethnic hair. Am Acad Dermatol. 2003;48(6, Supplement):S115–9.

45. Thibaut S, Bernard BA. The biology of hair shape. Int J Dermatol. 2005;44(S1):2–3.

46. Thibaut S, Gaillard O, Bouhanna P, Cannell DW, Bernard BA. Human hair shape is programmed from the bulb. Br J Dermatol. 2005;152(4):632–8.

47. Norton HL, Friedlaender JS, Merriwether DA, Koki G, Mgone CS, Shriver MD. Skin and hair pigmentation variation in Island Melanesia. Am J Phys Anthropol. 2006;130(2):254–68.

48. Norton HL, Edwards M, Krithika S, Johnson M, Werren EA, Parra EJ. Quantitative assessment of skin, hair, and iris variation in a diverse sample of individuals and associated genetic variation. Am J Phys Anthropol. 2016;160(4):570–81.

49. Shekar SN, Duffy DL, Frudakis T, Montgomery GW, James MR, Sturm RA, et al. Spectrophotometric methods for quantifying pigmentation in human hair—influence of MC1R genotype and environment. Photochem Photobiol. 2008;84(3):719–26.

50. Shekar SN, Duffy DL, Frudakis T, Sturm RA, Zhao ZZ, Montgomery GW, et al. Linkage and association analysis of spectrophotometrically quantified hair color in Australian adolescents: the effect of OCA2 and HERC2. J Investigative Dermatol. 2008;128(12):2807–14.

51. Aryiku SA, Salam A, Dadzie OE, Jablonski NG. Clinical and anthropological perspectives on chemical relaxing of afro-textured hair. J Eur Acad Dermatol Venereol. 2015;29(9):1689–95.

52. Porter CE, Diridollou S, Holloway Barbosa V. The influence of African–American hair's curl pattern on its mechanical properties. Int J Dermatol. 2005;44(s1):4–5.

53. Syed AN, Kuhajda A, Ayoub H, Ahmad K, Frank EM. African–American hair: its physical properties and differences relative to caucasian hair. Cosmetics Toiletries. 1995;110(10): 39–48.

54. Khumalo NP, Doe PT, Dawber RPR, Ferguson DJP. What is normal black African hair? A light and scanning electron-microscopic study. Am Acad Dermatol. 2000;43(5, Part 1): 814–20.

55. Perez Perez GI, Gao Z, Jourdain R, Ramirez J, Gany F, Clavaud C, et al. Body site is a more determinant factor than human population diversity in the health skin microbiome. PLoS ONE. 2016;11(4):e0151990.

56. Salam A, Aryiku S, Dadzie OE. Hair and scalp disorders in women of African descent: an overview. Br J Dermatol. 2013;169(Suppl 3):19–32.
57. Dadzie OE, Salam A. The hair grooming practices of women of African descent in London, United Kingdom: findings of a cross-sectional study. J Eur Acad Dermatol Venereol. 2016;30 (6):1021–4.

Chapter 19
Alopecias and Disorders of the Hair Follicle

Yunyoung C. Chang and Lynne J. Goldberg

Human hair has commonly been classified based on ethnic origin, with three conventional subgroups recognized, including Caucasian, Asian, and African hair [1–3]. These ethnic subgroups have compositional and structural variations, as well as distinct hair-grooming practices [4]. Such broad classification does not account for the great complexity of human hair but provides a basic framework for description. These ethnic differences are important to comprehend the pathophysiology of scalp and hair disorders in the context of ethnicity.

Ethnic Hair: Biochemical Diversity

There is a wide diversity of hair worldwide [3]. Briefly, the color of hair is determined by the type of pigment. Eumelanin gives darker colors to hair while pheomelanin confers lighter color to hair. Afro-ethnic hair characteristically contains more eumelanin than pheomelanin and is, thus, darker [5].

In terms of diameter and section, Asian hair has a larger diameter with circular geometry in cross section while African hair demonstrates a high degree of irregularity in diameter along the hair shaft and an elliptical cross section [1]. Caucasian hair has an intermediate diameter and section shape. In terms of the shape, African hair has a curved hair follicle bulb and the hair shaft shows frequent twists with random reversals in direction and pronounced flattening, a shape resembling a twisted oval rod. Caucasian and Asian hairs are more cylindrical. African hair

Y.C. Chang · L.J. Goldberg (✉)
Department of Dermatology, Boston University School of Medicine,
609 Albany St, Boston, MA 02118, USA
e-mail: lynngold@bu.edu

© Springer International Publishing AG 2017
N.A. Vashi and H.I. Maibach (eds.), *Dermatoanthropology of Ethnic Skin and Hair*, DOI 10.1007/978-3-319-53961-4_19

generally is more difficult to comb than Caucasian hair because of its extremely curly configuration. It also has less moisture content, less tensile strength, grows more slowly, and breaks more easily than Caucasian hair [1].

Hair Care Practices

Awareness of hair care and grooming practices in ethnic populations is important in understanding common hair complaints and hair disorders.

Hairstyles used by African Americans are typically divided into those that are "natural" and those that involve straightening. Examples of natural styles include braids or cornrows, twists, locks, afros, and other curly styles. Braiding is the interlocking of three or more hairpieces. Cornrowing is a form of small, tight braids very close to the scalp, sometimes with attached hair pieces, beads, or decorations [6]. Extensions or weaves of synthetic hair may also be attached to extend the length and provide fullness to the hair [6] (Fig. 19.1). Twists are short pieces of hair twisted together, that are removed and retwisted on a regular basis. Twists that are not removed become "locks", intentionally matted, sculpted ropes of hair that are irreversible. Curly styles are becoming increasingly popular.

Hair restructuring techniques are commonly used by African Americans. Hair straightening, with either heat or chemicals, is used to make the hair more manageable and easier to style. Hot combing was one of the first methods, which started in the early twentieth century in France [2]. This technique consists of use of a metal comb heated to high temperatures (150–500 °sF), either with a direct heat source or electrically, and slowly pulling it through portions of hair [2, 7]. This process causes disruption of disulfide bonds in the hair shaft and straightens the hair temporarily [6]. The hair returns to its normal state with water or moisture. Pre-application of oils or emollients is used to protect the scalp and hair from excess heat [6].

Hot combing became less popular after the introduction of chemical relaxers, which typically contain sodium, potassium, or guanine hydroxides, sulfites, or thioglycolates [2]. These agents permanently disrupt disulfide bonds and reset the hair in a straighter form; they are not reversed by water [6]. Use of the stronger agents is typically done by professionals, while treatment with others (such as guanine hydroxides) can be performed at home.

There are potential side effects to all types of hair styling, particularly in African Americans. Ethnic hairstyling techniques, including braids and extensions, have been recognized more recently to cause excess tension and traction on the hair and may lead to a scarring alopecia, especially when used in conjunction with relaxers (described below) [8]. Extensions may be very heavy and attach to a few fragile hair shafts causing traction damage [6]. In addition, there has been concern about allergic contact reactions of skin to some extension materials, including the adhesives used [6]. Gathers and Lim have also found an association between central centrifugal cicatricial alopecia (CCCA) and hair weaves and braids [9].

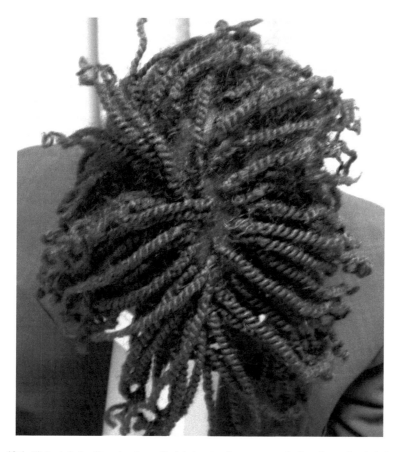

Fig. 19.1 Hair styled with extensions. Twisted extensions are attached to the patient's hair

Common complications from thermal straightening include moderate to severe burns from accidental contact with the hot comb, overheating of hair shaft causing weakening and breakage, and severe damage to the hair shaft [2]. To prevent against damage, one should counsel on using hot comb treatment at a maximum of once weekly, making sure the hair is completely dry, and regularly trimming split ends. In addition, moisturizing shampoos and conditioners should be used regularly and application of thick emollients to coat the hair can protect against further damage from heat [2].

Side effects of chemical relaxers include local contact irritation, chemical burns, hair shaft dryness, loss of hair shaft tensile strength, increased hair shaft fragility, and scarring alopecia [6]. Potassium and sodium hydroxides as well as thioglycolates tend to be the most damaging to scalp and hair [2]. Using a thick, protective emollient on the scalp during relaxer application ("basing the scalp") may lessen skin irritation [2]. Also, regular trimming and keeping relaxer applications to minimum interval of every 6 weeks can decrease damage to the hair shaft [2]. Other hair-care practices commonly used by African-American patients include use of blow dryers, hood dryers, and curling irons, which may cause fragility and loss of tensile strength as well as scalp damage.

Finally, emollients are commonly used in African Americans of all ages to help manageability of hair. Solid emollients, including pomades, are used on curly or kinky hair to allow for sheen hairstyles or facilitate braiding of hair. These thick products contain mixtures of petrolatum, lanolin, vegetable, mineral, or animal oils, waxes, and resins [2]. Liquid emollients are made primarily of oils, but sometimes, liquid lanolin is added. Common side effects of emollient use include both allergic and irritant contact dermatitis. In addition, thick hair emollients may mask or worsen common dermatologic conditions such as seborrheic dermatitis (SD) and acne. Patients should be counseled on regularly cleansing out the products, frequent pillowcase washing, clean scarf use on hair at nighttime to protect the face, and minimization of product use [2].

Hair Disorders

Hair loss disorders may be categorized broadly into nonscarring or scarring alopecias, hair shaft abnormalities, and inflammatory hair conditions.

Approach to the Alopecia Patient

Hair loss is a common presenting complaint, and a clinical diagnosis is typically based on a thorough history and focused physical examination. Some patients require laboratory tests and a punch biopsy.

A hair loss history should elucidate several factors. The provider should ascertain the duration of hair loss, the acuity of hair loss, and the course of hair loss (i.e., gradual vs flares). Clinical characteristics including whether there is complete baldness or hair thinning, the distribution of hair loss (i.e., generalized vs localized), the presence of hair shedding, the presence of scalp symptoms, including pruritus, pain, burning, and the presence of pustules or nodules, should be taken into account. Alleviating or triggering factors may also be elucidated.

The delineation of hair care practices, including frequency of washing, use of relaxers or heating combs, hairstyles like tight braids, weaves, or extensions, and use of topical hair products, is essential information, especially in the ethnic population.

A full medical history, including history of pregnancy, acne, hirsutism, thyroid disease, and lupus, should be obtained. In addition, a full medication list to determine if drugs may be triggering the hair loss should be reviewed. Family history is very important in alopecia patients, including family history of hair loss, thyroid disease, and other autoimmune diseases. Social history, including recent hospitalizations and recent emotional stressors, should be obtained given these may trigger acute telogen effluvium (TE).

The physical exam should focus on the head and neck, and all quadrants of the scalp should be examined. Physicians should take into account hair length, hair density, and presence of hair breakage. The presence of pustules, perifollicular erythema, perifollicular scaling as well as exclamation point hairs should be noted. The scalp exam should look for presence or absence of follicular orifices, though this may be difficult to distinguish by the naked eye and is best done with a dermatoscope. A dermatoscope is an essential tool for the hair clinician; in addition to looking at the scalp surface, one can more readily appreciate subtle perifollicular erythema, pigmentary alterations and scale, tufting, exclamation point hairs, and thin hair shaft diameters. One should also examine the eyebrows, eyelashes, and other body parts for hair loss, as well as the nails and oral mucosa to look for any associated findings.

Laboratory examination may, at times, be warranted. For example, in TE with no clear triggering cause, iron studies and thyroid studies, may be obtained. A punch biopsy of the scalp may be obtained if diagnosis is uncertain, especially when trying to distinguish between a scarring or nonscarring alopecia. In addition, biopsy can give clues to specific entities, as described below.

Nonscarring Alopecias: Androgenetic Alopecia (Pattern Hair Loss)

The most common nonscarring alopecia is male and female pattern hair loss (MPHL and FPHL), or androgenetic alopecia (AGA). This is a type of nonscarring hair loss that occurs worldwide. The overall prevalence of MPHL and FPHL varies significantly based on ethnicity and race [10]. The prevalence appears to be the highest for Caucasian males, ranging around 50–53% in middle-aged to older males [10, 11], and Caucasian females, around 19% [10], whereas prevalence in South African males is around 14.5% and females is around 3.5% [10]. In Asians, the prevalence in Korean and Chinese males is 14 and 19.21%, respectively, whereas higher prevalence is seen in Thai and Singaporean counterparts, 38.5 and 63%, respectively [11]. The mechanisms behind these ethnic variations have yet to be elucidated but may be due to distinct genetic predispositions, as described below. Overall, the prevalence of AGA increases with age in all populations, and AGA occurs more commonly in men than women [10, 11].

Clinically, MPHL is characterized by gradual hair thinning that typically begins in the bitemporal and midfrontal scalp, with the major complaint being hairline recession. Hair loss may also be seen in the vertex of the scalp [11]. The severity of involvement in these three areas is highly variable. Of note, bitemporal hairline recession may be seen in many postpubertal men but does not necessarily signify MPHL and is unlikely to reverse with treatment. A deeper bitemporal recession of greater than 1 inch from the frontal hairline is part of MPHL and may respond to treatment if treated early [12]. FPHL manifests as gradual central thinning of the crown with preservation of the frontal hairline and occipital hair [13]. Some women can exhibit bitemporal thinning and miniaturization, similar to men (Fig. 19.2). The major complaint for women may be increased central part width due to increased spacing between hairs and a "thinner" ponytail due to generalized thinning [14]. Frontal accentuation of hair loss is said to resemble a "Christmas tree" [15, 16]. AGA is a continuous process that progresses over the course of many years, and the rate of disease progression varies from person to person [12].

On physical exam, follicular miniaturization is one of the earliest and diagnostic signs of AGA. Variations in hair follicle caliber and length can be observed by examining the hair fibers against a background or with a dermatoscope [17, 18]. Dermoscopy may also show peripilar brown halos, yellow dots, and honeycomb-like scalp pigmentation [18, 19].

Histopathologic examination is not usually necessary but may have distinctive features to help with diagnosis. Horizontal (transverse) sectioning of punch biopsies allows visualization of more follicles as well as quantification of follicular number and size, and tends to yield more useful results than vertical sectioning [20]. Horizontal sections show increased numbers of telogen follicles as well as increased vellus hairs, with a terminal to vellus hair ratio of less than 4:1 (normal scalp ratio 7:1) [21]. There is miniaturization of terminal hair follicles with variation in size of follicles [21]. Although it is characterized as a noninflammatory form of hair loss,

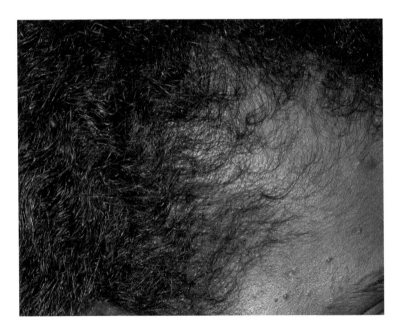

Fig. 19.2 Female pattern hair loss. Bitemporal thinning with fine, miniaturized hairs

inflammation is not uncommon, and a mild perifollicular lymphohistiocytic infiltrate may be present in one-third of biopsies [20]. In later stages, mild perifollicular fibrosis and decreased density of follicular structures may be seen [20].

The major differential diagnoses of AGA are diffuse alopecia areata and TE. Diffuse alopecia areata tends to be more acute in onset than AGA and does not follow a patterned distribution [22]. In addition, it tends to occur at an earlier age, is more severe, may be associated with hair loss in other body sites, and may be associated with pitting of the nails [22]. TE leads to diffuse hair loss over the entire scalp, which may or may not result in reduced hair volume [23]. It is usually associated with an acute event. Both diffuse AA and TE are associated with a positive pull test [23]. The pull test is performed by grasping approximately 40–60 hairs between the thumb and index fingers, applying steady traction proximally to distally along the length of the hair. A normal or "negative" pull test extracts three or fewer hairs while a positive pull test extracts six or more hairs from a single area (>10% hairs). Typically, at least three separate areas of the scalp are tested. Of note, both AA and TE may coexist with AGA, further challenging the diagnosis [23].

AGA is influenced by both genetic and hormonal factors [11]. It is mediated by high levels of potent androgen dihydrotestosterone (DHT) and increased expression of the androgen receptor (AR) gene [11]. AGA is likely under the control of multiple genes, such as genes for AR, insulin-like growth factor-1, and DHT regulations [24, 25]. The AR gene is a member of the nuclear receptor superfamily located on the X chromosome at Xq11-12 [11]. Its amino terminal domain is required for transcriptional activation and contains a region of polyglutamine that is encoded by CAG trinucleotide repeats that are important in human disease [24, 26, 27]. AR polymorphisms, including Stu1 restriction fragment length polymorphism, as well as shorter CAG and GGC triplet repeat lengths, are associated with MPHL [24, 26, 27]. Zhuo et al. [27] suggested that AR Stu I polymorphism might be a risk factor for AGA, especially in the European population. On the other hand, Jung et al. found no significant correlation between CAG repeat numbers and AGA in the Korean AGA population [28], suggesting that this polymorphism may not play a major role in AGA susceptibility in this specific population. Unlike males in which hair loss is likely androgen dependent, the role of androgens in FPHL is less clear, and the term FPHL is preferred over female AGA by some authors [29]. More recently, neurotrophic factors, including brain-derived nerve factor, were found to have potential importance in mediating effects of androgens on hair follicles and may serve as negative regulatory control signals [30].

Interestingly, in African-American men as well as non-African-American men, early onset AGA has been associated with prostate cancer [31]. A case-control study of African-American men with prostate cancer demonstrated that baldness was associated with increased odds of prostate cancer. In particular, frontal balding was associated with high stage and high grade prostate cancer [31]. There may be a genetic link between androgen metabolism and both early pattern baldness and prostate cancer [31]. In fact, a population study from China suggested that shorter CAG and GGC trinucleotide repeat lengths, more specifically <23 repeats, in the AR gene may be associated with increased risk of both AGA and prostate cancer

[32]. The *AR*-E211 > A allele has been associated with lower risk of metastatic prostate cancer and lower risk of AGA [26, 33]. Further studies are needed in this area to confirm this association.

AGA has also been associated with increased risk in cardiovascular disease, including metabolic syndrome and atherosclerosis [34, 35]. In addition, a lower number of CAG repeats in the AR gene were also associated with low HDL and decreased endothelial responsivity to ischemia [36]. This suggests cardiovascular screening, including lipid panels, should be done on AGA patients to enable early detection of at-risk individuals [34, 35].

AGA is often associated with poor self-image and low self-esteem in the ethnic population [12]. This is especially the case in individuals who have a thick baseline of hair or in ethnic populations where thick hair is a symbol of status. It is the role of the dermatologist to counsel on the genetic and physiological basis of AGA as well as the goals of various treatments. For example, it is important to counsel that available medical treatments are not curative and continuous treatment of AGA is needed to ensure sustained benefits. Patients should be counseled that treatment for AGA will not restore hair to prepubertal density and that the aim of treatment is to prevent progression of disease, rather than regrowth. Currently, topical 5% minoxidil solution and foam and oral finasteride at a dose of 1 mg are the only Food and Drug Administration (FDA)-approved medications for treatment of MPHL, and 2% minoxidil solution and 5% foam are the only approved medications for FPHL [12]. For minoxidil, the recommended dose is 1 mL (25 drops) for both 2 and 5% solutions, or half a cap of foam, applied twice daily to a dry scalp and left in place at least for 4 h [12]. For women, many physicians recommend using the higher dose of minoxidil once or twice daily over the 2% formulation given studies demonstrating superiority in increasing hair growth and earlier response to treatment [37]. Minoxidil takes about 6–12 months for effect. Patients should be warned that during the initial 2–8 weeks of treatment, a temporary TE with increased hair shedding may occur, but is self-limited and subsides when anagen regrowth begins [12]. The mechanism of action is unknown, but it appears to prolong the anagen phase and hair shaft diameter [12, 38]. Minoxidil likely causes the opening of potassium channels leading to vasodilation, stimulates prostaglandin E2 (PGE2) synthesis, stimulates vascular endothelial growth factor (VEGF) synthesis by dermal papilla cells promoting angiogenesis, and leads to cell growth [38].

Oral finasteride, a potent type II 5a-reductase inhibitor, is FDA approved for treatment of MPHL [12, 39]. It is prescribed as 1 mg daily dosage for males and is relatively well tolerated with durable improvements in scalp hair growth. Side effects are infrequent occurring at a rate of 2.1–3.8% [40] and are typically mild. Erectile dysfunction is the most common side effect, followed by ejaculatory dysfunction and loss of libido [41]. These effects occur early in therapy and are typically reversible with discontinuation of drug or while continuing use of the drug over a period of time. However, an initial report [42], followed by several others, have documented long lasting sexual side effects after use despite stopping. The role of the nocebo effect, an adverse effect resulting from the psychological awareness of the possibility of the side effect rather than a direct result from the medication [40], in sexual dysfunction due to finasteride has been investigated and demonstrated to be present [40]. The only causal relation between finasteride and sexual side effects is low ejaculatory volume, because of the action of DHT on the prostate gland [40].

The role of anti-androgenic agents in FPHL in both pre and post-menopausal women remains to be fully defined, and they are not FDA approved. Oral finasteride was ineffective at dose of 1 mg daily in females [43]. However, case series have shown efficacy at higher doses than used in males (2.5 mg daily or more) [44, 45]. For females, other anti-androgen medications such as spironolactone [46] can be used. While not extensively studied, spironolactone can be used as a second line agent after minoxidil given its long history and good tolerability of use. Other antiandrogens are not typically used due to their side effect profile (flutamide) or lack of availability in the United States (cyproterone acetate) [47, 48].

The use of low-level laser light was approved by the US FDA for the treatment of MPHL in 2007 and FPHL in 2011 [49, 50]. Many devices are currently available, ranging from hand held units to wearable helmets. The laser phototherapy is assumed to stimulate anagen re-entry in telogen hair follicles, prolong duration of anagen phase, increase rates of proliferation in active anagen hair follicles and to prevent premature catagen development [50]. In a double-blind, sham device-controlled, multicenter, 26-week trial randomized study among 110 male AGA patients, use of a device three times per week for 15 min for a total of 26 weeks was associated with significantly greater increase in mean terminal hair density, overall hair regrowth, slowing of hair loss, thicker feeling hair, and better scalp health [51]. Another multicenter, randomized double-blind study demonstrated use of a hand held comb three times per week for 26 weeks increased terminal hair density in both men and women with pattern hair loss [49].

Despite advances in medical therapy, hair transplantation remains the only means of permanent hair restoration in cases of severe AGA. However, it is used in combination with medical therapies as it does not prevent progression of disease.

Platelet-rich plasma (PRP) is a relatively new treatment for AGA. It involves removal of blood, centrifugation, and return of the plasma fraction to the scalp via multiple repeated injections. A recent randomized placebo-controlled blinded study of 25 AGA patients demonstrated benefit in increasing hair density [52], but further studies and standardized protocols are needed.

Nonmedical approaches may also provide cosmetic relief in ethnic skin patients, and may be used as an adjunct to, or independent of, medical therapy. Camouflage agents like fibers, and powder makeup can give the illusion of thicker hair, and prostheses such as wigs and hairpieces are invaluable in patients with severe hair loss.

Scarring Alopecias

Skin of color patients often present with permanent or scarring hair disorders. These are divided into those found in all skin types such as lichen planopilaris and frontal fibrosing alopecia, and those with a predilection for this population such as CCCA, dissecting cellulitis of the scalp (DCS), folliculitis decalvans (FD), pseudofolliculitis barbae (PFB), traction alopecia (TA), and acne keloidalis (AK) [53]. A classification scheme was created by Sperling encompassing these scarring alopecias [54], which are associated with permanent hair loss, disfigurement, emotional distress, and decreased quality of life. Hair-grooming practices, as described previously, have been associated with the pathophysiology of some of these conditions, and thus, patient education and behavior modifications are critical to the management of these disorders. Because many of these entities are discussed elsewhere, this chapter will focus on CCCA and TA, a typically nonscarring alopecia which often results in secondary scarring. We will then briefly discuss other entities.

Central Centrifugal Cicatricial Alopecia

CCCA is the most common scarring alopecia in females of African descent. It was formerly referred to as "hot comb alopecia," "follicular degeneration syndrome," and "chemically induced scarring alopecia." Studies demonstrate a prevalence ranging from 5.6 to 59% [55, 56, 58] in African-American populations, with higher prevalence in females and with age [8, 56, 57]. The reported prevalence is lower in African females, 2.7% [58]. However, large-scale epidemiologic studies need to be performed.

The etiology of CCCA is unclear and is most likely multifactorial, involving genetics and hair care practices. Hair care practices of African-American women have been implicated since 1968 [59]. It was purported that during hot combing, the hot lubricant travels down the hair shaft to the scalp and burns the follicle. They believed this repetitive injury caused scarring [59]. Later reports have failed to support a direct link with hot combing and have associated it with other grooming techniques, including chemical relaxers [60, 61] and traction hairstyles like extensions, weaves, and tight braids [8, 9]. Kyei et al. [8] demonstrated that hairstyles associated with traction, i.e., braids and weaves, but not heat or chemical relaxers were associated with CCCA. Hair care in individuals of color frequently involves multiple styling practices at the same time, contributing to difficulty in identifying independent risk factors. Kyei et al. [8] also demonstrated that bacterial scalp infections and diabetes mellitus two were significantly higher in those with CCCA, suggesting that CCCA may be a manifestation of metabolic dysregulation.

Genetics likely play a role in the pathogenesis of CCCA. Dlova et al. [62] reported 2 families with natural hair and evidence of CCCA. In addition, a recent study of 14 index South African families demonstrated a possible autosomal dominant mode of inheritance of CCCA with partial penetrance and strong modifying effect of gender and hairstyling [63]. While this study found a positive correlation between use of traction-inducing hairstyles, i.e., braids and weaving, and severity of CCCA, 6 of 31 participants (19.4%) did not have history of chemical processing or traction hairstyles, suggesting a genetic etiology [63].

Clinically, CCCA is a chronic, progressive condition characterized by a symmetric, roughly circular patch of scarring alopecia at the vertex or mid scalp that slowly expands centrifugally [53] (Fig. 19.3). It typically occurs in middle-aged females, in the third to fifth decade of life [64]. In the early inflammatory stage, the scalp may appear normal or exhibit hair breakage and/or decreased hair density localized to the vertex. There may be an active erythematous border or follicular pustules early in the course [64]. Many patients are asymptomatic, but some may experience pruritus, scalp tenderness, and dysesthesia [65]. The hair loss may be present for years before noticed by patients. Some patients have only breakage; however, biopsies may reveal histologic findings typical of CCCA [65]. Most patients present in late stage when clinical inflammation is lacking and scarring has already occurred. CCCA manifests as a symmetric area of hair loss on the vertex or mid scalp with smooth scalp devoid of hair follicles [64]. Dermoscopy shows peripilar white gray halo around remaining emerging hair follicles in 94% patients and is highly specific and sensitive for CCCA in all clinical stages [66]. These can be differentiated from pin-point white dots in normal black scalp, which are smaller and interfollicularly distributed in a "starry sky"-like pattern. In addition, broken

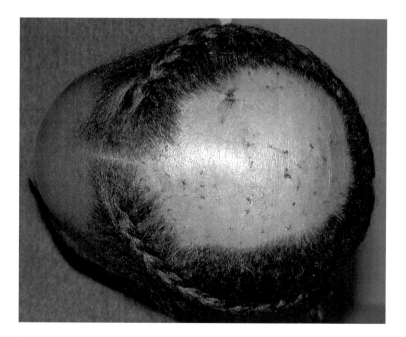

Fig. 19.3 Central centrifugal cicatricial alopecia. A large area of scarring hair loss on the crown

hairs, follicular dropout, and white patches representing follicular scarring can be found on dermoscopy [66].

Early histologic changes include perifollicular lymphocytic infiltrate and perifollicular fibroplasia [64]. Concentric lamellar fibroplasia occurs around mid and upper follicles [64], corresponding to the white gray halo seen on dermoscopy [66]. The lymphocytic infiltrate extends from the lower follicular infundibulum down to the upper isthmus. There is considerable reduction in terminal hair follicles with reciprocal increase in fibrous tracts as well as a loss of sebaceous epithelium [64]. With progression of disease, one finds disintegration of the inner root sheath, which has been emphasized as a diagnostic finding [21, 54, 67], but is not always found and not unique to CCCA [68]. The end-stage changes are indistinguishable from other scarring alopecias, with end-stage fibrosis and little inflammation [66]. Interface changes, dyskeratosis, pigment incontinence, and mucin are absent, differentiating it from other scarring alopecias like discoid lupus [9].

The differential diagnoses include AGA, lichen planopilaris, FD, discoid lupus erythematosus (DLE), and TA. Both AGA and CCCA can occur on vertex and crown of scalp with retention of frontal hairline; in AGA, the hair thinning tends to be more diffuse, nonscarring, asymptomatic, and exhibits miniaturization of hairs [69]. Hairs of varying lengths and diameters are characteristic of AGA. A biopsy can be performed to distinguish between these identities, however, AGA and CCCA may occur in the same patient [55, 70]. Lichen planopilaris may start at the vertex and spread centrifugally but can occur in all areas of the scalp; in addition, it is typically associated with perifollicular erythema and scale [64]. FD also involves the crown and vertex but typically presents as follicular pustules within or surrounding areas of alopecia. TA commonly occurs in the frontotemporal region and presents as alopecia surrounded by retained hairs.

Treatment of CCCA aims at reducing associated symptoms and preventing disease progression. Early intervention is crucial because hair loss is typically permanent once scarring has occurred [53, 70]. Patients should be educated about realistic treatment goals. To prevent expansion, mainstay of therapy is the use of anti-inflammatory agents. This may begin with potent to super potent, class 1 topical steroids, and/or intralesional corticosteroids (triamcinolone acetonide 2.5–10 mg/ml every 4–8 weeks). Target areas for injections should include the periphery of the hair loss at the edge of normal hair to prevent further expansion outwards [53]. Care should be taken to use lowest effective dose possible to minimize possible side effects, including dyspigmentation.

Systemic anti-inflammatory agents including oral tetracyclines and antimalarials have shown mixed effectiveness but may be the appropriate next step for those refractory to topical and intralesional steroids [53]. Topical minoxidil may be added to the regimen once inflammation is controlled and condition is stable to help increase the density of the remaining hair follicles and aid in hair growth [53].

Given the likely association with damaging hair styling practices, natural hairstyles should be encouraged. Hair care practices including traction hairstyles, excessive heat, and chemical relaxers should be avoided or limited [53]. Ethnic patients may be resistant to these modifications. If so, relaxers should be applied by a professional and their frequency decreased to once every 8–12 weeks. Chemical treatments, such as dyes, should not be applied to relaxed hair. In addition, the stylist should use mild formulations, apply a protective base to the scalp, and neutralize after no more than 20 min [53, 71].

Traction Alopecia

TA is a nonscarring alopecia associated with secondary scarring, caused by hairstyle practices that produce prolonged tension or stress on hair follicles [70]. TA is most common in ethnicities with afro-textured hair but all ethnicities can be affected; one study showed 29% of 41 TA patients were Hispanic [72]. Other case reports have shown TA in Sikh males [73, 74], Sudanese females [75], as well as white and Japanese females who wear distinct hairstyles [76, 77]. The prevalence is higher in African schoolgirls than boys (17.1 vs. 0%) and increases with age [57, 58].

TA, as its name suggests, is caused by prolonged or repetitive tension on the hair due to certain hairstyles, particularly tight ponytails or braids as a child. African Americans may be at particular risk given their use of hair weaves, braids, cornrows, extensions, and chemical relaxers [70, 78–81]. The risk of TA increases with symptomatic traction, like pain, pimples, and crusts [57], and is highest in combined hairstyles [57, 58]. For example, traction hairstyles like braids and weaves performed on relaxed hair increases the risk [58]. In its early form, TA may be nonscarring and initially reversible, but repeated damage and perifollicular inflammation eventually leads to miniaturized hairs, reduced hair density, and scarring [72].

Clinically, the hair thinning and loss typically occurs on the frontal and temporal scalp above the ears [70]. The manifestations depend on the stage and severity of disease. In early stages, hair loss may be absent or limited to a subtle decrease in hair density. Patient may have only noninflammatory hair thinning, or have folliculitis, characterized by perifollicular erythema, papules, and sterile pustules in sites of traction [2, 82]. Scalp scaling and pruritus may also occur.

With persistent traction, clinically noticeable hair loss occurs, progressing from decreased hair density to patches of alopecia. The most common manifestation is marginal TA, affecting the frontal and temporal scalp above the ears (Fig. 19.4). However, hair loss in the occiput may also be seen [83]. The scalp eventually shows loss of follicular openings, often with minimal amounts of short, fragile, intermediate hairs in the area of loss. The presence of retained fine or miniaturized hairs along the anterior frontal and/or temporal hairline with loss posteriorly, termed the "fringe sign" is a finding seen in both early and late TA and is a useful clinical marker of the condition [72, 84].

Nonmarginal TA, however, may affect other areas of the scalp and have varying clinical presentations depending on different ethnicities and hairstyle practices used [84]. For example, linear, curved, or horseshoe patterns of hair loss can occur on the crown or even in an ophiasis pattern when hair is tightly braided on the scalp in

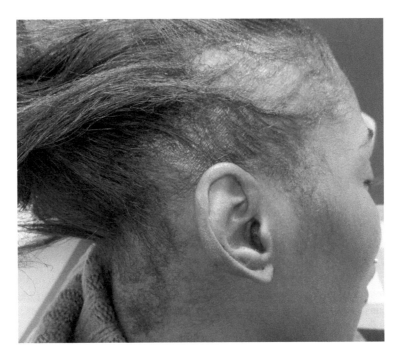

Fig. 19.4 Traction alopecia. Severe marginal hair loss with retained terminal hairs

preparation for the attachment of sewn-in or glued-in curtain-like hair extensions, as is often done for hair weaves [85, 86]. Frontal alopecia has been described in Sikh males secondary to wearing a turban on the head; this involves twisting uncut hair tightly into a knot resting on the frontal scalp for longer than 24 h periods [73]. TA can also arise in the submandibular area in Sikh males due to the practice of knotting the long, uncut beard [73, 74]. Females who frequently wear their hair in a tight chignon or bun, like ballerinas, may develop TA confined to the occipital or temporal scalp [76, 77]. Given the various clinical presentations, TA may be a diagnostic challenge, especially when appropriate history is not obtained.

Dermoscopic findings are similar to those found in trichotillomania. In black patients, dermoscopy shows elongation and linearization of follicular ostia in the frontal area, reflecting the traction process.

Histopathology in early TA may be similar to trichotillomania as well, demonstrating trichomalacia (twisted or deformed anagen hair shaft), increased number of telogen and catagen hairs, a normal number of terminal follicles, and preserved sebaceous glands [72]. There may be mild perifollicular inflammation in the dermis. Long-standing TA characteristically will demonstrate follicular miniaturization, decreased terminal hairs, fibrotic fibrous tracts, and absent or minimal dermal inflammation [72, 87, 88].

Differential diagnoses for TA include ophiasis pattern alopecia areata and frontal fibrosing alopecia. Clinical clues include follicular markings, which are retained in

AA, often decreased in TA (especially late stage), and absent in FFA [72]. The color of the scalp is normal in TA, may be peach-colored in AA, and is pale and atrophic in FFA. AA may have broken or miniaturized hairs that mimics the fringe sign, but is not usually symmetric or bilateral as in TA. Eyebrows are not affected in TA, whereas they may be affected in AA or FFA [72]. Biopsy is important in definitively distinguishing between these entities.

Treatment of TA is anecdotal and essentially involves prevention. Patient education is the key to prevention and should begin in childhood. Patients should be encouraged to wear loose hairstyles, avoiding tight ponytails, buns, braids, and weaves. In particular, pain with the traction hairstyles should be avoided. In addition, patients should avoid chemical relaxers or heat, especially in children because hair damage increases with exposure duration [72]. In particular, traction hairstyles on relaxed hair should be avoided or performed at least two weeks after processing as relaxed hair is weak and prone to breakage [84]. If cultural reasons prevent avoiding relaxing, relaxers should be applied professionally and according to package instructions, specifically only processing new hair growth while avoiding previously relaxed hair. In addition, the hair should be thoroughly rinsed and neutralized after processing or if scalp tingling or burning occurs [72]. If heat is used, air dry or low-heat hairdryer setting should be used. Conditioners and petroleum-free moisturizers for dry hair may reduce the risk of hair breakage. Even if TA has already developed, hairstyle modification should be emphasized to prevent scarring and progression of disease. Once scarring develops, hair loss is irreversible.

If behavioral modification is enforced, medical therapies may further decrease inflammation and slow or prevent progression. For early TA, topical and intralesional steroids are first-line therapies, directed at the periphery of hair loss [71]. Oral antibiotics may also be used in early stages of disease for their anti-inflammatory effect [71]. Topical minoxidil has also been reported to promote hair growth [89]. In long-standing disease, surgical options like hair transplants may be considered. For cosmesis, prostheses like hairpieces and clip-ons can be very helpful. Care must be taken with clip-ons to avoid further traction.

Chronic Cutaneous (Discoid) Lupus Erythematosus

DLE causes a primary scarring alopecia, characterized by well-defined erythematous plaques of alopecia with follicular plugging and adherent scale [70]. A "carpet tack" sign may be observed as keratotic spikes with retraction of the scale [90]. With long-standing disease, dyspigmentation with central hypopigmentation and surrounding hyperpigmentation, atrophic depigmented plaques, and scarring is seen (Fig. 19.5). The risk of progression to systemic lupus erythematosus is estimated to be 5–11% [90]. Treatment of DLE on the scalp is similar to other DLE lesions, including topical and intralesional steroids and oral antimalarials [70, 91, 92]. Topical calcineurin inhibitors have also been shown to have benefit [93, 94]. Oral steroids should be reserved for acute induction phase while awaiting therapeutic

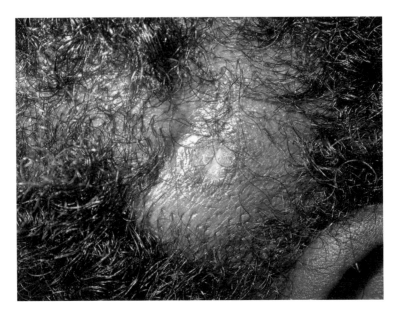

Fig. 19.5 Discoid lupus erythematosus. An area of hair loss with central scarring and peripheral hyperpigmentation

effect of other drugs or for severe cases [70]. In addition, photoprotection is critical in the prevention and treatment of this disease. This condition is described in more detail in other chapters.

Neutrophilic Scarring Alopecias

FD is a rare chronic and relapsing neutrophilic scarring alopecia [95] that is more common in African Americans compared to Caucasians [96]. FD predominantly occurs in middle-aged adults with slight preference of the male gender [95, 96]. The etiology of FD is unclear, but *Staphylococcus aureus* infection and immune dysfunction is thought to play a role. *S. aureus* can often be isolated from the pustules [97–99]. FD primarily involves the vertex and occipital scalp. It is characterized by follicular pustules, diffuse, and perifollicular erythema, loss of follicular ostia, and oftentimes hemorrhagic crusts and erosions [95]. It may be associated with pain, itching, burning, and spontaneous bleeding. In later lesions, variably sized, irregularly shaped atrophic patches of scarring alopecia develop. "Tufted hairs" is a common finding in FD, characterized by multiple hairs (5–20) emerging from a single dilated follicular orifice. Although suggestive of neutrophilic scalp disorders like FD, tufted hairs can be found in several forms of cicatricial alopecia, such as discoid lupus, lichen planopilaris, CCCA, AK, and dissecting cellulitis [96, 98]. Eyelashes and other body hairs are not affected in FD, though eyebrows and beard may rarely be involved [95].

For diagnosis, along with history and thorough scalp examination, bacterial cultures should be taken from an intact pustule or from a scalp swab and tested for antibiotic sensitivities [96]. A nasal swab can be performed to identify *S. aureus* colonization [96]. Biopsy from an active hair-bearing margin can be helpful for diagnosis of FD. Early lesions show keratin aggregation and dilation of the infundibulum along with numerous intraluminal neutrophils [96]. Sebaceous glands are destroyed early in the process. An intrafollicular and perifollicular predominantly neutrophilic infiltrate is found. In advanced lesions, the infiltrate may be mixed, consisting of neutrophils, lymphocytes, and numerous plasma cells [96]. Granulomatous inflammation with foreign-body giant cells is also common. Follicular tufts can be seen on biopsy. End-stage lesions demonstrate fibrous tracts and interstitial dermal fibrosis [96].

FD causes significant suffering from severe symptoms and extensive involvement and tends to be resistant to treatment. Anti-staphylococcal antibiotics, including doxycycline, minocycline, erythromycin, trimethoprim/sulfamethoxazole, and clindamycin, are the first-line therapy, although a recent report suggests isotretinoin might be more effective [100]. Combination of anti-staphylococcal antibiotics with rifampin has shown additional benefits [97]. Oral rifampin 300 mg twice daily and clindamycin 300 mg twice daily for 10–12 weeks has been used in resistant cases with possibility of long-term remission [95, 97, 98]. Patients should be warned that secretions, like urine, tears, and saliva, may turn red-orange with rifampin. Relapse is common after discontinuation of antibiotic therapy, and patients may have to stay on low-dose antibiotics for many years [97, 98, 101]. A recent study found that over half of patients required long term antibiotics [101]. Potent topical or intralesional triamcinolone acetonide at a concentration 10 mg/mL every 4–6 weeks [96, 101], topical antibiotics [95], oral dapsone [102, 103], oral isotretinoin [100], and photodynamic therapy [104] have also been used with some success. The patient must be educated that scarred areas may not regrow and that long-term treatment may be necessary. Patients should also be advised about different camouflage techniques. However, caps, hats, weaves, and hair pieces may be problematic as they may serve as a reservoir for *S. aureus*. These devices should be cleaned with antiseptics regularly [96].

Other neutrophilic scalp disorders include dissecting cellulitis and AK, which are both more common in African-American males. Dissecting cellulitis is a chronic inflammatory condition characterized by fluctuant cysts, boggy nodules, draining sinus tracts, and subsequent scarring alopecia, typically on the occipital or vertex of the scalp [70, 105] (Fig. 19.6). It may be seen in association with pilonidal cysts, acne conglobata, and hidradenitis suppurativa, known as the "follicular tetrad," suggesting a common mechanism consisting of abnormal follicular keratinization, occlusion, secondary bacterial infection and follicular destruction [2, 70]. First-line treatment includes antibiotics, typically of the tetracycline class, which may be combined with topical antibiotic or antiseptics, like chlorhexidine or benzoyl peroxide, as well as topical and intralesional steroids [2, 70]. Oral isotretinoin [106–109], dapsone [110], and more recently TNFα inhibitors [111–113] have also been used in treatment. Surgical options include lesional aspiration, incision and

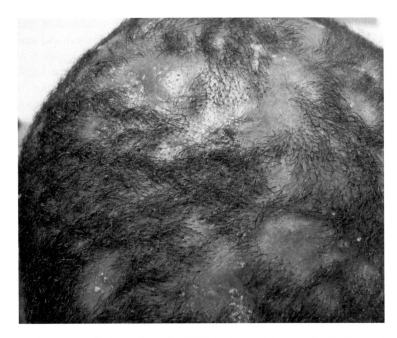

Fig. 19.6 Dissecting cellulitis of the scalp. Multiple deep nodules associated with crusting and drainage

drainage, excision with skin grafting [114], laser therapies [115, 116], and photo-dynamic therapy [117]. Patients should be made aware of an increased risk of squamous cell carcinoma with long-standing disease [118].

AK is a common scarring alopecia typically occurring in African males, with a prevalence of 1.6–16.1% [57, 80, 119–123]. Peak prevalence occurs in men aged 25–34 years [119]. It is characterized by skin-colored to hyperpigmented follicular papules and pustules which can coalesce into firm hypertrophic plaques and nodules at the nape of the neck and occipital scalp [124, 125]. Severe keloid formation is often observed [2]. The alopecia is often painful and disfiguring. The etiology is likely multifactorial, including hormonal factors, friction and shaving behaviors, resulting in inflammation, and secondary infection [119]. It has been noted that Africans have a genetic predisposition for curly hair which readily produces in growing hairs after it is cut short, which has also been implicated in the patho-genesis of AK [119]. Treatment includes topical steroids, intralesional steroids, topical antibiotics, and oral antibiotics. Surgical approaches include excision with primary or secondary closure, excision with skin grafting, and hair removal lasers [124]. In addition, physicians should counsel on avoiding manipulation of lesions, shirts with tight collars or friction to affected areas, and avoiding shaving or close hair cutting.

Lichen Planopilaris

Lichen planopilaris is a type of chronic lymphocytic scarring alopecia that is considered a variant of lichen planus affecting the hair follicle [126]. It is seen more commonly in Caucasians than in ethnic populations, and the female to male ratio is 1.8:112 [6]. The scalp lesions are characterized by irregularly shaped atrophic patches of alopecia with loss of follicular orifices, commonly involve the vertex and parietal regions [126]. The active borders reveal perifollicular erythema, scale, and occasionally, groups of keratotic follicular papules [126]. There may be associated hair shedding, itching, scaling, and burning. Skin, nail, and mucous membrane lichen planus may also be seen [126].

Frontal fibrosing alopecia is a variant of lichen planopilaris that presents with progressive band-like scarring alopecia [126, 127]. FFA primarily occurs in Caucasian patients, but may uncommonly occur in patients of Asian and African descent [105], when it can be confused or coexist with TA [128]. Clinical findings include progressive recession of frontotemporal hairline with loss of follicular ostia, follicular hyperkeratosis, and perifollicular erythema, as seen in lichen planopilaris. Fifty-two percent of affected patients also have eyebrow hair loss [126]. Follicular ostia can be retained in African patients [128]. Histopathology varies with the stage of disease. Early stages will show a lichenoid lymphocytic infiltrate affecting the infundibulum and isthmus with the lower portion of the hair follicle being spared [126]. Sebaceous glands are lost and root sheaths of the hair follicles are destroyed. With progression of disease, extensive perifollicular lamellar fibrosis, especially around the isthmus, will occur with eventual destruction of hair follicle and replacement by fibrous tracts [126].

First-line treatment of both disorders includes application of high-potency topical steroids and intralesional triamcinolone acetate, while oral steroids are reserved for more aggressive, severe disease [126]. Oral antimalarials, including hydroxychloroquine, are also used for its anti-inflammatory effects, though it takes about 2–3 months for efficacy to be seen [126]. For refractory disease, cyclosporine and mycophenolate mofetil have been used for treatment of LPP [126]. More recently, finasteride and dutasteride have been supported for use in FFA [127].

Hair Shaft Disorders

Acquired trichorrhexis nodosa (ATN) occurs when hair is so fragile that minor trauma to the proximal end causes breakage. The etiology of ATN include years of use of chemicals or heat devices [129], or excessive combing or brushing with stiff brushes and plastic combs [105, 129, 130], which cause cuticular disruption and weakening of the hair shaft. Some patients with ATN go on to develop CCCA [65], suggesting a similar pathophysiology. Clinically, the hair appears lusterless and dry, and patients may complain of "whitish spots" along the hair. Light microscopy will show small, beaded swellings (likened to two paintbrushes crushed against each

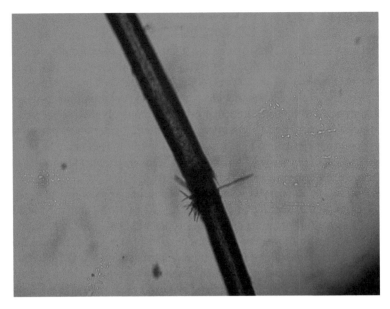

Fig. 19.7 Trichorrhexis nodosa. Fracture of the cuticle leads to hair shaft fragility and breakage

other) along the hair shaft along with loss of cuticle (Fig. 19.7) [2, 105]. Treatment mainly focuses on behavioral changes, including avoiding hair relaxers (or limiting them to every 8–12 weeks), straightening of hair with heat, excessive combing of hairs, and massaging or rubbing the hair [130].

Inflammatory Scalp Conditions

SD is a common chronic inflammatory scalp disorder frequently confronted in the ethnic population. SD is common in children between weeks 2–6 years of life, and it is often referred to as "cradle cap." The prevalence of SD in African-American children ranges from 1 to 6.7% [70]. SD is rare in toddlers or prepubescent children, but may recur during or after puberty and is quite common in African-American adults [70]. It presents with scalp dryness, dandruff and flaking, which may also involve the face and chest [70]. Scalp pruritus may be an associated symptom. Given the decreased tensile strength of African hair, aggressive scratching of the scalp may result in short, broken hair [105]. Treatment includes antifungal shampoos, often in combination with topical steroids. Although frequent washing is well tolerated in Caucasian and Asian patients, this may not be optimal in African patients because styling hair may take hours and is not practical [105], and because washing and drying can further damage an already weakened hair shaft [2]. Thus, in this patient population, washing can be recommended once to twice weekly [105].

Alternating dandruff shampoos with moisturizing shampoos can be helpful, and conditioners should be used. Because both over the counter and prescription shampoos may dry the hair shaft in ethnic patients, topical steroids are often recommended, especially those with moderate to severe disease. The vehicle of the medication is determined by patient preference, ethnicity, and hairstyle. For example, solution and foam formulations may be used in most hair types, including African Americans with "natural" hairstyles. In patients with chemically or heat processed hair, ointments are preferred [105]. Dyspigmentation from topical steroids is of particular concern in African patients and should be monitored for. Patients should be encouraged use emollients to coat the hair and not the scalp, as they can cause scalp irritation and worsen the dermatitis [2].

Conclusion

Structural differences in ethnic hair, specifically African hair, lead to decreased hair shaft strength, difficulties in combing, and may account for higher incidence of certain hair disorders like AK nuchae. African patients also practice traumatic hairstyles including weaves, extensions, and relaxing, which may contribute to scarring hair loss. Certain scarring alopecias, such as CCCA, are unique to the African-American population. Treatment of these hair diseases requires specific considerations as to skin type, for example, the avoidance of hypopigmentation from topical and intralesional steroid use. Dermatologists must have a clear knowledge of the basic hair care practices and hair disorders that occur in the ethnic population in order to properly diagnose and manage these patients.

References

1. Franbourg A, Hallegot P, Baltenneck F, Toutain C, Leroy F. Current research on ethnic hair. J Am Acad Dermatol. 2003;48(6 Suppl):S115–9.
2. McMichael AJ. Hair and scalp disorders in ethnic populations. Dermatol Clin. 2003;21 (4):629–44.
3. Loussouarn G, Garcel AL, Lozano I, Collaudin C, Porter C, Panhard S, Saint-Leger D, de La Mettrie R. Worldwide diversity of hair curliness: a new method of assessment. Int J Dermatol. 2007;46(Suppl 1):2–6.
4. Rook A. Racial and other genetic variations in hair form. Br J Dermatol. 1975;92(5): 599–600.
5. Blume-Peytavi U, Tosti A, Whiting DA, Trüeb RM. Hair growth and disorders. Berlin: Springer; 2008. p. 590.
6. McMichael AJ. Ethnic hair update: past and present. J Am Acad Dermatol. 2003;48(6 Suppl):S127–33.
7. Byrd AD, Tharps, LL. Hair story: untangling the roots of black hair in America. New York: St. Martin's Press; 2001 p. 20.

8. Kyei A, Bergfeld WF, Piliang M, Summers P. Medical and environmental risk factors for the development of central centrifugal cicatricial alopecia: a population study. Arch Dermatol. 2011;147(8):909–14.

9. Gathers RC, Lim HW. Central centrifugal cicatricial alopecia: past, present, and future. J Am Acad Dermatol. 2009;60(4):660–8.

10. Alexis AF, Barbosa VH. Skin of color: a practical guide to dermatologic diagnosis and treatment. New York: Springer; 2013. p. 355–6.

11. Lee WS, Lee HJ. Characteristics of androgenetic alopecia in asian. Ann Dermatol. 2012;24 (3):243–52.

12. Banka N, Bunagan MJ, Shapiro J. Pattern hair loss in men: diagnosis and medical treatment. Dermatol Clin. 2013;31(1):129–40.

13. Ludwig E. Classification of the types of androgenetic alopecia (common baldness) occurring in the female sex. Br J Dermatol. 1977;97(3):247–54.

14. Price VH. Treatment of hair loss. N Engl J Med. 1999;341(13):964–73.

15. Olsen EA. The midline part: an important physical clue to the clinical diagnosis of androgenetic alopecia in women. J Am Acad Dermatol. 1999;40(1):106–9.

16. Venning VA, Dawber RP. Patterned androgenic alopecia in women. J Am Acad Dermatol. 1988;18(5 pt 1):1073–7.

17. Olsen EA. Androgenetic alopecia. In: Olsen EA, editor. Disorders of hair growth: diagnosis and treatment. New York: McGraw-Hill; 1994. p. 257–83.

18. Ramos LD, Santili MC, Bezerra FC, Ruiz Mde F, Petri V, Patriarca MT. Dermoscopic findings in female androgenetic alopecia. An Bras Dermatol. 2012;87(5):691–4.

19. Tosti A, Torres F. Dermoscopy in the diagnosis of hair and scalp disorders. Actas Dermosifiliogr. 2009;100(Suppl 1):114–9.

20. Whiting DA. Diagnostic and predictive value of horizontal sections of scalp biopsy specimens in male pattern androgenetic alopecia. J Am Acad Dermatol. 1993;28(5):755–63.

21. Stefanato CM. Histopathology of alopecia: a clinicopathological approach to diagnosis. Histopathology. 2010;56(1):24–38.

22. Werner B, Mulinari-Brenner F. Clinical and histological challenge in the differential diagnosis of diffuse alopecia: female androgenetic alopecia, telogen effluvium and alopecia areata—part II. An Bras Dermatol. 2012;87(6):884–90.

23. Torres F, Tosti A. Female pattern alopecia and telogen effluvium: figuring out diffuse alopecia. Semin Cutan Med Surg. 2015;34(2):67–71.

24. Nyholt DR, Gillespie NA, Heath AC, Martin NG. Genetic basis of male pattern baldness. J Invest Dermatol. 2003;121:1561–4.

25. Tang L, Bernardo O, Bolduc C, Lui H, Madani S, Shapiro J. The expression of insulin-like growth factor 1 in follicular dermal papillae correlates with therapeutic efficacy of finasteride in androgenetic alopecia. J Am Acad Dermatol. 2003;49:229–33.

26. Ellis JA, Stebbing M, Harrap SB. Polymorphism of the androgen receptor gene is associated with male pattern baldness. J Invest Dermatol. 2001;116:452–5.

27. Zhuo FL, Xu W, Wang L, Wu Y, Xu ZL, Zhao JY. Androgen receptor gene polymorphisms and risk for androgenetic alopecia: a meta-analysis. Clin Exp Dermatol. 2012;37:104–11.

28. Jung JG, Park JW, Kim MH, Cinn YW. A study on CAG repeat polymorphisms of the androgen receptor in Korean androgenetic alopecia: preliminary report. Korean J Dermatol. 2009;47:772–6.

29. Olsen EA. Female pattern hair loss. J Am Acad Dermatol. 2001;45(3 Suppl):S70–80.

30. Panchaprateep R, Korkij W, Asawanonda P. Brain-derived nerve factor and neurotrophins in androgenetic alopecia. Br J Dermatol. 2011;165:997–1002.

31. Zeigler-Johnson C, Morales KH, Spangler E, Chang BL, Rebbeck TR. Relationship of early-onset baldness to prostate cancer in African-American men. Cancer Epidemiol Biomarkers Prev. 2013;22(4):589–96.

32. Hsing AW, Gao YT, Wu G, Wang X, Deng J, Chen YL, Sesterhenn IA, Mostofi FK, Benichou J, Chang C. Polymorphic CAG and GGN repeat lengths in the androgen receptor

gene and prostate cancer risk: a population-based case-control study in China. Cancer Res. 2000;60(18):5111–6.

33. Hayes VM, Severi G, Eggleton SA, Padilla EJ, Southey MC, Sutherland RL, et al. The E211 G> A androgen receptor polymorphism is associated with a decreased risk of metastatic prostate cancer and androgenetic alopecia. Cancer Epidemiol Biomarkers Prev. 2005;14:993–6.

34. Arias-Santiago S, Gutierrez-Salmeron MT, Castellote-Caballero L, Buendia-Eisman A, Naranjo-Sintes R. Androgenetic alopecia and cardiovascular risk factors in men and women: a comparative study. J Am Acad Dermatol. 2010;63(3):420–9.

35. Sasmaz S, Senol M, Ozcan A, Dogan G, Tuncer C, Akyol O, Sener S. The risk of coronary heart disease in men with androgenetic alopecia. J Eur Acad Dermatol Venereol. 1999;12 (2):123–5.

36. Zitzmann M, Brune M, Kornmann B, Gromoll J, von Eckardstein S, von Eckardstein A, et al. The CAG repeat polymorphism in the AR gene affects high density lipoprotein cholesterol and arterial vasoreactivity. J Clin Endocrinol Metab. 2001;86:4867–73.

37. Olsen EA, Dunlap FE, Funicella T, Koperski JA, Swinehart JM, Tschen EH, Trancik RJ. A randomized clinical trial of 5% topical minoxidil versus 2% topical minoxidil and placebo in the treatment of androgenetic alopecia in men. J Am Acad Dermatol. 2002;47 (3):377–85.

38. Messenger AG, Rundegren J. Minoxidil: mechanisms of action on hair growth. Br J Dermatol. 2004;150(2):186–94.

39. Kaufman KD, Olsen EA, Whiting D, et al. Finasteride in the treatment of men with androgenetic alopecia. J Am Acad Dermatol. 1998;39:578–89.

40. Mysore V. Finasteride and sexual side effects. Indian Dermatol Online J. 2012;3(1):62–5.

41. Mella JM, Perret MC, Manzotti M, Catalano HN, Guyatt G. Efficacy and safety of finasteride therapy for androgenetic alopecia: a systematic review. Arch Dermatol. 2010;146(10):1141–50.

42. Traish AM, Hassani J, Guay AT, Zitzmann M, Hansen ML. Adverse side effects of 5α-reductase inhibitors therapy: persistent diminished libido and erectile dysfunction and depression in a subset of patients. J Sex Med. 2011;8(3):872–84.

43. Price VH, Roberts JL, Hordinsky M, Olsen EA, Savin R, Bergfeld W, et al. Lack of efficacy of finasteride in postmenopausal women with androgenetic alopecia. J Am Acad Dermatol. 2000;43(5 Pt 1):768–76.

44. Yeon JH, Jung JY, Choi JW, Kim BJ, Youn SW, Park KC, et al. 5 mg/day finasteride treatment for normoandrogenic Asian women with female pattern hair loss. J Eur Acad Dermatol Venereol. 2011;25:211–4.

45. Trüeb RM; Swiss Trichology Study Group. Finasteride treatment of patterned hair loss in normoandrogenic postmenopausal women. Dermatology. 2004;209(3):202–7.

46. Rathnayake D, Sinclair R. Innovative use of spironolactone as an antiandrogen in the treatment of female pattern hair loss. Dermatol Clin. 2010;28(3):611–8.

47. Yazdabadi A, Sinclair R. Treatment of female pattern hair loss with the androgen receptor antagonist flutamide. Australas J Dermatol. 2011;52(2):132–4.

48. Scheinfeld N. A review of hormonal therapy for female pattern (androgenic) alopecia. Dermatol Online J. 2008;14(3):1.

49. Jimenez JJ, Wikramanayake TC, Bergfield W, Hordinsky M, Hickman JG, Hamblin MR, Schachner LA. Efficacy and safety of a low-level laser device in the treatment of male and female pattern hair loss: a multicenter, randomized, sham device-controlled, double-blind study. Am J Clin Dermatol. 2014;15(2):115–27.

50. Wikramanayake TC, Rodriguez R, Choudhary S, Mauro LM, Nouri K, Schachner LA, Jimenez JJ. Effects of the Lexington LaserComb on hair regrowth in the C3H/HeJ mouse model of alopecia areata. Lasers Med Sci. 2012;27(2):431–6.

51. Leavitt M, Charles G, Heyman E, Michaels D. HairMax LaserComb laser phototherapy device in the treatment of male androgenetic alopecia: a randomized, double-blind, sham device-controlled, multicentre trial. Clin Drug Investig. 2009;29(5):283–92.

52. Alves R, Grimalt R. Randomized Placebo-controlled, double-blind, half-head study to assess the efficacy of platelet-rich plasma on the treatment of androgenetic alopecia. Dermatol Surg. 2016;42(4):491–7.

53. Madu P, Kundu RV. Follicular and scarring disorders in skin of color: presentation and management. Am J Clin Dermatol. 2014;15(4):307–21.

54. Sperling LC. Scarring alopecia and the dermatopathologist. J Cutan Pathol. 2001;28:333–42.

55. Olsen EA, Bergfeld WF, Cotsarelis G, et al. Workshop on Cicatricial Alopecia. Summary of North American Hair Research Society (NAHRS)-sponsored Workshop on Cicatricial Alopecia, Duke University Medical Center, February 10 and 11, 2001. J Am Acad Dermatol. 2003;48(1):103–10.

56. Olsen EA, Callender V, McMichael A, Sperling L, Anstrom KJ, Shapiro J, et al. Central hair loss in African American women: incidence and potential risk factors. J Am Acad Dermatol. 2011;64(2):245–52.

57. Khumalo NP, Jessop S, Gumedze F, Ehrlich R. Hairdressing and the prevalence of scalp disease in African adults. Br J Dermatol. 2007;157(5):981–8.

58. Khumalo NP, Jessop S, Gumedze F, Ehrlich R. Determinants of marginal traction alopecia in African girls and women. J Am Acad Dermatol. 2008;59(3):432–8.

59. LoPresti P, Papa CM, Kligman AM. Hot comb alopecia. Arch Dermatol. 1968;98(3):234–8.

60. Sperling LC, Sau P. The follicular degeneration syndrome in black patients: 'hot comb alopecia' revisited and revised. Arch Dermatol. 1992;128(1):68–74.

61. Nicholson AG, Harland CC, Bull RH, Mortimer PS, Cook MG. Chemically induced cosmetic alopecia. Br J Dermatol. 1993;128(5):537–41.

62. Dlova NC, Forder M. Central centrifugal cicatricial alopecia: possible familial aetiology in two African families from South Africa. Int J Dermatol. 2012;51(Suppl 1):17–20, 23.

63. Dlova NC, Jordaan FH, Sarig O, Sprecher E. Autosomal dominant inheritance of central centrifugal cicatricial alopecia in black South Africans. J Am Acad Dermatol. 2014;70 (4):679–82.

64. Whiting DA, Olsen EA. Central centrifugal cicatricial alopecia. Dermatol Ther. 2008;21 (4):268–78.

65. Callender V, Wright D, Davis E, Sperling L. Hair breakage as a presenting sign of early or occult central centrifugal cicatricial alopecia. Clinicopathological findings in 9 patients. Arch Dermatol. 2012;148(9):1047–52.

66. Miteva M, Tosti A. Dermatoscopic features of central centrifugal cicatricial alopecia. J Am Acad Dermatol. 2014;71(30):443–9.

67. Sperling LC, Shelton HG III, Smith KJ, et al. Follicular degeneration syndrome in men. Arch Dermatol. 1994;130:763–9.

68. Headington JT. Cicatricial alopecia. Dermatol Clin. 1996;14(4):773–82.

69. Davis EC, Reid SD, Callender VD, Sperling LC. Differentiating central centrifugal cicatricial alopecia and androgenetic alopecia in African American men: report of three cases. J Clin Aesthet Dermatol. 2012;5(6):37–40.

70. Semble AL, McMichael AJ. Hair loss in patients with skin of color. Semin Cutan Med Surg. 2015;34(2):81–8.

71. Callender VD, McMichael AJ, Cohen GF. Medical and surgical therapies for alopecias in black women. Dermatol Ther. 2004;17(2):164–76.

72. Samrao A, Price VH, Zedek D, Mirmirani P. The, "Fringe Sign"- A useful clinical finding in traction alopecia of the marginal hair line. Dermatol Online J. 2011;17(11):1.

73. James J, Saladi RN, Fox JL. Traction alopecia in Sikh male patients. J Am Board Fam Med. 2007;20(5):497–8.

74. Kanwar AJ, Kaur S, Basak P, Sharma R. Traction alopecia in Sikh males. Arch Dermatol. 1989;125(11):1587.

75. Olsen EA. Disorders of hair growth: diagnosis and treatment. New York: McGraw-Hill Companies, 2003. Pp. 99–100, 508–9.

76. Samrao A, Chen C, Zedek D, Price VH. Traction alopecia in a ballerina: clinicopathologic features. Arch Dermatol. 2010;146(8):930–1.

77. Trueb RM. "Chignon alopecia": a distinctive type of nonmarginal traction alopecia. Cutis. 1995;55(3):178–9.
78. Rudolph RI, Klein AW, Decherd JW. Corn-row alopecia. Arch Dermatol. 1973;108(1):134.
79. Lipnik MJ. Traumatic alopecia from brush rollers. Arch Dermatol. 1961;84:493–5.
80. Khumalo NP, Jessop S, Gumedze F, Ehrlich R. Hairdressing is associated with scalp disease in African schoolchildren. Br J Dermatol. 2007;157(1):106–10.
81. Yang A, Iorizzo M, Vincenzi C, Tosti A. Hair extensions: a concerning cause of hair disorders. Br J Dermatol. 2009;160(1):207–9.
82. Fox GN, Stausmire JM, Mehregan DR. Traction folliculitis: an underreported entity. Cutis. 2007;79(1):26–30.
83. Goldberg LJ. Cicatrical marginal alopecia: is it all traction? Br J Dermatol. 2009;160:62–8.
84. Khumalo NP. The "fringe sign" for public education on traction alopecia. Dermatol Online J. 2012;18(9):16.
85. Heath CR, Taylor SC. Alopecia in an ophiasis pattern: traction alopecia versus alopecia areata. Cutis. 2012;89(5):213–6.
86. Ahdout J, Mirmirani P. Weft hair extensions causing a distinctive horseshoe pattern of traction alopecia. J Am Acad Dermatol. 2012;67(6):e294–5.
87. Sperling LC, Lupton GP. Histopathology of non-scarring alopecia. J Cutan Pathol. 1995;22 (2):97–114.
88. Miteva M, Tosti A. "A detective look" at hair biopsies from African-American patients. Br J Dermatol. 2012;166(6):1289–94.
89. Khumalo NP, Ngwanya RM. Traction alopecia: 2% topical minoxidil shows promise. Report of two cases. J Eur Acad Dermatol Venereol. 2007;21(3):433–4.
90. Hordinsky M. Cicatricial alopecia: discoid lupus erythematosus. Dermatol Ther. 2008;21 (4):245–8.
91. Ross E, Tan E, Shapiro J. Update on primary cicatricial alopecias. J Am Acad Dermatol. 2005;53:1–37.
92. Mirmirani P. Cicatricial alopecia. In: McMichael A, Hordinsky M, editors. Hair and scalp diseases: medical, surgical, and cosmetic treatments (basic and clinical dermatology). New York: Informa Healthcare; 2008. p. 137–48.
93. Milam EC, Ramachandran S, Franks AG Jr. Treatment of scarring alopecia in discoid variant of chronic cutaneous lupus erythematosus with tacrolimus lotion, 0.3. JAMA Dermatol. 2015;151(10):1113–6.
94. Sugano M, Shintani Y, Kobayashi K, Sakakibara N, Isomura I, Morita A. Successful treatment with topical tacrolimus in four cases of discoid lupus erythematosus. J Dermatol. 2006;33(12):887–91.
95. Vaño-Galvan S, Molina-Ruiz AM, Fernanez-Crehuet P, Rodrigues-Barata AR, Arias-Santiago S, Serrano-Falcon C, Martorell-Calatayud A, Barco D, Perez B, Serrano S, Requena L, Grimalt R, Paoli J, Jaen P, Camacho FM. Folliculitis decalvans: a multicentre review of 82 patients. J Eur Acad Dermatol Venereol. 2015;29(9):1750–7.
96. Otberg N, Kang H, Alzolibani AA, Shapiro J. Folliculitis decalvans. Dermatol Ther. 2008;21 (4):238–44.
97. Brooke RC, Griffiths CE. Folliculitis decalvans. Clin Exp Dermatol. 2001;26:120–2.
98. Powell JJ, Dawber RP, Gatter K. Folliculitis decalvans including tufted folliculitis: clinical, histological and therapeutic findings. Br J Dermatol. 1999;140:328–33.
99. Annessi G. Tufted folliculitis of the scalp: a distinctive clinicohistological variant of folliculitis decalvans. Br J Dermatol. 1998;138:799–805.
100. Tietze JK, Heppt MV, von PreuBen A, Wolf U, Ruzicka T, Wolff H, Sattler EC. Oral isotretinoin as the most effective treatment in folliculitis decalvans: a retrospective comparison of different treatment regimens in 28 patients. J Eur Acad Dermatol Venereol. 2015;29(9):1816–21.
101. Bunagan MJ, Banka N, Shapiro J. Retrospective review of folliculitis decalvans in 23 patients with course and treatment analysis of long-standing cases. J Cutan Med Surg. 2015;19(1):45–9.

102. Kunte C, Loeser C, Wolff H. Folliculitis spinulosa decalvans: successful therapy with dapsone. J Am Acad Dermatol. 1998;39(5):891–3.
103. Paquet P, Pierard GE. Dapsone treatment of folliculitis decalvans. Ann Dermatol Venereol. 2004;131(2):195–7.
104. Miguel-Gomez L, Vano-Galvan S, Perez-Garcia B, Carrillo-Gijon R, Jaen-Olasolo P. Treatment of folliculitis decalvans with photodynamic therapy: results in 10 patients. J Am Acad Dermatol. 2015;72(6):1085–7.
105. Rodney IJ, Onwudiwe OC, Callender VD, Halder RM. Hair and scalp disorders in ethnic populations. J Drugs Dermatol. 2013;12(4):420–7.
106. Georgala S, Korfitis C, Ioannidou D, Alestas T, Kylafis G, Georgala C. Dissecting cellulitis of the scalp treated with rifampicin and isotretinoin: case reports. Cutis. 2008;82(3):195–8.
107. Khaled A, Zeglaoui F, Zoghlami A, Fazaa B. Kamoun Mr. Dissecting cellulitis of the scalp: response to isotretinoin. J Eur Acad Dermatol Venereol. 2007;21(10):1430–1.
108. Taylor AE. Dissecting cellulitis of the scalp: response to isotretinoin. Lancet. 1987;2 (8552):225.
109. Koudoukpo C, Abdennader S, Cavelier-Balloy B, Gasnier C, Yedomon H. Dissecting cellulitis of the scalp: a retrospective study of 7 cases confirming the efficacy of oral isotretinoin. Ann Dermatol Venereol. 2014;141(8–9):500–6.
110. Bolz S, Jappe U, Hartschuh W. Successful treatment of perifolliculitis abscedens et suffodiens with combined isotretinoin and dapsone. J Dtsch Dermatol Ges. 2008;6:44–7.
111. Navarini AA, Trueb RM. 3 cases of dissecting cellulitis of the scalp treated with adalimumab: control of inflammation within residual structural disease. Arch Dermatol. 2010;146(5):517–20.
112. Brandt HR, Malheiros AP, Teixeira MG, Machado MC. Perifolliculitis abscedens et suffodiens successfully controlled with infliximab. Br J Dermatol. 2008;159:506–7.
113. Wollina U, Gemmeke A, Koch A. Dissecting cellulitis of the scalp responding to intravenous tumor necrosis factor-alpha antagonist. J Clin Aesthet Dermatol. 2012;5(4): 36–9.
114. Bellew SG, Nemerofsky R, Schwartz RA, Granick MS. Successful treatment of recalcitrant dissecting cellulitis of the scalp with complete scalp excision and split-thickness skin graft. Dermatol Surg. 2003;29(10):1068–70.
115. Krasner BD, Hamzavi FH, Murakawa GJ, Hamzavi IH. Dissecting cellulitis treated with the long-pulsed Nd:YAG laser. Dermatol Surg. 2006;32(8):1039–44.
116. Boyd AS, Binhlam JQ. Use of an 800-nm pulsed-diode laser in the treatment of recalcitrant dissecting cellulitis of the scalp. Arch Dermatol. 2002;138(10):1291–3.
117. Liu Y, Ma Y, Xiang LH. Successful treatment of recalcitrant dissecting cellulitis of the scalp with ALA-PDT: case report and literature review. Photodiagnosis Photodyn Ther. 2013;10 (4):410–3.
118. Curry SS, Gaither DH, King LE Jr. Squamous cell carcinoma arising in dissecting perifolliculitis of the scalp. A case report and review of secondary squamous cell carcinomas. J Am Acad Dermatol. 1981;4:673–8.
119. Ogunbiyi A, Adedokun B. Perceived aetiological factors of folliculitis keloidalis nuchae (acne keloidalis) and treatment options among Nigerian men. Br J Dermatol. 2015;173 (Suppl 2):22–5.
120. Salami T, Omeife H, Samuel S. Prevalence of acne keloidalis nuchae in Nigerians. Int J Dermatol. 2007;46:482–4.
121. George AO, Akanji AO, Nduka EU, et al. Clinical biochemical and morphologic features of acne keloidalis in a black population. Int J Dermatol. 1993;32:714–6.
122. Ogunbiyi AO, Daramola OO, Alese OO. Prevalence of skin diseases in Ibadan, Nigeria. Int J Dermatol. 2004;43:31–6.
123. Child FJ, Fuller LC, Higgind EM, Du Vivier AW. A study of the spectrum of skin disease occurring in the black population in South East London. Br J Dermatol. 1991;141:512–7.
124. Bajaj V, Langtry JA. Surgical excision of acne keloidalis nuchae with secondary intention healing. Clin Exp Dermatol. 2008;33(1):53–5.

125. Dinehart SM, Herzberg AJ, Kerns BJ, Pollack SV. Acne keloidalis: a review. J Dermatol Surg Oncol. 1989;15(6):642–7.
126. Kang H, Alzolibani AA, Otberg N, Shapiro J. Lichen planopilaris. Dermatol Ther. 2008;21 (4):249–56.
127. Vañó-Galván S, Molina-Ruiz AM, Serrano-Falcón C, Arias-Santiago S, Rodrigues-Barata AR, Garnacho-Saucedo G, Martorell-Calatayud A, Fernández-Crehuet P, Grimalt R, Aranegui B, Grillo E, Diaz-Ley B, Salido R, Pérez-Gala S, Serrano S, Moreno JC, Jaén P, Camacho FM. Frontal fibrosing alopecia: a multicenter review of 355 patients. J Am Acad Dermatol. 2014;70(4):670–8.
128. Dlova NC, Jordaan HF, Skenjane A, Khoza N, Tosti A. Frontal fibrosing alopecia: a clinical review of 20 black patients from South Africa. Br J Dermatol. 2013;169(4):939–41.
129. Halder RM. Hair and scalp disorders in blacks. Cutis. 1983;32:378–80.
130. Tanus A, Oliveira CC, Villarreal DJ, Sanchez FA, Dias MF. Black women's hair: the main scalp dermatoses and aesthetic practices in women of African ethnicity. An Bras Dermatol. 2015;90(4):450–65.

Chapter 20
Adnexal Disorders

Andrew F. Alexis and Bridget P. Kaufman

Pseudofolliculitis Barbae

Pseudofolliculitis barbae (PB) is a chronic, noninfectious inflammatory condition that occurs in shaven areas. Also referred to as shave bumps, razor bumps, ingrown hairs, and chronic sycosis barbae, this disorder results from a foreign body reaction to the growing hair shaft, especially when the hair is thick and tightly curled [1].

Epidemiology

PB most often affects males of African ancestry with a prevalence ranging from 43 to 83% [2, 3]. This condition also is seen in other ethnic groups, including Hispanic and Middle Eastern populations, although with lesser frequency. Men aged 14–25 are most frequently affected [4]. Women may also develop PB in shaven or plucked areas, including the chin and the groin [4].

A.F. Alexis (✉) · B.P. Kaufman
Department of Dermatology, Mount Sinai St. Luke's
and Mount Sinai West, 1090 Amsterdam Ave Ste 11B,
New York, NY 10025, USA
e-mail: aalexis@chpnet.org

B.P. Kaufman
e-mail: bkaufman@chpnet.org

© Springer International Publishing AG 2017
N.A. Vashi and H.I. Maibach (eds.), *Dermatoanthropology of Ethnic
Skin and Hair*, DOI 10.1007/978-3-319-53961-4_20

Pathophysiology

PB is thought to develop when closely shaven hairs reenter the epidermis or dermis as they grow. The hair may enter the skin in one of two manners: extrafollicular penetration or transfollicular penetration [5]. In extrafollicular penetration, the hair grows normally within the follicular shaft. Upon reaching the skin surface, the hair curls back upon itself and enters the epidermis about 1–2 mm away from the follicular opening. Transfollicular penetration occurs when the shaved hair curls while still within the follicle, breaks through the follicular wall, and enters the dermis without ever exiting the skin. The presence of hair within the dermis or epidermis triggers a foreign body reaction around the tip of the hair [4].

Several hypotheses explain why this occurs. Pulling the skin taut while shaving allows for the hair to be cut shorter than it otherwise could in the resting position. Once the skin is released, the short hair retracts beneath the skin surface where it can curl and pierce the follicular wall [6, 7]. The weaker the follicular the wall, the more likely the hair will be to break through and initiate an inflammatory reaction. A substitution mutation in the 1A α-helical segment of the hair follicle-specific keratin 75 (formerly K6hf), which is expressed in a layer between the inner and outer root sheath of the hair follicle, is found in 36% of PB cases compared to 9% of controls [1, 8]. It is hypothesized that the structurally weaker hair sheath conferred by this mutation, in combination with curly hair and close shaving, increases the risk of transfollicular penetration and ultimately the inflammatory cascade leading to PB [1, 8]. African Americans and other populations of African ancestry are particularly predisposed to this condition because of the curvature of the hair shaft.

Clinical Features

Individuals with PB typically develop firm, follicular and perifollicular papules in frequently shaved areas, most commonly the anterior neck followed by the cheeks (Fig. 20.1). The mustache and nuchal areas tend to be spared despite repetitive shaving. Women who pluck or shave hair-bearing areas may develop papules on the chin [9]. Other possible locations include the axilla, groin, legs, and scalp [10–12].

The papules may be hyperpigmented, skin-colored, or erythematous. In some cases, pustules and papulopustules develop due to secondary infection. Patients with longstanding disease are at risk for developing hypertrophic scars and keloids. Postinflammatory hyperpigmentation is a common complication. PB may resemble several other conditions, including acne vulgaris and bacterial folliculitis (Table 20.1).

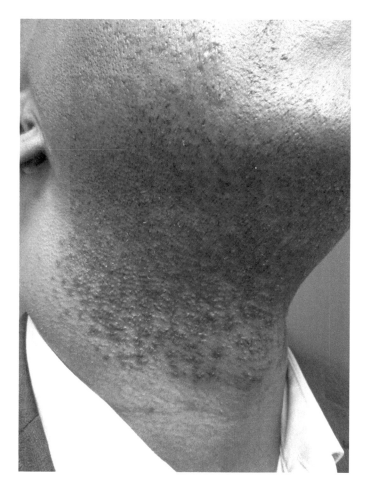

Fig. 20.1 Pseudofolliculitis barbae of the chin in an African-American male that occurred after shaving beard hairs

Table 20.1 Differential diagnosis of pseudofolliculitis barbae

Condition	Differentiating factors
Acne vulgaris	Presence of comedones and pustules Involves non-hair bearing areas of face
Traumatic folliculitis	Disappears within 24–48 h No evidence of ingrown hair
Bacterial folliculitis	Prominence of pustules Positive bacterial cultures
Tinea barbae	Unilateral facial involvement Scaling, annular

Treatment

Although there are several treatments that improve the appearance of PB, only discontinuation of shaving is curative [5]. Growing a beard typically results in resolution of PB within 2–6 weeks [12]. Therefore, as a first-line option, patients with PB can be advised to grow a beard for at least 1 month. When shaving is necessary or preferred, modification of the grooming regimen may help decrease the severity of the condition (Table 20.2).

Prior to shaving, the beard area should be washed with water and a gentle soap-free face cleanser. Washcloths, brushes, or scrubs can be used to gently remove trapped beard hairs [13]. Then, shaving cream should be applied.

Historically, single-blade razors have been recommended over multi-blade razors due to the risk of transfollicular penetration associated with close shaving [13]. However, newer razors with closer spacing of the blades may be safely used without exacerbation of PB, especially when used in combination with optimal technique (e.g., shaving with the grain) and a pre- and post-shave regimen [2, 14, 15]. Foil-guarded manual razors specifically designed for use in patients with PB may also help improve this condition [2]. Their stainless steel, polymer-coated, single blade is covered with a foil guard that prevents a close shave and reduces the risk of transfollicular penetration. Similarly, electric razors that cut beard hairs to an ideal length of 0.5–1 mm prevent transfollicular and extrafollicular penetration and, therefore, decrease the number of ingrown hairs after shaving [16]. Regardless of what type of razor is used, the blades should be kept clean and sharp so that less force is needed to cut through the hair. Each area should be shaved only once using soft strokes. The skin should be relaxed rather than pulled taut.

Pharmacological treatments of PB include topical tretinoin, topical and oral antibiotics, topical low-dose corticosteroids, and topical eflornithine hydrochloride cream (Table 20.3). These treatments reduce the severity of PB; however, none of them completely cure the condition. Once the treatment is stopped, the follicular papules and erythema recur, especially if the prior shaving regimen is continued [17].

For those willing to try alternative methods of hair removal, chemical depilatories containing barium sulfide and calcium thioglycolate may effectively remove hair without exacerbating PB. However, side effects including contact dermatitis and skin irritation may limit their use in some patients. Laser therapy has been used for treatment of PB with good results [18–23]. In patients with Fitzpatrick Skin Types IV to VI, the neodymium: yttrium aluminum garnet (Nd:YAG 1064 nm) laser has the best safety profile and, therefore, is typically preferred [24]. The diode laser (800–810 nm) is another option for patients with darker phototypes. This treatment should be used with caution as it may cause erythema, burning, and dyspigmentation of the skin [12].

Table 20.2 Shaving modifications for treatment of pseudofolliculitis barbae

Pre-shave regimen		
	Wash face with water and mild soap-free cleanser	– Washing face softens hairs making them easier to cut – Loosens and reduces the number of trapped and ingrown beard hairs [14]
	Gently rub face in circular motion with a washcloth, cleansing pad, scrub, or brush	– Scrub releases trapped beard hairs [13]
	Apply shaving cream	– Shaving cream creates an antifriction layer and smoother shave [14]
Hair removal practices		
Shaving method	Electric razor	– Electric razors that leave 0.5–1 mm of hair are very successful at decreasing PFB [16]
	Single-blade razor versus Multi-blade razor	– Single-blade razors are generally recommended; however, recent studies demonstrate that multi-blade razors may not exacerbate PFB [170]
	Razors with guards, i.e., foil-guarded manual razor	– Guards prevent hair from being cut too close thereby reducing transfollicular penetration [2, 5]
	Chemical Depilatories (i.e., barium sulfide powder or calcium thioglycolate cream)	– Depilatories are associated with decreased severity of PFB but greater irritant contact dermatitis [171]
Frequency of shaving	Daily versus 2–3 times per week	– There is no difference in papule or pustule count – Reduced frequency of shaving is associated with a significant reduction in ingrown hairs – Daily shaving is associated with patient perceived better response to treatment and decreased itching [15]
Blade characteristics	Sharp blade	– Use of a sharp blade decreases force of shaving and minimizes trauma to the hair follicle
Direction of shaving	With or against hair growth	– Shaving in the direction of hair growth is generally recommended; however, one study found that men who shaved against the grain had lower papule counts [15]
Post-shaving		
Practices after shaving	Aftershave preparation	– Rehydrates and soothes the skin
	Release ingrown hairs (with toothpick or sterile needle)	– Releasing ingrown hairs helps prevent PFB

Table 20.3 Treatment of pseudofolliculitis barbae

Lifestyle			
	Shaving modification	Only in mild cases see Table 20.1	
	Discontinue shaving	Mild—1 month Moderate—2–3 months Severe—3–6 months [33]	PFB may worzen within the first week
	Compresses Warm tap water Warm Saline Burow's solution	10–15 min 3 times daily	Soothe lesions, reduce drainage, and soften epidermis to allow for release of ingrown hairs
Pharmacologic			
Topical Treatment	Low- to mid-potency topical steroids	Daily application for 2 weeks or 1–3 times per week	
	Topical antibiotics	Twice daily benzoyl peroxide 5%/ clindamycin 1% gel	Significant reduction in combined papule and pustule counts compared to vehicle [172]
	Topical retinoids	Apply nightly	Significant improvement in clinical lesions and post-inflammatory hyperpigmentation [17, 173] Relapse after 2 weeks [17]
	Eflornithine hydrochloride cream 13.8%	Apply twice daily, rinse off 4 h after application	Decreases the number of hairs and inflammatory papules [174] Eflornithine + laser is more effective than laser alone
Oral treatment	Systemic antibiotics	Based on bacterial cultures	Can be used if PFB is secondarily infected
	Oral steroids	Prednisone 45–60 mg daily 7–10 days	May be effective in treatment of relcalcitrant disease
Intra-lesional treatment	Intra-lesional corticosteroids		
Procedural			
Laser Hair Removal	Diode laser (800–810 nm) Long-pulse Nd:YAG (1064 nm)	4–5 treatments spaced 4–6 weeks apart	Significant improvement in PFB [18–22] Nd:YAG has the safest profile [24] Lower fluence treatment significantly reduces PFB while mitigating pain, pigmentation alteration, crusting, and blistering [23]
Other procedures	Electrolysis Chemical peels Photodynamic therapy	Glycolic acid [175, 176] Salicylic acid ALA + PDT [177]	

Acne Keloidalis Nuchae

Acne keloidalis nuchae (AKN) is a chronic, scarring follicular disorder that affects the occipital scalp and posterior neck. Also called sycosis nuchae, dermatitis papillaris capillitii, keloidal folliculitis, and folliculitis keloidalis nuchae, AKN often presents with chronic fibrotic papules that may coalesce into keloidal plaques. The plaques enlarge over many years and become disfiguring.

Epidemiology

AKN predominately affects African-American males with a prevalence ranging from 1.6 to 16.1% [25–30]. This condition also can be observed in females, although it is 20 times more common in males [25, 31]. Typically AKN develops after puberty with a peak around ages 25–34 [32]. By age 55, the condition usually improves and, in some cases, even resolves due to reduction in hair shaft thickness, density, sebum production, and other hormonal factors [32].

Pathophysiology

The etiology of AKN is unclear [33]. AKN is frequently seen in patients who get close haircuts, which may contribute to the popular belief that AKN is due to an infection from barber's instruments [32, 34]. However, this condition is not an infectious process. Some believe that it is a mechanically induced folliculitis resulting in extensive scarring, while others suggest that AKN is a form of primary cicatricial alopecia, transepithelial elimination disorder resembling perforating folliculitis, or variant form of lichen simplex chronicus with follicular scarring [35–38].

The development of AKN is usually attributed to chronic trauma to the follicular scalp. The most common predisposing factor is frequent, close haircuts. The risk is particularly high when the patient or a barber uses blunted and poorly maintained blades, which requires increased force to cut the hair and may lead to irritation and bleeding of the scalp [34]. Chronic irritation and friction from collared shirts, sports helmets, cosmetics or Afro-pick use may also exacerbate AKN [26]. Seborrheic dermatitis, staphylococcus aureus infection, and elevated serum testosterone levels have also been reported to play a role [39]. These diverse triggers result in perifollicular inflammation [36].

It has been postulated that the posterior neck and occipital scalp are most affected due to an increased number of mast cells and dilated dermal capillaries in these areas [26]. The posterior neck and occipital scalp have almost twice the number of mast cells compared to other areas of the scalp, leading to an increased itch sensation [35]. By itching and touching the scalp, patients potentially traumatize and further irritate the scalp leading to the eruption of inflammatory papules and hypertrophic scars.

Clinical Features

AKN initially presents with small, firm follicular papules on the occipital scalp and the nape of the neck (Fig. 20.2). Early in the disease course, patients may be asymptomatic or may begin to experience pruritus. Over time, the papules increase in number and may coalesce into large, hairless fibrotic plaques or nodules that resemble keloids. There may be hair shafts exiting the lesion at first, but as the hair

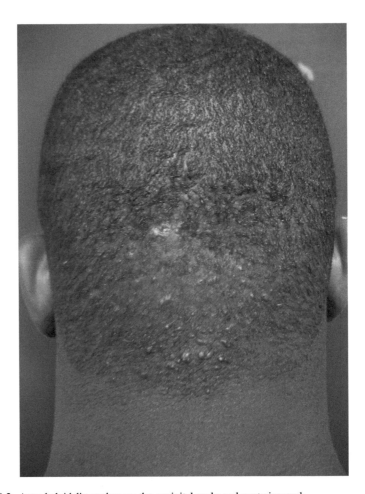

Fig. 20.2 Acne keloidalis nuchae on the occipital scalp and posterior neck

Table 20.4 Differential diagnosis of acne keloidalis nuchae

Condition	Differentiating factors
Folliculitis/perifolliculitis	Primary bacterial infection
Pseudofolliculitis barbae	Typically also affects the beard area
Keloid	Temporally related to trauma or inflammation
Acne mechanica	Usually associated with use of head gear
Folliculitis decalvans	Primarily on the vertex and parietal scalp Erythema and pustules/crusting
Dissecting cellulitis	Suppurative nodules and abscesses

follicles rupture and begin to scar, patchy scarring alopecia develops with little chance for hair regrowth [40]. Progression of the disease to the plaque-stage is associated with increasing pruritus, pain, and bleeding [32].

If the scalp becomes secondarily infected, crusted papules and pustules can be observed. In severe cases, patients may develop large abscesses and draining sinuses. When pustules are present, bacterial cultures should be obtained in order to guide antibiotic therapy. AKN may be mistaken for folliculitis, PB, and folliculitis decalvans (Table 20.4).

Treatment

The most important initial step in the management of AKN is the avoidance of potential triggers including close haircuts and mechanical irritation from clothing and hats. Patients should be instructed to avoid cutting hair on the occipital scalp with razors or clippers. Topical antimicrobial cleansers such as chlorhexidine or povidone iodine can be used to reduce the risk of bacterial super-infection [41].

Once preventative measures have been taken, various pharmacological, procedural, and surgical treatments may be indicated depending on the severity of disease. Mild and moderate cases of AKN (with predominately papules and minimal scarring) may be treated with potent and superpotent topical corticosteroids, topical immunomodulators, intralesional corticosteroids, topical and systemic antibiotics, and laser therapy (Table 20.5) [40, 41]. Short-term systemic corticosteroids can be considered for severely inflamed cases [4]. Unfortunately, the lesions recur within weeks to months after discontinuation.

Once large fibrotic plaques (≥ 3 cm) develop, AKN is often resistant to topical and systemic treatments. For these cases, surgical excision with either primary or secondary intention closure provides the best chance for cure [42, 43]. Typically, a horizontal ellipse containing the fibrotic lesion is removed along the posterior hairline. The excision must extend into the subcutaneous fat to reduce risk for recurrence of AKN. If primary closure is chosen, care must be taken to avoid neck flexion, as this may extend the size of the scar. Carbon dioxide laser, electrosurgery, or electrodessication can be used [44, 45].

Table 20.5 Treatment of mild to moderate acne keloidalis nuchae

Treatment	Dose	Considerations
Class I or II topical steroids	Clobetasol propionate 0.05% foam twice daily, two weeks on/two weeks off. Betamethasone diproprionate 0.05% or desoximetasone gel 0.05% twice daily	Decreased number of papules, improvement in itching, burning, and pain, improvement in physician/patient global assessments [40]. Combine with retinoic acid gel to help decrease pruritus and flatten lesions [4]
Intralesional corticosteroids	20–40 mg/ml triamcinolone acetonide injected at 3 week intervals [41]	May develop hypopigmentation at the injection site lasting up to 1.5 years [4]
Topical antibiotics	Clindamycin (Cleocin-T) gel BID	Used when there is evidence of infection i.e. pustules
Topical immunomodulators	Imiquimoid plus pimecrolimus twice daily for 8 weeks [178]. Imiquimod alone 5 days on and 2 days off for 8 weeks [33]	Associated with decreased lesion count and improvement in itching
Oral medications	Minocycline or doxycycline	Anti-inflammatory and antimicrobial. Choose based on bacterial culture
Punch biopsy	Removal of each papule with a hair transplant punch	May allow for second-intention healing or close with sutures. Must punch into subcutaneous tissue to decrease risk of recurrence
Laser therapy	Carbon dioxide laser	High risk of dyspigmentation generally outweighs potential benefits in patients with skin of color
	Nd:YAG laser-assisted hair removal	Destroys the hair follicle, thereby removing nidus of inflammation and reducing number of papules plaques [179]. May remove trapped hairs
UVB therapy	UVB therapy up to 3 times weekly for 16 weeks	UV-induced collagen breakdown and matrix remodeling decreases lesion count, improves patient self-assessment. Decreases the size of larger lesions and eliminates smaller lesions [180]
Cryotherapy	Freeze for 20 s, then thaw, and then freeze for another 20 s [4]	Freezing for >25 s destroys melanocytes and causes hypopigmentation

Dissecting Cellulitis

Dissecting cellulitis (DC), also called perifollicular capitis abscedens et suffodiens or Hoffman disease, is a chronic inflammatory condition of the scalp and a form of primary neutrophilic cicatricial alopecia. It may be observed as part of the follicular occlusion tetrad with hidradenitis suppurativa (HS), acne conglobata, and pilonidal cyst [46]. Abnormal follicular keratinization leads to occlusion and destruction of the hair follicle. Secondary bacterial infection and scarring alopecia can occur [47–49].

Epidemiology

DC predominately affects African American males between ages 15 and 62, with a mean age of onset of 26.6 years [50]. Approximately 84% of cases are observed in males, and 48–65% in African Americans [50]. However, it has been reported in various different ethnic groups, women, and pediatric populations [47, 50–52].

Pathophysiology

The exact etiology of DC is unknown, but the condition appears to be due to follicular occlusion in specific areas of the scalp. When keratin debris enters the pilosebaceous unit, it causes follicular expansion, inflammation, and eventually dilation of the follicle [53]. Bacteria such as Staphylococcus aureus, Pseudomonas aeruginosa, and anaerobes can in some cases enter the follicle and cause a secondary bacterial infection (e.g. folliculitis). Follicular occlusion leads to follicular rupture and precipitates a neutrophilic and granulomatous response to foreign material, creating an abscess [47–50]. Since follicular occlusion precipitates the development of DC, removal of the hair follicle by laser hair removal (or historically, by scalpectomy) improves the disease.

Clinical Features

DC initially resembles folliculitis with follicular and perifollicular pustules appearing on the vertex and occipital scalp [50]. The pustules increase in number and painful nodules develop, followed by abscesses and boggy plaques with interconnecting sinus tracts (Fig. 20.3) [54]. Purulent or keratinaceous fluid may drain spontaneously or with applied pressure, and pushing on one abscess may lead to drainage of a distant area due to interconnecting tracts. A foul odor may be present when the lesions become secondarily infected.

DC is characterized by a chronic waxing and waning course. Early in the disease, hair loss is nonscarring and may be temporary. However, the progressive inflammation in chronic and severe DC can lead to scarring alopecia with irreversible loss of hair [55]. Long-term severe cases have been associated with increased risk of squamous cell carcinoma and skull osteomyelitis [56, 57].

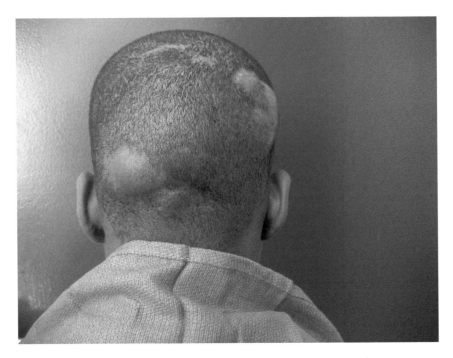

Fig. 20.3 Dissecting cellulitis of the scalp in an African-American male

DC may occur with the other diseases of the follicular occlusion tetrad (HS, acne conglobata, and pilonidal cyst) or present independently. Marginal keratitis, arthritis, spondyloarthropathy, and sternoclavicular hyperostosis have also been reported in association with DC [58–61].

The differential diagnosis includes bacterial folliculitis, folliculitis decalvans, AKN, tinea capitis, and cutis verticis gyrata (Table 20.6). Typically, DC can be diagnosed clinically, although a definitive diagnosis may be achieved with a 4 mm punch biopsy of a suppurative and tender nodule.

Treatment

The preferred treatment for DC depends on the severity of the condition. For mild to moderate DC, the first-line treatment is oral antibiotics, whether or not bacterial infection is present (Table 20.7). Commonly used antibiotics include tetracyclines, ciprofloxacin, trimethropim/sulfamethazole, or a combination of clindamycin and rifampin [59, 62–66]. A bacterial culture should be obtained prior to treatment and, if positive, antibiotic choice should be tailored to causative bacteria.

High dose oral zinc sulfate, with doses ranging from 135 to 220 mg three times per day, has been associated with complete healing of DC and long-term remission

Table 20.6 Differential diagnosis of dissecting cellulitis

Condition	Differentiating factors
Acne keloidalis nuchae	Fibrotic, keloid-like nodules and plaques No sinus tracts, suppurative nodules, or cicatricial alopecia
Tinea capitis or kerion	Positive KOH preparation or fungal culture
Folliculitis decalvans	No sinus tracts or nodules
Cutis verticis gyrata	Asymptomatic, no sinus tracts or suppurative nodules
Bacterial folliculitis	Absence of boggy nodules and sinus tracts

Table 20.7 Treatment of dissecting cellulitis

First line therapy
- Antibiotics (for at least 3 months)
  - Ciprofloxacin 250–500 mg BID [63, 64][a]
  - Clindamycin 300 mg BID with rifampin 300 mg BID [59, 65][a]
  - Trimethroprim/sulfamethoxazole DS BID [59]
  - Minocycline 100 mg BID[a]
    With antiandrogens [66]
- Zinc Sulfate
  - High dose zinc sulfate 135–220 mg TID for months [54, 67, 68]
- Improved scalp hygiene [84]
  - Avoid cosmetic products
  - Topical antibiotic soaps, i.e., chlorhexidine and benzoyl peroxide

Second line therapy
- Oral retinoids
  - Isotretinoin 0.5–1 mg/kg for 3–12 months [71–74][a]
  - Isotretinoin with dapsone 50–100 mg [181]
  - Acitretin 10 mg with oral prednisolone, zinc, and topical tacrolimus/glucocorticoids [54]

Third line therapy
- Biologics
  - Adalimumab 80 mg loading dose → 40 mg week 1 → 40 mg every other week [70]
  - Infliximab 5 mg/kg every 8 weeks [69]

Fourth line therapy
- Laser Hair Removal
  - Long-pulsed Nd:YAG laser (1064 nm) [76]
  - Diode Laser (800 nm) [75]
- Surgery [80–83]
  - Wide local excision with split-thickness skin graft
  - Full scalpectomy with skin grafting
- Radiation beam therapy [79]
- CO_2 laser ablation of scalp [78]

Adjunct treatments
- Intralesional Corticosteroids
  - Intralesional triamcinolone acetate 5–10 mg/kg every 2–4 weeks in combination with first, second, or third line therapies [84]
- Oral Prednisone
  - Prednisone 40–60 mg/day followed by taper [85]

[a]Preferred therapies
Modified from: Scheinfeld [59]

of more than 5 years [54, 67, 68]. In one patient with acne conglobata and DC, nodules began flattening within four weeks and hair regrowth was evident at three months; long-term low-dose oral zinc was necessary to prevent relapse of the condition [67]. Adalimumab and infliximab (anti-TNF agents) have been associated with improvement in symptoms in small case reports and series; however, DC may return after discontinuing treatment [69, 70].

For more severe cases or those resistant to topical antibiotics, isotretinoin is the treatment of choice. Isotretinoin 0.5–1.0 mg/kg is associated with complete remission in 92% of patients, usually within the first three months of treatment [71–74]. Isotretinoin should be continued for 6 months to 1 year. Unfortunately, relapse frequently occurs after discontinuation, although the severity may be decreased [50].

For any cases refractory to medications, procedural therapies should be considered. Incision and drainage can result in temporary relief of symptoms and reduction of nodule size. Laser-assisted epilation using the 800 nm diode laser and 1064 nm long-pulsed Nd:YAG laser have been reported in DC patients with skin of color [75–77]. For severe recalcitrant cases, surgical excision can be considered [78–83].

Although they do not alter the course of disease, intralesional injections of triamcinolone acetonide 5–10 mg/kg every 2–4 weeks in combination with other therapies may assist with symptomatic relief [84]. Prednisone 40–60 mg/day followed by a taper may also improve the symptoms of DC in the acute setting but has no long-term effect of the disease course [85]. In addition, use of topical antibiotic soaps including chlorhexidine and benzoyl peroxide help reduce the risk of secondary infection [84].

Hidradenitis Suppurativa

HS, also called acne inversa (OMIM 142690), is a chronic inflammatory disorder of the follicular epithelium in apocrine-gland bearing areas [86]. The condition is characterized by recurrent papules, nodules, abscesses, and sinus tracts most commonly found in the axilla, groin, and buttocks [87]. HS often is very distressing to patients and has a significant impact on quality of life [88].

Epidemiology

HS affects all ethnicities with an overall prevalence ranging from <1 to 4%, but may be more common in African Americans according to some reports [86, 89–91]. One retrospective chart review suggested that 6.4% of black patients versus 3.9% of white patients have HS [92]. Based on data from the 1990–2009 National Ambulatory Medical Care Survey (NAMCS), African Americans have 1.5 times more visits than non-Hispanic whites and 3.5 times more visits than Hispanics for HS [93]. This may be due to an increased number of apocrine sweat glands in African-American individuals [94]. Females are more commonly affected with a ratio of 3:1 [90]. HS usually develops between the onset of puberty and age 40, with the highest incidence during the third decade of life [95].

Pathophysiology

The pathogenesis of HS is not well understood. Although there are many theories for why the condition occurs, it is generally accepted that the primary event in the development of HS is follicular occlusion, followed by follicular rupture, and ultimately an aberrant immune response leading to chronic inflammation.

Initially there is a hormonally mediated increase in proliferation of ductal keratinocytes and decrease in keratinocyte shedding. The follicle duct becomes occluded and progressively expands [96]. One hypothesis suggests that a fragile sebofollicular junction allows for leakage, trauma, and rupture of the occluded follicle [97]. As a result, keratin fibers deposit in the epidermis triggering an innate inflammatory response [98]. Over time, the acute inflammation may progress to chronic granulomatous inflammation. In addition, stem cells released from the ruptured hair follicle may proliferate within the dermis and lead to the formation of sinus tracts [97].

Alternatively, the chronic inflammation may be the result of a dysfunctional immune response to microbial products [99]. Instead of initiating a protective response, keratinocytes may activate a chronic inflammatory pathway that damages the host tissue instead of eliminating the bacteria [100]. Overexpression of toll-like receptors, tumor necrosis factor α interleukin 23/T helper 17 (IL-23/Th17) pathway, and interleukin 1β all have been implicated in the development of HS [101–103]. The effectiveness of immunomodulatory agents such as oral steroids, cyclosporine, and anti-tumor necrosis factor α therapy in treating HS helps support the latter hypothesis [104]. Further, antibiotic therapy decreases bacterial colonization and, perhaps by abating the immunological impetus, helps reduce the severity of inflammation [105–107].

Genetics may also predispose patients to the development of HS. As many as one-third of affected individuals have a first-degree relative with the condition [107–109]. Chromosome 1p21.1-1q25.3 is associated with increased risk in Chinese individuals and mutations of the γ-secretase complex are found in Caucasians and Asians with HS [87, 109–115]. There is only one case study reporting genetic predisposition in African Americans. This study demonstrated autosomal dominant transmission of HS through a heterozygous nonsense mutation in *NCSTN* (c.C349T; p.R117X) on chromosome 1 [116]. Other risk factors include bacterial colonization and infection, hormonal influences, smoking, obesity, and metabolic syndrome [117, 118].

Clinical Features

HS is a chronic, relapsing and remitting condition that presents with exquisitely painful comedones, subcutaneous nodules, abscesses, and draining sinus tracts in areas of the body that contain apocrine glands (Fig. 20.4). Typically affected sites include the axillae (most common), submammary folds, abdominal fold, groin, buttocks, and medial thighs. Patients often complain of unrelenting pain and frequent drainage of serous, purulent, or bloody material from the interconnecting sinuses. Longstanding disease can result in fibrosis, dermal contractures, scarring, fistula formation, and rarely malignant transformation to squamous cell carcinoma [119, 120].

HS is seen in conjunction with several other conditions. Notably, as a member of the follicular occlusion triad, HS often occurs with acne conglobata, DC of the scalp, and/or pilonidal cysts [46]. There is also an association between HS and Crohn's disease, acne vulgaris, and PAPASH syndrome (pyogenic arthritis, pyoderma gangrenosum, acne, and suppurative hidradenitis) [89, 121, 122].

HS resembles several other clinical conditions (Table 20.8). The diagnosis of HS can be made if a patient meets all three criteria of the modified Dessau definition [123]. These criteria are (1) Presence of typical lesions (painful nodules, i.e., "blind boils," abscesses, draining sinuses, bridged scars, "tombstone" double-ended pseudocomedones) (2) Involvement of ≥ 1 classically involved body site (axillae, buttocks, groin, infra- and intermammary folds) and (3) Clear history of chronicity and recurrence (often defined as two recurrences within six months). A skin biopsy

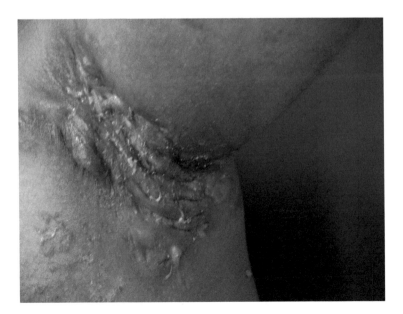

Fig. 20.4 Hidradenitis suppurativa on the axilla

Table 20.8 Differential diagnosis of hidradenitis suppurativa

Condition	Differentiating factors
Acne vulgaris	Primarily on face, chest, back No sinus tracts or extensive scarring
Folliculitis, carbuncles, furuncles	Transient lesions Usually respond to appropriate antibiotics No comedones, sinus tracts, hypertrophic scars
Pilonidal cyst	Isolated to area of the natal cleft May occur in conjunction with HS
Granuloma inguinale	Enlarging ulcer with an undermined border Visualization of Donovan bodies
Perianal Crohn's disease	History of gastrointerstinal Crohn's disease Classic "knife-cut" ulcers Rectovaginal and rectoperineal fistulas

usually is not necessary but can be performed if the diagnosis is unclear. Once a definitive diagnosis of HS is made, there are several scoring systems that physicians can use to determine the severity. These include Hurley staging, Sartorius score, HS-specific Physician Global Assessment (PGA), Hidradenitis Suppurativa Severity Index (HSSI), and Hidradenitis Suppurativa Clinical Response (HiSCR) score [124].

Treatment

The approach to treatment of HS involves a combination of lifestyle changes, supportive measures, and pharmacological and procedural therapies. No definitive cure for HS exists and therapies that are very successful in some patients may have no effect in others. While mild to moderate disease can often be controlled with medications, more severe cases with fibrosis, scarring, and contractures may be resistant to most accepted treatments.

The first step in management of HS involves educating the patient on lifestyle modifications that may improve the condition (Table 20.9). Smoking cessation, weight loss, avoidance of tight-fitting clothing and topical irritants, and elimination of dairy products and high glycemic foods from the diet may be associated with improvement in symptoms [97, 125–129]. In addition, it is important that providers inquire about possible psychological symptoms and refer patients to mental health services or support groups if needed.

Choice of pharmacological agents depends on the severity of the condition. Mild to moderate cases often respond to topical therapies, whereas oral medications and surgery are often needed for more advanced lesions (Table 20.10). Clindamycin 1% solution twice daily is associated with improvement in mild inflammatory lesions, likely due to treatment of coexisting superficial secondary infection and mild anti-inflammatory effects [129–131]. Unfortunately, the lesions recur after stopping

Table 20.9 Patient education, support, and lifestyle modifications in the management of hidradenitis suppurativa

- Patient education and support [125]
  - Inquire about impact on quality of life and symptoms of depression
  - Provide psychological support or refer to qualified provider
- Avoid trauma to affected areas [125]
  - Wear loose-fitting clothing
  - Do not manipulate the lesions
  - Use perfume- and dye-free laundry detergent for clothing
- Gently clean and dress the lesions daily
  - Use gentle, soap-free cleansers
  - Avoid scrubbing the area
  - Cover draining lesions and post-surgical wounds with white petrolatum, absorbent dressing, and tubular net or mesh dressings
- Other Lifestyle modification
  - Smoking cessation [126, 127]
  - Weight loss [127]
  - Low glycemic and low dairy diet [127, 128]

the antibiotic. Topical resorcinol 15%, a chemical peeling agent, has been shown to reduce pain, improve healing, and promote resolution of abscesses when applied to acutely inflamed lesions once to twice daily [132]. Intralesional corticosteroids are frequently used as an adjunct to other therapies and can relieve symptoms in actively inflamed cases [86].

Patients with refractory mild to moderate disease are often started on oral doxycycline or minocycline 50–100 mg twice daily. Although anecdotal reports suggest that these antibiotics are effective, a randomized trial of oral tetracycline versus topical clindamycin showed no significant difference in improvement between the two treatments [130]. Acute flares of mild HS are typically treated for 7–10 days. Moderate cases usually require at least a 2- to 3-month course. Oral clindamycin and rifampin twice daily for 10 weeks has been shown to be very effective in patients who fail traditional therapy [105, 131, 133]. However, the majority of responders relapse within 5 months of stopping the medication [133]. Dapsone 50–200 mg is also associated with clinically significant improvement, but as with other antibiotics, symptoms tend to recur after treatment cessation [134, 135]. In one retrospective study, a combination of rifampin, moxifloxacin, and metronidazole was effective, but treatment was limited by side effects [106].

Other possible treatments for HS include oral retinoids, hormonal (anti-androgen) agents, targeted therapies, and immunosuppressants [136–141]. The effect of isotretinoin is limited in HS compared to acne vulgaris with only 24% of patients achieving full clearance and 49% achieving any improvement at all, but the relapse rate is significantly lower than other therapies [136, 142]. Acitretin is associated with better outcomes, although its use is limited due to side effects—including teratogenicity in women of childbearing potential—and the need for close monitoring [143]. Hormonal therapies that work to counteract the effects of androgens, including cyproterone acetate (not available in the US), oral contraceptive pills,

Table 20.10 Pharmacological and non-pharmacological treatment of hidradenitis suppurativa

- Local therapy
  - Benzoyl peroxide wash [125]
  - Topical clindamycin [129–131]
  - Topical resorcinol [132]
  - Intralesional corticosteroids [86]
- Systemic Therapy
  - Oral antibiotics
    Tetracyclines
      Doxycycline 50–100 mg BID
      Minocycline 50–100 mg BID
    Clindamycin 300 mg BID and rifampin 300–600 mg BID [105, 131, 133]
    Dapsone 50–200 mg daily
  - Hormonal therapy
    Anti-androgen medications i.e. cyproterone acetate + estrogen, oral contraceptives, oral contraceptives + spironolactone, finasteride
  - Targeted therapy
    Infliximab [146, 147]
    Adalimumab [104, 150]
    Ustekinumab [153, 154]
    Anakinra [155, 156]
    Etanercept (not currently recommended) [151, 152]
  - Immunosuppressants
    Systemic glucocorticoids [125]
    Cyclosporine [140, 141]
    Tacrolimus [157]
  - Oral retinoids
    Acitretin 0.6 mg/kg daily for 9–12 months [143]
    Isotretinoin 0.5–0.8 mg/kg for at least 4–6 months [136, 142]
  - Metformin [182]
  - Zinc supplementation [183, 184]
- Surgery
  - Punch debridement (mini-unroofing)
  - Incision and drainage [165]
  - Surgical unroofing
  - Carbon dioxide (CO_2) laser excision [167]
  - Wide excision [168, 169]
- Other procedures
  - 1064 nm long-pulsed Nd:YAG laser [158, 159]
  - Intense pulsed light [160]
  - External beam radiation [161]
  - Photodynamic therapy [162–164]

and finasteride are thought to be more effective than antibiotics alone [137–139, 144]. Oral contraceptive pills containing ethinyl estradiol or drospirenone are preferred and should be combined with spironolactone 50–100 mg if possible [145].

For severe, inflammatory HS, anti-TNFα inhibitors adalimumab and infliximab are associated with significant clinical improvement [104, 146–150]. Adalimumab is FDA (Food and Drug Administration) approved for moderate to severe HS. Infliximab appears to be more effective based on current evidence; however, more research is needed to directly compare different targeted therapies. Etanercept is not currently recommended due to inconclusive data on its efficacy [151, 152]. Newer therapies targeting IL-23/Th17, ustekinumab, and IL-1β, anakinra, are being actively studied and show promise for the treatment of HS [153–156]. Temporary improvement in symptoms also may be seen with cyclosporine, tacrolimus, and systemic corticosteroid taper [125, 140, 141, 157].

Laser and light therapy are another choice for refractory cases. The 1064 nm long-pulsed Nd:YAG laser is associated with a 64–73% decrease in severity for treated sites in the inguinal, axillary, and inframammary regions [158, 159]. Treatment of affected areas with intense pulsed light and external beam radiation has also been reported to be effective in HS [160, 161]. Mixed results with photodynamic therapy have been reported [162–164].

For severely debilitating disease with scarring and contractures, surgery can be considered. Possible surgical approaches include incision and drainage, punch debridement, unroofing, and surgical excision. Incision and drainage provides symptomatic relief without any effect on the long-term course of the disease, and therefore punch debridement is often preferred for treatment of acute nodules [165]. The initial surgical therapy for severe nodules, abscesses, and sinus tracts would be unroofing (also referred to as deroofing) [166]. This involves exploring lesions with a blunt probe and then using a scalpel to remove the top of each tract so that the base of the lesion can be scraped. The lesion then will heal by secondary intention. Surgical excision with carbon dioxide laser is extremely effective in treating HS, with recurrence seen in only 3% of patients upon follow-up of up to 19 years [167]. However, carbon dioxide laser is associated with a high risk of severe dyspigmentation in patients with higher Fitzpatrick Skin Types. Severe, recalcitrant cases can be cured with complete lesion resection [168, 169]. A limited number of expert surgical teams and the risks of delayed wound closure and wound dehiscence significantly limit a radical surgical approach.

Key Points

- PB presents as 2–4 mm papules and pustules, most commonly in the beard area of African-American males. The first step in management is discontinuation of close shaving. Topical medications, including antibiotics, steroids, and retinoids, as well as laser hair removal have been shown to be effective in treatment of this condition.
- AKN presents with inflammatory papules and pustules that coalesce into nodules and keloid plaques on the occipital scalp. Patients should be advised to avoid short haircuts and friction to the occipital scalp. Mild to moderate cases may be treated with class I/II topical corticosteroids, topical antibiotics, and intralesional corticosteroids, whereas large keloids may require procedural or surgical intervention.
- DC initially resembles folliculitis of the vertex and occiput and ultimately progresses to the formation of inflammatory pustules, cysts, abscesses, and draining sinus tracts. First-line treatments include improved scalp hygiene, oral

antibiotics, zinc sulfate, and laser hair removal. Refractory cases may require oral retinoids, biologics, or even surgical removal.

- HS is characterized by painful comedones, subcutaneous nodules, abscesses, and draining sinus tracts in areas of the body that contain apocrine glands, particularly the axilla, groin, and buttocks. Initial management involves counseling on lifestyle modifications and use of topical antibiotics. Refractory disease may be treated with systemic antibiotics, oral retinoids, hormonal (anti-androgen) agents, or laser therapy. Severe cases may require targeted therapy or surgical excision.

References

1. Winter H, Schissel D, Parry DAD, et al. An unusual Ala2Thr polymorphism in the 1A-Helical segment of the companion layer-specific keratin K6hf: evidence for a risk factor in the etiology of the common hair disorder pseudofolliculitis barbae. J Invest Dermatol. 2014;122(3):652–7.
2. Alexander AM, Delph WI. Pseudofolliculitis barbae in the military. A medical, administrative and social problem. J Natl Med Assoc. 1974;66(6):459–79.
3. Edlich RF, Haines PC, Nichter LS, et al. Pseudofolliculitis barbae with keloids. J Emerg Med. 1986;4(4):283–6.
4. Perry PK, Cook-Bolden FE, Rahman Z, et al. Defining pseudofolliculitis barbae in 2001: a review of the literature and current trends. J Am Acad Dermatol. 2002;46(2):S113–9.
5. Alexis A, Heath CR, Halder RM. Folliculitis keloidalis nuchae and pseudofolliculitis barbae: are prevention and effective treatment within reach? Dermatol Clin. 2014;32(2):183–91. doi:10.1016/j.det.2013.12.001.
6. Craig GE. Shaving; its relationship to diseases of the bearded area of the face. AMA Arch Derm. 1955;71(1):11–3.
7. Halder RM. Pseudofolliculitis barbae and related disorders. Dermatol Clin. 1988;6(3):407–12.
8. McLean WHI. 2004. Close shave for a keratin disorder-K6hf polymorphism linked to Pseudofolliculitis barbae. J Invest Dermatol. 2004;122(3): xi–xiii.
9. Garcia RL, White JW Jr. Pseudofolliculitis barbae in a woman. Arch Dermatol. 1978;114 (12):1856.
10. Dilaimy M. Pseudofolliculitis of the legs. Arch Dermatol. 1976;112(4):507–8.
11. Smith JD, Odom RB. Pseudofolliculitis capitis. Arch Dermatol. 1977;113(3):328–9.
12. Bridgeman-Shah S. The medical and surgical therapy of pseudofolliculitis barbae. Dermatol Ther. 2004;17(2):158–63.
13. Cowley K, Vanoosthuyze K. Insights into shaving and its impact on skin. Br J Dermatol. 2012;166(Suppl 1):6–12. doi:10.1111/j.1365-2133.2011.10783.x.
14. Gray J, McMichael J. Pseudofolliculitis barbae: understanding the condition and the role of facial grooming. Int J Costemic Science. 2016;38(Suppl 1):24–7. doi:10.1111/ics.12331.
15. Daniel A, Gustafson CJ, Zupkosky PJ, et al. Shave frequency and regimen variation effects on the management of pseudofolliculitis Barbae. J Drugs Dermatol. 2013;12(4):410–8.
16. Kuchabal S, Kuchabal D. Shaving. Internet. J Dermatol. 2010;8(2):1–7.
17. Kligman AM, Mills OH Jr. Pseudofolliculitis of the beard and topically applied tretinoin. Arch Dermatol. 1973;107(4):551–2.
18. Weaver SM, Sagaral EC. Treatment of pseudofolliculitis barbae using the long-pulse Nd: YAG laser on skin types V and VI. Dermatol Surg. 2003;29(12):1187–91.

19. Ross EV, Cooke LM, Oerstreet KA, et al. Treatment of pseudofolliculitis barbae in very dark skin with a long pulse Nd:YAG laser. J Natl Med Assoc. 2002;94(10):888–93.
20. Ross EV, Cooke LM, Timko AL, et al. Treatment of pseudofolliculitis barbae in skin types IV, V, and VI with a long-pulsed neodymium: yttrium aluminum garnet laser. J Am Acad Dermatol. 2002;47(2):263–70.
21. Greppi I. Diode laser hair removal of the black patient. Lasers Surg Med. 2001;28(2):150–5.
22. Smith EP, Winstanley D, Ross EV. Modified superlong pulse 810 nm diode laser in the treatment of pseudofolliculitis barbae in skin types V and VI. Dermatol Surg. 2005;31 (3):297–301.
23. Schulze R, Meehan KJ, Lopez A, et al. Low-fluence 1,064-nm laser hair reduction for pseudofolliculitis barbae in skin types IV, V, and VI. Dermatol Surg. 2009;35(1):98–107. doi:10.1111/j.1524-4725.2008.34388.x.
24. Alexis AF. Lasers and light-based therapies in ethnic skin: treatment options and recommendations for Fitzpatrick skin types V and VI. Br J Dermatol. 2013;169(Suppl 3):91–7. doi:10.1111/bjd.12526.
25. Salami T, Omeife H, Samuel S. Prevalence of acne keloidalis nuchae in Nigerians. Int J Dermatol. 2007;46(5):482–4.
26. George AO, Akanji AO, Nduka EU, et al. Clinical biochemical and morphologic features of acne keloidalis in a black population. Int J Dermatol. 1993;32(10):714–6.
27. Ogunbiyi AO, Daramola OO, Alese OO. Prevalence of skin diseases in Ibadan. Nigeria. Int J Dermatol. 2004;43(1):31–6.
28. Child FJ, Fuller LC, Higgins EM, et al. A study of the spectrum of skin disease occurring in a black population in south-east London. Br J Dermatol. 1991;141(3):512–7.
29. Khumalo NP, Jessop S, Gumedze F, et al. Hairdressing is associated with scalp disease in African schoolchildren. Br J Dermatol. 2007;157(1):106–10.
30. Khumalo NP, Jessop S, Gumedze F, et al. Hairdressing and the prevalence of scalp disease in African adults. Br J Dermatol. 2007;157(5):981–8.
31. Ogunbiyi A, George A. Acne keloidalis in females: case report and review of literature. J Natl Med Assoc. 2005;97(5):736–8.
32. Ogunbiyi A, Adedokun B. Perceived aetiological factors of folliculitis keloidalis nuchae (acne keloidalis) and treatment options among Nigerian men. Br J Dermatol. 2015;173 (Suppl 2):22–5. doi:10.1111/bjd.13422.
33. Kelly AP. Pseudofolliculitis barbae and acne keloidalis nuchae. Dermatol Clin. 2003;21 (4):645–53.
34. Khumalo NP, Gumedze F, Lehloenva R. Folliculitis keloidalis nuchae is associated with the risk for bleeding from haircuts. Int J Dermatol. 2011;50(10):1212–6. doi:10.1111/j.1365-4632.2010.04655.x.
35. Shapero J, Shapero H. Acne keloidalis nuchae is scar and keloid formation secondary to mechanically induced folliculitis. J Cutan Med Surg. 2011;15(4):238–40.
36. Sperling LC, Homoky C, Pratt L, et al. Acne keloidalis is a form of primary scarring alopecia. Arch Dermatol. 2000;136(4):479–84.
37. Goette DK, Berger TG. Acne keloidalis nuchae. A transepithelial elimination disorder. Int J Dermatol. 1987;26(7):442–4.
38. Burkhart CG, Burkhart C. Acne keloidalis is lichen simplex chronicus with fibrotic keloidal scarring. J Am Acad Dermatol. 1998;39:661.
39. Lee AH, Cho SY, Harris K, et al. Staphylococcus aureus and chronic folliculocentric pustuloses of the scalp—cause or association? Br J Dermatol. 2016;175(2):410–3.
40. Callender VD, Young CM, Haverstock CL, et al. An open label study of clobetasol propionate 0.05% and betamethasone valerate 0.12% foams in the treatment of mild to moderate acne keloidalis. Cutis. 2005;75(6):317–21.
41. Ramos-e-silva M, Pirmez R. Red face revisited: disorders of hair growth and the pilosebaceous unit. Clin Dermatol. 2014;32(6):784–99. doi:10.1016/j.clindermatol.2014.02.018.

42. Gloster HM Jr. The surgical management of extensive cases of acne keloidalis nuchae. Arch Dermatol. 2000;136(11):1376–9.
43. Glenn MJ, Bennett RG, Kelly AP. Acne keloidalis nuchae: treatment with excision and second-intention healing. J Am Acad Dermatol. 1995;33(2):243–6.
44. Kantor G, Ratz JL, Wheeland RG. Treatment of acne keloidalis nuchae with carbon dioxide laser. J Am Acad Dermatol. 1968;14(2):263–7.
45. Hollander L. Treatment of folliculitis keloidalis chronica nuchae (acne keloid). AMA Arch Derm Syphilol. 1951;64(5):639–40.
46. Chicarilli ZN. Follicular occlusion triad: hidradenitis suppurativa, acne conglobata, and dissecting cellulitis of the scalp. Ann Plast Surg. 1987;18(3):230–7.
47. Rodney IJ, Onwudiwe OC, Callender VD, et al. Hair and scalp disorders in ethnic populations. J Drugs Dermatol. 2013;12(4):420–7.
48. Ross EK, Shapiro J. Management of hair loss. Dermatol Clin. 2005;23(2):227–43.
49. Benvenuto ME, Rebora A. Fluctuant nodules and alopecia of the scalp. Perifolliculitis capitis abscedens et suffodiens. 1992;128(8):1115–9.
50. Badaoui A, Reygagne P, Cavelier-Balloy B, et al. Dissecting cellulitis of the scalp: a retrospective study of 51 patients and review of literature. Br J Dermatol. 2016;174(2):421–3. doi:10.1111/bjd.13999.
51. Arneja JS, Vashi CN, Gursel E, et al. Management of fulminant dissecting cellulitis of the scalp in the pediatric population: Case report and literature review. Can J Plast Surg. 2007;15 (4):211–4.
52. Koca R, Altinyazar HC, Ozen OI, et al. Dissecting cellulitis in a white male: response to isotretinoin. Int J Dermatol. 2002;41(8):509–13.
53. Madu P, Kundu RV. Follicular and scarring disorders in skin of color: presentation and management. Am J Clin Dermatol. 2014;15(4):307–21. doi:10.1007/s40257-014-0072-x.
54. Jacobs F, Metzler G, Kubiak J, et al. New approach in combined therapy of perifolliculitis capitis abscedens et suffodiens. Acta Derm Venereol. 2011;91(6):726–7. doi:10.2340/00015555-1146.
55. McMichael AJ. Hair and scalp disorders in ethnic populations. Dermatol Clin. 2003;21 (4):629–44.
56. Curry SS, Gaither DH, King LE. Squamous cell carcinoma arising in dissecting perifolliculitis of the scalp. A case report and review of secondary squamous cell carcinomas. J Am Acad Dermatol. 1981;4(6):673–8.
57. Ramasastry SS, Granick MS, Boyd JB, et al. Severe perifolliculitis capitis with osteomyelitis. Ann Plast Surg. 1987;18(3):241–4.
58. Prasad SC, Bygum A. Successful treatment with alitretinoin of dissecting cellulitis of the scalp in keratitis-ichthyosis-deafness syndrome. Acta Derm Venereol. 2013;93(4):473–4. doi:10.2340/00015555-1499.
59. Scheinfeld N. Dissecting cellulitis (Perifolliculitis Capitis Abscedens et Suffodiens): a comprehensive review focusing on new treatments and findings of the last decade with commentary comparing the therapies and causes of dissecting cellulitis to hidradenitis suppurativa. Dermatol Online J. 2014;20(5):22692.
60. Thein M, Hogarth MB, Acland K. Seronegative arthritis associated with the follicular occlusion tetrad. Clin Exp Dermatol. 2004;29(5):550–2.
61. Ongchi DR, Fleming MG, Harris CA. Sternocleidomastoid hyperostosis: two cases with differing dermatologic syndromes. J Rheumatol. 1990;17(10):1415–8.
62. Semble AL, McMichael AJ. Hair loss in patients with skin of color. Semin Cutan Med Surg. 2015;34(2):81–8. doi:10.12788/j.sder.2015.0145.
63. Greenblatt DT, Sheth N, Teixeira F. Dissecting cellulitis of the scalp responding to oral quinolones. Clin Exp Dermatol. 2008;33(1):99–100.
64. Onderdijk AJ, Boer J. Successful treatment of dissecting cellulitis with ciprofloxacin. Clin Exp Dermatol. 2010;35(4):440. doi:10.1111/j.1365-2230.2009.03514.x.
65. Brook I. Recovery of anaerobic bacteria from a case of dissecting cellulitis. Int J Dermatol. 2006;45(2):168–9.

66. Goldsmith PC, Dowd PM. Successful therapy of the follicular occlusion triad in a young woman with high dose oral antiandrogens and minocycline. J R Soc Med. 1993;86(12): 729–30.
67. Kobayashi H, Aiba S, Tagami H. Successful treatment of dissecting cellulitis and acne conglobata with oral zinc. Br J Dermatol. 1999;141(6):1137–8.
68. Berne B, Venge P, Ohman S. Perifolliculitis capitis abscedens et suffodiens (Hoffman). Complete healing associated with oral zinc therapy. Arch Dermatol. 1985;121(8):1028–30.
69. Wollina U, Gemmeke A, Koch A. Dissecting cellulitis of the scalp responding to intravenous tumor necrosis factor-alpha antagonist. J Clin Aesthet Dermato. 2012;5(4):36–9.
70. Navarini AA, Trüeb RM. 3 cases of dissecting cellulitis of the scalp treated with adalimumab: control of inflammation within residual structural disease. Arch Dermatol. 2010;146(5):517–20.
71. Taylor AE. Dissecting cellulitis of the scalp: response to isotretinoin. Lancet. 1987;2 (8552):225.
72. Bjellerup M, Wallengren J. Familial perifolliculitis capitis abscedens et suffodiens in two brothers successfully treated with isotretinoin. J Am Acad Dermatol. 1990;23(4):752–3.
73. Khaled A, Zeglaoui F, Zoghlami A, et al. Dissecting cellulitis of the scalp: response to isotretinoin. J Eur Acad Dermatol Venereol. 2007;21(10):1430–1.
74. Scerri L, Williams HC, Allen BR. Dissecting cellulitis of the scalp: response to isotretinoin. Br J Dermatol. 1996;134(6):1105–8.
75. Boyd AS, Binhlam JQ. Use of an 800-nm pulsed-diode laser in the treatment of recalcitrant dissecting cellulitis of the scalp. Arch Dermatol. 2012;138(10):1291–3.
76. Krasner BD, Hamzavi FH, Murakawa GJ. Dissecting cellulitis treated with the long-pulsed Nd:YAG laser. Dermatol Surg. 2006;32(8):1039–44.
77. Chui CT, Berger TG, Price VH, et al. Recalcitrant scarring follicular disorders treated by laser-assisted hair removal: a preliminary report. Dermatol Surg. 1999;25(1):34–7.
78. Glass LF, Berman B, Laub D. Treatment of perifolliculitis capitis abscedens et suffodiens with the carbon dioxide laser. J Dermatol Surg Oncol. 1989;159(6):673–6.
79. Chinnaiyan P, Tena LB, Brenner MJ, et al. Modern external beam radiation therapy for refractory dissecting cellulitis of the scalp. Br J Dermatol. 2005;152(4):777–9.
80. Moschella SL, Klein MH, Miller RJ. Perifolliculitis capitis abscedens et suffodiens. Report of a successful therapeutic scalping. Arch Dermatol. 1967;96(2):195–7.
81. Williams CN, Cohen M, Ronan SG, et al. Dissecting cellulitis of the scalp. Plast Reconstr Surg. 1986;77(3):378–82.
82. Housewright CD, Rensvold E, Tidwell J, et al. Excisional surgery (scalpectomy) for dissecting cellulitis of the scalp. Dermatol Surg. 2011;37(8):1189–91. doi:10.1111/j.1524-4725.2011.02049.x.
83. Hintze JM, Howard BE, Donald CB, et al. Surgical management and reconstruction of Hoffman's disease (dissecting cellulitis of the scalp). Case Rep Surg. 2016;2016:2123037. doi:10.1155/2016/2123037.
84. Scheinfeld NS. A case of dissecting cellulitis and a review of the literature. Dermatol Online J. 2003;9(1):8.
85. Adrian RM, Arndt KA. Perifolliculitis capitis: successful control with alternate-day corticosteroids. Ann Plast Surg. 1980;4(2):166–9.
86. Jemec GBE. Clinical practice. Hidradenitis suppurativa. New Engl J Med. 2012;366(2):158–64. doi:10.1056/NEJMcp1014163.
87. Pink AE, Simpson MA, Desai N, et al. γ-Secretase mutations in hidradenitis suppurativa: new insights into disease pathogenesis. J Invest Dermatol. 2013;133(3):601–7.
88. Onderdijk AJ, van der Zee HH, Esmann S, et al. Depression in patients with hidradenitis suppurativa. J Eur Acad Dermatol Venereol. 2013;27(4):473–478.
89. Alikhan A, Lynch PJ, Eisen DB. Hidradenitis suppurativa: a comprehensive review. J Am Acad Dermatol. 2009;60(4):539.

90. Vlassova N, Kuhn D, Okoye GA. Hidradenitis suppurativa disproportionately affects African Americans: a single-center retrospective analysis. Acta Derm Venereol. 2015;95 (8):990–1.
91. Cosmatos I, Matcho A, Weinstein R. Analysis of patient claims data to determine the prevalence of hidradenitis suppurativa in the United States. J Am Acad Dermatol. 2013;68 (3):412–9.
92. Reeder VJ, Mahan GM, Hamzavi IH. Ethnicity and hidradenitis suppurativa. J Invest Dermatol. 2014;134(11):2842–3.
93. Davis SA, Lin HC, Balrishnan R, et al. Hidradenitis Suppurativa management in the United States: An Analysis of the National Ambulatory Medical Care Survey and MarketScan Medicaid Databases. Skin Appendage Disord. 2015;1(2):65–73.
94. Attanoos RL, Appleton MA, Douglas-Jones AG. The pathogenesis of hidradenitis suppurativa: a closer look at apocrine and apoeccrine glands. Br J Dermatol. 1995;133 (2):254–8.
95. Vazquez BG, Alikhan A, Weaver AL, et al. Incidence of hidradenitis suppurativa and associated factors: a population-based study of Olmsted County, Minnesota. J Invest Dermatol. 2013;133(1):97–103.
96. von Laffert M, Stadie V, Wohlrab J, et al. Hidradenitis suppurativa/acne inversa: bilocated epithelial hyperplasia with very different sequelae. Br J Dermatol. 2011;164(2):367.
97. Danby FW, Jemec GB, Marsch WC, et al. Preliminary findings suggest hidradenitis suppurativa may be due to defective follicular support. Br J Dermatol. 2013;168(5):1034.
98. van der Zee HH, Laman JD, Boer J, et al. Hidradenitis suppurativa: viewpoint on clinical phenotyping, pathogenesis and novel treatments. Exp Dermatol. 2012;21(1):735–9.
99. Ring HC, Riis Mikkelsen P, Miller IM, et al. The bacteriology of hidradenitis suppurativa: a systematic review. Exp Dermatol. 2015;24(10):727–31. doi:10.1111/exd.12793.
100. Hotz C, Boniotto M, Guguin A, et al. Intrinsic defect in keratinocyte function leads to inflammation in Hidradenitis suppurativa. J Invest Dermatol. 2016. doi:10.1016/j.jid.2016.04.036.
101. van der Zee HH, de Ruiter L, van den Broecke DG, et al. Elevated levels of tumour necrosis factor (TNF)-α, interleukin (IL)-1β and IL-10 in hidradenitis suppurativa skin: a rationale for targeting TNF-α and IL-1β. Br J Dermatol. 2011;164:1292–8.
102. Schlapbach C, Hänni T, Yawalkar N, et al. Expression of the IL-23/Th17 pathway in lesions of hidradenitis suppurativa. J Am Acad Dermatol. 2011;65:790–8.
103. Hunger RE, Surovy AM, Hassan AS, et al. Toll-like receptor 2 is highly expressed in lesions of acne inversa and colocalizes with C-type lectin receptor. Br J Dermatol. 2008;158:691–7.
104. van Rappard DC, Leenarts MF, Meijerink-van't Oost L, et al. Comparing treatment outcome of infliximab and adalimumab in patients with severe hidradenitis suppurativa. J Dermatolog Treat. 2011;23(4):284–9. doi:10.3109/09546634.2011.571657.
105. Gener G, Canoui-Poitrine F, Revuz JE, et al. Combination therapy with clindamycin and rifampicin for hidradenitis suppurativa: a series of 116 consecutive patients. Dermatology. 2009;219(2):148–54. doi:10.1159/000228334.
106. Join-Lambert O, Coignard H, Jais JP, et al. Efficacy of rifampin-moxifloxacin-metronidazole combination therapy in hidradenitis suppurativa. Dermatology. 2011;222(1):49–58. doi:10.1159/000321716.
107. Fitzsimmons JS, Guilbert PR. A family study of hidradenitis suppurativa. J Med Genet. 1985;22:367–73.
108. Gao M, Wang PG, Cui Y, et al. Inversa acne (hidradenitis suppurativa): a case report and identification of the locus at chromosome 1p21.1-1q25.3. J Invest Dermatol. 2006;126 (6):1302–6.
109. Wang B, Yang W, Wen W, et al. Gamma-secretase gene mutations in familial acne inversa. Science. 2010;330(6007):1065.
110. Li CR, Jiang MJ, Shen DB, et al. Two novel mutations of the nicastrin gene in Chinese patients with acne inversa. Br J Dermatol. 2011;165(2):415–418.

111. Liu Y, Gao M, Lv YM, et al. Confirmation by exome sequencing of the pathogenic role of NCSTN mutations in acne inversa (hidradenitis suppurativa). J Invest Dermatol. 2011;131 (7):1570–2.
112. Pink AE, Simpson MA, Brice GW, et al. PSENEN and NCSTN mutations in familial hidradenitis suppurativa (acne inversa). J Invest Dermatol. 2011;131(7):1568–70.
113. Miskinyte S, Nassif A, Merabtene F, et al. Nicastrin mutations in French families with hidradenitis suppurativa. J Invest Dermatol. 2012;132:1728–30.
114. Zhang C, Wang L, Chen L, et al. Two novel mutations of the NCSTN gene in Chinese familial acne inverse. J Eur Acad Dermatol Venereol. 2012;27(12):1571–4.
115. Nomura Y, Nomura T, Sakai K, et al. A novel splice site mutation in NCSTN underlies a Japanese family with hidradenitis suppurativa. Br J Dermatol. 2012;68(1):206–9.
116. Chen S, Mattei P, You J, et al. γ-Secretase mutation in an African American family with hidradenitis Suppurativa. JAMA Dermatol. 2015;151(6):668–70.
117. Canoui-Poitrine F, Revuz JE, Wolkenstein P. Clinical characteristics of a series of 302 French patients with hidradenitis suppurativa, with an analysis of factors associated with disease severity. J Am Acad Dermatol. 2009;61(1):51–7. doi:10.1016/j.jaad.2009.02.013.
118. Thomas C, Rodby KA, Thomas J. Recalcitrant Hidradenitis Suppurativa: an investigation of demographics, surgical management, bacterial isolates, pharmacologic intervention, and patient-reported health outcomes. Am Surg. 2016;82(4):362–6.
119. Losanoff JE, Sochaki P, Khoury N, Levi E, Salwen WA, Basson MD. Squamous cell carcinoma complicating chronic suppurative hydradenitis. Am Surg. 2011;77(11):1449–53.
120. Rosen T. Squamous cell carcinoma: complication of chronic skin disorders in black patients. J Natl Med Assoc. 1986;78(12):1203–5.
121. Roussomoustakaki M, Dimoulios P, Chatzicostas C, et al. Hidradenitis suppurativa associated with Crohn's disease and spondyloarthropathy: response to anti-TNF therapy. J Gastroenterol. 2003;38(10):1000.
122. Marzano AV, Trevisan V, Gattorno M, et al. Pyogenic arthritis, pyoderma gangrenosum, acne, and hidradenitis suppurativa (PAPASH): a new autoinflammatory syndrome associated with a novel mutation of the PSTPIP1 gene. JAMA Dermatol. 2013;149(6):762.
123. Zouboulis CC, Desai N, Emtestam L, et al. European S1 guideline for the treatment of hidradenitis suppurativa/acne inversa. J Eur Acad Dermatol Venereol. 2015;29(4):619–44. doi:10.1111/jdv.12966.
124. van der Zee HH, Jemec GB. New insights into the diagnosis of hidradenitis suppurativa: clinical presentations and phenotypes. J Am Acad Dermatol. 2015;73(Suppl 5):S23–6. doi:10.1016/j.jaad.2015.07.047.
125. Micheletti RG (2015) An update on the diagnosis and treatment of hidradenitis suppurativa. Cutis. 2015;96(Suppl 6):7–12.
126. Simonart T. Hidradenitis suppurativa and smoking. J Am Acad Dermatol. 2010;62(1): 149–50.
127. Sartorius K, Emtestam L, Jemec GB, et al. Objective scoring of hidradenitis suppurativa reflecting the role of tobacco and obesity. Br J Dermatol. 2009;161(4):831.
128. Melnik BC, John SM, Schmitz G. Over-stimulation of insulin/IGF-1 signaling by western diet may promote diseases of civilization: lessons learnt from laron syndrome. Nutr Metab. 2011;8:41.
129. Clemensen OJ. Topical treatment of hidradenitis suppurativa with clindamycin. Int J Dermatol. 1983;22(5):325.
130. Jemec GB, Wendelboe P. Topical clindamycin versus systemic tetracycline in the treatment of hidradenitis suppurativa. J Am Acad Dermatol. 1998;39(6):971–4.
131. Mendonça CO, Griffiths CE. Clindamycin and rifampicin combination therapy for hidradenitis suppurativa. Br J Dermatol. 2006;154(5):977–8.
132. Boer J, Jemec GB. Resorcinol peels as a possible self-treatment of painful nodules in hidradenitis suppurativa. Clin Exp Dermatol. 2010;35(1):36.

133. van der Zee HH, Boer J, Prens EP, et al. The effect of combined treatment with oral clindamycin and oral rifampin in patients with hidradenitis suppurativa. Dermatology. 2009;219(2):143–7.
134. Yazdanyar S, Boer J, Ingvarsson G, et al. Dapsone therapy for hidradenitis suppurativa: a series of 24 patients. Dermatology. 2011;222(4):342–6.
135. Kaur MR, Lewis HM. Hidradenitis suppurativa treated with dapsone: a case series of five patients. J Dermatol Treat. 2006;17(4):211.
136. Boer J, van Gemert MJ. Long-term results of isotretinoin in the treatment of 68 patients with hidradenitis suppurativa. J Am Acad Dermatol. 1999;40(1):73–6.
137. Mortimer PS, Dawber RP, Gales MA, et al. A double-blind controlled cross-over trial of cyproterone acetate in females with hidradenitis suppurativa. Br J Dermatol. 1986;115 (3):263–8.
138. Farrell AM, Randall VA, Vafaee T, et al. Finasteride as a therapy for hidradenitis suppurativa. Br J Dermatol. 1999;141(6):1138–9.
139. Joseph MA, Jayaseelan E, Ganapathi B, et al. Hidradenitis suppurativa treated with finasteride. J Dermatol Treat. 2005;16(1):75–8.
140. Rose RF, Goodfield MJ, Clark SM. Treatment of recalcitrant hidradenitis suppurativa with oral ciclosporin. Clin Exp Dermatol. 2006;31(1):154–5.
141. Buckley DA, Rogers S. Cyclosporin-responsive hidradenitis suppurativa. J R Soc Med. 1995;88(5):289P–90P.
142. Soria A, Canoui-Poitrine F, Wolkenstein P. Absence of efficacy of oral isotretinoin in hidradenitis suppurativa: a retrospective study based on patients' outcome assessment. Dermatology. 2009;218(2):134–5.
143. Boer J, Nazary M. Long-term results of acitretin therapy for hidradenitis suppurativa. Is acne inversa also a misnomer? Br J Dermatol. 2011;164(1):170.
144. Kraft JN, Searles GE. Hidradenitis suppurativa in 64 female patients: retrospective study comparing oral antibiotics and antiandrogen therapy. J Cutan Med Surg. 2007;11:125–31.
145. Danby FW, Margesson LJ. Hidradenitis suppurativa. Dermatol Clin. 2010;28(4):779.
146. Grant A, Gonzalez T, Montgomery MO, et al. Infliximab therapy for patients with moderate to severe hidradenitis suppurativa: a randomized, double-blind, placebo-controlled crossover trial. J Am Acad Dermatol. 2010;62(2):205.
147. Lesage C, Adnot-Desanlis L, Perceau G, et al. Efficacy and tolerance of prolonged infliximab treatment of moderate-to-severe forms of hidradenitis suppurativa. Eur J Dermatol. 2012;22(5):640–4.
148. Delage M, Samimi M, Atlan M, et al. Efficacy of infliximab for hidradenitis suppurativa: assessment of clinical and biological inflammatory markers. Acta Derm Venereol. 2011;91 (2):169–71.
149. Shuja F, Chan CS, Rosen T. Biologic drugs for the treatment of hidradenitis suppurativa: an evidence-based review. Dermatol Clin. 2010;28(3):511.
150. Kimball AB, Kerdel F, Adams D, et al. Adalimumab for the treatment of moderate to severe Hidradenitis suppurativa: a parallel randomized trial. Ann Intern Med. 2012;157:846–55.
151. Lee RA, Dommasch E, Treat J, et al. A prospective clinical trial of open-label etanercept for the treatment of hidradenitis suppurativa. J Am Acad Dermatol. 2009;60:565–73.
152. Adams DR, Yankura JA, Fogelberg AC, et al. Treatment of hidradenitis suppurativa with etanercept injection. Arch Dermatol. 2010;146:501–4.
153. Gulliver WP, Jemec GB, Baker KA. Experience with ustekinumab for the treatment of moderate to severe hidradenitis suppurativa. J Eur Acad Dermatol Venereol. 2012;26 (7):911.
154. Blok JL, Li K, Brodmerkel C, et al. Ustekinumab in hidradenitis suppurativa: clinical results and a search for potential biomarkers in serum. Br J Dermatol. 2016;174(4):839–46.
155. Leslie KS, Tripathi SV, Nguyen TV, et al. An open-label study of anakinra for the treatment of moderate to severe hidradenitis suppurativa. J Am Acad Dermatol. 2014;70:243–51.
156. Tzanetakou V, Kanni T, Giatrakou S, et al. Safety and efficacy of anakinra in severe hidradenitis suppurativa: a randomized clinical trial. JAMA Dermatol. 2016;152(1):52.

157. Ducroux E, Ocampo MA, Kanitakis J, et al. Hidradenitis suppurativa after renal transplantation: complete remission after switching from oral cyclosporine to oral tacrolimus. J Am Acad Dermatol. 2014;71(5):e210.
158. Mahmoud BH, Tierney E, Hexsel CL, et al. Prospective controlled clinical and histopathologic study of hidradenitis suppurativa treated with the long-pulsed neodymium: yttrium-aluminium-garnet laser. J Am Acad Dermatol. 2010;62:637–45.
159. Tierney E, Mahmoud BH, Hexsel C, et al. Randomized control trial for the treatment of hidradenitis suppurativa with a neodymium-doped yttrium aluminium garnet laser. Dermatol Surg. 2009;35(8):1188–98. doi:10.1111/j.1524-4725.2009.01214.x.
160. Highton L, Chan WY, Khwaja N, et al. Treatment of hidradenitis suppurativa with intense pulsed light: a prospective study. Plast Reconstr Surg. 2011;128(2):459–65.
161. Iwasaki J, Marra DE, Fincher EF, et al. Treatment of hidradenitis suppurativa with a nonablative radiofrequency device. Dermatol Surg. 2008;34(1):114–7.
162. Gold M, Bridges TM, Bradshaw VL, et al. ALA-PDT and blue light therapy for hidradenitis suppurativa. J Drugs Dermatol. 2004;3(Suppl. 1):S32–5.
163. Strauss RM, Pollock B, Stables GI, et al. Photodynamic therapy using aminolaevulinic acid does not lead to clinical improvement in hidradenitis suppurativa. Br J Dermatol. 2005;152(4):803.
164. Schweiger ES, Riddle CC, Aires DJ. Treatment of hidradenitis suppurativa by photodynamic therapy with aminolevulinic acid: preliminary results. J Drugs Dermatol 10(4):381–386.
165. Ellis LZ. Hidradenitis suppurativa: surgical and other management techniques. Dermatol Surg. 2012;38(4):517.
166. van der Zee HH, Prens EP, Boer J. Deroofing: a tissue-saving surgical technique for the treatment of mild to moderate hidradenitis suppurativa lesions. J Am Acad Dermatol. 2010;63:475–80.
167. Hazen PG, Hazen BP. Hidradenitis suppurativa: successful treatment using carbon dioxide laser excision and marsupialization. Dermatol Surg. 2010;36:208–13.
168. Menderes A, Sunay O, Vayvada H, et al. Surgical management of hidradenitis suppurativa. Int J Med Sci. 2010;7(4):240–47.
169. Rompel R, Petres J. Long-term results of wide surgical excision in 106 patients with hidradenitis suppurativa. Dermatol Surg. 2000;26:638–43.
170. Gillette. Advances in shaving technology: a review of the optimal shaving regimen for men highlighting technical advances associated with the fusion five-blade razor and its myth-bust- ing effect on pseudofolliculitis Barbae. Proctor & Gamble:1–24 http://www.pgdermatology.com/downloads/documents/Gillette_WhitePaper.pdf. Last accessed 30 May 2012.
171. Kindred C, Oresajo CO, Yatskayer M, et al. Comparative evaluation of men's depilatory composition versus razor in black men. Cutis. 2011;88(2):98–103.
172. Cook-Bolden FE, Barba A, Halder R, et al. Twice-daily applications of benzoyl peroxide 5%/clindamycin 1% gel versus vehicle in the treatment of pseudofolliculitis barbae. Cutis. 2004;73(Suppl 6):18–24.
173. Coley MK, Alexis AF. Dermatologic conditions in men of African ancestry. Expert Rev Dermatol. 2009;4:595–609.
174. Xia Y, Cho S, Howard RS, et al. Topical eflornithine hydrochloride improves the effectiveness of standard laser hair removal for treating pseudofolliculitis barbae: a randomized, double-blinded, placebo-controlled trial. J Am Acad Dermatol. 2012;67(4):694–9.
175. Perricone NV. Treatment of pseudofolliculitis barbae with topical glycolic acid: a report of two studies. Cutis. 1993;52(4):232–5.
176. Roberts WE. Chemical peeling in ethnic/dark skin. Dermatol Ther. 2004;17(2):196–205.
177. Diernaes JE, Bygum A. Successful treatment of recalcitrant folliculitis barbae and pseudofolliculitis barbae with photodynamic therapy. Photodiagnosis Photodyn Ther. 2013;10(4):651–3.

178. Barr J, Friedman A, Balwin H. Use of imiquimod and pimecrolimus cream in the treatment of acne keloidalis nuchae. J Am Acad Dermatol. 2005;52(suppl 3):P64.
179. Esmat SM, Abdel Hay RM, Abu Zeid OM, et al. The efficacy of laser-assisted hair removal in the treatment of acne keloidalis nuchae; a pilot study. Eur J Dermatol. 2012;22(5):645–50.
180. Okoye GA, Rainer BM, Leung SG, et al. Improving acne keloidalis nuchae with targeted ultraviolet B treatment: a prospective, randomized, split-scalp comparison study. Br J Dermatol. 2014;171(5):1156–63.
181. Bolz S, Jappe U, Hartschuh W. Successful treatment of perifolliculitis capitis abscedens et suffodiens with combined isotretinoin and dapsone. J Dtsch Dermatol Ges. 2008;6(1):44–7.
182. Verdolini R, Clayton N, Smith A, et al. Metformin for the treatment of hidradenitis suppurativa: a little help along the way. Eur Acad Dermatol Venereol. 2013;27(9):1101–8.
183. Brocard A, Knol AC, Khammari A, et al. Hidradenitis suppurativa and zinc: a new therapeutic approach. A pilot study. Dermatology. 2007;214(4):325.
184. Dréno B, Khammari A, Brocard A, et al. Hidradenitis suppurativa: the role of deficient cutaneous innate immunity. Arch Dermatol. 2012;148(2):182–6.

Chapter 21
Skin Aging in Individuals with Skin of Color

Daniel J. Callaghan III., Babu Singh and Kavitha K. Reddy

We have been fortunate as a global population that life expectancy continues to increase. With time, we have also seen an increased number of and availability of effective cosmetic treatments, along with increasing individual and cultural preferences for cosmetic improvement. These coalescing factors have increased our desire to understand the aging process and increased the demand for effective aging treatments. These trends affect all skin types, including those with skin of color.

Traditional discussions of skin aging and aging treatments focused primarily on white skin. However, more recently the discussion has been expanded to include the entire human family and all of its various skin colors. Those with skin of color comprised approximately 15% of patients undergoing cosmetic procedures in 1997; this number had increased to 22% by 2014 [1]. Today, cosmetic treatments are performed in skin of all colors with continued increases in the number of individuals seeking safe and effective treatment. As a clinician, it is important to understand aging not only to treat the elderly patient who may want to look a few years younger but also to be able to provide proper counseling to younger patients to help reduce preventable signs of aging. Additionally, a firm understanding of the changes seen in aging can allow a clinician to better counsel and treat any individual who simply would like to improve an aspect or aspects of their cosmetic appearance whether or not it is directly related to aging. Though it is informative to compare and contrast some of the differences in characteristics of aging seen in various skin colors, it is important to remember that while generalizations are easy

D.J. Callaghan III. · B. Singh · K.K. Reddy (✉)
Department of Dermatology, Boston University Medical Center,
609 Albany St., Boston, MA 02118, USA
e-mail: kreddy@bu.edu

D.J. Callaghan III.
e-mail: DanielJCallaghan3@gmail.com

B. Singh
e-mail: singhba@bu.edu

© Springer International Publishing AG 2017
N.A. Vashi and H.I. Maibach (eds.), *Dermatoanthropology of Ethnic Skin and Hair*, DOI 10.1007/978-3-319-53961-4_21

to make, a thoughtful reader will take into account population data while also realizing the limitations of such data to ultimately treat each and every patient individually.

Physiologic and Structural Properties of Skin

The vast majority of the elements of the skin are identical between races. However, there are some differences seen in skin of individuals of a variety of colors. The most noticeable difference is an increased melanin concentration. In terms of aging, this is significant because melanin serves as a natural defense against ultraviolet (UV) damage and photoaging, and is able to reduce, though not eliminate, photoaging. Melanin content in the epidermis of black individuals has been reported to provide on average a SPF protection of 13 compared with white skin and to block three times the amount of UVA transmission [2]. There has also been discussion that Asian and Black skin may be more compact and in some cases thicker as compared to white skin [3, 4]. People of color have also been reported to have more numerous, larger and more nucleated fibroblasts in the dermis [5]. Due to the role fibroblasts play in the production of collagen, it has been hypothesized that this may enable people of color to better preserve the structural integrity of their skin with aging [6]. More recently, Fantasia et al. have demonstrated that African-American skin has enhanced TGF-β signaling which is thought to increase the expression of elastin, ultimately providing additional protection against the changes seen in not only extrinsic but also intrinsic aging [7]. It should be kept in mind, however, that many of these studies are either quite dated or small in number, and until larger and more robust studies are completed, we cannot reliably assess these hypotheses and conclusions.

Features of Aging

Aging is a complex process of biologic and physiologic changes in the skin and other organs. Informally, the most rapid and common way those in society approximate another persons' age is by their appearance. The most common signs of aging across all skin types include wrinkles, loss of elasticity, loss of facial and subcutaneous fat volume, fat redistribution, changes in bone structure, and uneven skin color.

Intrinsic and Extrinsic Aging

Aging is often subdivided into intrinsic and extrinsic aging processes. In reality, these are often overlapping or mixed, since various intrinsically generated and extrinsically delivered assaults on the skin share some common endpoints. Intrinsic aging, also described as chronologic aging, is a natural process that occurs with time and is not related to external stressors such as ultraviolet damage or smoking. Features of intrinsic aging include fine wrinkles, fat atrophy, soft tissue redistribution, skin thinning, and bone remodeling [8]. Conversely, extrinsic aging is a result of one's lifestyle choices or environment. Tobacco use, diet and exercise habits, nutrition, and type and amount of alcohol use are all contributors to extrinsic aging. Ultraviolet light (sun) exposure has traditionally been considered the single largest driver of extrinsic aging. While this appears most true for light skin colors, as with all skin colors, the amount of contribution to individuals with skin of color likely varies with factors such as amount of lifetime UV exposure, use of sun protection, natural skin pigmentation level, and amount of exposure to other non-UV stressors.

Photoaging

Photoaging may manifest clinically as loss of elasticity leading to skin sagging, deep rhytids, propensity to senile purpura, telangiectasias, and pigmentary disorders [9]. While senile purpura and telangiectasias are less common in skin of color, one can immediately recognize that some photoaging signs can also be seen in intrinsic aging, and appear to be accelerated by the addition of UV exposure.

Changes of photoaging in people of color as a whole is generally believed to occur on average at a later age than Caucasians, typically not becoming apparent until the fifth or sixth decade of life [10]. A study by Hillebrand et al. which compared different ethnic groups in Los Angeles found that increased skin wrinkling was observed in the following order: Caucasian > Hispanic > African American > East Asian [11]. Though this is a single study which obviously cannot be generalized to entire populations, it is an interesting observation that less wrinkling was observed in East Asians compared to African Americans, which reinforces that there are likely additional factors beyond melanin content alone in providing protection from rhytids and aging. Cultural practices, sun safety/avoidance practices, and individual skin care regimens and lifestyles all sensibly contribute to skin aging.

Age-Associated Pigmentary Changes

The increased melanin that protects against photoaging also makes one more susceptible to problems with dyspigmentation. These changes may include mottled pigmentation and solar lentigines. In clinical practice, these are common concerns in those with skin of color. Photoaging was reported in one study to account for up to 17% of all dermatological diagnoses in Hispanic patients seen [12]. In another report, uneven skin tone was the chief complaint of darker skinned women more than 33% of the time [13]. Pigmentary concerns must be evaluated carefully and appropriately diagnosed to provide a more accurate prognosis and identify optimal treatment options. Common pigmentary concerns associated with skin aging are described below.

Dermatosis Papulosa Nigra/Seborrheic Keratoses

Seborrheic keratoses are common across all skin colors and types. They are clearly associated with age clinically, and appear to have a genetic or as yet unidentified environmental component, as some individuals are more prone to developing a large number of them compared with others. The precise etiology of seborrheic keratoses is not known. When present as medium to dark brown papules and plaques particularly grouped around the eyelids and upper cheeks in individuals of color, these are called dermatosis papulosa nigra (DPN) (Fig. 21.1). DPN are believed to represent a variant of seborrheic keratoses, as the histologies overlap. DPN are often particularly abundant in blacks, affecting upto one-third of African Americans.

Although these lesions are benign, treatment is often pursued for cosmetic purposes. Due to the risks of dyspigmentation and scarring, patients should be counseled with care about these risks before treating them. Treatment options include simple snipping, curettage, excision, or electrodesiccation. Cryotherapy or laser ablation are also available, though dyspigmentation may be of even greater concern with these modalities.

(a)   **(b)**

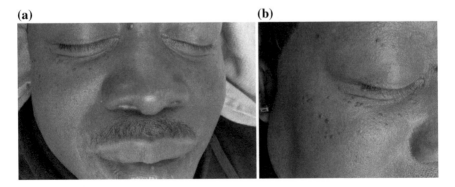

Fig. 21.1 **a** Bilateral brown periorbital waxy papules; **b** closer view

Maturational Hyperpigmentation

Maturational hyperpigmentation is a controversial term that has been described as ill-defined hyperpigmentation greatest on the lateral forehead and cheekbones. It is thought to be associated with chronic photodamage given the sun-exposed distribution [14].

Cherry Angiomas

Cherry angioma, also known as senile angioma or Campbell-De Morgan spot, is the most commonly acquired vascular proliferation with aging. Cherry angiomas may occasionally develop during adolescence, but usually first appear during the third decade or later of life. Murison et al. observed an incidence of 75% at age 60, and an increasing number and size of lesions with age [15]. Tindall et al. observed cherry angiomas in 73% of their elderly (age 64 and greater) study population [16]. Equal incidence of cherry angiomas in men and women has been reported [15, 16]. There has been no clear genetic inheritance of cherry angiomas observed to date. The etiology for developing cherry angiomas is unknown, but has been associated with pregnancy, occupational exposure to bromides and glycol ether solvent 2-butoxyethanol, and toxicity from sulfur mustard gas [17–20].

Clinically, cherry angiomas appear as asymptomatic flat, red macules or dome-shaped, red compressible papules, ranging in size from 1 to 5 mm (Fig. 21.2). Cherry angiomas are most frequently distributed on the trunk, although they are also often observed on the scalp [21–23]. Histologically, cherry angiomas consist of ectatic capillaries and venules in the papillary dermis and superficial reticular dermis.

Limited data exists on the incidence of cherry angiomas in different racial groups or skin types. Some have suggested that darker brown skin types may have lower incidences of cherry angiomas than skin types I and II. In a retrospective study performed with Indian subjects who were skin type IV, cherry angiomas were observed in 15.2% of the population studied [9]. Tindall et al. found that people of color had lower incidences of cherry angiomas (11% in men, 45% in women) compared to Caucasian men and men (77% in both men and women) [16]. Beauregard et al. reported that cherry angiomas were statistically associated with skin type III or less, but not with skin type VI [24]. In clinical practice, however, cherry angiomas are regularly seen on a variety of skin types, including type IV.

Evidence on the safe and effective treatment of cherry angiomas in skin of color is limited. Treatment modalities must be carefully selected in patients of color to prevent scar, keloid, and pigmentation changes. Cherry angiomas, although benign, may pose a cosmetic concern for some patients who request removal of lesions. Cryotherapy may cause undue scarring and pigmentation sequela if performed on skin of color [25]. Electrodessication can be considered though risks remain.

Fig. 21.2 *Cherry red* dome-shaped round papules on the chest

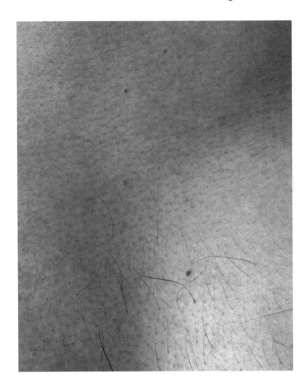

Sclerotherapy is not standard and does not show high efficacy rates [26]. The 532 nm KTP laser risks unnecessary dyspigmentation in darker skin types. The pulsed dye laser is an option, though also carries some risk of dyspigmentation or scarring. The 1064-nm neodymium-doped yttrium aluminum garnet (Nd:YAG) laser has been effective for many in treating cherry angiomas, though there is a risk of ulceration and scar [27]. Given the common nature of these lesions, more studies will be beneficial in documenting and providing optimal treatment options and parameters.

Periorbital Hyperpigmentation

Periorbital hyperpigmentation presents as bilateral round or semicircular, ill-defined hyperpigmentation around the eyes and eyelids. It is often attempted to be classified into pigmented (brown color), vascular (blue/pink/purple color), or mixed [28]. Although it is a common worldwide problem across all skin types, it is commonly seen in skin of color [29]. While its etiology remains unclear, it has been associated with genetics, sometimes with a history of excess pigmentation from a resolved or chronic contact or allergic dermatitis, history of chronic periorbital edema, and hormonal factors. Treatment is difficult and patients should be made aware of this. Adequate sleep, hydration, and sun protection remain the foundation of therapy, though additional cosmetic measures such as topical vitamin C, or daily antihistamine therapy, can be tried, sometimes with improvement [30].

Solar Lentigines

Solar lentigines are a result of sun exposure and appear more in the aged population. While they are reported to be more common in white skin, they remain a common complaint in those with skin of color [31]. Sun protection, combined with lightening agents and/or laser treatment, are the typical treatments.

Idiopathic Guttate Hypomelanosis

Idiopathic guttate hypomelanosis (IGH) is an aging condition presenting as discrete, round to oval hypopigmented light to white-appearing macules. These range in size from 2 to 5 mm in diameter. Congenital or childhood hypopigmented macules are usually of a different cause and should be evaluated by a dermatologist. IGH are often found in a photodistribution, with the arms, legs, trunk, and face possibly being affected. Its etiology remains unclear; however, causative factors that have been suggested include genetics, possible auto-immunity, and chronic sun exposure. The belief that photodamage plays a role is due to the observation that IGH often presents in sun-exposed areas. Conversely, Kim et al. were not able to find any histopathologic features of actinic damage in skin affected by IGH [32].

Changes in Facial Volume and Structure

It is useful to highlight the classic features of facial aging in all skin colors. These include increasing laxity of the skin of the upper eyelids. An increase in skin laxity leads to the lower eyelids to also transition from the 'single convexity' seen in a youthful face, to a frequent 'double convexity' [33]. In the lower face, sagging and jowling are commonplace, increasing the prominence of the nasolabial folds and blurring the cervico-mental angle. Rhytides are often seen on the forehead, glabella, periorally, and periorbitally. Additionally, there is typically a decrease in the volume of the lips [6, 34, 35].

African Americans have been suggested by some to have increased soft tissue of the mid-face, more prominent lips, and increased facial convexity as compared to Caucasians, though this would of course vary by individual. Mid-face volume changes are a prominent concern as with those of all skin colors. In general, the lips of African Americans have also been reported by some to more often be fuller than their Caucasian counterparts. Although lip atrophy with aging occurs, it has been reported less commonly as a concern at least in published literature [14].

In discussing aging in Asians, it is important to appreciate the differences between skin type and skeletal structure in individuals from East Asia compared with those from Southeast Asia. Individuals from East Asia often have a more delicate appearing facial skeletal framework. Despite this, some have reported there is a stronger support network for the muscles and skin. Nonetheless, like those of all skin types, over time almost all individuals succumb to some degree of facial sagging [36–38]. There is a paucity of studies examining the specific aging features in most groups with skin of color. This includes those of South Asian descent and those of several Latino or Hispanic backgrounds. From a structural point of view, individuals from these groups share more Caucasoid features, and facial volume changes can occur similarly as with all other individuals of any skin color.

We remind the reader that it is important to remember there is an incredible amount of heterogeneity and diversity within the different populations representing 'skin of color', and that data is limited. It is important to evaluate each patient individually.

Photoprotection and Aging Prevention

The increased melanin found in individuals of skin of color does provide some level of photoprotection. This has been estimated at an SPF of 13 for the African-American skin studied in an old study [2], though this clearly cannot be generalized with much accuracy to the large and diverse global population of individuals with skin of color. While melanin protection is certainly beneficial to protect against photoaging, it likely does not provide sufficient sun protection in and of itself to optimally reduce photoaging or pigmentary disorders. The common recommendation by dermatologists is to apply a broad spectrum, SPF 30 + sunscreen daily and avoid unnecessary sun exposure, particularly peak or prolonged exposures. This applies to individuals with skin of color as equally as those with lighter skins, provided that the individual is concerned with skin aging. Even if he/she is not, sun safety is of some concern as well, since skin cancer can also afflict those with skin of color. Vitamin D levels can be bolstered with oral supplementation when needed in those who may benefit from reducing sun exposure.

Despite this information, people of color and their physicians are often unaware of these recommendations. Many do not routinely practice photoprotection as they are often under the assumption that it does not apply to them, and in some cases, physicians may also erroneously believe that UV-related aging changes, dyspigmentation, or skin cancer are not of significant concern for patients of color [39]. It is appropriate to consider counseling individuals of color about sun protection. That includes the importance of daily broad-spectrum sunscreen of at least SPF 30 as well as other sun-protective behaviors such as UV protective clothing, use of wide-brimmed hats, and avoiding midday sun [40]. This not only helps combat the aging effects of the sun but also can help prevent skin cancers in susceptible individuals.

While sun protection remains the most commonly recommended preventive agent for the skin, exercise and healthy nutrition habits are also important to reduce signs of aging in all organs, including some important benefits for the skin.

Dermal Fillers

Dermal fillers are a popular option for treating the volume loss and soft tissue redistribution seen with aging. Features of mid-facial aging are most commonly treated. Other frequently treated areas of volume loss include the temporal region, chin, and lips [41]. Though there had initially been concerns that the use of fillers in skin of color could lead to dyspigmentation or the development of keloids, studies to date involving hyaluronic acid, cohesive polydensified matrix hyaluronic acid (HA), calcium hydroxyapetite, and poly-L-lactic acid have shown these risks to be minimal to nearly nonexistent. Common HA fillers used in clinical practice are as effective in skin of color patients as they are in Caucasians [42–50].

The most common side effects typically seen with fillers include injection-site related erythema and edema [42]. Techniques that may dissipate adverse events include slower injection rates and injection of smaller boluses [49, 51]. If post-injection erythema and bruising occurs, patients can be counseled that it typically resolves without sequelae. That being said, if the post-injection erythema is significant, the use of a mid- to high-potency topical corticosteroid may diminish the risk of PIH and can be considered [46].

Neuromodulators

Botulinum toxin is used to reduce muscle contraction, thereby reducing the wrinkles that form as a result of repeated movements. Botulinum is also sometimes used to shape or relax certain areas of the face by decreasing muscle size or strength. Available botulinum toxins include Onabotulinumtoxin A (Botox®), incobotulinumtoxin A (Xeomin®), and abobotulinumtoxin A (Dysport®). Botulinum toxin-type B includes rimabotulinumtoxin B, which at the time of publication has not been FDA approved for cosmetic usage. Botulinum toxin medications are routinely used on-label for rhytides, for example of the glabella, and often off-label for the treatment of a wide variety of indications including horizontal forehead lines, Crow's feet, nasal bunny lines, perioral rhytides, marionette lines, and masseter hypertrophy.

Botulinum toxin has been found to be equally well tolerated in skin of color as in white skin without any clear differences noted. Dosage, injection sites, injection techniques, response, and duration of response do not appear to differ. Onabotulinumtoxin A and abobotulinumtoxin A have been studied more extensively in skin of color patients and were found to have a similar side effect profile as with their use in Caucasian patients [44, 52, 53]. One study comparing the use of abobotulinumtoxin A in skin of color patients suggested a greater response rate at 30 days compared to lighter skinned counterparts being studied [52], but again larger studies would be needed to confirm this report. Incobotulinumtoxin A and rimabotulinumtoxin B have not been studied as extensively in skin of color, although one study out of South Korea with 22 patients found no increased adverse events with the use of rimabotulinumtoxin B as compared to onabotulinumtoxin A [54]. No difference would be expected based on clinical practice experience to date and on scientific and biologic theory.

Chemical Peels

Chemical peels are frequently used to treat photodamage and textural concerns. In light skin types, chemical peels are more often used to treat skin changes associated with photoaging; however, in darker skin types they are most often employed for dyschromias including PIH and melasma [55]. Chemical peels are broadly classified by the depth to which they penetrate. Superficial peels are often well tolerated in all skin types, and medium peels can also be used in skin of color with caution. Deep peels, however, should typically be avoided due to the high risk of side effects in skin of color [56].

In order to reduce the risk of PIH, pre-peel priming with hydroquinone and photoprotection may be beneficial. Post-peel instructions include emollients, sun protection, and sometimes restarting hydroquinone one week after the peel. Corticosteroids can also be used to reduce inflammation when there is significant erythema to reduce the risk of PIH [56].

Lasers

Lasers use light of a particular wavelength to target certain chromophores in the skin, including melanin, hemoglobin, and water. With the goal of selectively heating a target chromophore, the energy is absorbed by the chromophore(s) and then dispersed as heat. This allows for the controlled destruction of different types of tissue depending on which chromophore is abundant.

The melanin content within skin of color patients necessitates an appropriate knowledge of the proper selection and use of lasers in these individuals in order to provide safe and effective treatment. Many early-generation lasers were contraindicated in darker skin types or when used, caused adverse effects such as dyspigmentation and scarring. However, advances in technology within the last decade have provided more options for the use of lasers with relative safety in all skin colors, though this still depends very much on the laser type, settings, and technique.

The use of ablative resurfacing lasers, such as the carbon dioxide and erbium-doped yttrium aluminum garnet (Er:YAG), have been used for full face skin resurfacing in light-skinned patients for years. Due to the fact that by definition these lasers destroy the epidermis, these are most often either not used in skin of color or used with extreme caution by experienced operators because of the risk of PIH and scarring.

Nonablative lasers have provided a safer alternative though with milder effect for resurfacing in skin of color. These lasers reach the dermis while sparing the epidermis. This allows for tissue remodeling while reducing the side effect profile and time needed to heal.

Nonablative lasers are frequently employed to treat changes such as rough skin texture, fine and moderate rhytides, and aging-independent conditions such as scars.

Quality-Switched Lasers

Quality- or Q-switched (QS) lasers emit maximum energy output in nanosecond (ns) pulses. Due to the fact that their pulse time is significantly shorter than the thermal relaxation time of melanosomes, they provide a means to treat pigmented lesions and dyschromia. Frequently employed QS systems include the QS ruby (694 nm), alexandrite (755 nm), and Nd:YAG (1064 nm). The Nd:YAG laser can be used for all skin types and is safer in skin of color, while the alexandrite is best suited for lighter skin types including some lighter skin of color patients if the Nd:YAG is not available. The ruby should be reserved for white skin as the risk of dyspigmentation is very high.

Intense Pulsed Light

Intense Pulsed Light (IPL), which emits a broad band of visible light (400–1,200 nm), has been used for the treatment of dyschromia and pigmented lesions in a variety of lighter skin colors, including East Asian populations [57]. IPL carries a relatively high risk of PIH in the experience of many, and it should ideally not be used in patients with more than minimal skin pigmentation since safer alternatives are available.

Side Effects and Treatment Considerations

Despite the fact that the above modalities have been found to be well tolerated in skin of color patients, it is important to counsel patients on potential risks such as scarring and pigmentary changes, which can be temporary or permanent.

In order to minimize these risks, it is important for the clinician to take extra precautions when treating skin of color patients. Appropriate training, selection of treatment, and technique is paramount. The use of lower fluences and treatment densities should be considered. Properly chosen test spots also help the clinician determine how a patient will react to a given laser and settings. Counseling patients on vigilant sun protection is important. Use of hydroquinone 2 or 4% 2–4 weeks before and after each treatment is optional but may help reduce risks of dyspigmentation in some cases. The use of epidermal cooling devices and ice packs posttreatment are often beneficial. Finally, corticosteroids may be used to reduce inflammation on an as needed or individual basis.

Conclusion

Individuals with skin of color encompass a tremendously diverse group comprising billions of individuals in our global population. The differences seen in individuals with skin of color bring both benefits and some challenges. Ultimately, each patient must be evaluated on an individual basis to determine their personal cosmetic and aging-related goals, and to provide recommendations for safe and effective treatment while offering honest recommendations regarding risks and how they can be mitigated or avoided. Aging affects all humans, and indeed all beings, regardless of color. With continued study and efforts, we will continue to improve our understanding of the aging process and improve treatment options, with the ultimate goal of improving health and well-being.

References

1. American Society for Aesthetic Plastic Surgery. ASAPS 2014 Statistics. Cosmet Surg Natl Data Bank [Internet]. 2014.
2. Kaidbey KH, Agin PP, Sayre RM, Kligman AM. Photoprotection by melanin–a comparison of black and caucasian skin. J Am Acad Dermatol. 1979;1(3):249–60.
3. Weigand DA, Haygood C, Gaylor JR. Cell layers and density of negro and caucasian stratum corneum. J Investiative Dermatol. 1974;563–8.
4. Johnson LC, Corah NL. Racial differences in skin resistance. Science. 1963;139(3556):766–7.
5. Montagna W, Prota G, Kenney J. The structure of black skin. In: Montagna W, Prota G, Kenney J, editors. Black skin structure and function. Gulf Professional Publishing; 1993.
6. Vashi NA, de Castro Maymone MB, Kundu RV. Aging differences in ethnic skin. J Clin Aesthet Dermatol [Internet]. 2016;9(1):31–8.
7. Fantasia J, Lin CB, Wiwi C, Kaur S, Hu YP, Zhang J, et al. Differential levels of elastin fibers and TGF-β signaling in the skin of Caucasians and African Americans. J Dermatol Sci [Internet]. 2013;70(3):159–65.
8. Alam M, Bhatia A, Kundu R, Yoo S, Chan H. Cosmetic dermatology for skin of color. 1st ed. McGraw-Hill Education; 2009.

9. Durai PC, Thappa DM, Kumari R, Malathi M. Aging in elderly: chronological versus photoaging. Indian J Dermatol [Internet]. 2012;57(5):343–52.

10. R.M. H. The role of retinoids in the management of cutaneous conditions in blacks [Internet]. J Am Acad Dermatol. 1998;S98–S103.

11. Hillebrand G, Levine M, Miyamoto K. The age-dependent changes in skin conditions in African Americans, Asian Indians, Caucasians. East Asians and Latinos. IFSCC Mag. 2001;4:259–66.

12. Rawlings AV. Ethnic skin types: are there differences in skin structure and function? Int J Cosmet Sci [Internet]. 2006;28(2):79–93.

13. Baumann L, Rodriguez D, Taylor SC, Wu J. Natural considerations for skin of color. Cutis [Internet]. 2006;78(6 Suppl):2–19.

14. Taylor S, Kelly A, Lim H, Serrano A. Dermatology for skin of color. 2nd ed. McGraw-Hill Education; 2016.

15. Murison AR, Sutherland JW, Williamson AM. De Morgan's spots. Br Med J [Internet]. 1947;1(4505):634–6.

16. Tindall JP, Smith JG. Skin lesions of the aged and their association with internal changes. JAMA [Internet]. 1963;21(186):1039–42.

17. Barter RH, Letterman GS, Schurter M. Hemangiomas, in pregnancy. Am J Obstet Gynecol [Internet]. 1963;1(87):625–35.

18. Cohen AD, Cagnano E, Vardy DA. Cherry angiomas associated with exposure to bromides. Dermatology [Internet]. 2001;202(1):52–3.

19. Firooz A, Komeili A, Dowlati Y. Eruptive melanocytic nevi and cherry angiomas secondary to exposure to sulfur mustard gas. J Am Acad Dermatol [Internet]. 1999;40(4):646–7.

20. Raymond LW, Williford LS, Burke WA. Eruptive cherry angiomas and irritant symptoms after one acute exposure to the glycol ether solvent 2-butoxyethanol. J Occup Environ Med [Internet]. 1998;40(12):1059–64.

21. Kim J-H, Park H-Y, Ahn SK. Cherry angiomas on the scalp. Case Rep Dermatol [Internet]. 2009;1(1):82–6.

22. Köhn F-M. Penile cherry angiomas. MMW Fortschr Med [Internet]. 2014;156(19):65.

23. Odom R, James W, Berger T. Andrews' diseases of the skin: clinical dermatology. 9th ed. Saunders; 2000.

24. Beauregard S, Gilchrest BA. A survey of skin problems and skin care regimens in the elderly. Arch Dermatol [Internet]. 1987;123(12):1638–43.

25. Aversa AJ, Miller OF. Cryo-curettage of cherry angiomas. J Dermatol Surg Oncol [Internet]. 1983;9(11):930–1.

26. Jairath V, Dayal S, Jain VK, Jindal N, Gogna P, Sehrawat M, et al. Is sclerotherapy useful for cherry angiomas? Dermatol Surg [Internet]. 2014;40(9):1022–7.

27. Pancar GS, Aydin F, Senturk N, Bek Y, Canturk MT, Turanli AY. Comparison of the 532 nm KTP and 1064 nm Nd:YAG lasers for the treatment of cherry angiomas. J Cosmet Laser Ther [Internet]. 2011;13(4):138–41.

28. Huang YL, Chang SL, Ma L, Lee MC, Hu S. Clinical analysis and classification of dark eye circle. Int J Dermatol. 2014;53(2):164–70.

29. Roberts WE. Periorbital hyperpigmentation: review of etiology, medical evaluation, and aesthetic treatment. J Drugs Dermatol [Internet]. 2014;13(4):472–82.

30. Sheth PB, Shah HA, Dave JN. Periorbital hyperpigmentation: a study of its prevalence, common causative factors and its association with personal habits and other disorders. Indian J Dermatol [Internet]. 2014;59(2):151–7.

31. Rhodes AR, Harrist TJ, Momtaz-T K. The PUVA-induced pigmented macule: a lentiginous proliferation of large, sometimes cytologically atypical, melanocytes. J Am Acad Dermatol [Internet]. 1983;9(1):47–58.

32. Kim SK, Kim EH, Kang HY, Lee E-S, Sohn S, Kim YC. Comprehensive understanding of idiopathic guttate hypomelanosis: clinical and histopathological correlation. Int J Dermatol [Internet]. 2010;49(2):162–6.

33. Brissett AE, Naylor MC. The aging african-american face. Facial Plast Surg. 2010;26(2): 154–63.
34. Alexis AF, Alam M. Racial and ethnic differences in skin aging: implications for treatment with soft tissue fillers. J Drugs Dermatol [Internet]. 2012;11(8):s30–2; discussion s32.
35. McCann JD, Pariseau B. Lower eyelid and midface rejuvenation. Facial Plast Surg [Internet]. 2013;29(4):273–80.
36. Liew S. Ethnic and gender considerations in the use of facial injectables: Asian patients. Plast Reconstr Surg [Internet]. 2015;136(5 Suppl):22S–7S.
37. Sykes JM. Management of the aging face in the Asian patient. Facial Plast Surg Clin North Am [Internet]. 2007;15(3):353–60, vi–vii.
38. Shirakabe Y, Suzuki Y, Lam SM. A new paradigm for the aging Asian face. Aesthetic Plast Surg [Internet];27(5):397–402.
39. Pourciau CY, Eide MJ, Mahan M, Lim HW. Photoprotection counseling of non-white ethno-racial groups: a survey of the practice of expert dermatologists. Photodermatol Photoimmunol Photomed [Internet]. 2012;28(6):335–7.
40. Agbai ON, Buster K, Sanchez M, Hernandez C, Kundu RV, Chiu M, et al. Skin cancer and photoprotection in people of color: a review and recommendations for physicians and the public. J Am Acad Dermatol [Internet]. 2014;70(4):748–62.
41. Davis EC, Callender VD. Aesthetic dermatology for aging ethnic skin. Dermatol Surg. 2011;901–17.
42. Downie JB, Grimes PE, Callender VD. A multicenter study of the safety and effectiveness of hyaluronic acid with a cohesive polydensified matrix for treatment of nasolabial folds in subjects with Fitzpatrick skin types IV, V, and VI. Plast Reconstr Surg [Internet]. 2013; 132(4 Suppl 2):41S–7S.
43. Taylor SC, Burgess CM, Callender VD. Safety of nonanimal stabilized hyaluronic acid dermal fillers in patients with skin of color: a randomized, evaluator-blinded comparative trial. Dermatol Surg [Internet]. 2009;35(Suppl 2):1653–60.
44. Grimes PE, Thomas JA, Murphy DK. Safety and effectiveness of hyaluronic acid fillers in skin of color. J Cosmet Dermatol [Internet]. 2009;8(3):162–8.
45. Marmur ES, Taylor SC, Grimes PE, Boyd CM, Porter JP, Yoo JY. Six-month safety results of calcium hydroxylapatite for treatment of nasolabial folds in Fitzpatrick skin types IV–VI. Dermatol Surg [Internet]. 2009;35(Suppl 2):1641–5.
46. Odunze M, Cohn A, Few JW. Restylane and people of color. Plast Reconstr Surg [Internet]. 2007;120(7):2011–6.
47. Talarico S, Meski AP, Buratini L, Manela-Azulay M, Simpson H, Sidou F, et al. High patient satisfaction of a hyaluronic acid filler producing enduring full-facial volume restoration: an 18-month open multicenter study. Dermatol Surg [Internet]. 2015;41(12):1361–9.
48. Narins RS, Baumann L, Brandt FS, Fagien S, Glazer S, Lowe NJ, et al. A randomized study of the efficacy and safety of injectable poly-L-lactic acid versus human-based collagen implant in the treatment of nasolabial fold wrinkles. J Am Acad Dermatol [Internet]. 2010;62 (3):448–62.
49. Burgess C, Awosika O. Ethnic and gender considerations in the use of facial injectables: African-American patients. Plast Reconstr Surg [Internet]. 2015;136(5 Suppl):28S–31S.
50. Montes JR. Ethnic and gender considerations in the use of facial injectables: latino patients. Plast Reconstr Surg [Internet]. 2015;136(5 Suppl):32S–9S.
51. Heath CR, Taylor SC. Fillers in the skin of color population. J Drugs Dermatol [Internet]. 2011;10(5):494–8.
52. Taylor SC, Callender VD, Albright CD, Coleman J, Axford-Gatley RA, Lin X. AbobotulinumtoxinA for reduction of glabellar lines in patients with skin of color: post hoc analysis of pooled clinical trial data. Dermatol Surg [Internet]. 2012;38(11):1804–11.
53. Wu Y, Zhao G, Li H, Zheng Z, Zhong S, Yang Z, et al. Botulinum toxin type A for the treatment of glabellar lines in Chinese: a double-blind, randomized, placebo-controlled study. Dermatol Surg [Internet]. 2010;36(1):102–8.

54. Lee DH, Kang SM, Feneran A, Youn CS, Kim JK, Cho S, et al. RimabotulinumtoxinB versus onabotulinumtoxinA for the treatment of forehead lines: an evaluator-blind, randomized, pilot study. J Eur Acad Dermatol Venereol [Internet]. 2013 Jan;27(1):e1–7.
55. Roberts WE. Chemical peeling in ethnic/dark skin. Dermatol Ther [Internet]. 2004;17(2): 196–205.
56. Salam A, Dadzie OE, Galadari H. Chemical peeling in ethnic skin: an update. Br J Dermatol. 2013;82–90.
57. Alexis AF. Lasers and light-based therapies in ethnic skin: Treatment options and recommendations for Fitzpatrick skin types 5 and 6. Br J Dermatol. 2013;91–7.

Chapter 22
Common Cosmetic Concerns and Approaches

Shalini B. Reddy, Pedro Zancanaro and Neelam A. Vashi

As cosmetic treatments have become more widely accessible, there is an increased demand among all patients, including patients with skin of color. While cosmetic treatments are relatively similar among all races and ethnicities, there are subtle nuances to treating patients with ethnic skin. Treatment can be challenging because these patients often are more vulnerable to side effects of common dermatologic procedures, including hyperpigmentation and scarring. It is also important to understand that ethnic populations may seek cosmetic treatments for different reasons as standards of beauty may differ by cultural background. This chapter will provide an overview of the common cosmetic concerns of individuals with skin of color, including treatment of hyperpigmentation, dermatosis papulosa nigra (DPN), unwanted hair, photoaging, varicosities, acne scars, and striae.

S.B. Reddy · P. Zancanaro
Department of Dermatology, Boston University Medical Center,
609 Albany Street, J-205, Boston, MA 02118, USA
e-mail: sreddy87@bu.edu

P. Zancanaro
e-mail: pedroz@bu.edu

N.A. Vashi (✉)
Department of Dermatology, Center for Ethnic Skin, Boston University,
Boston, MA, USA
e-mail: nvashi419@gmail.com

N.A. Vashi
Boston University School of Medicine, Boston Medical Center,
Boston, MA, USA

© Springer International Publishing AG 2017
N.A. Vashi and H.I. Maibach (eds.), *Dermatoanthropology of Ethnic Skin and Hair*, DOI 10.1007/978-3-319-53961-4_22

Hyperpigmentation

Hyperpigmentation is one of the most common concerns among women with skin of color [1]. In a survey-based study looking at cosmetic concerns in women with skin of color including African Americans, Hispanics, and Asians, 86% of women endorsed hyperpigmentation or dark spots and 80% reported blotchy or uneven skin as cosmetic concerns. Dyspigmentation can be a result of post-inflammatory hyperpigmentation (PIH) or melasma among others causes [2]. Treatment includes photoprotection, topical therapies including hydroquinone, topical retinoids, azelaic acid, triple combination therapy, and other modalities such as chemical peels, microdermabrasion, and laser treatments. A detailed review of treatment options for hyperpigmentation is discussed in a separate chapter.

Periorbital Hyperpigmentation

Periorbital hyperpigmentation (POH), also known as periorbital melanosis, periorbital circles, dark circles, dark eye circles, under eye circles, periocular pigmentation, periocular melanosis, and idiopathic cutaneous hyperchromia of the orbital region, is a commonly reported cosmetic concern that is more prevalent among women, particularly in those with skin of color [3–5]. Patients seek treatment due to complaints of lesions making them appear sad, tired, stressed, or older than their reported age [6]. The etiology of POH is thought to be multifactorial and can include genetics, hormones, photoaging, an underlying systemic disorder, allergic contact dermatitis, nutritional deficiency, and sleep disturbance [7].

Although POH is often refractory to treatment, numerous treatment modalities have been tried with variable success, including hydroquinone and non-hydroquinone skin bleaching and brightening agents, topical retinoids, ascorbic acid, botanicals, microdermabrasion, chemical peels, lasers, radiofrequency, injectable fillers, surgery, and fat transfer [7, 8]. In addition, adequate sleep, hydration, and sun protection are advised to prevent progression of POH [9].

While chemical peels have been effectively used to treat a variety of facial pigmentary disorders, there is little published data specifically regarding treatment of POH. One study looked at the effectiveness of trichloroacetic acid 3.75% and lactic acid 15% chemical peels for the treatment of POH in 30 patients with skin types II–IV. Peels were performed in a staged approach every week for a series of 4 weeks. Almost all patients showed significant improvement for at least 4–6 months based on patient's and physician's global assessment scores and photodocumentation. Some patients experienced temporary side effects including erythema, edema, frosting, dryness, and telangiectasia [10].

Nonablative fractionated 1550 nm erbium-doped fiber laser and combination therapy with topical hydroquinone, tretinoin and Q-switched ruby laser (694 nm) have been reported as effective treatments for POH [7, 11, 12]. In addition, injectable hyaluronic acid fillers have been shown to improve tear trough deformities, which may be an important contributing factor in some cases of POH [7]. Roh et al. reported 78% improvement of POH in ten patients who underwent autologous fat transplantation [13]. Blepharoplasty is a surgical procedure that aims to restore natural eye anatomy by removing excess periocular skin and fat. As a result, it is thought to decrease the shadow effect caused by excess skin thereby decreasing the appearance of POH.

Cosmetic camouflaging agents are a useful adjunctive treatment as treatment of POH is often prolonged and sometimes ineffective [7]. Thick cream concealers that match the skin color, such as Dermablend® or CoverFx®, may be applied to help mask the appearance of POH. Patients with an erythematous or violaceous component to their POH may benefit from a green concealer, such as Physicians Formula Gentle Cover Concealer Stick®, as it neutralizes these hues and can help cover patients' underlying POH [7].

Dermatosis Papulosa Nigra

Dermatosis papulosa nigra (DPN) are benign epithelioid tumors that are more common in patients with skin of color, particularly African Americans. DPN are thought to be a variant of seborrheic keratoses and are characterized by small hyperpigmented papules that are often grouped on the forehead, malar cheeks, around the eyelids, neck, or chest. The etiology is unknown; however, there appears to be a strong genetic predisposition with more than 50% of patients reporting a family history of DPN [14–16]. Patients often request removal of DPN for cosmetic purposes. Treatment options include snip excision with scissors, electrodessication, curettage, cryotherapy, laser ablation, and microdermabrasion [14–20]. The preferred treatments in skin of color are snip excision and electrodessication on its lowest setting to minimize the potential side effects of scarring and dyspigmentation. Cryotherapy and laser ablation should generally be avoided due to the significant risk of pigmentary changes in skin of color [21]. However, in a randomized split-face study, potassium-titanyl-phosphate (KTP) laser was found to be equally as effective as electrodessication in treating DPN in patients with skin types IV–VI. In addition, KTP was found to be less painful for patients, but given its limited availability and cost, snip excision, and electrodessication are still the more commonly used treatments [22].

Unwanted Hair

The removal of unwanted hair is a common practice in many cultures across the world and has been performed since ancient times. Treatment has evolved from temporary methods of removal to procedures that provide more permanent hair reduction. Temporary treatments include shaving, chemical depilatories, waxing, tweezing, threading, and "sugaring" [23]. Treatments aimed at permanent hair reduction include electrolysis and laser hair removal.

Though electrolysis has been available for many years, it is a difficult procedure particularly in those with curlier hair and darker skin phototypes (IV–VI) as they are susceptible to a higher risk of scarring, dyspigmentation, and exacerbation of inflammation [23]. Before the introduction of longer wavelengths and longer pulse durations, laser hair removal was recommended only for patients with phototypes I–III with dark terminal hairs. Now, laser hair removal is recognized as a safe and effective method of permanent hair reduction in all patients.

Laser hair removal is based on the principal of selective photothermolysis that specifically targets the pigmented chromophore, melanin, within the hair matrix [24]. In darker-skinned patients, there is an increased risk of damaging epidermal melanin as energy can be absorbed by the heavily pigmented basal layer [25]. At specific wavelengths near the red to near-infrared range (600–1100 nm), the absorbed energy is effectively converted to thermal energy in the hair follicle. The long-pulsed neodymium-doped yttrium aluminum garnet (Nd:YAG) 1064 nm laser is considered the safest in treating patients with phototypes IV–VI [23, 25]. By using a longer wavelength, such as 1064 nm, the tissue destruction is limited to deeper structures, such as the hair follicle, with limited absorption by epidermal melanin [25]. As a result, the Nd:YAG laser poses less risk of burns or dyspigmentation in darker-skinned patients [23, 25]. The 810-nm diode laser can also be used in patients with skin of color, but long pulse durations and aggressive cooling are recommended to minimize side effects such as transient blistering and dyspigmentation [26].

Overall, longer wavelengths, conservative fluences, longer pulse durations, and appropriate cooling methods with laser treatments are recommended in patients with skin of color to maximize efficacy and minimize unwanted epidermal damage [23, 25]. The most common side effects of laser treatment include pain, transient erythema, perifollicular edema, and hypo- or hyperpigmentation [27]. Rare, more severe, side effects include thermal burns, blisters, and permanent scarring. These side effects can be limited by ensuring use of the right laser, limiting fluences, using post-treatment cooling, and ensuring there is no residue left on the face (e.g., makeup) prior to treatment, which can act as a competing chromophore [27].

One rare side effect of laser hair removal is paradoxical hypertrichosis at previously treated areas, which is seen in 0.6–10% of patients [28, 29]. Although the exact etiology is still unclear, studies have shown that several factors may contribute to this adverse effect including: thick hair, dark hair color, presence of underlying untreated hormonal conditions (e.g., polycystic ovarian syndrome), use of hormone supplements or medications, presence of post-treatment side effects, suboptimal treatment fluences (which can trigger follicles to convert from telogen phase to anagen phase), laser use on the face or neck, female sex, and darker skin types (III–VI) [30]. It has been reported to be more common in those of Mediterranean descent [31] and, in the experience of the senior author, also in South East Asians. Treatment largely consists of repeated laser hair removal with optimal fluences and using cold packs post-treatment to prevent low energies from stimulating peripheral follicles [30].

Of note, topical eflornithine hydrochloride 13.9% cream, which is an irreversible inhibitor of ornithine decarboxylase, has been shown to be safe and effective in slowing hair growth. A randomized control trial that compared the efficacy of laser hair removal alone to combination therapy with laser hair removal and topical eflornithine hydrochloride 13.9% cream showed that combination therapy resulted in more rapid hair removal, but at 34 weeks, no significant differences were seen between the two treatment groups [32, 33].

Photoaging

Although photoaging is often more prominent and manifests earlier in lighter skin compared to darker skin phototypes, signs of photoaging, including dynamic and static rhytids, skin sagging, volume loss and telangiectasias, can still be seen in skin of color [34]. For this reason, the number of cosmetic procedures using botulinum toxin type A, soft tissue augmentation, and lasers has increased in darker racial and ethnic groups. For a detailed review of treatment options for photoaging, refer to the chapter on aging in skin of color.

Varicosities

Varicose veins are enlarged, tortuous, superficial veins of the legs. Varicose dilation is caused by poorly functioning (incompetent) valves and decreased vein wall elasticity that results in pooling of blood within the veins [35]. The prevalence of varicose veins in the Western population is estimated to be between 25–30% in women and 10–20% in men and as a result, is a common cosmetic complaint [35]. Treatment of varicosities includes compression stockings, superficial vein ligation, phlebectomy, surgical stripping, endothermal radiofrequency ablation, laser therapy, and sclerotherapy [36, 37]. Surgical treatment methods are more commonly used to treat larger or deeper varicosities. Sclerotherapy is the primary treatment for small varicosities including venules, reticular veins, and telangiectasias [38]. It involves the injection of a liquid or foam chemical into a vein causing damage to the endothelium, vessel occlusion, and production of a fibrous chord [38–40]. Sclerotherapy is not only thought to improve the cosmetic appearance of varicosities and telangiectasias, but it has also been shown to relieve associated leg pain and discomfort [41]. Sclerosing agents can be classified into detergents, chemical irritants, and osmotic agents. Detergents destroy the vein wall through protein denaturation and they include: polidocanol, sodium tetradecyl sulfate, sodium morrhuate, and ethanolamine oleate. Chemical irritants cause destruction of the vein wall through direct toxicity to the endothelium and include: polyiodinated iodine, chromated glycerin, alcoholic solution of zein, OK 432, and bleomycin. Osmotic agents draw water out of the endothelial cells and cause dehydration and denaturation of the endothelium. Osmotic agents include hypertonic sodium chloride solution and sodium chloride solution with dextrose [37, 40]. Polidocanol, chromated glycerin, and sodium tetradecyl sulfate are the most commonly used sclerosants because of their safety and efficacy profiles [39]. Chromated glycerin, a popular treatment in Europe that has not been approved by the Food and Drug Administration (FDA) in the United States, has been reported to have lower rates of post-therapy hyperpigmentation, bruising and swelling, when compared to sodium tetradecyl sulfate [42]. Although used heavily in the past, hypertonic saline is a less favored treatment given the side effects of pain, burning, and risk of necrosis with extravasation [39]. There is limited data regarding the safety and efficacy of sclerotherapy in patients with skin of color. In a randomized control trial looking at the treatment of varicose veins with polidocanol versus placebo, Zhang et al. showed that polidocanol 0.5, 1, and 3% solution was safe and effective in Chinese patients [43]. The most common side effects of sclerotherapy are hyperpigmentation and telangiectatic matting. Hyperpigmentation can be transient or permanent and is a result of increased melanin and dermal hemosiderin deposition. Transient hyperpigmentation most commonly presents 6–8 weeks post-therapy and persists for several months. The incidence of transient hyperpigmentation ranges from 10 to 30%. Spontaneous resolution occurs in 70% of patients in 6 months and 99% of patients in 1 year. Permanent hyperpigmentation affects 1–2% of patients [40]. Telangiectatic matting occurs in approximately 15–20% of patients and usually resolves between 3 and 12 months after treatment.

Long-pulsed Nd:YAG 1064 nm lasers have been shown to be successful in treating telangiectasias on the leg. When used at high fluences, the 1064 nm wavelength is selectively absorbed by hemoglobin/deoxyhemoglobin within leg telangiectasias. The most common side effect of treatment is transient PIH. In a head-to-head pilot study, Levy et al. demonstrated no statistical significance in efficacy and safety between long-pulsed Nd:YAG laser alone, sclerotherapy alone, and combination therapy in the treatment of 0.5–2 mm leg telangiectasias [44].

Acne Scars

Acne scarring, a common sequela of acne vulgaris, can present with macular, atrophic, or hypertrophic scars. There are three main categories of atrophic scars: rolling, boxcar, and ice pick scars [45]. Treatment options include chemical peels, microdermabrasion, microneedling, photodynamic therapy, laser therapy, silicone gel dressings, subcision, excision, radiofrequency, fillers, fat transplantation, and combination therapy [45, 46]. When deciding which treatment to use, it is important to first determine the type, size, and severity of the scar.

While chemical peels are commonly used for treatment of PIH, they are not as frequently used for treatment of atrophic scars given low rates of efficacy and high rates hyperpigmentation and scarring. However, the CROSS (chemical reconstruction of skin scars) technique, which uses high concentrations of trichloracetic acid, has been reported to be highly effective in treatment of ice pick scars [47, 48]. In a case series, Khunger et al. treated ice pick scars in thirty patients with skin types IV and V via the CROSS technique with 100% trichloracetic acid. Patients were primed with hydroquinone 4% cream and tretinoin 0.025% cream and subsequently treated with four sessions of the CROSS technique at 2 week intervals. Over 90% of patients had significant improvement of their acne scars. Two patients experienced transient hyperpigmentation, and one patient had transient hypopigmentation, but overall the treatment was well tolerated without any prolonged adverse effects, such as dyspigmentation or scarring [49].

Microneedling treats acne scars through stimulation of collagen and elastin production. Several studies have looked at the safety and efficacy of microneedling in patients with skin types III–VI and have found that there is minimal risk of dyspigmentation [50].

Ablative and nonablative lasers are commonly used in the treatment of acne scarring. Ablative lasers are generally more effective than nonablative lasers in the treatment of atrophic scars, however, as a result of epidermal destruction, there is a much higher risk of adverse effects including PIH, hypopigmentation, prolonged erythema and scarring so, overall, are not advised [45, 51]. Compared to traditional ablative lasers, fractional non-ablative laser resurfacing has been associated with a lower risk of PIH in patients with skin types IV–VI when conservative parameters are used. The 1450 nm diode laser has been shown to be effective for the treatment of atrophic acne scars in Asians with skin types IV and V, but post-therapy, transient hyperpigmentation has been reported [51]. Preliminary data on the treatment of atrophic scars in skin types IV–VI with the 1064 nm Nd:YAG laser shows significant improvement of skin texture, scarring, and PIH [52].

Silicone gel dressings are topical sheets that can be applied daily to hypertrophic scars. They inhibit fibroblast production of collagen and have been reported to decrease hypertrophic scar size in 60–80% of patients. Side effects are minimal and include local skin maceration and pruritus. Given that acne scars are common in highly visible locations such as the face, compliance may be a problem [53].

Subcision involves the use of a small needle that is inserted into the base of a scar to release fibrotic strands that contribute to the depressed, atrophic appearance of the scar. Subcision has a reported success rate of 50–60% in the treatment of rolling scars. Few patients develop a nodule at the site of treatment, which can be treated with intralesional corticosteroids.

Soft tissue augmentation with hyaluronic acid, calcium hydroxylapatite, poly-L-lactic acid, silicone, polymethylmethacrylate, and autologous fat are effective treatments in the treatment of atrophic acne scars. Hyaluronic acid has been reported to be effective in treating rolling scars but given its temporary results, patients often require repeated treatments [45].

Striae Distensae

Striae distensae (SD) or stretch marks are a common dermatologic condition that is characterized by epidermal and dermal skin thinning or atrophy. SD initially present as raised, erythematous plaques (striae rubra) that then progress to linear, white, atrophic scars over time (striae alba). There are many physiologic and pathologic conditions associated with SD including adolescent growth spurts, pregnancy, obesity, Cushing's syndrome, Marfan's syndrome, and long-term systemic or topical corticosteroid use. Mechanical stress, hormones, and genetics are thought to play a role in the development of SD [54]. Although SD are a common aesthetic complaint across all racial and ethnic populations, they have been reported to be more severe in African American women compared to Caucasian women [55]. To date, there is no consistently effective treatment modality for SD. Generally, striae rubra are more responsive to therapy than striae alba. Numerous treatments have been tried with variable results, including topical retinoids, microdermabrasion, chemical peels, radiofrequency, microneedling, platelet rich plasma, intense pulse light, and ablative and non-ablative lasers [56].

Topical 0.1% tretinoin cream daily for 6 months has been shown to decrease the length and width of SR [57]. In the first 2 months of treatment, some patients experienced erythema and scaling. In a prospective, randomized, open-label study comparing topical 0.05% tretinoin cream and microdermabrasion, both treatments were shown to be effective without any statistically significant difference between the two groups [58]. In a double blind, randomized control trial of 40 women with SD, 70% topical glycolic acid applied weekly for 6 months resulted in a significant decrease in furrow width and erythema in striae rubra, and it similarly resulted in a significant decrease in furrow width and an increase in melanin in striae alba, compared to placebo [59].

Microdermabrasion, intense pulse light, and radiofrequency have been shown to be effective in treating SD by increasing type 1 collagen [60, 61]. Several ablative and nonablative lasers have been shown to be effective in treating SD including the pulsed-dye laser (for striae rubra), 308 nm excimer laser (for striae alba), 1064 nm Nd:YAG laser, short-pulsed 10,600 nm CO_2 laser, and fractional CO_2 laser [54, 61, 62]. The long-pulsed Nd:YAG laser demonstrates a low risk of hyperpigmentation (2.2%), while the ablative, short-pulsed, 10,600 nm CO_2 laser presents the greatest risk of hyperpigmentation, particularly in darker skin types [56, 61].

Prominent Mandible

As a result of racial differences in facial architecture and differing cultural standards of beauty, certain ethnic populations are more likely to present with specific cosmetic concerns. For example, Asian women often seek treatment for prominent mandibular angles and hypertrophic masseter muscles [63, 64]. Compared to

Caucasian women, Asian women have an increased mandibular width that results in an angular facial shape [64]. Neurotoxin injection with botulinum toxin type A can be used to relax the masseter and soften the mandibular angle leading to a softer ovoid facial shape that is more culturally desired [63, 64].

Conclusion

With a growing worldwide ethnic population and an increased desire for and availability of cosmetic therapy, it is becoming ever more important to understand the cosmetic concerns of patients with skin of color. Treatment plans for patients should be individualized to their cosmetic goals and expectations. It is important to note that side effects may differ by skin type and should be considered in selection of therapy.

References

1. Grimes PE. Skin and hair cosmetic issues in women of color. Dermatol Clin. 2000;18(4):659–65.
2. Desai SR. Hyperpigmentation therapy: a review. J Clin Aesthet Dermatol. 2014;7(8):13–7.
3. Grimes PE. Aesthetic and cosmetic surgery for darker skin types. New York: Lippincott; 2007.
4. Maruri CA, Diaz LA. Dark Circles around the eyes. Cutis. 1969;5:979.
5. Cestari T, Freitag FM, Cestari TF. What causes dark circles under the eyes? J Cosmet Dermatol. 2007;6:211–5.
6. Gendler EC. Treatment of periorbital hyperpigmentation. Aesthet Surg J. 2005;25(6):618–24.
7. Roberts WE. Periorbital hyperpigmentation: review of etiology, medical evaluation, and aesthetic treatment. J Drugs Dermatol. 2014;13(4):472–82.
8. Saedi N, Ganesan AK. Treating hyperpigmentation in darker-skinned patients. J Drugs Dermatol. 2013;12(5):563–7.
9. Sheth PB, Shah HA, Dave JN. Periorbital hyperpigmentation: a study of its prevalence, common causative factors and its association with personal habits and other disorders. Indian J Dermatol [Internet]. 2014;59(2):151–7.
10. Vavouli C, Katsambas A, Gregoriou S, Teodor A, Salavastru C, Alexandru A, et al. Chemical peeling with trichloroacetic acid and lactic acid for infraorbital dark circles. J Cosmet Dermatol. 2013;12(3):204–9.
11. Momosawa A, Kurita M, Ozaki M, Miyamoto S, Kobayashi Y, Ban I, Harii K. Combined therapy using Q-switched ruby laser and bleaching treatment with tretinoin and hydroquinone for periorbital skin hyperpigmentation in Asians. Plast Reconstr Surg. 2008;121(1):282–8.
12. Manuskiatti W, Fitzpatrick RE, Goldman MP. Treatment of facial skin using combinations of CO_2, Q-switched alexandrite, flashlamp-pumped pulsed dye, and Er:YAG lasers in the same treatment session. Dermatol Surg. 2000;26(2):114–20.
13. Ciuci PM, Obagi S. Rejuvenation of the periorbital complex with autologous fat transfer: current therapy. J Oral Maxillofac Surg. 2008;66(8):1686–93.
14. Grimes PE, Arora S, Minus HR, Kenney JA Jr. Dermatosis papulosa nigra. Cutis. 1983;32 (4):385–386, 392.
15. Hairston MA Jr, Reed RJ, Derbes VJ. Dermatosis papulosa nigra. Arch Dermatol. 1964;89:655–8.

16. Alam M, et al. Cosmetic dermatology for skin of color. New York, NY: McGraw-Hill Medical; 2009.

17. Coley MK, Alexis AF. Managing common dermatoses in skin of color. Semin Cutan Med Surg. 2009;28(2):63–70.

18. Kundu RV, Joshi SS, Suh KY, et al. Comparison of electrodesiccation and potassium-titanyl-phosphate laser for treatment of dermatosis papulosa nigra. Dermatol Surg. 2009;35(7):1079–83.

19. Garcia MS, Azari R, Eisen DB. Treatment of dermatosis papulosa nigra in 10 patients: a comparison trial of electrodesiccation, pulsed dye laser, and curettage. Dermatol Surg. 2010;36(12):1968–72.

20. Kauh YC, et al. A surgical approach for dermatosis papulosa nigra. Int J Dermatol. 1983;22 (10):590–2.

21. Lupo MP. Dermatosis papulosa nigra: treatment options. J Drugs Dermatol. 2007;6:29–30.

22. Shah S, Alster TS. Laser treatment of dark skin: an updated review. Am J Clin Dermatol. 2010;11(6):389–97.

23. Battle EF. Advances in laser hair removal in skin of color. J Drugs Dermatol. 2011;10 (11):1235–9.

24. Anderson RR, Parrish JA. Selective photothermolysis: precise microsurgery by selective absorption of pulsed radiation. Science. 1983;220145961:524–7.

25. Chan CS, Dover JS. Nd:YAG laser hair removal in Fitzpatrick skin types IV to VI. J Drugs Dermatol. 2013;12(3):366–7.

26. Greppi I. Diode laser hair removal of the black patient. Lasers Surg Med. 2001;28(2):150–5.

27. Gan S, Graber E. Laser hair removal: a review. Dermatol Surg. 2013;36:823–38.

28. Alajlan A, Shapiro J, Rivers JK, et al. Paradoxical hypertrichosis after laser epilation. J Am Acad Dermatol. 2005;53:85–8.

29. Moreno-Arias G, Castelo-Branco C, Ferrando J. Paradoxical effect after IPL photoepilation. Dermatol Surg. 2002;28:1013–6.

30. Desai S, Mahmoud BH, Bhatia AC, Hamzavi IH. Paradoxical hypertrichosis after laser therapy: a review. Dermatol Surg. 2010;36(3):291–8.

31. Hirsch RJ, Farinelli WA, Laughlin SA, et al. Hair removal induced by laser hair removal. Lasers Surg Med. 2003;32(Suppl 15):63.

32. Hamzavi I, Tan E, Shapiro J, Lui H. A randomized bilateral vehicle-controlled study of eflornithine cream combined with laser treatment versus laser treatment alone for facial hirsutism in women. J Am Acad Dermatol. 2007;57(1):54–9.

33. Smith SR, Piacquadio DJ, Beger B, Littler C. Eflornithine cream combined with laser therapy in the management of unwanted facial hair growth in women: a randomized trial. Dermatol Surg. 2006;32(10):1237–43.

34. Halder RM. The role of retinoids in the management of cutaneous conditions in blacks. J Am Acad Dermatol. 1998;39(2);S98–103.

35. Tisi PV. Varicose veins. BMJ Clin Evid. 2011;5:2011.

36. Onida S, Lane TR, Davies AH. Improving the management of varicose veins. Practitioner. 2013;257(1766);21–4, 2–3.

37. Weiss RA, Weiss MA. Treatment of varicose and telangiectatic veins. In: Freedberg JM, Eisen AZ, Wolff K, Austen KF, Goldsmith LA, Katz SI, editors. Fitzpatrick's dermatology in general medicine, 6th ed. USA: McGraw Hill Publishers; 2009. p. 2549–56.

38. Tisi PV, Beverley C, Rees A. Injection sclerotherapy for varicose veins. Cochrane Database Syst Rev. 2006;4;CD001732.

39. Khunger N, Sacchidanand S. Standard guidelines for care: sclerotherapy in dermatology. Indian J Dermatol Venereol Leprol. 2011;77(2);222–31.

40. Yiannakopoulou E. Safety concerns for sclerotherapy of telangiectases, reticular and varicose veins. Pharmacology. 2016;98:62–9.

41. Weiss RA, Weiss MA. Resolution of pain associated with varicose and telangiectatic leg veins after compression sclerotherapy. J Dermatol Surg Oncol. 1990;16(4):333–6.

42. Leach BC, Goldman MP. Comparative trial between sodium tetradecyl sulfate and glycerin in the treatment of telangiectatic leg veins. Dermatol Surg. 2003;29(6):612–4; discussion 615.
43. Zhang J, Jing Z, Schliephake DE, Otto J, Malouf GM, Gu YQ. Efficacy and safety of Aethoxysklerol(R) (polidocanol) 0.5, 1 and 3% in comparison with placebo solution for the treatment of varicose veins of the lower extremities in Chinese patients (ESA-China Study). Phlebology. 2012;27(4):184–90.
44. Levy JL, Elbahr C, Jouve E, Mordon S. Comparison and sequential study of long pulsed Nd: YAG 1064 nm laser and sclerotherapy in leg telangiectasias treatment. Lasers Surg Med. 2004;34(3):273–6.
45. Lanoue J, Goldenberg G. Acne scarring: a review of cosmetic therapies. Cutis. 2015;95 (5):276–81.
46. Goodman GJ. Treatment of acne scarring. Int J Dermatol. 2011;50(10):1179–94.
47. Lee JB, Chung WG, Kwahck H, et al. Focal treatment of acne scars with trichloroacetic acid: chemical reconstruction of skin scars method. Dermatol Surg. 2002;28:1017–21.
48. Bhardwaj D, Khunger N. An assessment of the efficacy and safety of CROSS technique with 100% TCA in the management of ice pick acne scars. J Cutan Aesthet Surg. 2010;3:93–6.
49. Khunger N, Bhardwaj D, Khunger M. Evaluation of CROSS technique with 100% TCA in the management of ice pick acne scars in darker skin types. J Cosmet Dermatol. 2011;10 (1):51–7.
50. Cohen BE, Elbuluk N. Microneedling in skin of color: a review of uses and efficacy. J Am Acad Dermatol. 2016;74(2):348–55.
51. Yin NC, McMichael AJ. Acne in patients with skin of color: practical management. Am J Clin Dermatol. 2014;15(1):7–16.
52. Badawi A, Tome MA, Atteya A, Sami N, Morsy IA. Retrospective analysis of non-ablative scar treatment in dark skin types using the sub-millisecond Nd:YAG 1064 nm laser. Lasers Surg Med. 2011;43(2):130–6.
53. Puri N, Talwar A. The efficacy of silicone gel for the treatment of hypertrophic scars and keloids. J Cutan Aesthet Surg. 2009;2:104–6.
54. El Taieb MA, Ibrahim AK. Fractional CO_2 laser versus intense pulsed light in treating striae distensae. Indian J Dermatol. 2016;61(2):174–80.
55. Elbuluk N, Kang S, Hamilton T. Differences in clinical features and risk factors for striae distensae in African American and white women. J Am Acad Dermatol. 2009;60(Suppl 1); AB56.
56. Elsaie ML, Hussein MS, Tawfik AA, Emam HM, Badawi MA, Fawzy MM, et al. Comparison of the effectiveness of two fluences using long-pulsed Nd:YAG laser in the treatment of striae distensae. Histological and morphometric evaluation. Lasers Med Sci. 2016;31(9):1845–53.
57. Kang S, Kim KJ, Griffiths CE, et al. Topical tretinoin (retinoic acid) improves early stretch marks. Arch Dermatol. 1996;132:519–26.
58. Hexsel D, Soirefmann M, Porto MD, et al. Superficial dermabrasion versus topical tretinoin on early striae distensae: a randomized, pilot study. Dermatol Surg. 2014;40:537–44.
59. Mazzarello V, Farace F, Ena P, et al. A superficial texture analysis of 70% glycolic acid topical therapy and striae distensae. Plast Reconstr Surg. 2012;129:589e–90e.
60. Abdel-Latif AM, Albendary AS. Treatment of striae distensae with microdermabrasion: a clinical and molecular study. J Egyptian Women Dermatol Soc. 2008;5:24–30.
61. Al-Himandi S, Ud-Din S, Gilmore S, Bayat A. Striae distensae: a comprehensive review and evidence-based evaluation of prophylaxis and treatment. Br J Dermatol. 2014;170(3):527–47.
62. Suh DH, Chang KY, Son HC, et al. Radiofrequency and 585-nm pulsed dye laser treatment of striae distensae: a report of 37 Asian patients. Dermatol Surg. 2007;33:29–34.
63. Ahn J, Horn C, Blitzer A. Botulinum toxin for masseter reduction in Asian patients. Arch Facial Plast Surg. 2004;6(3):188–91.
64. Alexis AF, Alam M. Racial and ethnic differences in skin aging: implications for treatment with soft tissue fillers. J Drugs Dermatol. 2012;11(8);s30–2; discussion s32.

Chapter 23
Treatment Strategies for Hyperpigmentation

Judy Cheng and Neelam A. Vashi

Dyschromia is an increasingly common disorder, especially among darker skinned ethnic groups [1]. Despite the arsenal of treatment options available for pigmentary disorders, treating hyperpigmentation remains a clinical challenge. There are no standardized protocols and few randomized controlled trials studying the efficacy and safety of treatments. In addition, although skin of color patients are at greatest risk for developing undesired treatment-related dyspigmentation, there exists no algorithm to predict which particular patient is more prone to side effects. Given the refractory nature of disease and the evolving population from increases in migration, hyperchromic complaints are likely to rise. Providing a treatment framework for hyperpigmentation would, therefore, be beneficial [2].

Evaluation of Hyperpigmentation

Ruling out an underlying cause for hyperpigmentation is vital when first evaluating a patient with dyschromia. Diffuse hyperpigmentation suggests a metabolic (i.e., Addison's disease), malignant, medication-related, or infectious etiology [3]. For medication-related hyperpigmentation (i.e., minocycline, amiodarone, oral contraceptives), the offending agent should be discontinued first and time permitted

J. Cheng
Department of Dermatology, Boston University Medical Center,
609 Albany Street, J-205, Boston, MA 02118, USA
e-mail: judy.cheng@bmc.org

N.A. Vashi (✉)
Department of Dermatology, Center for Ethnic Skin, Boston University,
Boston, MA, USA
e-mail: nvashi419@gmail.com

N.A. Vashi
Boston University School of Medicine, Boston Medical Center, Boston, MA, USA

© Springer International Publishing AG 2017
N.A. Vashi and H.I. Maibach (eds.), *Dermatoanthropology of Ethnic Skin and Hair*, DOI 10.1007/978-3-319-53961-4_23

for natural pigmentation to return. For metabolic disorders, appropriate supplementation to correct the deficiency should be provided (i.e., vitamin B12, folic acid, levothyroxine) [3].

Localized disease suggests other etiologies, including post-inflammatory hyperpigmentation (PIH) or melasma, which are two of the most common causes of hyperpigmentation [3]. For PIH, underlying dermatoses, such as acne, should be treated first before pursuing post-inflammatory pigmentation therapeutics. Melasma is typically categorized into types depending on the pigmentation deposition: (i) epidermal—brown colored with basal or suprabasal pigment, (ii) dermal—blue-gray color with upper and deep dermal pigment, (iii) mixed—brown-gray color with epidermal and dermal pigment, and (iv) inapparent or indeterminate, which is seen more in darker skin types. Distinguishing pigment location is important as it informs likelihood of response to topical treatment, with dermal type being less likely to respond [4]. Under Wood's lamp, only the epidermal component intensifies, which can be useful in determining disease extent, although the utility of this is controversial as all subtypes will show some amount of increased pigment deposition in both dermal and epidermal layers of the skin [5].

Treatment of these most common acquired causes of hyperpigmentation is based on two key principles: photoprotection and the use of agents that both disrupt melanogenesis and remove melanin. Topical lightening agents, chemical peels, oral agents, microdermabrasion, microneedling, and laser therapy are all potential treatment modalities.

Topical Therapies

The induction of melanin production and, therefore, pigmentation has been demonstrated with ultraviolent (UV) in the UVA (290–320 nm), UVB (320–340 nm), and visible light (400–760 nm) spectrums. Sun-protective strategies, therefore, are crucial in the treatment and prevention regimen for hyperpigmentation disorders. The American Academy of Dermatology (AAD) recommends sunscreens with a sun protection factor (SPF) of 30 or higher, that offer broad-spectrum coverage, and are water resistant for 40 or 80 min [6]. In addition, patients should practice sun-protective behavior including seeking shade whenever possible, wearing sun-protective clothing (wide-brimmed hats, sunglasses with UV protection), avoiding indoor tanning beds, applying sunscreen 15–30 min before going outdoors, and reapplying every 2 hours [7]. Darker skinned ethnic groups may furthermore benefit from vitamin D supplementation as their higher melanin content inherently predisposes them to vitamin D deficiency [7, 8].

Most individuals apply sunscreen at a quarter to a half of the FDA-mandated amount of 2 mg/cm^2 used in SPF testing [6, 9]. SPF, a measure of UVB, is the ratio of the minimal erythema dose in sunscreen-protected skin over the minimal erythema dose in non-sunscreen-protected skin [10]. Consequently, to achieve a 10–15-fold protection, a sunscreen with SPF 30–50 should be applied [11].

Sunscreens can be categorized into two types based on mechanism of action—physical (inorganic) versus chemical (organic). Chemical sunscreens absorb light and convert it to heat energy, while physical sunscreens (i.e., titanium dioxide, zinc oxide) reflect or scatter light [10]. Micronized forms of metal oxides, though often classified as physical sunscreens, actually act as chemical sunscreens by absorbing UV radiation and emitting it as longer-wave heat radiation [12]. Unfortunately, physical blockers are often less cosmetically acceptable, especially among darker skin types due to the white sheen they leave on the skin. Consequently, new physical blockers (i.e., iron oxide) have been developed that better simulate natural skin tones and can now be obtained as tinted products in different shades. Iron oxide also has the ability to block against visible light, which has been shown to be etiologic in melasma [13–15]. There are currently 17 FDA-approved active sunscreen ingredients (Table 23.1) [6, 10].

Aside from sunscreen, first-line treatment for hyperpigmentation disorders consists of topical lightening agents [16]. There are currently only a handful of prescription agents (i.e., hydroquinone (HQ), retinoids, and azelaic acid) in comparison to a plethora of over-the-counter lightening formulations (i.e., kojic acid, licorice extract, arbutin, ascorbic acid, soy, niacinamide, and N-acetyl glucosamine) (Table 23.2). The most commonly used agents are HQ, triple combination cream, azelaic acid, retinoids, and kojic acid. All other agents have demonstrated limited efficacy in clinical investigations but are used in practice with varying response.

Table 23.1 FDA-approved sunscreen ingredients (as of December 7, 2009)

UV spectrum coverage	Ingredient	
UVA1 (340–380 nm)	**Chemical**	**Physical**
	Avobenzone	Zinc oxide
	Ecamsule (terephthalydene dicamphor sulfonic acid)	
UVA2 (320–340 nm)	**Chemical**	**Physical**
	Oxybenzone	Titanium dioxide
	Sulisobenzone	
	Dioxybenzone	
	Meradimate (menthyl anthranilate)	
UVB (290–320 nm)	**Chemical**	**Physical**
	PABA	Zinc oxide
	Padimate O	Titanium dioxide
	Octinoxate (octyl methoxycinnamates)	
	Cinoxate	
	Octisalate (octyl salicylate)	
	Homosalate	
	Trolamine salicylate	
	Octylocrylene	
	Ensulizole (phenylbenzimidazole sulfonic acid)	

From Wang and Lim [6]

Table 23.2 Strengths and weaknesses of various topical hypopigmenting agents

Drug	Mechanism	Strengths	Weaknesses
Hydroquinone	• Inhibits tyrosinase [17] • Inhibits formation of melanosomes [18] • Promotes degradation of melanocytes [18] • Promotes necrosis of melanocytes [18]	• Long study record [19]	• Exogenous ochronosis [20] • Confetti leukoderma [21]

Retinoids
  Tretinoin
  Adapalene/tazarotene
	• Inhibits tyrosinase [22]
	• Enhances epidermopoiesis [22]
		• Can simultaneously treat comedonal acne [23]
		• Greater specificity for retinoic acid receptor compared to tretinoin [23]
		• Possibly fewer side effects compared to tretinoin [24]
			• Retinoid dermatitis [25]
			• Requires long treatment period [26]
			• More expensive than tretinoin [27]

Triple topical therapy (hydroquinone, retinoid, corticosteroid)	• Inhibits tyrosinase [17] • Inhibits formation of melanosomes [18] • Promotes degradation of melanocytes [18] • Promotes necrosis of melanocytes [18] • Enhances epidermopoiesis [22]	• Safe and effective in dark-skinned ethnic groups [28, 29] • More efficacious than constituent agents alone [30]	• Skin atrophy [31] • Telangiectasia [31]
Azelaic acid	• Inhibits tyrosinase activity [32] • Interferes with DNA synthesis [32]	• Cytotoxic effect specific to abnormally hyperactive melanocytes [33]	• Pruritus [19] • Transient erythema [19] • Scaling [19]
Mequinol	• Inhibits tyrosinase [33]	• Less irritating than hydroquinone [34]	• Limited studies in post-inflammatory hyperpigmentation
Kojic acid	• Inhibits tyrosine kinase by chelating copper [35]	• Pharmaceutically stable [36]	• More irritating compared to other topical agents [36] • High frequency of contact sensitivity [37]
Licorice	• Inhibits tyrosinase [38] • Disperses melanin [39] • Removes epidermal melanin [39]	• Minimal side effects [40]	• Few studies

(continued)

Table 23.2 (continued)

Drug	Mechanism	Strengths	Weaknesses
Arbutin	• Inhibits tyrosinase [41]	• Efficacious in light-skinned patients [41]	• May cause paradoxical hyperpigmentation [42] • Limited studies in darker Fitzpatrick skin types
Ascorbic acid	• Reduces oxidized dopaquinone [43] • Suppresses activation of NF-kβ and TNF-α [44] • Protects against phototoxic injury [45]	• 5% formulation has fewer side effects than 4% hydroquinone [46]	• Limited studies for PIH
Soy	• Blocks transfer of melanosomes to keratinocytes [47]	• Well-tolerated [48] • Efficacious in combination with other topicals [49]	• Few monotherapy studies
Niacinamide	• Decreases melanosome transfer to keratinocytes [50] • Interferes in cell-signaling pathway to decrease melanogenesis [50]	• Unaffected by light, moisture, acids, alkalis, oxidizers [43]	• Limited studies in darker skinned populations • Limited studies in post-inflammatory hyperpigmentation
N-acetyl glucosamine	• Inhibits tyrosinase glycosylation [51]	• Well-tolerated [51]	• Few studies among dark-skinned ethnic groups

Hydroquinone

HQ is one of the most popular agents given its efficacy. HQ blocks conversion of dihydroxyphenylalanine (DOPA) to melanin by inhibiting tyrosinase [17]. It also inhibits the formation of and promotes degradation of melanosomes, along with causing melanocyte necrosis [18]. HQ efficacy is proportional to its concentration, with lower concentrations having slower onset to action [52]. While over-the-counter preparations contain a maximum 2–3% concentration, depending on the formulation, higher concentrations can be obtained through prescription. HQ is efficacious when used as monotherapy or when used in conjunction with other topical agents [53, 54]. In a randomized, double-blind trial of 4% HQ and sunscreen versus sunscreen for 12 weeks ($n = 45$), Ennes et al. [53] demonstrated a significantly greater clearance rate of melasma among patients who used HQ compared to sunscreen alone (38% vs. 8%).

The most common acute side effect of HQ is irritant contact dermatitis, with up to 25% of users developing a pruritic eruption as evidenced by a single randomized study [21]. Other side effects include allergic contact dermatitis, PIH, and post-inflammatory hypopigmentation of surrounding skin—the "halo effect" [4, 21]. Fitzpatrick skin types (FST) V and VI are also more vulnerable to side effects including "confetti leukoderma," which refers to areas of focal depigmentation [21]. Long-term, rare side effects include ochronosis, nail discoloration, conjunctival melanosis, and corneal degeneration.

Exogenous ochronosis typically occurs in black patients and is secondary to the accumulation of homogentistic acid in the dermis. It presents as asymptomatic patches over bony prominences (i.e., face, neck, extensor surfaces) and sun-exposed sites coinciding with the application of topical lightening agents [20]. While it is more prevalent in Africa, where HQ is frequently combined with resorcinol or compounded in a hydroalcoholic lotion [20], many cases have been reported in the U.S., most often from patients using adulterated compounds from non-U.S. countries [55]. It is typically associated with the use of higher percentages of HQ; however, it has been reported with 2% formulations [56]. Clinicians should be prepared to recognize ochronosis as adulterated, and above FDA-recommended concentrations of hydroquinone are illicitly sold in ethnic stores and through websites [43, 55, 57]. Finally, although animal studies have shown an increased risk of cancer with the administration of high doses of oral HQ, there have been no human reports to date that show an increased risk of skin cancer or internal malignancies from topical application of HQ [33, 43, 58, 59].

Retinoids

Through the stimulation of keratinocyte turnover and reduction of melanosome transfer, retinoids (i.e., retinoic acid, tretinoin, adapalene, tazarotene) promote the loss of melanin [22]. Tretinoin (0.01–0.1%) has been shown to inhibit tyrosinase transcription and enhance epidermopoiesis, thereby decreasing contact time between keratinocytes and melanocytes [19, 60]. In a randomized, double-blind, vehicle-controlled study of African American patients with melasma ($n = 28$), 0.1% tretinoin for 40 weeks resulted in a 32% improvement in the Melasma Area and Severity Index (MASI) score compared to 10% in the placebo group [61]. Similarly, when used to treat PIH, 0.1% tretinoin cream applied daily for 40 weeks resulted in a significant lightening of lesions (40% vs. 18%) compared to vehicle cream [25]. However, 50% of patients developed retinoid dermatitis [25]. To minimize this side effect, retinoids can be started at lower concentrations and titrated up [62]. While tretinoin demonstrates good efficacy, it generally requires a long 20–40 week treatment period for maximal benefit [26].

Adapalene (0.1–0.3%) and tazarotene (0.05–0.1%) are synthetic retinoids that can be used to treat PIH and melasma as well [63, 64]. Compared to 0.05% tretinoin cream, 0.1% adapalene gel demonstrated similar efficacy in treating melasma among 30 Indian women. The adapalene gel was better tolerated as significantly more patients in the tretinoin group experienced pruritus, burning, dryness, erythema, and scaling compared to the adapalene group (63% vs. 8%) [24]. Tazarotene 0.1% cream similarly reduced severity and intensity of hyperpigmentation in a randomized, double-blind, vehicle-controlled study among 74 acne patients of darker skin types. Erythema, burning, and peeling occurred minimally in both treatment groups [65]. Retinoids are able to increase the epidermal penetration of other active ingredients and have, therefore, been found to be effective in combination products [29].

Combination Therapy

Hydroquinone is frequently combined with a retinoid, most commonly tretinoin, and a corticosteroid for synergistic effects. In addition to increasing keratinocyte proliferation, tretinoin increases pigment elimination by preventing oxidation of hydroquinone and improves epidermal penetration by causing mild irritation. Topical corticosteroids reduce irritation and inhibit melanin synthesis [4]. Combination therapy has been found to be more effective than any of its constituent agents alone [30]. The original Kligman's formula (5% hydroquinone, 0.1% tretinoin, 0.1% dexamethasone) was found to be effective in treating hyperpigmentation [19]. A subsequent formulation consisting of 4% hydroquinone, 0.05% tretinoin, and 0.01% fluocinolone acetonide has been shown to be safe and effective in dark-skinned ethnic groups. [28, 29] Two 8-week studies ($n = 161$, $n = 1042$) demonstrated good safety and efficacy for facial melasma across a wide range of FSTs with 75–77% of patients achieving "moderate or marked improvement," "almost clear," or "clear" results by week 8 [29, 66]. Two longer studies, a 12-month extension of a previous 8-week trial [31] ($n = 569$) and a 12-month multi-center study of patients with facial melasma ($n = 228$), demonstrated complete or nearly complete clearance of 80 and 90% of cases, respectively [31, 67]. Between the 2 long-term studies, 2 cases of skin atrophy and 29 cases of telangiectasia occurred [31]. These studies indicate that fixed triple combination agents are safe and effective [68].

Azelaic Acid

Azelaic acid is a dicarboxylic acid that inhibits tyrosinase activity and interferes with DNA synthesis. It is naturally found in *Malassezia furfur*, the etiologic agent for pityriasis versicolor [32]. Azelaic acid offers two advantages compared to other agents. First, azelaic acid's cytotoxic effect is specific to abnormally hyperactive melanocytes, and so normally pigmented skin does not become depigmented. Second, it has a good safety profile, with minimal side effects including pruritus, transient erythema, and scaling. [19, 52, 69, 70] However, a long treatment duration is required and improvement is not noticeable for several months.

In a study among FST IV-VI ($n = 52$), 20% azelaic acid cream significantly decreased the intensity of facial hyperpigmentation [71]. When compared to hydroquinone, results are mixed [72, 73]. A South American randomized, double-blind, multicenter study of melasma patients ($n = 243$) treated with 4% hydroquinone cream twice daily versus 20% azelaic acid cream twice daily yielded equivocal differences at 24 weeks [72]. In another randomized double-blind trial of melasma patients ($n = 155$) with FST III-V, 20% azelaic acid was more efficacious at decreasing lesion size and intensity compared to 2% hydroquinone at 24 weeks (73% vs. 19%) [73].

Mequinol

Mequinol (4-hydroxyanisole) is a derivative of hydroquinone and is postulated to induce depigmentation by inhibiting tyrosinase [33]. Although it is not as effective as hydroquinone, it is thought to be less irritating [34]. It is typically combined with 0.01% tretinoin, which can enhance penetration. Draelos et al. [74] demonstrated that 2% mequinol combined with 0.01% tretinoin can effectively treat solar lentigines in patients with FST II–V, with minimal adverse effects. However, few studies among dark-skinned ethnic groups have been conducted, and studies on its efficacy for PIH are still lacking.

Kojic Acid

Kojic acid, a fungal metabolite, inhibits tyrosine kinase by chelating copper [35]. It is available in gel or cream formulation with concentrations ranging from 1 to 4%. Kojic acid has marginal efficacy and can be irritating [30, 36]. It is typically used in combination products with studies showing mixed results. When combined with other lightening agents, 2% hydroquinone and 10% glycolic acid (GA), pigmentation was not significantly reduced with the addition of kojic acid ($n = 40$) [75]. Similarly, in a split-face study where a 4% HQ/5% GA gel was compared to 2% kojic acid/5% GA gel, there was no significant difference in pigmentation reduction between the two treatment arms [36]. Furthermore, kojic acid is highly sensitizing and is associated with a high frequency of contact sensitivity [37].

Licorice

Licorice extract contains glabridin, licochalcone A, and liquiritin, which exert skin-lightening effects [38, 39]. In a study of 20 Egyptian women with melasma, topical liquiritin cream decreased pigment intensity and lesion size in 70 and 60% of patients, respectively [40]. Side effects were minimal (i.e., mild irritation) and resolved with continuation of treatment [40].

Arbutin

Arbutin is a plant-derived derivative of hydroquinone that causes depigmentation by inhibiting tyrosinase activity and melanosome maturation. The more potent synthetic derivative, deoxyarbutin, has been effective in treating solar lentigines among light-skinned patients in a 3% formulation ($n = 34$) but not in dark-skinned populations ($n = 16$) [41]. It should be used with caution as higher concentrations may cause paradoxical hyperpigmentation [42].

Ascorbic Acid

Ascorbic acid exerts lightening effects through three mechanisms: reducing oxidized dopaquinone (a substrate in the melanin synthesis pathway), suppressing activation of NF-kβ and TNF-α (anti-inflammation), and protecting against UVA- and UVB-induced phototoxic injury (photoprotection) [44, 45]. As it is frequently combined with other lightening agents, few studies have examined its efficacy as monotherapy. In a small split-face study ($n = 16$) in a Latino population comparing 5% ascorbic acid cream versus 4% hydroquinone, there was no significant objective difference in improvement between the two treatment arms. However, there were fewer side effects among those treated with ascorbic acid. [46] When magnesium-L-ascorbyl-2-phosphage (a derivative of ascorbic acid) was used to treat chloasma or senile freckles in an Asian population, 56% of patients ($n = 34$) experienced "effective" or "fairly effective" improvement [76].

Soy

Soy blocks the transfer of melanosomes to nearby keratinocytes by inhibiting protease-activated receptor 2 (PAR-2) expressed on keratinocytes [47]. Few studies have examined the effect of soy extract alone in improving hyperpigmentation. However, in a 16-week study among FST III-V patients, soy combined with salicylic acid and retinol significantly improved PIH compared to placebo [49]. Soy is relatively well-tolerated, but more studies are needed to evaluate its efficacy among dark-skinned ethnic groups [43, 48].

Niacinamide

Niacinamide, the physiologically active form of niacin, decreases the transfer of melanosomes to keratinocytes [50]. In a study among 18 Asians, 5% niacinamide in a facial moisturizer compared to facial moisturizer alone significantly increased skin lightness at 4 weeks. Afterward, the effect plateaued, similar to other lightening agents (i.e., retinoids) [50]. The advantages of niacinamide are that it is generally well-tolerated and is unaffected by light, acids, alkalis, and oxidizers [77]. However, further studies are needed to evaluate its effect on disorders of hyperpigmentation.

N-Acetyl Glucosamine

N-acetyl glucosamine (NAG) is a precursor to hyaluronic acid and inhibits tyrosinase glycosylation—a step in the melanogenesis pathway [51]. When used as monotherapy for 8 weeks to treat hyperpigmentation in a Japanese population ($n = 50$), 2% NAG reduced the appearance of pigmentation, though not significantly. [51] When combined with 4% niacinamide, the improvement in hyperpigmentation was significantly greater, as demonstrated in 2 studies among Caucasian participants [51, 78]. The difference may be attributable to inhibiting 2 separate steps in the melanogenesis pathway [51]. Like niacinamide, NAG was well-tolerated in all studies [51]. However, few studies have evaluated its effect in dark-skinned ethnic groups.

Emerging Topical Agents

New promising agents include aloesin, linoleic acid, ellagic acid, resveratrol, 4-n-butylresorcinol, methimazole, and metformin. In a study among 7 Korean patients, aloesin, an inhibitor of tyrosinase, exerted an inhibitory effect on pigmentation after UV radiation in a dose-dependent manner [79, 80]. In a study using guinea pigs, linoleic acid demonstrated a lightening effect on UV-stimulated hyperpigmented skin by suppressing melanin production and promoting desquamation of pigment from the epidermis [81]. Ellagic acid, an inhibitor of melanin synthesis, demonstrated comparable efficacy to 4% hydroquinone when combined with 0.1% salicylic acid when treating hyperpigmentation in a multi-ethnic population ($n = 54$) [82]. The cosmetic use of resveratrol, another tyrosinase inhibitor, has been limited so far due to chemical instability [79]. However, Ryu et al. recently demonstrated that resveratrol triacetate (prodrug of resveratrol) decreases intensity of hyperpigmentation among FSTs III-IV without inducing skin irritation [83]. Similarly, 4-n-butylresorcinol, an inhibitor of tyrosinase and tyrosinase-related protein-1, has been shown to be efficacious in reducing melasma pigmentation after 8 weeks of use [84]. Topical methimazole cream was shown to inhibit melanin synthesis and significantly improve hyperpigmentation in two hydroquinone-resistant melasma patients [85]. Finally, topical metformin induced tail whitening in animal studies and exerted an anti-melanogenic effect on reconstituted human epidermis and human skin biopsies [86].

Chemical Peels

Chemical peels are an increasingly popular method to disperse unwanted pigment among those with more darkly pigmented skin tones [87]. They may be used as monotherapy or as an adjunct to topical agents. Superficial (epidermis to upper papillary dermis) and medium-depth (epidermis to upper reticular dermis) are the primary peels used in dark-skinned ethnic groups. Superficial peels include 30–50% glycolic acid (GA), 20–30% salicylic acid (SA), 10–35% trichloroacetic acid (TCA), and Jessner's solution [88]. Medium-depth peels include 50% TCA and 70% GA [87]. Deep peels are avoided in dark-skinned ethnic groups, due to the higher risk of hypopigmentation, hyperpigmentation, scarring, and keloid and milia formation [19, 89]. More details on patient selection, pre-and post-treatment care, and types of peels can be found in the chemical peels chapter.

Microdermabrasion

Microdermabrasion is a superficial skin resurfacing procedure that removes the stratum corneum. A negative pressure system pulls the skin into a handpiece connected to a vacuum pump that blows chemically inert crystals (usually aluminum oxide), which cause mechanical skin abrasion. Used crystals and abraded material are then suctioned off into a waste receptacle [90]. Alternative machines use less harsh sodium chloride and sodium bicarbonate crystals, and some employ diamond wand systems that are crystal-free [91].

Most studies have reported mild to moderate improvement (5–41%) in melasma after 6–8 weekly sessions [91, 92]. Compared to pre-treatment skin biopsies, post-treatment biopsies demonstrated decreased melanization and regular distribution of melanosomes in the epidermis [91, 93]. Of note, improvement can be enhanced when microdermabrasion sessions are combined with topical retinoid treatment (40% vs. 15% improvement) [92]. Similarly, Kauvar et al. demonstrated that a combination of microdermabrasion followed immediately by Q-switched neodymium-doped yttrium aluminium garnet (QS Nd:YAG) laser treatment yielded even higher improvement rates with 81% of participants achieving >75% clearance ($n = 27$) [94]. While there has been concern about potential adverse neurologic effects of aluminum oxide, there has been inconclusive evidence to date that long-term exposure to aluminum may be associated with cognitive impairment.

These findings have mainly been found in aluminum miners or factory workers and are specific to aluminum and not aluminum oxide [90].

In general, microdermabrasion is considered to be safe in all skin types with few side effects. Petechiae and purpura may develop depending on ablation speed and vacuum pressure, but lesions typically resolve by 3 days. Rarer side effects include acne and recurrent herpes simplex outbreaks. It should be performed with caution in darker skin types (i.e., III–VI) due to the risk of PIH, and those with rosacea as telangiectasias and erythema may be permanently worsened [92].

Microneedling

Microneedling is accomplished by rolling an instrument studded with rows of microneedles over the skin multiple times. The microneedles penetrate through the epidermis and into the upper dermis (0.5 mm), inducing a wound-healing response. For hyperpigmentary disorders, microneedling has been explored as a means of augmenting transepidermal drug delivery [95]. Fabbrocini et al. [95] conducted a split-face study among women with melasma ($n = 20$, FST III–V) wherein a serum containing rucinol and sophora-alpha was applied to skin with and without prior microneedling. Compared to the serum alone group, the MASI score decreased significantly more in the combination group (7.1 vs. 10.1 points). Lima Ede reported similar improvement with a combination of microneedling and triple combination cream (0.05% tretinoin, 4% hydroquinone, 1% fluocinolone acetonide), with preserved results at 2 years follow-up [96]. In a prospective randomized trial, microinjections of tranexamic acid with and without microneedling were administered among patients with melasma ($n = 60$, FST IV–V). After the third treatment session, there was greater improvement in the microneedling group compared to the microinjection alone group (44.41% vs. 35.72%). Furthermore, 41% of patients in the microneedling group showed >50% improvement [97]. Based on these studies, the augmented response to treatment with microneedling may be attributable to deeper and more uniform penetration of medication.

Microneedling is generally well-tolerated with no adverse effects reported in most studies [95–97]. Furthermore, as the epidermis remains largely intact, risks of scarring and infection are limited [98].

Lasers

Lasers are typically used as third-line agents for disorders of hyperpigmentation, as data is still limited, and there is an increased risk of scarring and dyspigmentation. Lasers that have been extensively explored in the treatment of pigmented disease, albeit with variable success include Q-switched Ruby (695 nm), Q-switched Alexandrite (755 nm), QS Nd:YAG (1064 nm), intense pulsed light, pulsed dye laser, and fractional photothermolysis. For pigmentary disorders, the target chromophore is melanin (630–1100 nm), so ideally lasers with wavelengths within this range are used [99]. Lasers that produce pulses of light shorter than the thermal relaxation time (time necessary for the target tissue to lose 50% of its initial heated temperature) of melanosomes (250–1000 ns) must be used in order to selectively destroy melanin. Consequently, the QS Nd:YAG 1064 nm laser which emits long wavelengths in ultra short pulse durations is most commonly used [100]. Further details on patient selection, pre-and post-treatment care, and types of lasers can be found in the laser chapter.

Oral Agents

Oral agents are generally considered third-line agents for treatment of dyschromia after topical agents and/or chemical peels have failed. However, some authors use it as second-line agents [101].

Tranexamic Acid

Originally marketed as a fibrinolytic agent, tranexamic acid has recently demonstrated efficacious off-market use in treating melasma [102]. Unlike other treatments, which aim to decrease melanogenesis (majority of topical agents) or remove pre-existing melanin (peels, lasers), tranexamic acid is postulated to prevent activation of melanocytes by blocking plasminogen binding to keratinocytes [102]. Tranexamic acid may also modulate angiogenic factors involved in the development of melasma [101]. In the largest retrospective study to date of melasma patients with a median follow-up of 4 months ($n = 561$), 89.7% of patients showed improvement while on tranexamic acid 250 mg twice a day [101]. These promising findings are consistent with multiple previous studies based on Asian populations; however, studies are lacking in other patient populations [103, 104]. Common side effects included nausea, diarrhea, and orthostasis [102].

Prior to initiating treatment, clinicians should screen for a history of thrombosis, angina, and stroke, and consider obtaining monthly coagulation labs. Lightening effects should be expected after 2 months of treatment [101]. If no response is observed, increasing treatment duration is more effective than increasing dosage [101, 102]. Finally, like other topical agents, patients should be counseled on the risk of relapse, as 27% of patients in the Lee et al. study relapsed on cessation of oral treatment [101].

Botanical Agents

Botanical products, such as procyanidin, pycnogenol, and *Polypodium leucotomos* (*P. leucotomos*), are increasingly attractive to consumers because they are inexpensive, easily accessible without prescription, and perceived to be "more safe" than pharmaceuticals. They inhibit hyperpigmentation by exerting antioxidant or anti-inflammatory effects [105]. Only a few studies have been conducted to date and although they found these agents (procyanidin 48 mg/day with vitamins A, C, E, or pycnogenol 75 mg/day) to be safe and efficacious in treating melasma, they are limited by different factors including very short follow-up periods (i.e., 1 or 2 months). Studies on *P. leucotomos* have demonstrated mixed results with respect to efficacy, but one small study showed that it may prevent UVA-induced pigmentary changes [106–110]. Of note, no studies have examined their efficacy in PIH and overall improvement in skin of color. In the interim, while further studies are conducted, clinicians should be aware that botanicals carry an inherent risk of allergic and phototoxic reactions and do not require rigorous safety testing by the Food and Drug Administration (FDA) before marketing. They may also be adulterated with corticosteroids, putting users at risk of steroid-induced atrophy and dyspigmentation [105].

Emerging Oral Treatments

Oral grape seed extract can reduce the appearance of melasma by inhibiting melanin synthesis and UV-induced hyperpigmentation [111]. To date, there have been limited studies in humans, but in one study among Japanese women ($n = 12$), 6 months of oral grape seed extract therapy led to a reduction in the melanin-index score that persisted during the next 6 months [112]. Although it was well-tolerated, more studies with larger sample sizes are needed to further evaluate its efficacy.

Intravenous Agents

Glutathione (GSH) is an endogenously produced antioxidant that is found naturally in food (i.e., watermelon, avocado, spinach) and also commercially, in oral and intravenous formulations. It is more commonly used in Asian countries (i.e., Thailand, Philippines, India), where "fair" skin is highly desired as a symbol of social ranking [113]. While GSH initially appeared promising through its multi-faceted inhibition of melanogenesis—inactivating tyrosinase, mediating the switch from eumelanin to pheomelanin, and quenching formation of free radicals—few studies have examined its efficacy and safety in skin whitening [113]. These agents are currently not recommended or FDA-approved for this purpose. The FDA has banned injectable versions due to the risk of Stevens Johnson syndrome, toxic epidermal necrolysis, and abnormalities in thyroid and renal function [114]. Injectable formulations are furthermore likely to be counterfeit and administered by untrained personnel, which raises the risk of sepsis, air embolism, and transmission of infectious disease [114]. Finally, it is unknown whether switching from eumelanin (protective against UV radiation) to pheomelanin (potentially photosensitizing to UVA in melanocyte cultures) may result in an increased risk of skin cancer [115].

Conclusion

By 2050, more than half of the U.S. population will be composed of darker ethnic skin types. Consequently, clinicians should be prepared to treat a higher volume of disorders of hyperpigmentation (i.e., melasma, PIH).

Topical agents are generally first-line treatment, with hydroquinone and triple combination therapy often used initially given their long history of safety and efficacy. Chemical peels are considered a second-line agent as they are both more expensive and carry a higher risk of side effects. Oral tranexamic acid demonstrates excellent efficacy but is still limited by a high relapse rate and warrants more study in non-Asian populations. Microdermabrasion, microneedling, and laser treatments are third-line options given the limited data to date and the higher risks of side effects. Finally, maintenance therapy with sunscreen and topical agents are crucial to prevent relapse.

References

1. Alexis AF, Sergay AB, Taylor SC. Common dermatologic disorders in skin of color: a comparative practice survey. Cutis. 2007;80(5):387–94.
2. Day J. Population projection of the US by age, sex, race, and Hispanic origin: 1995–2050, US Bureau of Census, Current Population Report. Washington, DC: US Government Printing Office; 1996. p. 25–1130.
3. Desai SR. Hyperpigmentation therapy: a review. J Clin Aesthet Dermatol. 2014;7(8):13–7.
4. Lynde CB, Kraft JN, Lynde CW. Topical treatments for melasma and postinflammatory hyperpigmentation. Skin Therapy Lett. 2006;11(9):1–6.
5. Grimes PE, Yamada N, Bhawan J. Light microscopic, immunohistochemical, and ultrastructural alterations in patients with melasma. Am J Dermatopathol. 2005;27(2):96–101.
6. Wang SQ, Lim HW. Current status of the sunscreen regulation in the United States: 2011 Food and Drug Administration's final rule on labeling and effectiveness testing. J Am Acad Dermatol. 2011;65(4):863–9.
7. Agbai ON, Buster K, Sanchez M, Hernandez C, Kundu RV, Chiu M, et al. Skin cancer and photoprotection in people of color: a review and recommendations for physicians and the public. J Am Acad Dermatol. 2014;70(4):748–62.

8. Nesby-O'Dell S, Scanlon KS, Cogswell ME, Gillespie C, Hollis BW, Looker AC, et al. Hypovitaminosis D prevalence and determinants among African American and white women of reproductive age: third National Health and Nutrition Examination Survey, 1988–1994. Am J Clin Nutr. 2002;76(1):187–92.

9. Azurdia RM, Pagliaro JA, Diffey BL, Rhodes LE. Sunscreen application by photosensitive patients is inadequate for protection. Br J Dermatol. 1999;140(2):255–8.

10. Sambandan DR, Ratner D. Sunscreens: an overview and update. J Am Acad Dermatol. 2011;64(4):748–58.

11. Diffey B. Sunscreens: expectation and realization. Photodermatol Photoimmunol Photomed. 2009;25(5):233–6.

12. Wolf R, Tüzün B, Tüzün Y. Sunscreens. Dermatol Ther. 2001;14(3):208–14.

13. Kullavanijaya P, Lim HW. Photoprotection. J Am Acad Dermatol. 2005;52(6):937–58.

14. Stark KEG. Method for creating custom blended cosmetics. Google Patents; 2009.

15. Castanedo-Cazares JP, Hernandez-Blanco D, Carlos-Ortega B, Fuentes-Ahumada C, Torres-Álvarez B. Near-visible light and UV photoprotection in the treatment of melasma: a double-blind randomized trial. Photodermatol Photoimmunol Photomed. 2014;30(1):35–42.

16. Vashi NA, Kundu RV. Facial hyperpigmentation: causes and treatment. Br J Dermatol. 2013;169(Suppl 3):41–56.

17. Palumbo A, d'Ischia M, Misuraca G, Prota G. Mechanism of inhibition of melanogenesis by hydroquinone. Biochim Biophys Acta. 1991;1073(1):85–90.

18. Jimbow K, Obata H, Pathak MA, Fitzpatrick TB. Mechanism of depigmentation by hydroquinone. J Invest Dermatol. 1974;62(4):436–49.

19. Grimes PE. Management of hyperpigmentation in darker racial ethnic groups. Semin Cutan Med Surg. 2009;28(2):77–85.

20. Levin CY, Maibach H. Exogenous ochronosis. An update on clinical features, causative agents and treatment options. Am J Clin Dermatol. 2001;2(4):213–7.

21. Haddad AL, Matos LF, Brunstein F, Ferreira LM, Silva A, Costa D Jr. A clinical, prospective, randomized, double-blind trial comparing skin whitening complex with hydroquinone vs. placebo in the treatment of melasma. Int J Dermatol. 2003;42(2):153–6.

22. Ortonne JP. Retinoid therapy of pigmentary disorders. Dermatol Ther. 2006;19(5):280–8.

23. Bikowski J. Mechanisms of the comedolytic and anti-inflammatory properties of topical retinoids. J Drugs Derm. 2004;4(1):41–7.

24. Dogra S, Kanwar AJ, Parsad D. Adapalene in the treatment of melasma: a preliminary report. J Dermatol. 2002;29(8):539–40.

25. Bulengo-Ransby SM, Griffiths CE, Kimbrough-Green CK, Finkel LJ, Hamilton TA, Ellis CN, et al. Topical tretinoin (retinoic acid) therapy for hyperpigmented lesions caused by inflammation of the skin in black patients. N Engl J Med. 1993;328(20):1438–43.

26. Griffiths CE, Finkel LJ, Ditre CM, Hamilton TA, Ellis CN, Voorhees JJ. Topical tretinoin (retinoic acid) improves melasma. A vehicle-controlled, clinical trial. Br J Dermatol. 1993;129(4):415–21.

27. Fleckman P. Management of the ichthyoses. Skin Therapy Lett. 2003;8(6):3–7.

28. Chan R, Park KC, Lee MH, Lee ES, Chang SE, Leow YH, et al. A randomized controlled trial of the efficacy and safety of a fixed triple combination (fluocinolone acetonide 0.01%, hydroquinone 4%, tretinoin 0.05%) compared with hydroquinone 4% cream in Asian patients with moderate to severe melasma. Br J Dermatol. 2008;159(3):697–703.

29. Grimes P, Kelly AP, Torok H, Willis I. Community-based trial of a triple-combination agent for the treatment of facial melasma. Cutis. 2006;77(3):177–84.

30. Cayce KA, McMichael AJ, Feldman SR. Hyperpigmentation: an overview of the common afflictions. Dermatol Nurs. 2004;16(5):401–6, 13–6; quiz 17.

31. Torok H, Taylor S, Baumann L, Jones T, Wieder J, Lowe N, et al. A large 12-month extension study of an 8-week trial to evaluate the safety and efficacy of triple combination (TC) cream in melasma patients previously treated with TC cream or one of its dyads. J Drugs Derm. 2005;4(5):592–7.

32. Fitton A, Goa KL. Azelaic acid. A review of its pharmacological properties and therapeutic efficacy in acne and hyperpigmentary skin disorders. Drugs. 1991;41(5):780–98.
33. Draelos ZD. Skin lightening preparations and the hydroquinone controversy. Dermatol Ther. 2007;20(5):308–13.
34. Fleischer AB Jr, Schwartzel EH, Colby SI, Altman DJ. The combination of 2% 4-hydroxyanisole (Mequinol) and 0.01% tretinoin is effective in improving the appearance of solar lentigines and related hyperpigmented lesions in two double-blind multicenter clinical studies. J Am Acad Dermatol. 2000;42(3):459–67.
35. Ortonne JP, Passeron T. Melanin pigmentary disorders: treatment update. Dermatol Clin. 2005;23(2):209–26.
36. Garcia A, Fulton JE Jr. The combination of glycolic acid and hydroquinone or kojic acid for the treatment of melasma and related conditions. Dermatol Surg. 1996;22(5):443–7.
37. Nakagawa M, Kawai K, Kawai K. Contact allergy to kojic acid in skin care products. Contact Dermatitis. 1995;32(1):9–13.
38. Yokota T, Nishio H, Kubota Y, Mizoguchi M. The inhibitory effect of glabridin from licorice extracts on melanogenesis and inflammation. Pigment Cell Res. 1998;11(6):355–61.
39. Fu B, Li H, Wang X, Lee FS, Cui S. Isolation and identification of flavonoids in licorice and a study of their inhibitory effects on tyrosinase. J Agric Food Chem. 2005;53(19):7408–14.
40. Amer M, Metwalli M. Topical liquiritin improves melasma. Int J Dermatol. 2000;39(4):299–301.
41. Boissy RE, Visscher M, DeLong MA. DeoxyArbutin: a novel reversible tyrosinase inhibitor with effective in vivo skin lightening potency. Exp Dermatol. 2005;14(8):601–8.
42. Maeda K, Fukuda M. Arbutin: mechanism of its depigmenting action in human melanocyte culture. J Pharmacol Exp Ther. 1996;276(2):765–9.
43. Davis EC, Callender VD. Postinflammatory hyperpigmentation: a review of the epidemiology, clinical features, and treatment options in skin of color. J Clin Aesthet Dermatol. 2010;3(7):20–31.
44. Carcamo JM, Pedraza A, Borquez-Ojeda O, Golde DW. Vitamin C suppresses TNF alpha-induced NF kappa B activation by inhibiting I kappa B alpha phosphorylation. Biochemistry. 2002;41(43):12995–3002.
45. Darr D, Combs S, Dunston S, Manning T, Pinnell S. Topical vitamin C protects porcine skin from ultraviolet radiation-induced damage. Br J Dermatol. 1992;127(3):247–53.
46. Espinal-Perez LE, Moncada B, Castanedo-Cazares JP. A double-blind randomized trial of 5% ascorbic acid vs. 4% hydroquinone in melasma. Int J Dermatol. 2004;43(8):604–7.
47. Paine C, Sharlow E, Liebel F, Eisinger M, Shapiro S, Seiberg M. An alternative approach to depigmentation by soybean extracts via inhibition of the PAR-2 pathway. J Invest Dermatol. 2001;116(4):587–95.
48. Finkey MB, Herndon J, Stephens T, Appa Y. Soy moisturizer SPF15 improves dyschromia. J Am Acad Dermatol. 2005;52(3):P170.
49. Sah A, Stephens TJ, Kurtz ES. Topical acne treatment improves postacne postinflammatory hyperpigmentation (PIH) in skin of color. J Am Acad Dermatol. 2005;52(3):P25.
50. Hakozaki T, Minwalla L, Zhuang J, Chhoa M, Matsubara A, Miyamoto K, et al. The effect of niacinamide on reducing cutaneous pigmentation and suppression of melanosome transfer. Br J Dermatol. 2002;147(1):20–31.
51. Bissett DL, Robinson LR, Raleigh PS, Miyamoto K, Hakozaki T, Li J, et al. Reduction in the appearance of facial hyperpigmentation by topical N-acetyl glucosamine. J Cosmet Dermatol. 2007;6(1):20–6.
52. Halder RM, Richards GM. Topical agents used in the management of hyperpigmentation. Skin Therapy Lett. 2004;9(6):1–3.
53. Ennes S, Paschoalick R, Alchorne MMDA. A double-blind, comparative, placebo-controlled study of the efficacy and tolerability of 4% hydroquinone as a depigmenting agent in melasma. J Dermatolog Treat. 2000;11(3):173–9.

54. Rendon M, Dryer L. Investigator-blinded, single-center study to evaluate the efficacy and tolerability of a 4% hydroquinone skin care system plus 0.02% tretinoin cream in mild-to-moderate melasma and photodamage. J Drugs Derm. 2016;15(4):466–75.

55. Simmons BJ, Griffith RD, Bray FN, Falto-Aizpurua LA, Nouri K. Exogenous ochronosis: a comprehensive review of the diagnosis, epidemiology, causes, and treatments. Am J Clin Dermatol. 2015;16(3):205–12.

56. Hoshaw RA, Zimmerman KG, Menter A. Ochronosislike pigmentation from hydroquinone bleaching creams in American blacks. Arch Dermatol. 1985;121(1):105–8.

57. Andersen FA, Bergfeld WF, Belsito DV, Hill RA, Klaassen CD, Liebler DC, et al. Final amended safety assessment of hydroquinone as used in cosmetics. Int J Toxicol. 2010;29(6 Suppl):274s–87.

58. Nordlund JJ, Grimes PE, Ortonne JP. The safety of hydroquinone. J Eur Acad Dermatol Venereol. 2006;20(7):781–7.

59. Kari FW, Bucher J, Eustis SL, Haseman JK, Huff JE. Toxicity and carcinogenicity of hydroquinone in F344/N rats and B6C3F1 mice. Food Chem Toxicol. 1992;30(9):737–47.

60. Ortonne JP. Retinoic acid and pigment cells: a review of in-vitro and in-vivo studies. Br J Dermatol. 1992;127(Suppl 41):43–7.

61. Kimbrough-Green CK, Griffiths CE, Finkel LJ, Hamilton TA, Bulengo-Ransby SM, Ellis CN, et al. Topical retinoic acid (tretinoin) for melasma in black patients: a vehicle-controlled clinical trial. Arch Dermatol. 1994;130(6):727–33.

62. Callender VD. Acne in ethnic skin: special considerations for therapy. Dermatol Ther. 2004;17(2):184–95.

63. Jacyk WK, Mpofu P. Adapalene gel 0.1% for topical treatment of acne vulgaris in African patients. Cutis. 2001;68(4 Suppl):48–54.

64. Rivas S, Pandya AG. Treatment of melasma with topical agents, peels and lasers: an evidence-based review. Am J Clin Dermatol. 2013;14(5):359–76.

65. Grimes P, Callender V. Tazarotene cream for postinflammatory hyperpigmentation and acne vulgaris in darker skin: a double-blind, randomized, vehicle-controlled study. Cutis. 2006;77(1):45–50.

66. Taylor SC, Torok H, Jones T, Lowe N, Rich P, Tschen E, et al. Efficacy and safety of a new triple-combination agent for the treatment of facial melasma. Cutis. 2003;72(1):67–72.

67. Torok HM, Jones T, Rich P, Smith S, Tschen E. Hydroquinone 4%, tretinoin 0.05%, fluocinolone acetonide 0.01%: a safe and efficacious 12-month treatment for melasma. Cutis. 2005;75(1):57–62.

68. Torok HM. A comprehensive review of the long-term and short-term treatment of melasma with a triple combination cream. Am J Clin Dermatol. 2006;7(4):223–30.

69. Nguyen QH, Bui TP. Azelaic acid: pharmacokinetic and pharmacodynamic properties and its therapeutic role in hyperpigmentary disorders and acne. Int J Dermatol. 1995;34(2):75–84.

70. Breathnach AS. Melanin hyperpigmentation of skin: melasma, topical treatment with azelaic acid, and other therapies. Cutis. 1996;57(1 Suppl):36–45.

71. Lowe NJ, Rizk D, Grimes P, Billips M, Pincus S. Azelaic acid 20% cream in the treatment of facial hyperpigmentation in darker-skinned patients. Clin Ther. 1998;20(5):945–59.

72. Balina LM, Graupe K. The treatment of melasma. 20% azelaic acid versus 4% hydroquinone cream. Int J Dermatol. 1991;30(12):893–5.

73. Verallo-Rowell VM, Verallo V, Graupe K, Lopez-Villafuerte L, Garcia-Lopez M. Double-blind comparison of azelaic acid and hydroquinone in the treatment of melasma. Acta Derm Venereol. 1989;143(Suppl):58–61.

74. Draelos ZD. The combination of 2% 4-hydroxyanisole (mequinol) and 0.01% tretinoin effectively improves the appearance of solar lentigines in ethnic groups. J Cosmet Dermatol. 2006;5(3):239–44.

75. Lim JT. Treatment of melasma using kojic acid in a gel containing hydroquinone and glycolic acid. Dermatol Surg. 1999;25(4):282–4.

76. Kameyama K, Sakai C, Kondoh S, Yonemoto K, Nishiyama S, Tagawa M, et al. Inhibitory effect of magnesium L-ascorbyl-2-phosphate (VC-PMG) on melanogenesis in vitro and in vivo. J Am Acad Dermatol. 1996;34(1):29–33.
77. Badreshia-Bansal S, Draelos ZD. Insight into skin lightening cosmeceuticals for women of color. J Drugs Derm. 2007;6(1):32–9.
78. Kimball AB, Kaczvinsky JR, Li J, Robinson LR, Matts PJ, Berge CA, et al. Reduction in the appearance of facial hyperpigmentation after use of moisturizers with a combination of topical niacinamide and N-acetyl glucosamine: results of a randomized, double-blind, vehicle-controlled trial. Br J Dermatol. 2010;162(2):435–41.
79. Briganti S, Camera E, Picardo M. Chemical and instrumental approaches to treat hyperpigmentation. Pigment Cell Res. 2003;16(2):101–10.
80. Choi S, Lee SK, Kim JE, Chung MH, Park YI. Aloesin inhibits hyperpigmentation induced by UV radiation. Clin Exp Dermatol. 2002;27(6):513–5.
81. Ando H, Ryu A, Hashimoto A, Oka M, Ichihashi M. Linoleic acid and alpha-linolenic acid lightens ultraviolet-induced hyperpigmentation of the skin. Arch Dermatol Res. 1998;290 (7):375–81.
82. Dahl A, Yatskayer M, Raab S, Oresajo C. Tolerance and efficacy of a product containing ellagic and salicylic acids in reducing hyperpigmentation and dark spots in comparison with 4% hydroquinone. J Drugs Derm. 2013;12(1):52–8.
83. Ryu JH, Seok JK, An SM, Baek JH, Koh JS, Boo YC. A study of the human skin-whitening effects of resveratryl triacetate. Arch Dermatol Res. 2015;307(3):239–47.
84. Huh SY, Shin JW, Na JI, Huh CH, Youn SW, Park KC. Efficacy and safety of liposome-encapsulated 4-n-butylresorcinol 0.1% cream for the treatment of melasma: a randomized controlled split-face trial. J Dermatol. 2010;37(4):311–5.
85. Malek J, Chedraoui A, Nikolic D, Barouti N, Ghosn S, Abbas O. Successful treatment of hydroquinone-resistant melasma using topical methimazole. Dermatol Ther. 2013;26(1):69–72.
86. Lehraiki A, Abbe P, Cerezo M, Rouaud F, Regazzetti C, Chignon-Sicard B, et al. Inhibition of melanogenesis by the antidiabetic metformin. J Invest Dermatol. 2014;134(10):2589–97.
87. Roberts WE. Chemical peeling in ethnic/dark skin. Dermatol Ther. 2004;17(2):196–205.
88. Quarles FN, Brody H, Johnson BA, Badreshia S. Chemical peels in richly pigmented patients. Dermatol Ther. 2007;20(3):147–8.
89. Stratigos AJ, Katsambas AD. Optimal management of recalcitrant disorders of hyperpigmentation in dark-skinned patients. Am J Clin Dermatol. 2004;5(3):161–8.
90. Spencer JM. Microdermabrasion. Am J Clin Dermatol. 2005;6(2):89–92.
91. El-Domyati M, Hosam W, Abdel-Azim E, Abdel-Wahab H, Mohamed E. Microdermabrasion: a clinical, histometric, and histopathologic study. J Cosmet Dermatol. 29 June 2016 [epub before print].
92. Bhalla M, Thami GP. Microdermabrasion: reappraisal and brief review of literature. Dermatol Surg. 2006;32(6):809–14.
93. Shim EK, Barnette D, Hughes K, Greenway HT. Microdermabrasion: a clinical and histopathologic study. Dermatol Surg. 2001;27(6):524–30.
94. Kauvar AN. Successful treatment of melasma using a combination of microdermabrasion and Q-switched Nd:YAG lasers. Lasers Surg Med. 2012;44(2):117–24.
95. Fabbrocini G, De Vita V, Fardella N, Pastore F, Annunziata MC, Mauriello MC, et al. Skin needling to enhance depigmenting serum penetration in the treatment of melasma. Plast Surg Int. 2011;2011:158241.
96. Lima Ede A. Microneedling in facial recalcitrant melasma: report of a series of 22 cases. An Bras Dermatol. 2015;90(6):919–21.
97. Budamakuntla L, Loganathan E, Suresh DH, Shanmugam S, Suryanarayan S, Dongare A, et al. A randomised, open-label, comparative study of tranexamic acid microinjections and tranexamic acid with microneedling in patients with melasma. J Cutan Aesthet Surg. 2013;6 (3):139–43.

98. Cohen BE, Elbuluk N. Microneedling in skin of color: a review of uses and efficacy. J Am Acad Dermatol. 2016;74(2):348–55.
99. Arora P, Sarkar R, Garg VK, Arya L. Lasers for treatment of melasma and post-inflammatory hyperpigmentation. J Cutan Aesthet Surg. 2012;5(2):93.
100. Vashi NA. Cosmetic interventions for dyschromia: lasers. Aestheticians J. 2014;4(5):16–20.
101. Lee HC, Thng TG, Goh CL. Oral tranexamic acid (TA) in the treatment of melasma: a retrospective analysis. J Am Acad Dermatol. 2016;75(2):385–92.
102. Tse TW, Hui E. Tranexamic acid: an important adjuvant in the treatment of melasma. J Cosmet Dermatol. 2013;12(1):57–66.
103. Zhu H, Yang X. The clinical study of acidum tranexamicum on melasma. Pharm Prog. 2001;3:178–81.
104. Wu S, Shi H, Wu H, Yan S, Guo J, Sun Y, et al. Treatment of melasma with oral administration of tranexamic acid. Aesthetic Plast Surg. 2012;36(4):964–70.
105. Fisk WA, Agbai O, Lev-Tov HA, Sivamani RK. The use of botanically derived agents for hyperpigmentation: a systematic review. J Am Acad Dermatol. 2014;70(2):352–65.
106. Handog EB, Galang DA, de Leon-Godinez MA, Chan GP. A randomized, double-blind, placebo-controlled trial of oral procyanidin with vitamins A, C, E for melasma among Filipino women. Int J Dermatol. 2009;48(8):896–901.
107. Ni Z, Mu Y, Gulati O. Treatment of melasma with Pycnogenol. Phytother Res. 2002;16(6):567–71.
108. Ahmed AM, Lopez I, Perese F, Vasquez R, Hynan LS, Chong B, et al. A randomized, double-blinded, placebo-controlled trial of oral Polypodium leucotomos extract as an adjunct to sunscreen in the treatment of melasma. JAMA Dermatol. 2013;149(8):981–3.
109. Martin L, Caperton C, H W-L, editors. A randomized double-blind placebo controlled study evaluating the effectiveness and tolerability of oral Polypodium leucotomos in patients with melasma. American Academy of Dermatology Annual Meeting; March 15–20, 2012; San Diego, California.
110. Middelkamp-Hup MA, Pathak MA, Parrado C, Garcia-Caballero T, Rius-Diaz F, Fitzpatrick TB, et al. Orally administered Polypodium leucotomos extract decreases psoralen-UVA-induced phototoxicity, pigmentation, and damage of human skin. J Am Acad Dermatol. 2004;50(1):41–9.
111. Yamakoshi J, Otsuka F, Sano A, Tokutake S, Saito M, Kikuchi M, et al. Lightening effect on ultraviolet-induced pigmentation of guinea pig skin by oral administration of a proanthocyanidin-rich extract from grape seeds. Pigment Cell Res. 2003;16(6):629–38.
112. Yamakoshi J, Sano A, Tokutake S, Saito M, Kikuchi M, Kubota Y, et al. Oral intake of proanthocyanidin-rich extract from grape seeds improves chloasma. Phytother Res. 2004;18(11):895–9.
113. Malathi M, Thappa DM. Systemic skin whitening/lightening agents: what is the evidence? Indian J Dermatol Venereol Leprol. 2013;79(6):842–6.
114. Food and Drug Administration. DOH-FDA Advisory No. 2011–004: Safety on the off-label use of glutathione solution for injection (IV). Department of Health, editor. Republic of the Philippines 2011.
115. Wenczl E, Van der Schans GP, Roza L, Kolb RM, Timmerman AJ, Smit NP, et al. (Pheo) melanin photosensitizes UVA-induced DNA damage in cultured human melanocytes. J Invest Dermatol. 1998;111(4):678–82.

Chapter 24
Chemical Peels in Ethnic Skin

Judy Cheng and Neelam A. Vashi

Chemical peels have been used for decades to improve the cosmetic appearance of skin. Chemical peels create a superficial injury to the epidermis with the goal of stimulating new epidermal growth with more even melanin distribution [1]. Among darker skinned ethnic groups, common indications include lentigines, post-inflammatory hyperpigmentation (PIH), melasma, acne vulgaris, scarring, and pseudofolliculitis barbae [1] (Table 24.1).

Prior to peel initiation, pre-procedure protocols should be utilized. Procedures including laser hair removal, waxing, and facials should be stopped 1 week prior to peel initiation. Benzoyl peroxide and retinol products should be stopped 2–5 days beforehand. Photographic documentation, including full-face and areas of special interest, should be obtained prior to initiation of peels with patient consent. A pre-peel (priming) regimen consisting of glycolic acid (8–12%), hydroquinone, azelaic acid, kojic acid, or triple combination cream should be initiated, optimally 2–4 weeks before the first peel. The regimen should be discontinued 3 days before the peel [1, 31, 32]. Skin priming is important as it reduces healing time and risk of hyperpigmentation, as well as enabling more uniform penetration of the peeling agent [31]. Performing a test spot prior to initiating a series of peels may also be helpful to establish skin reactiveness. For PIH patients, test spots at specific, distinct sites of

J. Cheng
Department of Dermatology, Boston University Medical Center,
609 Albany Street, J-205, Boston 02118, MA, USA
e-mail: judy.cheng@bmc.org

N.A. Vashi (✉)
Department of Dermatology, Center for Ethnic Skin, Boston University,
Boston, MA, USA
e-mail: nvashi419@gmail.com

N.A. Vashi
Boston University School of Medicine, Boston Medical Center, Boston, MA, USA

© Springer International Publishing AG 2017
N.A. Vashi and H.I. Maibach (eds.), *Dermatoanthropology of Ethnic Skin and Hair*, DOI 10.1007/978-3-319-53961-4_24

Table 24.1 Chemical peel options for various dermatologic disorders

Condition	Alpha-hydroxy acids					Beta-hydroxy acids		Trichloroacetic acid	Jessner's solution	Retinoids
	Glycolic acid	Lactic acid	Phytic acid	Pyruvic acid	Salicylic-mandelic acid	Salicylic acid	β-Lipo-hydroxyacid			
Melasma	^[2]	^[3]	^a[4]	^[5]	^[4]	^[6]	*[7]	^[8]	^[9]	^[10]
Post-inflammatory hyperpigmentation	^[11]	*[7]		*[12]	^[13]	^b[6]	*[7]	*d[7]	*[7, 14]	
Acne	^[15]	^[16]		^[17]	^[13]	^[18]	^[19]	^e[20, 21]	^f[21, 22]	*[23]
Photoaging	^[24]			^[25]		^c[26]	^[27]	^e[28, 29]	^f[28, 29]	^[30]

Reference citations in square brackets
^Support of use demonstrated in literature
*Support of use by expert opinion
a In combination with glycolic acid, lactic acid, mandelic acid
b In combination with hydroquinone
c In combination with hydroquinone and glycolic acid
d In combination with glycolic acid
e In combination with Jessner's solution
f In combination with trichloroacetic acid

hyperpigmentation are a viable technique as different locations of the face are prone to behave uniquely [32, 33].

The following variables determine the depth of peeling: agent used, concentration, volume applied, time of contact, force of contact, frequency of application, integrity of the stratum corneum, and skin thickness [34]. Make-up is first removed and the eyes protected with moistened cotton pads or eye shields. Ear openings are covered with cottons balls, and the lips are protected with petrolatum [32]. Before applying a peeling agent, the area to be treated must first be degreased to facilitate even penetration of the agent. Degreasing agents include acetone or isopropyl alcohol and should be applied until no yellow residue is left on the gauze [1, 32]. Peeling agent solutions are usually started at a low concentration and titrated up to assess for tolerability. Gel formulations limit the harshness of solutions and allow for delivery of higher concentrations of acid with a lower risk of adverse events (i.e., scarring and dyspigmentation) [35]. Application tools include gauze, sponges, or brushes, but gauze may allow for more sensitive tactile pressure. Cotton-tipped applicators may facilitate direct placement of peeling agent onto acneiform lesions and areas of hyperpigmentation [32]. After the peeling agent is applied, hand-held fans can reduce intra-procedural discomfort. Patients typically experience a burning or tingling sensation for 2–5 min. The peel is then terminated with copious amounts of cold water or neutralizing agent, if indicated. A mild steroid or emollient cream can be applied afterwards as needed (i.e., erythema) [31].

Peeling Agents

Despite the many types of peels that are available today, limited studies have been conducted in the skin of color population. Given the tremendous variability in responses to chemical peels, it is up to the clinician to carefully select a peeling agent based on the patient, disorder under treatment, and safety and efficacy profiles of the agent.

Alpha-hydroxy Acids

Alpha-hydroxy acids (AHAs) are naturally occurring or synthetic carboxylic acids that have been used anecdotally since ancient Egyptian times for cosmetic purposes [1, 36]. They suppress melanin formation and accelerate epidermal turnover, thereby expediting pigment dispersion [37].

Glycolic Acid

Glycolic acid (GA) is naturally found in sugar cane and is the most commonly used AHA for chemical peeling [34]. At low concentrations (20%), it causes corneocyte detachment and desquamation, while at higher concentrations (70%), it induces epidermolysis below the level of the stratum corneum [31, 38]. It also thins the stratum corneum, disperses melanin in the basal layer, and increases collagen synthesis within the dermis [39, 40]. Indications for use include acne, acne scars, melasma, PIH, photoaging, and seborrhea [41]. It may be beneficial to place patients on a pre-peel regimen with a topical GA product to acclimatize the skin to a low pH and induce a preliminary desquamation before the peel. Frosting indicates epidermolysis and detachment from the papillary dermis. The peel is then terminated with sodium bicarbonate solution (8–15%). Post-peel erythema will then ensue, followed by desquamation [31]. In general, serial peels with partially buffered solutions starting at a lower percentage of 30–35% with upward titration allow for the best ability to improve pigmentation while avoiding side effects [42].

GA peels have repeatedly demonstrated efficacy in treating melasma in skin of color [11, 38, 43–45]. Javaheri et al. treated 25 Indian women with melasma with 50% GA peels. After 3 sessions, the Melasma Area Severity Index (MASI) score improved in 91% of patients, with a better response in epidermal-type melasma [2]. Multiple studies have investigated the combined efficacy of GA peels with topical therapies with the hypothesis that improvement in melasma may be expedited by removing the superficial layer of epidermis through chemical peeling. In 1 study, 31 patients (FST III–V) with melasma were treated with modified Kligmans formula (5% hydroquinone, 0.05% tretinoin, 1% hydrocortisone acetate) with or without serial GA (30–40%) peels. The peel group demonstrated more rapid and greater improvement compared to the topical treatment alone group [38]. Similar results were obtained by other studies using topical regimens of 2% hydroquinone/10% GA gel/0.05% tretinoin or 10% azelaic acid cream/0.1% adapalene gel, and peel concentrations ranging from 20 to 70% [11, 46].

Through similar reasoning, chemical peels may augment the effects of laser treatment by helping to remove the upper epidermis and allowing long wavelength lasers to better reach deeper dermal melanophages without side effects. Park et al. conducted a split-face trial among 16 Korean women with melasma wherein both sides of the face were treated with Q-switched neodymium-doped yttrium–aluminum–garnet laser (1064 QS Nd:YAG) at weekly intervals, with one side of the face additionally receiving a 30% GA peel immediately after laser treatment every 2 weeks. While both sides improved, there was greater improvement in the combination side (37.4 vs. 16.7%), with results maintained through a 5-month follow-up period [45]. GA peels are generally well tolerated in studies; there may be focal erythema and burning during the peeling process and some may develop superficial vesiculation afterwards, but these side effects generally self-resolve [11]. Superficial GA peels are an effective adjunct to topical agents or laser therapy to expedite clinical response.

Finally, GA peels have been successfully used to treat acne and PIH in skin of color [15, 22, 41, 47]. Sharad et al. demonstrated 20–35% GA peels performed every 15 days for 8–10 sessions can effectively clear PIH secondary to acne (FST

III–IV) [41]. For acne, 70% GA peels can improve comedonal acne rapidly, while papulopustular acne and nodulocystic lesions require more sessions [47].

Lactic Acid

Lactic acid, an AHA found in sour milk, is effective in treating melasma among skin types IV–V [36, 48]. In these studies, 82–92% lactic acid peels applied every 2 weeks for 12 weeks resulted in a significant decrease in MASI scores [36, 48]. Treatment efficacy and time to achieve results were similar compared to 70% GA [36, 44]. Lactic acid is furthermore well tolerated, with little to no side effects [36].

Lactic acid has also been successfully used to treat Lifa disease (frictional dermal melanosis). Although the pathogenesis of Lifa disease is still not completely understood, it is postulated that squeezing of the basal layer by the lifa (loofah) and underlying bone causes damage to melanocytes, leading to dyspigmentation. In a small study ($n = 52$), 92% lactic acid improved hyperpigmentation in all patients with no relapses in a follow-up period of 3 months [49].

Mandelic Acid

Mandelic acid is a widely used AHA that suppresses pigmentation and rejuvenates skin [50]. Compared to other AHAs, it has a larger molecular size, which allows it to more slowly and evenly penetrate the epidermis [50]. Combination 20% salicylic/10% mandelic acid peels have been shown to be as efficacious as 35% GA peels in treating melasma and may be better tolerated than the latter in Indian skin [4]. For PIH, 20% salicylic/10% mandelic acid peels were more efficacious than 35% GA ($p < 0.001$) in 1 study among FSTs IV–VI [13]. Furthermore, 30 and 50% mandelic acid peels may result in fewer side effects compared to GA peels (i.e., erythema, blistering) [50].

Phytic Acid

Phytic acid is a newer peel with a low pH that is often included as an ingredient in combination AHA peels. A commonly used formulation is a mixture of glycolic acid, lactic acid, mandelic acid, and phytic acid, offering two advantages compared to other AHA peels. First, it does not require neutralization, which eliminates the risk of overpeeling. Second, it does not cause a burning sensation. The peel is left on the face until the following morning and can be applied up to twice a week for a greater effect. In general, 5–6 peels are required before effects are appreciated [51]. Few studies have investigated its efficacy to date. Sarkar et al. demonstrated that a series of six 50% phytic combination peels (phytic acid, GA, lactic acid, mandelic acid) in Indian women ($n = 30$) reduced the MASI score by 44%. However, it was less efficacious compared to 35% GA and 20% salicylic/10% mandelic acid peels [4]. Given the scarcity of literature published, more studies are needed.

Pyruvic Acid

Pyruvic acid is an alpha-keto acid that physiologically converts to lactic acid. It is considered a potent medium-depth chemical peeling agent that penetrates to the upper papillary dermis [25]. Ghersetich et al. treated 20 patients (FST II–III) with signs of photoaging (i.e., freckles and lentigines) with 50% pyruvic acid peels. After 4 sessions, there was lightening of hyperpigmented lesions, and some lesions completely faded, though no statistical analyses were conducted [25]. Berardesca et al. similarly treated 20 women (FST II–III) with photodamage, superficial scarring, or melasma with a 50% pyruvic acid peel ($n = 20$) and achieved significant improvement in skin elasticity, hyperpigmentation, and wrinkling ($p < 0.05$). Furthermore, no subjects developed persistent erythema or PIH [5]. While some clinicians report pyruvic acid peels are associated with intense pain that subsides after neutralization with 10% sodium bicarbonate, pain has not been a significant adverse effect reported in the above studies [5, 25, 31]. Patients should expect erythema to last for 15 min, with a subsequent desquamation that lasts 3 days. There is no systemic toxicity associated with pyruvic acid, but vapors are pungent [31].

Of note, while pyruvic acid peels appear promising, no studies have been conducted in skin of color to date, and the associated intense burning has limited its use. Caution should be exercised since it is classified as a medium-depth chemical agent and, consequently, may cause PIH in more richly pigmented skin types.

Given the multitude of options for AHA peels, it is up to the clinician to choose an agent that is safe and efficacious for the condition under treatment. AHA peels are generally well tolerated in darker skinned people based on the limited studies to date.

Beta-hydroxy Acids

Salicylic Acid

SA is a naturally occurring compound found in willow tree bark that can be formulated in a variety of vehicles. It is commonly used to treat acne due to its lipophilic properties. It also induces desquamation of the upper layers of the stratum corneum and activates underlying fibroblasts. At lower concentrations (3–5%), it acts as a keratolytic agent, improving the penetration of other peeling agents, and, at higher concentrations (20–30%), it is used as a peeling agent [1, 31]. Given its anti-inflammatory effects, SA can decrease PIH caused from peeling itself [51]. Consequently, it is also used to treat melasma and PIH [1, 6, 31]. When applied to the face, patients may initially experience a burning sensation that soon decreases as salicylic acid causes a superficial anesthesia. One of the advantages of SA is the ability to monitor uniformity of application as a white precipitate (representing crystalline precipitation rather than protein agglutination that occurs with deep peels) forms upon evaporation of the vehicle (hydroethanolic or polyethylene glycol). For this reason, some clinicians prefer to spot-treat focal areas of PIH rather than applying the agent to the entire face. Spot treatment of PIH also allows greater matching between hyperpigmented skin and normal skin, unlike full-face treatment, which may cause a diffuse lightening of skin [1]. The peel can then be terminated with water as no neutralization solution is necessary. Desquamation occurs 2–3 days later and lasts for up to 7 days. Although it is generally well tolerated, there is a risk of systemic toxicity, salicylism, so caution should be exercised if extensive areas are to be treated [31].

Several studies have documented the efficacy of SA peels in treating acne in ethnic populations. Lee et al. treated 35 Korean women with facial acne with 30% SA peels biweekly for 12 weeks and noted a reduction in inflammatory and non-inflammatory acne in proportion to treatment duration. Side effects included dryness that responded to emollients, and intense exfoliation that cleared by 10 days. There was no persistent PIH or scarring [52]. These results mirror those of Ahn et al., who treated a similar population and noted improvement in skin lightness and decreased redness [53].

Results have been more mixed with respect to efficacy of treating hyperpigmentary disorders. Joshi et al. conducted a split-face study comparing 20–30% SA peels with no treatment among 10 patients with PIH (FST IV–VI). After five peels, there was no significant improvement as rated by blinded dermatologists, but the peels were well tolerated [54]. Conversely, in a study by Grimes et al. ($n = 25$, FST V–VI), 20–30% SA peels in combination with 4% hydroquinone resulted in >50% improvement in 100% of PIH and 66% of melasma patients. Side effects were minimal and included transient dryness and hyperpigmentation [6]. However, when 20–30% SA peels were examined as an adjunctive agent to hydroquinone in a split-face study, the authors found no additional improvement with peels [55].

β-lipohydroxy Acid

β-lipohydroxy acid (LHA) is a derivative of SA that is widely used in Europe and has recently been introduced in the U.S. [56]. Compared to SA, it has an extra fatty chain, which increases its lipophilic properties and ability to target pilosebaceous units [57]. Unlike SA and GA, where there is partial detachment of cells causing uneven exfoliation, LHA detaches individual corneosomes in a uniform manner that mimics the natural turnover of skin. This may contribute to the smooth appearance of skin after LHA peels. LHA (up to 10%) is furthermore well tolerated given that its pH is similar to that of normal skin (pH 5.5) [56].

Levesque et al. conducted a split-face trial comparing LHA and SA peels among 20 patients with comedonal acne. Both showed a significant reduction in non-inflammatory lesions, but there was no difference in efficacy between the two [19]. In another study, 43 patients with signs of photoaging were randomized to receive LHA (5–10%) or GA (20–50%) peels. After 6 sessions, there was a significant reduction in fine lines, wrinkles, and hyperpigmentation. Furthermore, the efficacy of the 4 LHA peels was equivalent to that achieved by GA after 6 peels [7, 58]. This suggests that LHA may potentially offer higher efficacy compared to traditional AHA peels. More studies are needed, though, especially in skin of color.

Trichloroacetic Acid

TCA, an inorganic compound found in crystalline form, is an acetic acid that induces destruction of the epidermis and upper papillary dermis, followed by epidermal and dermal rejuvenation [1]. It produces a white frost whose intensity correlates with depth of penetration. For instance, a superficial TCA peel may only show erythema or irregular light frost.

When used to treat melasma, 1 study found that 10–15% TCA acted more rapidly than 55–75% GA peels [8]. However, TCA was associated with more side effects including tingling, burning sensation, post-peel cracking, as well as a higher relapse rate [8]. A subsequent study confirmed the initial faster response to TCA but showed no significant difference between TCA and GA at the end of 12 weeks [59]. Based on these studies, GA may be the agent of choice if fewer side effects are desired, while TCA is the preferable agent if a rapid response is desired.

Practically, treating lentigines may best be accomplished with TCA compared to GA. TCA produces an even frost over a discrete area, while GA spreads diffusely across the face and has no color to facilitate treatment monitoring [1]. Conversely, mottled pigmentation that typically affects large portions of the face may benefit from GA or SA peels [1].

Jessner's Solution

Jessner's solution is composed of a combination of resorcinol (14 g), SA (14 g), lactic acid (85%), and ethanol (95%) [1]. These keratolytic compounds work synergistically to expedite keratinocyte turnover, with resorcinol (phenol) additionally serving as a hypopigmenting agent. It is used with caution in skin types V and VI as it may cause depigmentation, with some clinicians asserting that it should never be used in skin type VI [1, 60]. Jessner's solution and TCA peels are both more efficacious than topical hydroquinone with kojic acid in treating melasma among skin types III and IV. However, TCA was shown to have a more long-term effect compared to Jessner's solution and topical agents [61]. Furthermore, Jessner's solution can add significant adjunctive benefit when used with 15% TCA

[9]. Compared to lactic acid, Jessner's solution has demonstrated similar efficacy and is also well tolerated [3].

Retinoids

In two studies ($n = 10$, $n = 63$) among darker skin types, 1% tretinoin peels were as efficacious as 70% GA peels in treating melasma and were, furthermore, less irritating to the skin [62, 63]. Time to therapeutic response was also similar [63]. Compared to topical tretinoin, tretinoin peels have more rapid therapeutic response (24 vs. 12 weeks, respectively) [62].

Retinoic acid peels (5–10%), also known as the yellow peel, can be used for facial melanosis, acne, and photoaging. As it is a superficial peel, it has few side effects. Retinoic acid is applied until a uniform yellow frost appears (usually 2–3 layers), and the patient can wash it off at home after 6–8 hours. This procedure may be repeated bimonthly [23].

Recently, interest has grown over whether microdermabrasion can augment the effects of peeling agents. In one study, participants were treated with a 5% retinoic acid peel with or without pre-treatment with microdermabrasion. Patients who underwent microdermabrasion reported greater satisfaction in skin texture and pigmentation compared to participants who received the peel alone [64, 65].

Post-treatment

After completing a chemical peel, patients can resume normal cleansing with gentle agents after 24 hours [1]. Emollients and mild steroids can be used as needed, but tretinoin and AHAs should be avoided for at least 1 week. Meticulous sunscreen protection with SPF ≥ 30 is critical during the post-peel period [31]. A 3–6 week interval between peels is appropriate for an effective response.

Conclusion

Chemical peels are an efficacious tool to treat a myriad of dermatologic disorders in skin of color patients. While there exists a higher risk of post-procedural hyperpigmentation and scar formation, these risks can be minimized with judicious choice of peels and candidate selection. Multiple peels are usually needed to obtain the desired clinical effect, and a maintenance regimen should be followed after to prevent relapse. Of note, to avoid complications, deeper peels should be avoided.

References

1. Roberts WE. Chemical peeling in ethnic/dark skin. Dermatol Ther. 2004;17(2):196–205.
2. Javaheri SM, Handa S, Kaur I, Kumar B. Safety and efficacy of glycolic acid facial peel in Indian women with melasma. Int J Dermatol. 2001;40(5):354–7.
3. Sharquie KE, Al-Tikreety MM, Al-Mashhadani SA. Lactic acid chemical peels as a new therapeutic modality in melasma in comparison to Jessner's solution chemical peels. Dermatol Surg. 2006;32(12):1429–36.
4. Sarkar R, Garg V, Bansal S, Sethi S, Gupta C. Comparative evaluation of efficacy and tolerability of glycolic acid, salicylic mandelic acid, and phytic acid combination peels in melasma. Dermatol Surg. 2016;42(3):384–91.
5. Berardesca E, Cameli N, Primavera G, Carrera M. Clinical and instrumental evaluation of skin improvement after treatment with a new 50% pyruvic acid peel. Dermatol Surg. 2006;32(4):526–31.
6. Grimes PE. The safety and efficacy of salicylic acid chemical peels in darker racial-ethnic groups. Dermatol Surg. 1999;25(1):18–22.
7. Berson DS, Cohen JL, Rendon MI, Roberts WE, Starker I, Wang B. Clinical role and application of superficial chemical peels in today's practice. J Drugs Derm. 2009;8(9):803–11.
8. Kalla G, Garg A, Kachhawa D. Chemical peeling-glycolic acid versus trichloroacetic acid in melasma. Indian J Dermatol Venereol Leprol. 2001;67(2):82–4.
9. Safoury OS, Zaki NM, El Nabarawy EA, Farag EA. A study comparing chemical peeling using modified Jessner's solution and 15% trichloroacetic Acid versus 15% trichloroacetic acid in the treatment of melasma. Indian J Dermatol. 2009;54(1):41–5.
10. Kligman DE. Tretinoin peels versus glycolic acid peels. Dermatol Surg. 2004;30(12 Pt 2):1609.
11. Burns RL, Prevost-Blank PL, Lawry MA, Lawry TB, Faria DT, Fivenson DP. Glycolic acid peels for postinflammatory hyperpigmentation in black patients. A comparative study. Dermatol Surg. 1997;23(3):171–4; discussion 5.
12. De Padova M, Tosti A. Types of chemical peels: advantages/disadvantages, an illustrated algorithm. In: Tosti A, Grimes PE, De Padova M, editors. Color atlas of chemical peels. 2nd ed. Berlin: Springer; 2012.
13. Garg VK, Sinha S, Sarkar R. Glycolic acid peels versus salicylic-mandelic acid peels in active acne vulgaris and post-acne scarring and hyperpigmentation: a comparative study. Dermatol Surg. 2009;35(1):59–65.
14. Soriano T, Grimes P. Postinflammatory hyperpigmentation. In: Tosti A, Grimes P, De Padova M, editors. Color atlas of chemical peels. 2nd ed. Berlin: Springer; 2012.
15. Wang CM, Huang CL, Hu CT, Chan HL. The effect of glycolic acid on the treatment of acne in Asian skin. Dermatol Surg. 1997;23(1):23–9.
16. Sachdeva S. Lactic acid peeling in superficial acne scarring in Indian skin. J Cosmet Dermatol. 2010;9(3):246–8.
17. Cotellessa C, Manunta T, Ghersetich I, Brazzini B, Peris K. The use of pyruvic acid in the treatment of acne. J Eur Acad Dermatol Venereol. 2004;18(3):275–8.
18. Kessler E, Flanagan K, Chia C, Rogers C, Anna Glaser D. Comparison of α-and β-hydroxy acid chemical peels in the treatment of mild to moderately severe facial acne vulgaris. Dermatol Surg. 2008;34(1):45–51.
19. Levesque A, Hamzavi I, Seite S, Rougier A, Bissonnette R. Randomized trial comparing a chemical peel containing a lipophilic hydroxy acid derivative of salicylic acid with a salicylic acid peel in subjects with comedonal acne. J Cosmet Dermatol. 2011;10(3):174–8.
20. Fabbrocini G, De Padova M, Cacciapouti S, Tosti A. Acne. In: Tosti A, Grimes P, De Padova M, editors. Color atlas of chemical peels. 2nd ed. Berlin: Springer; 2012.
21. Al-Waiz MM, Al-Sharqi AI. Medium-depth chemical peels in the treatment of acne scars in dark-skinned individuals. Dermatol Surg. 2002;28(5):383–7.

22. Kim SW, Moon SE, Kim JA, Eun HC. Glycolic acid versus Jessner's solution: which is better for facial acne patients? A randomized prospective clinical trial of split-face model therapy. Dermatol Surg. 1999;25(4):270–3.
23. Nagaraju U, AS S. Practical problems in chemical peels. In: Pai GS, editor. Complications in cosmetic dermatology: crafting cures. 1st ed. USA: Jaypee Medical Inc; 2016.
24. Newman N, Newman A, Moy LS, Babapour R, Harris AG, Moy RL. Clinical improvement of photoaged skin with 50% glycolic acid. A double-blind vehicle-controlled study. Dermatol Surg. 1996;22(5):455–60.
25. Ghersetich I, Brazzini B, Peris K, Cotellessa C, Manunta T, Lotti T. Pyruvic acid peels for the treatment of photoaging. Dermatol Surg. 2004;30(1):32–6.
26. Gladstone HB, Nguyen SL, Williams R, Ottomeyer T, Wortzman M, Jeffers M, et al. Efficacy of hydroquinone cream (USP 4%) used alone or in combination with salicylic acid peels in improving photodamage on the neck and upper chest. Dermatol Surg. 2000;26(4):333–7.
27. Oresajo C, Yatskayer M, Hansenne I. Clinical tolerance and efficacy of capryloyl salicylic acid peel compared to a glycolic acid peel in subjects with fine lines/wrinkles and hyperpigmented skin. J Cosmet Dermatol. 2008;7(4):259–62.
28. Monheit GD. Combination medium-depth peeling: the Jessner's+ TCA peel. Facial Plast Surg. 1996;12(2):117–24.
29. Kadhim K, Al-Waiz M. Treatment of periorbital wrinkles by repeated medium-depth chemical peels in dark-skinned individuals. J Cosmet Dermatol. 2005;4(1):18–22.
30. Cucé LC, Bertino M, Scattone L, Birkenhauer MC. Tretinoin peeling. Dermatol Surg. 2001;27(1):12–4.
31. Zakopoulou N, Kontochristopoulos G. Superficial chemical peels. J Cosmet Dermatol. 2006;5(3):246–53.
32. Vashi NA. Cosmetic interventions for dyschromia: chemical peels. Aestheticians J. 2014;30–2.
33. Swinehart JM. Test spots in dermabrasion and chemical peeling. J Dermatol Surg Oncol. 1990;16(6):557–63.
34. Gupta RR, Mahajan BB, Garg G. Chemical peeling-evaluation of glycolic acid in varying concentrations and time intervals. Indian J Dermatol Venereol Leprol. 2001;67(1):28–9.
35. Cook KK, Cook WR. Chemical peel of nonfacial skin using glycolic acid gel augmented with TCA and neutralized based on visual staging. Dermatol Surg. 2000;26(11):994–9.
36. Sharquie KE, Al-Tikreety MM, Al-Mashhadani SA. Lactic acid as a new therapeutic peeling agent in melasma. Dermatol Surg. 2005;31(2):149–54.
37. Kornhauser A, Coelho SG, Hearing VJ. Applications of hydroxy acids: classification, mechanisms, and photoactivity. Clin Cosmet Investig Dermatol. 2010;3:135–42.
38. Sarkar R, Kaur C, Bhalla M, Kanwar AJ. The combination of glycolic acid peels with a topical regimen in the treatment of melasma in dark-skinned patients: a comparative study. Dermatol Surg. 2002;28(9):828–32; discussion 32.
39. Van Scott EJ, Yu RJ. Hyperkeratinization, corneocyte cohesion, and alpha hydroxy acids. J Am Acad Dermatol. 1984;11(5 Pt 1):867–79.
40. Tung RC, Bergfeld WF, Vidimos AT, Remzi BK. Alpha-hydroxy acid-based cosmetic procedures. Guidelines for patient management. Am J Clin Dermatol. 2000;1(2):81–8.
41. Sharad J. Glycolic acid peel therapy—a current review. Clin Cosmet Investig Dermatol. 2013;6:281–8.
42. Grimes P. Chemical peels in dark skin. In: Tosti A, Grimes PE, De Padova M, editors. Color atlas of chemical peels. 2nd ed. Berlin: Springer; 2012.
43. Sehgal VN, Luthra A, Aggarwal AK. Evaluation of graded strength glycolic acid (GA) facial peel: an Indian experience. J Dermatol. 2003;30(10):758–61.
44. Lawrence N, Cox SE, Brody HJ. Treatment of melasma with Jessner's solution versus glycolic acid: a comparison of clinical efficacy and evaluation of the predictive ability of Wood's light examination. J Am Acad Dermatol. 1997;36(4):589–93.
45. Park KY, Kim DH, Kim HK, Li K, Seo SJ, Hong CK. A randomized, observer-blinded, comparison of combined 1064-nm Q-switched neodymium-doped yttrium-aluminium-garnet

laser plus 30% glycolic acid peel vs. laser monotherapy to treat melasma. Clin Exp Dermatol. 2011;36(8):864–70.

46. Erbil H, Sezer E, Tastan B, Arca E, Kurumlu Z. Efficacy and safety of serial glycolic acid peels and a topical regimen in the treatment of recalcitrant melasma. J Dermatol. 2007;34 (1):25–30.

47. Atzori L, Brundu MA, Orru A, Biggio P. Glycolic acid peeling in the treatment of acne. J Eur Acad Dermatol Venereol. 1999;12(2):119–22.

48. Singh R, Goyal S, Ahmed QR, Gupta N, Singh S. Effect of 82% lactic acid in treatment of melasma. Int Sch Res Notices. 2014;2014(407142):1–7.

49. Sharquie KE, Al-Dhalimi MA, Noaimi AA, Al-Sultany HA. Lactic acid as a new therapeutic peeling agent in the treatment of lifa disease (frictional dermal melanosis). Indian J Dermatol. 2012;57(6):444–8.

50. Taylor MB. Summary of mandelic acid for the improvement of skin conditions. Cosmet Dermatol. 1999;12:26–8.

51. Sarkar R, Bansal S, Garg VK. Chemical peels for melasma in dark-skinned patients. J Cutan Aesthet Surg. 2012;5(4):247–53.

52. Lee HS, Kim IH. Salicylic acid peels for the treatment of acne vulgaris in Asian patients. Dermatol Surg. 2003;29(12):1196–9; discussion 9.

53. Ahn HH, Kim IH. Whitening effect of salicylic acid peels in Asian patients. Dermatol Surg. 2006;32(3):372–5; discussion 5.

54. Joshi SS, Boone SL, Alam M, Yoo S, White L, Rademaker A, et al. Effectiveness, safety, and effect on quality of life of topical salicylic acid peels for treatment of postinflammatory hyperpigmentation in dark skin. Dermatol Surg. 2009;35(4):638–44; discussion 44.

55. Kodali S, Guevara IL, Carrigan CR, Daulat S, Blanco G, Boker A, et al. A prospective, randomized, split-face, controlled trial of salicylic acid peels in the treatment of melasma in Latin American women. J Am Acad Dermatol. 2010;63(6):1030–5.

56. Rendon MI, Berson DS, Cohen JL, Roberts WE, Starker I, Wang B. Evidence and considerations in the application of chemical peels in skin disorders and aesthetic resurfacing. J Clin Aesthet Dermatol. 2010;3(7):32–43.

57. Saint-Leger D, Leveque JL, Verschoore M. The use of hydroxy acids on the skin: characteristics of C8-lipohydroxy acid. J Cosmet Dermatol. 2007;6(1):59–65.

58. LaRoche-Posay. Data on file. Scientific File; 2008.

59. Kumari R, Thappa DM. Comparative study of trichloroacetic acid versus glycolic acid chemical peels in the treatment of melasma. Indian J Dermatol Venereol Leprol. 2010;76 (4):447.

60. Quarles FN, Brody H, Johnson BA, Badreshia S. Chemical peels in richly pigmented patients. Dermatol Ther. 2007;20(3):147–8.

61. Azzam OA, Leheta TM, Nagui NA, Shaarawy E, Hay RM, Hilal RF. Different therapeutic modalities for treatment of melasma. J Cosmet Dermatol. 2009;8(4):275–81.

62. Khunger N, Sarkar R, Jain RK. Tretinoin peels versus glycolic acid peels in the treatment of melasma in dark-skinned patients. Dermatol Surg. 2004;30(5):756–60.

63. Faghihi G, Shahingohar A, Siadat AH. Comparison between 1% tretinoin peeling versus 70% glycolic acid peeling in the treatment of female patients with melasma. J Drugs Derm. 2011;10(12):1439–42.

64. Grimes PE. Combination of microdermabrasion and chemical peels. Color atlas of chemical peels. Berlin: Springer; 2011. p. 81–6.

65. Briden E, Jacobsen E, Johnson C. Combining superficial glycolic acid (alpha-hydroxy acid) peels with microdermabrasion to maximize treatment results and patient satisfaction. Cutis. 2007;79(1 Suppl Combining):13–6.

Chapter 25
Laser Treatment in Ethnic Skin

Judy Cheng and Neelam A. Vashi

Lasers (Light Amplification by Stimulated Emission of Radiation) are an important addition to the arsenal of treatment options for dermatologic conditions. Currently, conditions that are frequently treated with lasers include pigmentary disorders, nevi, unwanted hair, vascular lesions, scars, and photoaging (Table 25.1) [1]. While there is an abundance of literature on its use in lighter skin types (Fitzpatrick skin types (FST) I-II), there remains a paucity of data in darker skin types. This disparity is due in part to patient candidacy and also clinician hesitancy to try laser therapy on ethnic patients due to the risk of scarring and dyspigmentation. At the same time, the demand for laser procedures in darker skin types continues to grow [49]. By providing an understanding of laser principles and efficacy data for various dermatologic conditions in skin of color, clinicians may be equipped with the tools to provide safe laser treatment for ethnic patients.

Laser Principles

Laser light therapy relies on the absorption of light energy by target chromophores in the skin. There exist 3 main endogenous chromophores (melanin, hemoglobin/ oxyhemoglobin, and water) and several exogenous chromophores (i.e., psoralens,

J. Cheng
Department of Dermatology, Boston University Medical Center,
609 Albany Street, J-205, Boston, MA 02118, USA
e-mail: judy.cheng@bmc.org

N.A. Vashi (✉)
Department of Dermatology, Center for Ethnic Skin, Boston University,
Boston, MA, USA
e-mail: nvashi419@gmail.com

N.A. Vashi
Boston University School of Medicine, Boston Medical Center,
Boston, MA, USA

© Springer International Publishing AG 2017
N.A. Vashi and H.I. Maibach (eds.), *Dermatoanthropology of Ethnic Skin and Hair*, DOI 10.1007/978-3-319-53961-4_25

Table 25.1 Studies of Treatment indications of various types of lasers

Conditions	Q-switched ruby	Q-switched alexandrite	Q-switched Nd:YAG	Intense pulsed light	Pulsed dye laser	Fractional photothermolysis
Nevus of Ota	[2]	[15, 16]				
Acquired bilateral nevus of Ota-like macules			[3]			
Hori nevi	[4]					
Exogenous ochronosis	[5]	[6]				
Minocycline-induced hyperpigmentation	[8, 9]	[10, 11]	[7]			[12]
Chloroquine-induced hyperpigmentation	[13]					
Hydroxychloroquine-induced hyperpigmentation	[13]					
Amiodarone-induced hyperpigmentation	[14]		[15]			
Melasma	[16, 17][a]		[18, 19]	[20, 21]	[22]	[23, 24]
Photoaging			[19]			[25]
Periorbital rhytides						[26]
Post-inflammatory hyperpigmentation	[16, 27][a]		[28]			[29]
Café au lait macules	[30][a]					
Tattoos		[31]	[32, 33]			
Lentigines		[34]		[34]	[35]	
Ephelides		[34]		[34]		
Unwanted hair		[36–38] (long pulse)		[39][a]		

(continued)

Table 25.1 (continued)

Conditions	Q-switched ruby	Q-switched alexandrite	Q-switched Nd: YAG	Intense pulsed light	Pulsed dye laser	Fractional photothermolysis
Dermatosis papulosa nigra			[40]			[41]
Poikiloderma of Civatte				[42, 43]		
Port-wine stain					[44, 45]	
Hemangiomas					[46]	
Scars					[47]	[48]

[a]Treatment ineffective or caused worsening of lesions

tattoo ink), in which each has unique absorption spectrums. Delivery to the skin occurs via a continuous, quasi-continuous, or pulsed mode (long duration in milliseconds, short duration in nanoseconds, or ultra-short duration in picoseconds). When light of a specific wavelength is absorbed by a chromophore, it undergoes a photochemical reaction whereby light energy is converted to heat energy, causing destruction of the chromophore. In the process, heat diffuses to the cooler surrounding tissue in a process called thermal relaxation. The time it takes for the target chromophore to cool down to 50% of its initial temperature is analogously called the thermal relaxation time (TRT). By the theory of selective photothermolysis, when light of a certain wavelength is emitted in a period of time shorter than the TRT of the target chromophore, the target can be selectively destroyed without damage to surrounding tissue. Clinicians can therefore vary wavelength, pulse duration (exposure time to the laser), and fluence (amount of energy delivered to an area of skin; J/cm^2) parameters to selectively destroy targets [49, 50].

Special Considerations in Skin of Color

Differences in skin color between darker and lighter skin types are due to the amount, density, and distribution of melanin [51]. As melanin has a broad absorption spectrum (250–1200 nm), light intended to reach dermal targets may be competitively absorbed by the highly melanized epidermis in richly pigmented skin types and cause scarring and dyspigmentation. This competitive absorption also decreases the efficacy of lasers in darker skin types when using equivalent fluences in lighter skin types [51].

However, longer wavelengths, longer pulse durations, and wider, yet conservative, fluence ranges can circumvent these difficulties. Longer wavelengths (>600 nm) enable deeper dermal penetration and more selective absorption of dermal chromophores [52]. Longer pulse durations permit slower heating and more efficient cooling of the epidermis, but higher energies must be used to obtain efficacious treatment [51]. The TRT of melanosomes is in nanoseconds, and so pulse durations in the milliseconds prevent melanosome destruction [49]. Using efficient cooling devices (i.e., sapphire cooled tip, cryogen spray cooling (CSC), forced air cooling) may also prevent overheating of the epidermis and reduce adverse effects [51]. Finally, choosing the lowest fluence necessary to achieve results should be used. Test spots should be conducted in representative yet non-visible areas to identify the ideal fluence for each patient [49].

Laser Consultation

Determining if a patient would be an appropriate candidate for laser therapy first involves a detailed medical history, focusing on conditions that may affect postoperative healing. Patients with a tendency to form keloids or hypertrophic scars should not undergo laser treatment deeper than the papillary dermis [53]. Patients with a history of herpes simplex virus should be placed on a prophylactic course of antiviral therapy and continued on it until complete re-epithelialization of the skin has occurred. Lastly, it is crucial that patient goals and realistic treatment expectations be in alignment. Potential side effects and post-treatment expectations should be reviewed [49].

Pretreatment

Before treatment, patients may benefit from a topical priming regimen with skin lightening properties (i.e., hydroquinone, azelaic acid, kojic acid). Photographic documentation should be obtained of the full-face as well as specific treatment areas to better appreciate improvement.

Test spots, typically performed in the post-auricular area, can be conducted to identify optimal laser settings. 2 to 4 fluences are usually tested, with a 48 hour wait time afterwards to assess for side effects. Of note, test spots are not always predictive of outcome as different areas of the face and body may respond uniquely given intrinsic skin differences and involved treatment sites of sun-protected versus sun-exposed areas [51].

Types of Lasers

Ruby Laser (694 nm)

Q-switched (QS) lasers emit high-energy light in short pulses. This contrasts with continuous wave lasers, which emit a continuous output of light. Pulses of light energy provide the advantage of limiting thermal necrosis to a target thus limiting damage to surrounding tissue [54]. The QS ruby laser (QSRL) emits light at 694 nm and can be used to treat pigmented lesions with limited bruising, as it is not absorbed by hemoglobin [52]. The QSRL is more selective for melanin compared to the QS neodymium-doped yttrium aluminum garnet (Nd:YAG) laser (1064 nm), and so theoretically, should be more effective. However, results have been mixed, and its role in treating melasma is controversial and overall not recommended. Taylor et al. found QSRLs ineffective in treating melasma and post-inflammatory hyperpigmentation (PIH) ($n = 8$) and furthermore caused darkening in some cases [16]. Similarly, in a small study comparing QSRL with QS Nd:YAG, neither laser was effective in treating melasma ($n = 3$), and both caused PIH after only 1 treatment session [17]. Jang et al. [55] investigated whether repeat low-dose fractional-mode QSRL may better treat melasma with the hypothesis that a sublethal cumulative dose of energy will fragment melanin but not destroy cells

(n = 15, FST III-IV). While the majority experienced a 30% improvement in the Melasma Area and Severity Index (MASI) score after 6 sessions, 2 developed a higher MASI score and 2 had no change [55].

QSRL has also been used successfully to treat a variety of drug-induced hyperpigmentation. Minocycline-induced hyperpigmentation has responded well to QSRL, clearing all cases in 2 studies with no side effects [8, 9]. One case of chloroquine and hydroxychloroquine-induced gray-blue hyperpigmentation was treated with QSRL for 3 sessions with significant improvement. Post-laser biopsy revealed reduced melanin deposits in the papillary and mid-dermis [13]. QSRL and QS Nd:YAG have both successfully treated amiodarone-induced hyperpigmentation, with complete resolution using the QSRL [14, 15].

Nevus of Ota and acquired bilateral nevus of Ota-like macules (ABNOM) can also be treated with QSRL. In a large-scale study, Watanabe and Takahashi treated 114 Asian patients with nevus of Ota with QSRL (fluence 6 J/cm^2, pulse duration 30 ns) at 3–4 month intervals. Ninety-four percent of patients who received 4 or 5 treatments had $\geq 70\%$ of lightening of lesions. No patients developed hypertrophic or atrophic scarring [2]. These results mirror the previous results of Taylor et al. and Geronemus et al. [56, 57]. For ABNOM, 1 study treated 140 patients with QSRL (fluence 7–10 J/cm^2, 1 Hz), and 93% of patients achieved complete clearance. Unfortunately, 3 patients developed long-term hypopigmentation [4].

QSRL is less effective in treating café au lait macules and PIH. In a study comparing QSRL and QS Nd:YAG-treated café au lait macules, both lasers yielded variable responses, including causing lightening and darkening of lesions. Histologic subtypes of these lesions furthermore did not predict response to laser treatment [30]. Two studies have found QSRL to be ineffective in treating PIH [16, 27].

Although QSRL is a mainstay in the treatment of dyschromias (i.e., nevus of Ota/Ito, Hori nevi) among skin of color patients with lighter FSTs, its overall use is not recommended in the ethnic population.

Alexandrite (755 nm)

Alexandrite lasers at a wavelength of 755 nm can be used in short- and long-pulsed modalities. QS alexandrite lasers (QSAL) have been used to treat nevus of Ota, drug-induced hyperpigmentation, tattoos, lentigines, and ephelides. Although the sample sizes were small (n = 3 and n = 4), the picosecond alexandrite laser was successful in treating nevus of Ota with >50% improvement in 2 studies [58, 59]. In another small study, 3 patients with minocycline-induced facial pigmentation were successfully treated with the picosecond alexandrite in 1 to 2 sessions [10]. Vangipuram et al. [11] achieved 100% clearance of minocycline-induced facial pigmentation with nonablative photothermolysis followed by 1 session with the alexandrite laser.

Few studies have investigated the role of alexandrite lasers in the removal of unwanted tattoos and hair. In 1 study among 20 Arabic patients (FST III-IV), QSAL (fluence 4–7.5 J/cm^2, pulse duration 100 ns) in 6–12 week treatment intervals led to >75% lightening in 75% of patients after 3–6 sessions. None developed dyspigmentation or scarring [31]. For the treatment of lentigines and ephelides, 1 study compared the efficacy of intense pulsed light (IPL) therapy versus QSAL. While ephelides responded more rapidly to IPL compared to QSAL, there was no difference in efficacy in the treatment of lentigines. PIH furthermore occurred more frequently among patients treated with QSAL [34]. Long- pulsed alexandrite lasers can safely destroy hair follicles without damage to epidermal melanin in some darker skinned populations. This treatment modality for unwanted hair in the skin of color population is typically limited to FSTs III/IV [36–38]. Overall, alexandrite lasers should be used with caution in FST IV-VI as it can lead to PIH [34].

Nd:YAG (1064 nm)

Nd:YAG lasers at a wavelength of 1064 nm can be used in short- and long-pulsed modalities. The QS Nd:YAG laser produces light at a wavelength of 1064 nm but can be frequency-doubled to emit green light at 534 nm. The long wavelength is more suitable for treating dermal lesions, while the 532 nm light is better for epidermal pigmentation [60]. This section will focus on the 1064 nm QS Nd:YAG. The 1064 nm long-pulsed modality can be used for other dermatologic conditions (i.e., unwanted hair, scars, vascular lesions) and will be covered in another chapter.

The QS Nd:YAG (1064 nm) is the most popular laser choice for the treatment of pigmentation disorders, and the most commonly employed laser for the treatment of melasma. Its long wavelength provides two advantages. First, it can target dermal melanin while limiting damage to the epidermis. Second, it can target the upper dermal vascular plexus, which can be a pathologic factor in melasma [52]. In a review of 10 studies among darker skinned ethnic groups, Arora et al. reported that the majority of patients with melasma treated with QS Nd:YAG laser improved, even in cases of refractory and dermal melasma [52]. Settings used include fluence <5 J/cm^2, 6 mm spot size, and a frequency of 10 Hz [61]. Common side effects included mottled hypopigmentation, erythema, and burning. However, they can be minimized by avoiding too frequent (weekly) and too many laser sessions (>6–10 sessions) [52].

"Laser toning" is an increasingly popular method for nonablative skin rejuvenation and treatment of melasma in East Asia. It involves repetitive low-fluence (1.6–3.5 J/cm^2), large spot size (6–8 mm), multiple-passed treatment with the QS Nd:YAG laser. It is repeated every 1-2 weeks for a total treatment duration ranging from weeks to months [62]. Laser toning is postulated to improve melasma through sublethal injury to melanosomes and melanocytes, which causes fragmentation of melanin granules into surrounding cytoplasm without cellular destruction [19]. Cho et al. treated 25 Korean patients with low pulse energy 1064 QS Nd:YAG laser;

specifically, 2.5 J/cm^2 to the whole face, followed by an additional 4–5 J/cm^2 over melasma lesions. After 1 to 5 treatment sessions, 44% of patients showed marked improvement and 28% near-total improvement [18]. These results were echoed by Choi et al., who demonstrated lightening of melasma and tightening of wrinkles after five treatments at 1 week intervals with low-fluence QS Nd:YAG ($n = 20$, fluence 2–3.5 J/cm^2) [19]. When low-fluence QS Nd:YAG was combined with microdermabrasion in 1 study ($n = 27$, FST II-V), 81% of patients had >75% clearance with remission lasting through 6 months. Of the 9 patients who were followed up at 12 months, 89% maintained their clearance [63].

Of note, prolonged use of low-fluence QS Nd:YAG has been associated with the development of punctate leukoderma, described as white, round, confetti-like macules [18, 61, 64]. Wattanakrai et al. [61] reported 8 out of 22 patients treated with QS Nd:YAG (3.0–3.8 J/cm^2) developed punctate leukoderma after multiple treatment sessions. Kim et al. used lower fluences (1.6 J/cm^2 to the face and 2.2– 2.5 J/cm^2 for melasma lesions) and reported 3 out of 259 patients with punctate leukoderma. Possible mechanisms for laser-induced depigmentation include cumulative subthreshold additive effects, excessive fluences causing direct photo-toxicity and cellular damage to melanocytes, intrinsic unevenness of skin, and non-uniform laser energy output [62]. More studies are needed to determine the optimal number of treatment sessions and interval period. In the interim, patients should be monitored for the earliest sign of hypopigmentation and laser treatment terminated upon development.

QS Nd:YAG has also been used to successfully treat other pigmentary disorders including PIH, ABNOM, tattoos, exogenous ochronosis, and dermatosis papulosa nigra (DPN) [3, 7, 28, 32, 33, 40]. In two small studies, the QS Nd:YAG completely cleared charcoal tattoos in FST V-VI ($n = 4$) and lightened the majority of black-pigmented tattoos by >75% in FST IV ($n = 8$, 8/15 tattoos) [32, 33]. Tan et al. treated 6 Chinese patients with exogenous ochronosis using the QS Nd:YAG laser (fluence 1.2 J/cm^2 on first pass, 4–6 J/cm^2 on second to fourth pass). All patients exhibited improvement, especially those with Dogliotti stage II (hyperpigmentation, black colloid milia) and III (papulonodules) disease [7, 65]. The longer wavelength in the QS Nd:YAG laser likely enabled deeper penetration into the dermis to ablate homogentisic acid deposits [66]. Spoor et al. treated 34 patients of Asian, African American, and Hispanic descent with QS Nd:YAG. DPN lesions cleared after one treatment session in 90% of patients, and only one patient developed transient hypopigmentation [40]. The QS Nd:YAG laser is a popular and effective laser choice in treating pigmentary disorders in skin of color. However, it can cause hypopig-mentation and clinicians should remain vigilant for signs of pigmentary complications.

Intense Pulsed Light

IPL uses a xenon-chloride lamp to emit short, intense, incoherent pulses of light energy in the spectrum of 500–1200 nm [21]. While it can treat a variety of dermatological conditions, it is not the recommended treatment of choice for FST V-VI. For the treatment of melasma, it is postulated that light energy is absorbed by melanin in keratinocytes and melanocytes, which leads to photothermolysis and epidermal coagulation. Micro-crust containing melanin forms and is eventually sloughed off, with a subsequent decrease in pigmentation [67].

In one study among melasma patients ($n = 38$) with FST III-IV, IPL achieved 80–100% clearance in 47% of patients after four–five sessions [21]. These results echo previous findings in a study among FST II-IV, which demonstrated a 76–100% clearance rate for epidermal melasma, but <25% clearance for mixed type [20]. When used adjunctively with topical 4% hydroquinone (FST III-IV) or triple combination cream (FST II-V), IPL can augment response rates, including clearance [68, 69]. Unfortunately, there is a high relapse rate once IPL sessions are completed [69], which suggests the need for additional treatments to maintain improvements.

IPL has also been used to treat solar lentigines and ephelides. Sixty Asian patients with solar lentigines or ephelides were treated with IPL (fluence 20–24 J/cm², double or triple pulses of 2.6–5.0 ms with pulse delays of 20 ms, cutoff filters of 560) at 2–3 week intervals for a total of 3–5 treatments. Forty, 71, and 75% of patients with lentigines, ephelides, and lentigines and ephelides, respectively showed >50% improvement. None developed PIH or scarring afterwards [70, 71]. IPL has also been used to treat other UV-related pigmentary disorders, such as poikiloderma of Civatte, but it has not been well studied in skin of color [42, 43].

IPL is not recommended for laser hair removal in skin of color. One split-body study compared laser hair removal with long-pulsed Nd:YAG (20–25 ms, fluence 35–42 J/cm²) versus IPL (600 nm, 5 and 40 ms, fluence 12–14 J/cm²) among FST IV-VI ($n = 11$). After 1 treatment, 45% of participants (5/11) experienced PIH on the IPL-treated side, whereas none developed hyperpigmentation on the Nd:YAG-treated side. Of the five participants who experienced PIH, four were FST IV and 1 was FST VI [39].

Although the risk of hyperpigmentation with IPL may be reduced by using low fluences [52], given the risk of post-procedural dyspigmentation, treatment with IPL should be limited to skin of color patients with lighter skin types and refractory dermal pigmentation.

Pulsed Dye Laser

Pulsed dye lasers (PDL) deliver yellow light that is well absorbed by superficial blood vessels. They are commonly used for vascular lesions (i.e., port-wine stains (PWS) and hemangiomas) but have also been used for pigmentation disorders. Specifically, it can target the dermal vascular component of melasma and decrease melanocyte stimulation [52]. Melanocytes express endothelial growth factor receptors 1 and 2, which are involved in the pigmentation process [72]. Passeron et al. demonstrated that PDL, when used adjunctively with triple topical treatment, can significantly improve melasma, particularly among lighter skin types (FST II-III). The improvement persisted even at 2 months follow-up. However, among darker skin types, PDL was associated with development of PIH ($n = 3$) [22]. Similarly, PDL has also been used to successfully treat lentigines. In a study among 21 Iranian patients with solar lentigines, 57% of participants demonstrated >75% improvement. Although it caused transient hyperpigmentation in some patients, there were no recurrences at 6 months follow-up [35].

Interestingly, in 1 case report, a woman treated with PDL developed relapse of melasma 3 years later in areas that completely spared the laser-treated areas. These areas furthermore showed decreased vascularization compared to areas of melasma, suggesting that decreased vascularization from PDL may prevent recurrence of melasma [73].

Vascular lesions, such as PWS and superficial hemangiomas, respond well to PDL. The main complications include PIH and scarring. Sommer and Sheehan-Dare treated 13 patients (FST V) with PWS with PDL (585 nm, fluence 6–7.25 J/cm^2) at bimonthly intervals for a mean number of 7.5 treatments. While two patients achieved complete or near-complete clearance after three and eleven treatments, respectively, 46% ($n = 6/13$) of participants developed PIH. In addition, 15% of patients developed atrophic scarring ($n = 2/13$) [45]. However, these side effects may be minimized by combining PDL with a cryogen spray cooling CSC device. In a study among Asian patients ($n = 196$), those treated with PDL-CSC (fluence 8–10 J/cm^2) had higher improvement scores and could tolerate higher fluences than those treated with PDL alone (fluence 5–7 J/cm^2). Furthermore, none of the patients treated with PDL-CSC incurred scarring or PIH [44].

For superficial hemangiomas, a 10-year single-institution retrospective analysis of 657 cases among Chinese infants treated with PDL (595 nm, pulse duration 10–20 ms, fluence 9–13 J/cm^2, dynamic cooling duration of 40 ms and delay of 20 ms, 1–14 treatment sessions at 4–6 week intervals) revealed an overall effectiveness rate of 91.17%. Lesions on the extremities responded particularly well, with complete clearance seen after 2-3 treatment sessions. The most common side effects were pigmentary changes (increase or decrease) and skin atrophy, which resolved in 3–6 months [46].

Data for the use of PDL in the treatment of hypertrophic scars have been mixed, with some showing improvement and some no difference [74, 75]. Differences may be attributable to different laser fluence settings, with some studies suggesting higher fluences leading to better responses. However, higher fluences must be tempered with the risk of causing nonspecific thermal injury in patients of higher FSTs [74]. A recent study investigated whether the use of a CSC device concurrently with laser treatment can minimize the risk. Fifteen Asian patients with 22 hypertrophic scars were treated with 2 PDL treatments spaced 4 weeks apart (595 nm, fluence 9–10 J/cm^2, pulse duration 1.5–10 ms, cryogen spurt duration 30 ms with a 30 ms delay between coolant spray and laser pulse). All treated sites demonstrated a significant decrease in scar thickness and erythema, and no participants developed permanent pigmentary changes or ulceration [47]. The mechanism by which PDL improves erythematous hypertrophic scars is unknown, but hypotheses include laser-induced tissue hypoxia from damage of the microvasculature causing early scar maturation, collagen fiber heating causing subsequent collagen fiber realignment, and activation of mast cells and cytokines leading to matrix degrading products that promote collagen remodeling [47, 76, 77].

Fractional Photothermolysis

Resurfacing using ablative methods causes a controlled destruction of the epidermis with subsequent re-epithelialization, a process known to improve dyschromia and photoaging. Although traditional methods using the carbon dioxide (CO_2) and erbium-doped yttrium aluminum garnet (er:YAG) have shown striking results, especially in FSTs I-II, these procedures have been associated with scarring and further pigment alteration. Because of this, ablative methods are typically not employed in the skin of color population. Nonablative, fractional lasers allow for effective treatment of multiple skin disorders including rhytides, vascular lesions, scarring, and dyschromias with a much higher safety profile [78].

Fractional light therapy uses an infrared laser to induce multiple microcolumns of thermal damage [microthermal treatment zones (MTZ)] in a pixelated pattern [79]. Microscopic epidermal necrotic debris (MEND), including pigment from the basal layer and dermal material, are then removed through the columns of damage, termed the "melanin shuttle" [79, 80]. The surrounding unaffected tissue then serves as a reservoir to repopulate the damaged areas with keratinocytes and melanocytes [79, 81]. As the majority of skin remains intact and the stratum corneum is unperturbed, recovery time is relatively fast [80, 81]. Currently, both the 1550 nm erbium-doped and QS Nd:YAG lasers are FDA-approved for the treatment of melasma [82, 83]. The former is also FDA-approved for the treatment of pigmented lesions, periorbital rhytides, and scars [83, 84].

Multiple studies including 2 randomized controlled trials have explored the efficacy of fractional photothermolysis in treating melasma [23, 24, 85–88]. Wind et al. compared fractional photothermolysis (2000–2500/cm^2, 15 mJ/microbeam) to topical triple combination cream in the treatment of melasma. Unfortunately, 31% of laser-treated patients developed PIH after 2 or more treatments (FST III or higher). At 6 months follow-up, the majority of patients preferred triple topical treatment [24]. In a subsequent randomized controlled trial, Kroon et al. found no significant difference between patients treated with fractional photothermolysis (2000–2500 MTZ/cm^2, 10 mJ/microbeam) compared to triple topical therapy, and no patients developed PIH [23]. The difference in PIH rates may be partially attributable to the higher energy level used in the Wind et al. study (15 mJ/microbeam) [52]. However, patients in several other studies where even lower energy levels (i.e., 6–12 mJ/MTZ) were used still developed PIH [86, 89].

Additional uses of fractional photothermolysis include scar treatment and photoaging [48, 78]. Cho et al. compared the efficacy of a 1550 nm er:Glass fractional laser (200 spots/cm^2, 25–32 mJ/MTZ) versus a 10,600 nm CO_2 fractional laser

(100–150 mJ fluence, 100–120 spots/cm^2) in treating surgical scars ($n = 36$), posttraumatic scars ($n = 42$), burn scars ($n = 10$), acne scars ($n = 5$), and scars after cutaneous diseases ($n = 7$) in a Korean population (FST III-IV). Follow-up at 3 months after the last treatment sessions (1–12 sessions at 1.5–2 month intervals) revealed that 57.5 and 11.3% of patients showed marked or near-total improvement, respectively. There were no significant differences in efficacy between the 2 types of lasers, and side effects included only transient PIH and erythema. Interestingly, the results did not differ by scar type, but scars <3 years old responded better [48].

Two small studies ($n = 10$, 20) conducted in an East Asian population using a 1440 nm fractional diode-based laser, and a 1550- and 1565-nm er:glass fractional laser, respectively found these devices to be effective in treating signs of photoaging. The 1440 nm fractional diode-based laser resulted in mild improvement in texture, pigmentation, and wrinkles, with only one case of transient PIH [25]. Similarly, both the 1550- and 1565-nm er:glass fractional laser were equally efficacious in decreasing the area and degree of periorbital rhytides [26].

Anecdotal evidence from case reports suggests that fractional photothermolysis can also treat PIH, minocycline-induced hyperpigmentation, and DPNs. One patient (FST IV) with PIH achieved near-complete clearance (>95%) after 3 treatment sessions (15 mJ/microbeam, 880–1100 MTZ/cm^2) [29]. Another patient with minocycline-induced facial pigmentation was almost completely cleared after 4 sessions without any complications [12]. Lastly, a Pakistani woman with DPNs experienced 75% improvement after 3 treatment sessions with no post-procedural complications at 1-month follow-up [41]. Although these case reports are promising for future applications of fractional photothermolysis, they are limited by small sample sizes and short follow-up periods.

As PIH is one of the main drawbacks to fractional photothermolysis in darker skinned populations, Chan et al. studied the risk factors that predispose toward the development of PIH among Asians treated with fractional resurfacing. The authors found that high treatment density, high energy level, small anatomical treatment site, and inadequate epidermal cooling were associated with PIH. These risks can be reduced by using adjunctive cooling methods, decreasing treatment density, reducing the number of passes, and lengthening treatment intervals (i.e., 4–6 weeks vs. 1–2 weeks) [90].

Overall, fractional photothermolysis should be used with caution as it carries a high risk of PIH in skin of color and can have lower tolerability [91]. It may also cause acneiform eruptions, herpes simplex virus outbreaks, erosions, and prolonged erythema and edema [92].

Post-treatment

After laser treatment, topical corticosteroids can be prescribed to reduce inflammation and prevent PIH. Potentially irritating topicals (i.e., tretinoin, alpha hydroxy acids) should be avoided during the immediate posttreatment period. As always, photoprotection with sunscreen SPF $\geq$ 30 is essential to maintaining results and preventing relapse of UV-related dyschromias.

Conclusion

Laser therapy can be an effective treatment for dyschromias, photoaging, vascular lesions, scars, hair removal, and epidermal pigmented lesions in skin of color. In particular, hyperpigmentation continues to be a major concern for the skin of color population. While lightening agents and chemical peels remain first- and second-line agents, respectively, lasers can be an effective third-line agent when used appropriately. Adherence to pretreatment regimens, along with the use of appropriate laser and laser parameters can help reduce the risk of adverse events. Although it is often challenging for clinicians to provide laser therapy to darker skinned individuals, with proper patient selection and appropriate laser parameter settings, safe and effective treatment can be rendered.

References

1. Chan HH, Alam M, Kono T, Dover JS. Clinical application of lasers in Asians. Dermatol Surg. 2002;28(7):556–63.
2. Watanabe S, Takahashi H. Treatment of nevus of Ota with the Q-switched ruby laser. N Engl J Med. 1994;331(26):1745–50.
3. Cho SB, Park SJ, Kim MJ, Bu TS. Treatment of acquired bilateral nevus of Ota-like macules (Hori's nevus) using 1064-nm Q-switched Nd:YAG laser with low fluence. Int J Dermatol. 2009;48(12):1308–12.
4. Kunachak S, Leelaudomlipi P, Sirikulchayanonta V. Q-Switched ruby laser therapy of acquired bilateral nevus of Ota-like macules. Dermatol Surg. 1999;25(12):938–41.
5. Kramer KE, Lopez A, Stefanato CM, Phillips TJ. Exogenous ochronosis. J Am Acad Dermatol. 2000;42(5 Pt 2):869–71.
6. Bellew SG, Alster TS. Treatment of exogenous ochronosis with a Q-switched alexandrite (755 nm) laser. Dermatol Surg. 2004;30(4 Pt 1):555–8.
7. Tan SK. Exogenous ochronosis - successful outcome after treatment with Q-switched Nd:YAG laser. J Cosmet Laser Ther. 2013;15(5):274–8.
8. Collins P, Cotterill JA. Minocycline-induced pigmentation resolves after treatment with the Q-switched ruby laser. Br J Dermatol. 1996;135(2):317–9.
9. Tsao H, Busam K, Barnhill RL, Dover JS. Treatment of minocycline-induced hyperpigmentation with the Q-switched ruby laser. Arch Dermatol. 1996;132(10):1250–1.
10. Rodrigues M, Bekhor P. Treatment of minocycline-induced cutaneous pigmentation with the picosecond alexandrite (755-nm) laser. Dermatol Surg. 2015;41(10):1179–82.
11. Vangipuram RK, DeLozier WL, Geddes E, Friedman PM. Complete resolution of minocycline pigmentation following a single treatment with non-ablative 1550-nm fractional resurfacing in combination with the 755-nm Q-switched alexandrite laser. Lasers Surg Med. 2016;48(3):234–7.

12. Izikson L, Anderson RR. Resolution of blue minocycline pigmentation of the face after fractional photothermolysis. Lasers Surg Med. 2008;40(6):399–401.
13. Becker-Wegerich PM, Kuhn A, Malek L, Lehmann P, Megahed M, Ruzicka T. Treatment of nonmelanotic hyperpigmentation with the Q-switched ruby laser. J Am Acad Dermatol. 2000;43(2 Pt 1):272–4.
14. Karrer S, Hohenleutner U, Szeimies RM, Landthaler M. Amiodarone-induced pigmentation resolves after treatment with the Q-switched ruby laser. Arch Dermatol. 1999;135(3):251–3.
15. Bernstein EF. Q-switched laser treatment of amiodarone pigmentation. J Drugs Dermatol. 2011;10(11):1316–9.
16. Taylor CR, Anderson RR. Ineffective treatment of refractory melasma and postinflammatory hyperpigmentation by Q-switched ruby laser. J Dermatol Surg Oncol. 1994;20(9):592–7.
17. Tse Y, Levine VJ, McClain SA, Ashinoff R. The removal of cutaneous pigmented lesions with the Q-switched ruby laser and the Q-switched neodymium: yttrium-aluminum-garnet laser. A comparative study. J Dermatol Surg Oncol. 1994;20(12):795–800.
18. Cho SB, Kim JS, Kim MJ. Melasma treatment in Korean women using a 1064-nm Q-switched Nd:YAG laser with low pulse energy. Clin Exp Dermatol. 2009;34(8):e847–50.
19. Choi M, Choi JW, Lee SY, Choi SY, Park HJ, Park KC, et al. Low-dose 1064-nm Q-switched Nd:YAG laser for the treatment of melasma. J Dermatol Treat. 2010;21(4):224–8.
20. Moreno Arias GA, Ferrando J. Intense pulsed light for melanocytic lesions. Dermatol Surg. 2001;27(4):397–400.
21. Zoccali G, Piccolo D, Allegra P, Giuliani M. Melasma treated with intense pulsed light. Aesthetic Plast Surg. 2010;34(4):486–93.
22. Passeron T, Fontas E, Kang HY, Bahadoran P, Lacour JP, Ortonne JP. Melasma treatment with pulsed-dye laser and triple combination cream: a prospective, randomized, single-blind, split-face study. Arch Dermatol. 2011;147(9):1106–8.
23. Kroon MW, Wind BS, Beek JF, van der Veen JP, Nieuweboer-Krobotova L, Bos JD, et al. Nonablative 1550-nm fractional laser therapy versus triple topical therapy for the treatment of melasma: a randomized controlled pilot study. J Am Acad Dermatol. 2011;64(3):516–23.
24. Wind BS, Kroon MW, Meesters AA, Beek JF, van der Veen J, Nieuweboer-Krobotová L, et al. Non-ablative 1,550 nm fractional laser therapy versus triple topical therapy for the treatment of melasma: a randomized controlled split-face study. Lasers Surg Med. 2010;42 (7):607–12.
25. Marmon S, Shek SY, Yeung CK, Chan NP, Chan JC, Chan HH. Evaluating the safety and efficacy of the 1,440-nm laser in the treatment of photodamage in Asian skin. Lasers Surg Med. 2014;46(5):375–9.
26. Jung JY, Cho SB, Chung HJ, Shin JU, Lee KH, Chung KY. Treatment of periorbital wrinkles with 1550- and 1565-nm Er:glass fractional photothermolysis lasers: a simultaneous split-face trial. J Eur Acad Dermatol Venereol. 2011;25(7):811–8.
27. Kopera D, Hohenleutner U. Ruby laser treatment of melasma and postinflammatory hyperpigmentation. Dermatol Surg. 1995;21(11):994.
28. Cho SB, Park SJ, Kim JS, Kim MJ, Bu TS. Treatment of post-inflammatory hyperpigmentation using 1064-nm Q-switched Nd:YAG laser with low fluence: report of three cases. J Eur Acad Dermatol Venereol. 2009;23(10):1206–7.
29. Katz TM, Goldberg LH, Firoz BF, Friedman PM. Fractional photothermolysis for the treatment of postinflammatory hyperpigmentation. Dermatol Surg. 2009;35(11):1844–8.
30. Grossman MC, Anderson RR, Farinelli W, Flotte TJ, Grevelink JM. Treatment of cafe au lait macules with lasers. A clinicopathologic correlation. Arch Dermatol. 1995;131(12):1416–20.
31. Bukhari IA. Removal of amateur blue-black tattoos in Arabic women of skin type (III-IV) with Q-switched alexandrite laser. J Cosmet Dermatol. 2005;4(2):107–10.
32. Grevelink JM, Duke D, van Leeuwen RL, Gonzalez E, DeCoste SD, Anderson RR. Laser treatment of tattoos in darkly pigmented patients: efficacy and side effects. J Am Acad Dermatol. 1996;34(4):653–6.
33. Jones A, Roddey P, Orengo I, Rosen T. The Q-switched Nd: YAG laser effectively treats tattoos in darkly pigmented skin. Dermatol Surg. 1996;22(12):999–1001.

34. Wang CC, Sue YM, Yang CH, Chen CK. A comparison of Q-switched alexandrite laser and intense pulsed light for the treatment of freckles and lentigines in Asian persons: a randomized, physician-blinded, split-face comparative trial. J Am Acad Dermatol. 2006;54 (5):804–10.

35. Ghaninejhadi H, Ehsani A, Edrisi L, Gholamali F, Akbari Z, Noormohammadpour P. Solar lentigines: evaluating pulsed dye laser (PDL) as an effective treatment option. J Lasers Med Sci. 2013;4(1):33–8.

36. Jackson BA. Lasers in ethnic skin: a review. J Am Acad Dermatol. 2003;48(6 Suppl):S134–8.

37. Jackson B, Junkins-Hopkins J, editors. Effect of pulsewidth variation on laser hair removal in African-American skin. 1999 oral presentation ASDS meeting Miami, FL.

38. Jackson B. Lasers in skin of color. J Cosmet Dermatol. 2003;16:57–60.

39. Goh CL. Comparative study on a single treatment response to long pulse Nd:YAG lasers and intense pulse light therapy for hair removal on skin type IV to VI–is longer wavelengths lasers preferred over shorter wavelengths lights for assisted hair removal. J Dermatol Treat. 2003;14 (4):243–7.

40. Spoor T. Treatment of dermatosis papulosa nigra with the 532 nm diode laser. Cosmet Dermatol. 2001;14(10):21–3.

41. Katz TM, Goldberg LH, Friedman PM. Dermatosis papulosa nigra treatment with fractional photothermolysis. Dermatol Surg. 2009;35(11):1840–3.

42. Rusciani A, Motta A, Fino P, Menichini G. Treatment of poikiloderma of Civatte using intense pulsed light source: 7 years of experience. Dermatol Surg. 2008;34(3):314–9 (discussion 9).

43. Weiss RA, Goldman MP, Weiss MA. Treatment of poikiloderma of Civatte with an intense pulsed light source. Dermatol Surg. 2000;26(9):823–7 (discussion 8).

44. Chang CJ, Nelson JS. Cryogen spray cooling and higher fluence pulsed dye laser treatment improve port-wine stain clearance while minimizing epidermal damage. Dermatol Surg. 1999;25(10):767–72.

45. Sommer S, Sheehan-Dare RA. Pulsed dye laser treatment of port-wine stains in pigmented skin. J Am Acad Dermatol. 2000;42(4):667–71.

46. Chen W, Liu S, Yang C, Yang S. Clinical efficacy of the 595 nm pulsed dye laser in the treatment of childhood superficial hemangioma - analysis of 10-year application in Chinese patients. J Dermatol Treat. 2015;26(1):54–8.

47. Kono T, Ercocen AR, Nakazawa H, Nozaki M. Treatment of hypertrophic scars using a long-pulsed dye laser with cryogen-spray cooling. Ann Plast Surg. 2005;54(5):487–93.

48. Cho S, Jung JY, Shin JU, Lee JH. Non-ablative 1550 nm erbium-glass and ablative 10,600 nm carbon dioxide fractional lasers for various types of scars in Asian people: evaluation of 100 patients. Photomed Laser Surg. 2014;32(1):42–6.

49. Battle EF Jr, Hobbs LM. Laser therapy on darker ethnic skin. Dermatol Clin. 2003;21(4): 713–23.

50. Anderson RR, Parrish JA. Selective photothermolysis: precise microsurgery by selective absorption of pulsed radiation. Science. 1983;220(4596):524–7.

51. Vashi NA. Cosmetic interventions for dyschromia: lasers. Aestheticians J. 2014;4(5):16–20.

52. Arora P, Sarkar R, Garg VK, Arya L. Lasers for treatment of melasma and post-inflammatory hyperpigmentation. J Cutan Aesthet Surg. 2012;5(2):93.

53. Bernestein LJ, Geronemus RG. Keloid formation with the 585-nm pulsed dye laser during isotretinoin treatment. Arch Dermatol. 1997;133(1):111–2.

54. Alster TS, Tanzi EL. Complications in laser and light surgery. In: Goldberg LH, editor. Lasers and lights, vol. II. 2nd ed. USA: Saunders; 2008.

55. Jang WS, Lee CK, Kim BJ, Kim MN. Efficacy of 694-nm Q-switched ruby fractional laser treatment of melasma in female Korean patients. Dermatol Surg. 2011;37(8):1133–40.

56. Taylor CR, Flotte TJ, Gange RW, Anderson RR. Treatment of nevus of Ota by Q-switched ruby laser. J Am Acad Dermatol. 1994;30(5):743–51.

57. Geronemus RG. Q-switched ruby laser therapy of nevus of Ota. Arch Dermatol. 1992;128 (12):1618–22.

J. Cheng and N.A. Vashi

58. Chesnut C, Diehl J, Lask G. Treatment of nevus of Ota with a picosecond 755-nm alexandrite laser. Dermatol Surg. 2015;41(4):508–10.
59. Chan JC, Shek SY, Kono T, Yeung CK, Chan HH. A retrospective analysis on the management of pigmented lesions using a picosecond 755-nm alexandrite laser in Asians. Lasers Surg Med. 2016;48(1):23–9.
60. Alster TS, Lupton JR. Laser therapy for cutaneous hyperpigmentation and pigmented lesions. Dermatol Ther. 2001;14(1):46–54.
61. Wattanakrai P, Mornchan R, Eimpunth S. Low-fluence Q-switched neodymium-doped yttrium aluminum garnet (1,064 nm) laser for the treatment of facial melasma in Asians. Dermatol Surg. 2010;36(1):76–87.
62. Chan NP, Ho SG, Shek SY, Yeung CK, Chan HH. A case series of facial depigmentation associated with low fluence Q-switched 1,064 nm Nd:YAG laser for skin rejuvenation and melasma. Lasers Surg Med. 2010;42(8):712–9.
63. Kauvar AN. Successful treatment of melasma using a combination of microdermabrasion and Q-switched Nd:YAG lasers. Lasers Surg Med. 2012;44(2):117–24.
64. Kim MJ, Kim JS, Cho SB. Punctate leucoderma after melasma treatment using 1064-nm Q-switched Nd:YAG laser with low pulse energy. J Eur Acad Dermatol Venereol. 2009;23(8):960–2.
65. Dogliotti M, Leibowitz M. Granulomatous ochronosis - a cosmetic-induced skin disorder in Blacks. S Afr Med J. 1979;56(19):757–60.
66. Simmons BJ, Griffith RD, Bray FN, Falto-Aizpurua LA, Nouri K. Exogenous ochronosis: a comprehensive review of the diagnosis, epidemiology, causes, and treatments. Am J Clin Dermatol. 2015;16(3):205–12.
67. Kawada A, Asai M, Kameyama H, Sangen Y, Aragane Y, Tezuka T, et al. Videomicroscopic and histopathological investigation of intense pulsed light therapy for solar lentigines. J Dermatol Sci. 2002;29(2):91–6.
68. Figueiredo Souza L, Trancoso Souza S. Single-session intense pulsed light combined with stable fixed-dose triple combination topical therapy for the treatment of refractory melasma. Dermatol Ther. 2012;25(5):477–80.
69. Wang CC, Hui CY, Sue YM, Wong WR, Hong HS. Intense pulsed light for the treatment of refractory melasma in Asian persons. Dermatol Surg. 2004;30(9):1196–200.
70. Kawada A, Shiraishi H, Asai M, Kameyama H, Sangen Y, Aragane Y, et al. Clinical improvement of solar lentigines and ephelides with an intense pulsed light source. Dermatol Surg. 2002;28(6):504–8.
71. Lin J, Chan H. Pigmentary disorders in Asian skin: treatment with laser and intense pulsed light sources. Skin Ther Lett. 2006;11(8):8–11.
72. Plonka PM, Passeron T, Brenner M, Tobin DJ, Shibahara S, Thomas A, et al. What are melanocytes really doing all day long…? Exp Dermatol. 2009;18(9):799–819.
73. Passeron T. Long-lasting effect of vascular targeted therapy of melasma. J Am Acad Dermatol. 2013;69(3):e141–2.
74. Chan HH, Wong DS, Ho WS, Lam LK, Wei W. The use of pulsed dye laser for the prevention and treatment of hypertrophic scars in Chinese persons. Dermatol Surg. 2004;30(7):987–94 (discussion 94).
75. Kono T, Ercocen AR, Nakazawa H, Honda T, Hayashi N, Nozaki M. The flashlamp-pumped pulsed dye laser (585 nm) treatment of hypertrophic scars in Asians. Ann Plast Surg. 2003;51(4):366–71.
76. Gabbiani G, Badonnel MC. Early changes of endothelial clefts after thermal injury. Microvasc Res. 1975;10(1):65–75.
77. Ehrlich HP, Kelley SF. Hypertrophic scar: an interruption in the remodeling of repair–a laser Doppler blood flow study. Plast Reconstr Surg. 1992;90(6):993–8.
78. Chae WS, Seong JY, Jung HN, Kong SH, Kim MH, Suh HS, et al. Comparative study on efficacy and safety of 1550 nm Er: Glass fractional laser and fractional radiofrequency microneedle device for facial atrophic acne scar. J Cosmet Dermatol. 2015;14(2):100–6.

79. Tierney EP, Hanke CW. Review of the literature: Treatment of dyspigmentation with fractionated resurfacing. Dermatol Surg. 2010;36(10):1499–508.
80. Hantash BM, Bedi VP, Sudireddy V, Struck SK, Herron GS, Chan KF. Laser-induced transepidermal elimination of dermal content by fractional photothermolysis. J Biomed Opt. 2006;11(4):041115.
81. Manstein D, Herron GS, Sink RK, Tanner H, Anderson RR. Fractional photothermolysis: a new concept for cutaneous remodeling using microscopic patterns of thermal injury. Lasers Surg Med. 2004;34(5):426–38.
82. Food and Drug Administration. 510(k) summary for the Lutronic corporatoin Spectra laser system. In: Department of Health & Human Services, editor. Silver Spring, MD 2012.
83. Food and Drug Administration. Section 5: 510(k) summary statement. In: Department of Health & Human Services, editor. Silver Spring, MD 2013.
84. Sherling M, Friedman PM, Adrian R, Burns AJ, Conn H, Fitzpatrick R, et al. Consensus recommendations on the use of an erbium-doped 1,550-nm fractionated laser and its applications in dermatologic laser surgery. Dermatol Surg. 2010;36(4):461–9.
85. Tannous ZS, Astner S. Utilizing fractional resurfacing in the treatment of therapy-resistant melasma. J Cosmet Laser Ther. 2005;7(1):39–43.
86. Rokhsar CK, Fitzpatrick RE. The treatment of melasma with fractional photothermolysis: a pilot study. Dermatol Surg. 2005;31(12):1645–50.
87. Barysch MJ, Rummelein B, Kolm I, Karpova MB, Schonewolf N, Bogdan Allemann I, et al. Split-face study of melasma patients treated with non-ablative fractionated photothermolysis (1540 nm). J Eur Acad Dermatol Venereol. 2012;26(4):423–30.
88. Lee HS, Won CH, Lee DH, An JS, Chang HW, Lee JH, et al. Treatment of melasma in Asian skin using a fractional 1,550-nm laser: an open clinical study. Dermatol Surg. 2009;35 (10):1499–504.
89. Naito SK. Fractional photothermolysis treatment for resistant melasma in Chinese females. J Cosmet Laser Ther. 2007;9(3):161–3.
90. Chan HH, Manstein D, Yu CS, Shek S, Kono T, Wei WI. The prevalence and risk factors of post-inflammatory hyperpigmentation after fractional resurfacing in Asians. Lasers Surg Med. 2007;39(5):381–5.
91. Rivas S, Pandya AG. Treatment of melasma with topical agents, peels and lasers: an evidence-based review. Am J Clin Dermatol. 2013;14(5):359–76.
92. Graber EM, Tanzi EL, Alster TS. Side effects and complications of fractional laser photothermolysis: experience with 961 treatments. Dermatol Surg. 2008;34(3):301–5 (discussion 5–7).

Chapter 26
Cultural Considerations

Rechelle Z. Tull and Steven R. Feldman

The United States is becoming increasingly racially and ethnically diverse. Currently, 38% of the population, and the majority of immigrants are people of color. However, by 2044, ethnic and racial minorities will comprise over half of the population [1]. With this demographic shift and the resultant increase in people of color seeking dermatological care, it is important to consider how historical, socioeconomic, and cultural factors can hinder the delivery of care, leading to health disparities for these populations [2]. Treatment adherence greatly affects health outcomes; thus, it is an important factor in delivery of care. In addition, the common use of complementary and alternative medicine (CAM) among minority groups can alter medication utilization, impact treatment outcomes, and result in harmful sequelae [3]. Moreover, given the required continuous control necessary to treat many chronic dermatoses—including psoriasis, cutaneous lupus, and acne—treatment adherence is crucial to achieving positive clinical outcomes [4–6].

Cultural Competency in Dermatology

As the United States demographics evolve and the patient population becomes increasingly diverse, it is important for dermatologists to provide empathetic, equitable, and culturally competent care [7]. Cultural competency is defined as "the

R.Z. Tull
Department of Dermatology, Wake Forest University School of Medicine,
1 Medical Center Blvd, Winston-Salem, NC 27157, USA
e-mail: rtull@wakehealth.edu

S.R. Feldman (✉)
Department of Dermatology, Pathology and Public Health Sciences, Wake Forest University
School of Medicine, 1 Medical Center Boulevard, Winston-Salem, NC 27157, USA
e-mail: sfeldman@wakehealth.edu

© Springer International Publishing AG 2017
N.A. Vashi and H.I. Maibach (eds.), *Dermatoanthropology of Ethnic
Skin and Hair*, DOI 10.1007/978-3-319-53961-4_26

ability of an organization or an individual within the healthcare delivery system to provide effective, equitable, understandable, and respectful quality care and services that are responsive to diverse cultural health beliefs and practices, preferred languages, health literacy, and other communication needs of the patient" [8]. Culturally competent care not only enhances the patient–provider relationship but is also key to reducing ethnic and racial health disparities [8, 9].

Dermatologists should understand that culture can influence a patient's understanding of disease, physician trust, and treatment compliance. However, physician trainees are often not adequately trained in cultural competency [10]. Circumventing issues regarding culture, race, and/or ethnicity may seem prudent to avoid unwillingly offending a patient. However, cultural traditions, beliefs, and social norms can significantly impact health behaviors. Furthermore, historical factors, including immigration, assimilation, poverty, language barriers, and racism, can affect patient perspectives and practices [11]. Lack of cultural competency can negatively affect patient–physician communication leading to medical errors, decreased patient satisfaction, poor physician trust, and medication nonadherence [7].

Dermatologists should understand that certain health practices, beliefs, and concerns are more prevalent among specific cultural groups. However, culture is not always just defined by race or ethnicity, but rather explained within the context of a group of people, community, kin, or country [12]. In Latino and Asian communities, use of CAM, such as traditional herbal remedies, can lead to delays in seeking medical care, compromise prescribed treatment regimens, and result in hypersensitivity reactions [3, 13–16]. Specific CAM practices in Asian communities, including coining, cupping, and moxibustion, may be mistaken as abuse. In Asian cultures, fair skin is often desired as a sign of socioeconomic status. Patients in this group avidly use sunscreen, parasols, and seek treatment to lighten the skin [14]. Potentially damaging hair practices, including use of hotcombs, chemical relaxers, and high tractional styles, are prevalent among African American. These practices often begin in early childhood and are associated with scalp irritation, folliculitis, and alopecia [17].

Cultural competency is essential to providing quality health care and improving patient outcomes, especially among the growing minority patient population [7]. Open-minded acknowledgement of cultural differences and incorporation of cultural knowledge can advance patient–physician communication and patient compliance [7, 8]. Discussing, rather than dismissing, cultural health practices and beliefs can support a positive therapeutic relationship [11]. Patients may be reluctant to initiate this discussion and anticipate a negative response. However, asking open questions, showing nonjudgmental interest, and respectfully listening to patient concerns, is consistent with patient-centered practice. In this setting, patients are more likely to reveal perspectives regarding their health, discuss use of CAM, and participate in medical decision-making [18, 19].

Importance of Medication Adherence

Treatment adherence is defined as the extent to which patients use their medication as prescribed by their healthcare provider [20]. When patients take their medication as directed, they receive its full benefit, leading to improved clinical outcomes and reduced overall healthcare costs [20–22]. In contrast, poor adherence can have significant individual, public health, and economic implications, including disease exacerbation, adverse clinical events, increased healthcare costs, and mortality [2, 23]. Poor medication adherence is a relatively prevalent phenomenon. Researchers estimate 20–30% of medication prescriptions are never filled and average adherence to long-term therapy is 50% [24]. Estimated adherence rates for dermatological medication range from 55 to 66% [25]. Furthermore, adherence to topical medications is lower than to systemic medications [26, 27].

Improper medication adherence is a multifaceted behavioral problem heavily influenced by the patient. However, healthcare providers and healthcare systems also factor into this issue [20]. One patient factor that underlies nonadherence is cognitive dysfunction that impairs a patients' ability to understand the importance of following a prescribed regimen. Psychological problems, especially depression, can affect motivation and cause forgetfulness. A lack of medical insurance, an erratic daily schedule, and emotional factors can also cause patients to deviate from their prescription. Providers factor into poor treatment adherence by prescribing complex regimens; ineffectually educating patients about benefits, risks, and alternatives to medication; inadequately following-up with patients after medication initiation; cultivating poor patient–provider relationships; and not considering the cost of medication or patient preference. Health systems can contribute barriers to adherence by limiting access to health care and insurance coverage, establishing restricting formularies, and having prohibitively high medication costs and co-pays [6, 20].

Race, ethnicity, and socioeconomic status may not directly impact rates of medication adherence [5, 20]. However, cultural and ethnic differences that influence delivery of care can impact medication adherence. Furthermore, potential barriers to adherence may have varying impacts on medication adherence in different ethnic groups [28].

Barriers to Dermatologic Medication Adherence in Ethnic and Racial Minority Populations

Socioeconomic and Health Disparities

Socioeconomic disparities among ethnic and racial minority patients can impact medication adherence [29]. In 2014, 26% of African Americans, 23.6% of Hispanics, and 12% of Asians earned at or below the poverty level compared to

10% of non-Hispanic Whites [30]. Patients of a lower socioeconomic status (SES) may have fewer financial resources to pay for medications. In one study, lower SES patients with psoriasis exhibited higher rates of medication nonadherence, which was associated with worse clinical outcomes on biologic therapy compared to patients of a higher SES [29].

Furthermore, due to higher levels of poverty, minority patients are more likely to be uninsured or have less comprehensive insurance coverage [28, 31, 32]. In 2014, Hispanics had the highest uninsured rate, at 20%, followed by 11.8% of African Americans, and 9.3% of Asians compared to 7.6% of non-Hispanic Whites [31]. Patients with lower SES are more likely to have public insurance, such as Medicaid, which is associated with poorer health outcomes [13, 32–34].

Patients with limited financial resources and insurance coverage may have higher co-pays, which can contribute to missed medication doses [29]. In one study, factors that contributed to poor medication adherence in Black versus White patients were eliminated after controlling for substantial income disparities between the two racial groups [5]. More affordable co-pays have been linked to improved adherence [35].

Implementing the most affordable treatment plan possible may be helpful. Generic therapies should be utilized when available to decrease costs. The average retail price of a generic drug is 75% lower than its brand-name counterpart (though even generic prices have been rapidly increasing). One study revealed that the average wholesale price of topical corticosteroids is consistently higher than the mean copayment, regardless of potency and unit size [36]. Thus, patients with no insurance who resort to paying out of pocket may find medication cost prohibitive. Such patients may risk exacerbating their disease and developing complications because they cannot afford their prescriptions [37]. Physicians should inform patients of sources for affordable drugs and coverage programs so patients do not forgo treatment leading to possible morbidity and mortality.

Low Health Literacy and Limited English Proficiency

Health literacy is defined as the skillset needed to function in a healthcare system. Health literacy competencies—speaking and listening effectively, reading, and understanding printed material, such as prescription bottle labels, and using numeracy skills—are needed to assure adherence to medication regimens [38]. Approximately, 80 million Americans have some difficulty understanding and using health information. Furthermore, Black, Hispanic, and multiracial individuals display lower average health literacy scores compared to White adults [39]. Low health literacy can impact medication adherence [2, 38]. Patients with low literacy struggle to identify their medications, understand medication instructions, and comprehend prescription warning labels [38, 40, 41]. Limited health literacy in underserved populations is associated with unintentional nonadherence, such as forgetting to take medications. This contrasts with intentional adherence, in which patients make a conscious decision not to take their medication [42].

Patients with limited health literacy are likely to exhibit poor patient–physician communication, resulting in miscommunication regarding medication regimens and adverse side effects [42]. For minority patients, physician–patient discordance in race, ethnicity, or culture can contribute to miscommunication and subsequent nonadherence [28]. Ethnic and racial minorities report feeling less understood by their doctors, and Hispanic patients are twice as likely to leave the doctor with unanswered questions [43].

A major barrier to effective communication is patient–physician language discordance [44]. About 60.6 million Americans (21% of the U.S. population) speak a language other than English at home; about 42% (25.3 million) of these individuals have limited English proficiency (LEP), meaning they self-report speaking English less than "very well." The majority of the LEP population speak Spanish (16.2 million, 64% of LEP population). In addition, 6% speak Chinese (1.6 million), 3% speak Vietnamese (847,000), 2% speak Korean (599,000), and 2% speak Tagalog (509,000) [45, 46]. Language barriers can cause patients to misunderstand medication instruction, leading to decreased adherence [29].

Professional interpreters can help patients who have LEP. These patients are more likely to leave their health encounter with a poor understanding of their diagnosis and treatment plan [44]. In a fast-paced dermatology office where complex dosing regimens, such as an oral corticosteroid taper, are standard, a language barrier can cause poor communication, resulting in subsequent improper medication usage and poor clinical outcome.

Trained medical interpreters are preferred over ad hoc interpreters, including family members, children, friends, and untrained support staff. Ad hoc interpreters are not trained in medical terminology and confidentiality, often omit up to half of all physician questions, and are more likely to commit translation errors with clinical consequences. In addition, ad hoc interpreters may have motives that are not in the patient's best interest [44].

Dermatologists should prescribe medication regimens that suit patients' lifestyles and cultural preferences. Treatment plans should consist of the simplest dosing regimen and use the patients' desired medication vehicle [29]. Though ointments are thought to have higher potency due to their occlusive nature, patients who find an ointment cosmetically unacceptable will be less likely to use the medication as directed [47]. When prescribing scalp treatments for African American patients, dermatologists should be aware of cultural differences in hair care practices. For example, it may be difficult for African American female patients to use a regimen that requires washing their hair more than once per week as half (50%) of African American women wash their hair biweekly and a minority (43%) wash their hair weekly [48].

Behavioral and educational strategies should be used to maximize medication adherence in patients with limited health literacy. Dermatologists can use audiotapes, websites, YouTube videos, and language appropriate brochures as resources for patient education in routine clinical practice. Printed action plans that summarize the patient visit and detail the prescribed treatment plan remove the burden of trying to remember instructions [37]. Dermatologists should strive to cultivate physician–patient relationships built on patient participation in decision-making and care, clear explanations of medication benefits and risk, and physician trust. Furthermore, strong physician–patient relationships are associated with patient satisfaction, higher health status, and improved adherence [49].

When patients are nonadherent to their medication, dermatologists should avoid making global judgements based on patient health status, socioeconomic status, or providers' inherent cultural or ethnic biases [28]. Instead physicians should non-judgmentally ask patients how often they miss doses. An open approach may allow patients to feel comfortable while being forthright about poor adherence. Patients should be asked to identify barriers to adherence, such as experiencing medication side effects, patient misconceptions, and their understanding of medication benefits and risks [20].

Use of Complementary and Alternative Medicine

CAM is defined as healthcare systems, practices, and products that are not part of conventional modern medicine [50]. The National Health Interview Survey esti-mated that in 2012, 34% of adults in the United States used CAM [51]. However, use of complementary remedies is highly prevalent among ethnic and cultural minority groups. Hispanic women are three times more likely to use herbal remedies compared to the general population and more likely to use CAM in substitute of prescribed medications [52, 53]. CAM treatments are primarily paid for out of pocket and may take away from the patient's ability to pay for pre-scription co-pays or physician recommended over-the-counter dermatologic prod-ucts [43, 50].

CAM is commonly used as adjunctive therapy or replacement for conventional medical care. However, users are often unaware of possible side effects of CAM therapies or adverse interactions between complementary treatments and pharma-ceutical medications [51]. Many patients believe herbal medicines are harmless because they are "natural" [54]. Unlike prescription medications, alternative ther-apies are not highly regulated by government agencies. There may be no quality control measures in place to confirm the purity, concentration, and safety of some herbal supplements. Manufacturers are restricted from making claims of efficacy; however, there are no restrictions limiting claims about herbs alleviating issues not considered medical by regulatory authorities [55].

Fewer than half of CAM users discuss alternative therapy use with their doctor. African American, Hispanic, and Asian American patients are less likely to disclose their use of CAM compared to non-Hispanic White patients [56–59]. Major reasons patients refrain from discussing CAM use are physicians not inquiring and patients assuming it is unimportant [46]. Language barriers may also play a role in patients discussing treatment preferences and patient health. One study observed that among

Chinese- and Vietnamese-speaking patients at community health centers, fewer than 8% discussed their use of CAM with their provider [54]. Immigrants may not disclose information because they cannot find a provider who communicates in their preferred language and because they are unfamiliar with the American healthcare system. Patients are more likely to disclose use of CAM when they have a language-concordant physician [56].

African American patients may be distrustful of conventional medicine due to historical racial injustices, such as the Tuskegee syphilis study, and seek CAM as an alternative to the healthcare system [54, 60, 61]. African Americans, who as a group are more likely to rely on religion than Whites, often use religion as a means of coping with their disease. However, studies reveal this dependence on religion is used as a complement to conventional medicine instead of an alternative [28]. In contrast, many Hispanics believe illness to be a form of divine punishment. A new diagnosis may induce feeling of guilt or depression. Patients may pray or perform good deeds as penance in attempts to restore good health [62].

Use of alternative therapies and home remedies is very common within the Hispanic community. Due to the many healthcare barriers immigrant Hispanic communities encounter, including LEP, cultural differences, inadequate financial resources, unreliable transportation, lack of health insurance and documentation, and fear of the United States' medical system, Hispanics may turn to home remedies and over-the counter medicines [16, 63]. Hispanics also can access prescription-grade pharmaceuticals, such as antibiotics, steroids, and controlled substances, from Hispanic-owned convenience stores called "tiendas." In addition, patients may visit a curandero, or traditional folk healer, for treatment [62]. Although the use and belief in home remedies or curandero therapies over conventional medicine varies based on acculturation, education, and socioeconomic level, many Hispanics have a strong preference for alternative medicine [62]. In a study interviewing immigrants from Mexico and across South America, 39% favored physician medicine but 31% believed the curandero's medicine was more effective [64]. Studies reveal that most Hispanics patients (77–80.3%) use CAM to treat their illnesses because they prefer traditional remedies to conventional medical interventions [16, 65]. In one survey study of 620 Hispanic patients, over half (58%) believed that herbs were drugs and only about one-third (35%) believed herbs could interact with prescription medication [65].

When evaluating possible sequelae of herb use, physicians most also consider the vehicle and the possibility of contamination. Various substances are reported as contaminates of herbal medicines, including betamethasone, hydrocortisone, chlordiazepoxide, dexamethasone, mefenamic acid, methyltestosterone, thiamine, lead, and other heavy metals [55]. Patients can be exposed to inorganic arsenic from using alternative remedies. Cutaneous manifestations of chronic arsenic exposure include arsenical keratosis, macular hypopigmentation and an increased risk of developing Bowen's disease, squamous cell carcinoma, and basal cell carcinomas [66].

Physicians should directly ask patients about their use of alternative therapies in an open and nonjudgmental manner. It is important for physicians to be aware of commonly used alternative therapies and serious side effects so they can inform patients and possibly diagnose serious sequelae [55]. Racial and ethnic minority patients may benefit from patient–physician communication regarding CAM use as cultural beliefs about dermatologic conditions can affect patient decisions regarding medication use and traditional remedies.

Conclusion

As the United States becomes more diverse, cultural competence is increasingly an integral component of quality health care. Socioeconomic disparities, low health literacy, and LEP can negatively impact access to health care, patient–provider communication, and medication adherence. Furthermore, use of complementary remedies is highly prevalent among minorities and can alter medication efficacy, influence treatment adherence, and cause harmful sequelae. It is important for dermatologists to understand how culture, race, and ethnicity can directly and indirectly influence healthcare outcomes.

References

1. Colby SL, Jennifer JO. Projections of the size and composition of the U.S. population: 2014 to 2060. Curr Population Rep. 2014:25–1143. Available from: URL: https://www.census.gov/content/dam/Census/library/publications/2015/demo/p25-1143.pdf. Accessed 19 Apr 2016.
2. Viswanathan M, Golin CE, Jones CD, et al. Medication adherence interventions: comparative effectiveness. Closing the quality gap: revisiting the state of the science. Evidence Report No. 208. AHRQ Publication No. 12-E010-EF. Agency for Healthcare Research and Quality. September 2012. Available from: http://www.effectivehealthcare.ahrq.gov/reports/final.cfm. Accessed 10 May 2016.
3. Chao MT, Handley MA, Quan J, Sarkar U, Ratanawongsa N, Schillinger D. Disclosure of complementary health approaches among low income and racially diverse safety net patients with diabetes. Patient Educ Couns. 2015;98(11):1360–6.
4. Zschocke I, Mrowietz U, Karakasili E, Reich K. Non-adherence and measures to improve adherence in the topical treatment of psoriasis. J Eur Acad Dermatol Venereol. 2014;28(Suppl 2):4–9.
5. Farhangian ME, Huang WW, Feldman SR. Adherence to oral and topical medications in cutaneous lupus erythematosus is not well characterized. Dermatol Ther (Heidelb). 2015;5(2):91–105.
6. Ou HT, Feldman SR, Balkrishnan R. Understanding and improving treatment adherence in pediatric patients. Semin Cutan Med Surg. 2010;29(2):137–40.
7. Lorié Á, Reinero DA, Phillips M, Zhang L, Riess H. Culture and nonverbal expressions of empathy in clinical settings: a systematic review. Patient Educ Couns. 2016;S0738–3991(16):30446–3.
8. Alper J. Integrating health literacy, cultural competence, and language access services: workshop summary. Roundtable on health literacy; board on population health and public health practice; health and medicine division; National Academies of Sciences, Engineering, and Medicine.

9. Pandya AG, Alexis AF, Berger TG, Wintroub BU. Increasing racial and ethnic diversity in dermatology: a call to action. J Am Acad Dermatol. 2016;74(3):584–7.
10. Weissman JS, Betancourt J, Campbell EG, Park ER, et al. Resident physicians' preparedness to provide cross-cultural care. JAMA. 2005;294(9):1058–67.
11. Barbosa V. Cultural considerations in people of African descent. In: Alexis AF, Barbosa VH, editors. Skin of color: a practical guide to dermatologic diagnosis and treatment. New York, NY: Springer; 2013.
12. Smith G. Communication and culture. In: Holt RaW, editor. New York; 1966.
13. Rodriguez D. Cultural considerations in Latino patients. In: Alexis AF, Barbosa VH, editors. Skin of color: a practical guide to dermatologic diagnosis and treatment. New York, NY: Springer; 2013.
14. Wongpraparat C, Lim HW. Cultural considerations in Asian patients. In: Alexis AF, Barbosa VH, editors. Skin of color: a practical guide to dermatologic diagnosis and treatment. New York, NY: Springer; 2013.
15. Feldman SR1, Vallejos QM, Quandt SA, Fleischer AB Jr, Schulz MR, Verma A, Arcury TA. Health care utilization among migrant Latino farmworkers: the case of skin disease. J Rural Health. 2009 Winter;25(1):98–103.
16. Tafur MM1, Crowe TK, Torres E. A review of curanderismo and healing practices among Mexicans and Mexican Americans. Occup Ther Int. 2009;16(1):82–8.
17. Rucker Wright D, Gathers R, Kapke A, et al. Hair care practices and their association with scalp and hair disorders in African American girls. J Am Acad Dermatol. 2011;64:253–62.
18. Shelley BM, Sussman AL, Williams RL, Segal AR, Crabtree BF, et al. They don't ask me so I don't tell them: patient-clinician communication about traditional, complementary, and alternative medicine. Ann Fam Med. 2009;7(2):139–47.
19. Brown EA, Bekker HL, Davison SN, Koffman J, Schell JO. Supportive care: communication strategies to improve cultural competence in shared decision making. Clin J Am Soc Nephrol. 2016.
20. Osterberg L, Blaschke T. Adherence to medication. N Engl J Med. 2005;353(5):487–97.
21. Massanari MJ. Asthma management: curtailing costs and improving patient outcomes. J Asthma. 2000;37(8):641–51.
22. Valenti WM. Treatment adherence improves outcomes and manages costs. AIDS Read. 2001;11(2):77–80.
23. Simpson SH, Eurich DT, Majumdar SR, et al. A meta-analysis of the association between adherence to drug therapy and mortality. BMJ. 2006;333:15.
24. Nieuwlaat R, Wilczynski N, Navarro T, et al. Interventions for enhancing medication adherence. Cochrane Database Syst Rev. 2014;11:CD000011.
25. Serup J, Lindblad AK, Maroti M, et al. To follow or not to follow dermatological treatment–a review of the literature. Acta Derm Venereol. 2006;86:193–7.
26. van de Kerkhof PC, de Hoop D, de Korte J, Cobelens SA, Kuipers MV. Patient compliance and disease management in the treatment of psoriasis in the Netherlands. Dermatology. 2000;200:292–8.
27. Krejci-Manwaring J, McCarty MA, Camacho F, et al. Adherence with topical treatment is poor compared with adherence with oral agents: implications for effective clinical use of topical agents. J Am Acad Dermatol. 2006;54(5):S235–6.
28. Mosley-Williams A, Lumley MA, Gillis M, et al. Barriers to treatment adherence among African American and white women with systemic lupus erythematosus. Arthritis Rheum. 2002;47(6):630–8.
29. Sorensen EP, Algzlan H, Au SC, Garber C, et al. Lower socioeconomic status is associated with decreased therapeutic response to the biologic agents in Psoriasis patients. J Drugs Dermatol. 2016;15(2):147–53.
30. DeNavas-Walt C, Proctor BD. U.S. Census Bureau, current population reports, P60-252, income and poverty in the United States: 2014. Washington, DC: U.S. Government Printing Office; 2015.

31. Smith JC, Medalia C. Health insurance in the United States 2014. Current Population Reports. https://www.census.gov/content/dam/Census/library/publications/2015/demo/p60-253.pdf Issued September 2015. U.S. Census Bureau, Current Population Reports, P60-253, Health Insurance Coverage in the United States: 2014. Washington, DC: U.S. Government Printing Office; 2015.
32. Choi SE, Ngo-Metzger Q, Billimek J, et al. Contributors to patients' ratings of quality of care among ethnically diverse patients with type 2 diabetes. J Immigr Minor Health. 2016;18(2):382–9.
33. Churilla T, Egleston B, Dong Y, et al. Disparities in the management and outcome of cervical cancer in the United States according to health insurance status. Gynecol Oncol. 2016;141(3):516–23.
34. Fossati N, Nguyen DP, Trinh QD, et al. The impact of insurance status on tumor characteristics and treatment selection in contemporary patients with prostate cancer. J Natl Compr Canc Netw. 2015;13(11):1351–8.
35. Chernew ME, Shah MR, Wegh A, et al. Impact of decreasing copayments on medication adherence within a disease management environment. Health Aff (Millwood). 2008;27(1):103–12.
36. Skojec A, Foulke G, Kirby JS. Variation in the cost of generic Topical corticosteroids. JAMA Dermatol. 2015;151(11):1255–6.
37. Aslam I, Feldman SR. Practical strategies to improve patient adherence to treatment regimens. Dermatol Clin South Med J. 2015;108(6):325–31.
38. Berkman ND, Sheridan SL, Donahue KE, Halpern DJ, Crotty K. Low health literacy and health outcomes: an updated systematic review. Ann Intern Med. 2011;155(2):97–107.
39. Kutner M, Greenberg E, Jin Y, Paulsen C. The health literacy of America's adults: results from the 2003 national assessment of adult literacy (NCES 2006–483). U.S. Department of Education. Washington, DC: National Center for Education Statistics; 2006.
40. Kim S, Love F, Quistberg DA, et al. Association of health literacy with self-management behavior in patients with diabetes. Diabetes Care. 2004;27(12):2980–2.
41. Miller LG, Liu H, Hays RD, et al. Knowledge of antiretroviral regimen dosing and adherence: a longitudinal study. Clin Infect Dis. 2003;36(4):514–8.
42. Fan JH, Lyons SA, Goodman MS, Blanchard MS, Kaphingst KA. Relationship between health literacy and unintentional and intentional medication nonadherence in medically underserved patients with type 2 diabetes. Diabetes Educ. 2016;42(2):199–208.
43. Betancourt JR, Green AR, Carrillo JE. The challenges of cross-cultural healthcare-diversity, ethics, and the medical encounter. Bioethics Forum. 2000;16(3):27–32.
44. Flores G1. Language barriers to health care in the United States. N Engl J Med. 2006;355(3):229–31.
45. Ryan C. Language use in the United States: 2011. American Community Survey Reports. http://www.census.gov/content/dam/Census/library/publications/2013/acs/acs-22.pdf Issued August 2013. U.S. Census Bureau, American Community Survey Reports, P 1–16. Washington, DC: U.S. Government Printing Office; 2013.
46. Zong J, Batalova J. The limited English proficient population in the United States. Migration Information Source. July 2015. http://www.migrationpolicy.org/article/limited-english-proficient-population-united-states. Accessed 19 May 2016.
47. Sandoval LF1, Huang KE, Harrison J et al. Calcipotriene 0.005%-betamethasone dipropionate 0.064% ointment versus topical suspension in the treatment of plaque psoriasis: a randomized pilot study of patient preference. Cutis. 2014;94(6):304–9.
48. Lewallen R, Francis S, Fisher B, et al. Hair care practices and structural evaluation of scalp and hair shaft parameters in African American and Caucasian women. J Cosmet Dermatol. 2015;14(3):216–23.
49. Zolnierek KB, Dimatteo MR. Physician communication and patient adherence to treatment: a meta-analysis. Med Care. 2009;47(8):826–34.

50. Nahin RL1, Barnes PM, Stussman BJ, Bloom B. Costs of complementary and alternative medicine (CAM) and frequency of visits to CAM practitioners: United States, 2007. Natl Health Stat Report. 2009;18:1–14.
51. Clarke TC, Black LI, Stussman BJ, et al. Trends in the use of complementary health approaches among adults: United States, 2002-2012. Natl Health Stat Report. 2015;79:1–16.
52. Zenk SN, Shaver JLF, Peragallo N, et al. Use of herbal therapies among midlife Mexican women. Health Care Women Inter. 2001;22:585–97.
53. Nguyen H, Sorkin DH, Billimek J, Kaplan SH, Greenfield S, Ngo-Metzger Q. Complementary and alternative medicine (CAM) use among non-Hispanic white, Mexican American, and Vietnamese American patients with type 2 diabetes. J Health Care Poor Underserved. 2014;25(4):1941–55.
54. Barnes P, Powell-Griner E, McFann K et al. Complementary and alternative medicine use among adults: United States, 2002. Advance data from vital and health statistics. 343. Hyattsville, MD: National Center for Health Statistics; 2004.
55. Koo J1, Desai R. Traditional Chinese medicine in dermatology. Dermatol Ther. 2003;16 (2):98–105.
56. Chao MT1, Wade C, Kronenberg F. Disclosure of complementary and alternative medicine to conventional medical providers: variation by race/ethnicity and type of CAM. J Natl Med Assoc. 2008;100(11):1341–9.
57. Kuo GM, Hawley ST, Weiss LT, et al. Factors associated with herbal use among urban multiethnic primary care patients: a cross-sectional survey. BMC Complement Altern Med. 2004;4:18.
58. Graham RE, Ahn AC, Davis RD, et al. Use of complementary and alternative medical therapies among racial and ethnic minority adults: results from the 2002 National Health Interview Survey. J Natl Med Assoc. 2005;97:535–45.
59. Mehta DH, Phillips RS, Davis RB, et al. Use of complementary and alternative therapies by Asian Americans. Results from the National Health Interview Survey. J Gen Intern Med. 2007;22:762–7.
60. Franke N, Ohene-Frempong J. Health care for African Americans: availability, accessibility, and usability. In: Ma GX, Henderson G, editors. Rethinking ethnicity and health care: a sociocultural perspective. IL: Charles C. Thomas Publisher Ltd.; Springfield; 1999. p. 154–83.
61. Baer HA. Biomedicine and alternative healing systems in America: issues of class, race, ethnicity, & gender. Madison, WI: University of Wisconsin Press; 2001.
62. Moy JA, McKinley-Grant L, Sanchez MR. Cultural aspects in the treatment of patients with skin disease. Dermatol Clin. 2003;21(4):733–42.
63. Fishman B, Bobo L, Kosub K, Womeodu RJ. Cultural issues in serving minority populations: emphasis on Mexican Americans and African Americans. Am J Med Sci. 1993;306:160–6.
64. Risser AL1, Mazur LJ. Use of Folk Remedies in a Hispanic Population. Arch Pediatr Adolesc Med. 1995;149(9):978–81.
65. Howell L1, Kochhar K, Saywell R Jr, Zollinger T, Koehler J, Mandzuk C, Sutton B, Sevilla-Martir J, Allen D. Use of herbal remedies by Hispanic patients: do they inform their physician? J Am Board Fam Med. 2006;19(6):566–78.
66. Wong SS1, Tan KC, Goh CL. Cutaneous manifestations of chronic arsenicism: review of seventeen cases. J Am Acad Dermatol. 1998;38(2 Pt 1):179–85.

Index

© Springer International Publishing AG 2017
N.A. Vashi and H.I. Maibach (eds.), *Dermatoanthropology of Ethnic
Skin and Hair*, DOI 10.1007/978-3-319-53961-4